BIOMECHANICS OF THE UPPER LIMBS

Mechanics, Modeling, and Musculoskeletal Injuries

BIOMECHANICS OF THE UPPER LIMBS

Mechanics, Modeling, and Musculoskeletal Injuries

Andris Freivalds

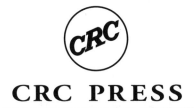

CRC PRESS

Boca Raton   London   New York   Washington, D.C.

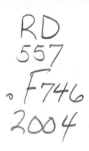

Library of Congress Cataloging-in-Publication Data

Freivalds, Andris.
    Biomechanics of the upper limbs : mechanics, modeling, and musculoskeletal injuries /
by Andris Freivalds.
      p. cm.
    Includes bibliographical references and index.
    ISBN 0-7484-0926-2 (alk. paper)
      1. Arm--Wounds and injuries. 2. Human mechanics. I. Title.

    RD557.F746 2004
    617.5'74044--dc22

                                            2004049376

Visit the CRC Press Web site at www.crcpress.com

© 2004 by CRC Press LLC

No claim to original U.S. Government works
International Standard Book Number 0-7484-0926-2
Library of Congress Card Number 2004049376
Printed in the United States of America 1 2 3 4 5 6 7 8 9 0
Printed on acid-free paper

Preface

What Is Biomechanics and Why Study It?

Biomechanics is the science that deals with forces and their effects, applied to biological systems. For this book, though, the focus will be exclusively on the upper limbs of the human. Over the last 20 years or so, there has been a tremendous increase in the number of work-related musculoskeletal disorders (WRMSDs) in the upper limbs. Not only do these preventable injuries produce unnecessary pain, suffering, and expense in workers, they also place an undue financial burden on industry in our tight economy. By better understanding the forces and their effects on the human body, the ergonomist may have a better insight into the role of various job stressors on the development of these disorders. With better control of these job stressors and the workplace environment, the current epidemic of WRMSDs may perhaps be brought under control. In so doing, both workers and companies will benefit. Although much effort has already been expended by NIOSH and the medical community in understanding WRMSDs and educating the practitioners, further work is still needed, and this book may help with the process.

Why Was This Book Written?

The objective of this book is to provide a practical up-to-date engineering-oriented graduate-level textbook on the biomechanics of the upper limbs. There are numerous other books providing general introductions to cumulative trauma disorders and medical management to the layperson and several serious texts on the biomechanics of manual material handling and low back problems; however, none focuses solely on the upper limbs, where most of the work-related musculoskeletal disorders seem to reside. Furthermore, this textbook emphasizes the musculoskeletal components involved, engineering models of these components, and measurement and prediction of injury potential based on these models.

For Whom Was This Book Written?

This book is primarily intended as a university textbook for graduate-level engineering or kinesiology students, the future practitioners in the WRMSD research area. A large amount of material was collected from various research literature sources and technical reports from very diverse disciplines. It is hoped that this material was distilled into a happy medium of medical and engineering expertise, at a technical level that is appropriate for the reader. The book may also prove useful to researchers, industrial ergonomists, industrial hygienists, and medical professionals as a reference text to supplement their professional material.

How Is the Book Organized?

The book is organized into ten chapters. Chapters 1 through 3 provide an introduction to the human musculoskeletal system, neuromuscular physiology, and the motor control system. Chapters 4 and 5 present the mechanics and models of the various components of the neuromuscular systems as well as models of larger systems. Chapter 6 discusses the various WRMSDs and their associated risk factors. Chapters 7 and 8 present the types of instruments and analysis tools that can be used to identify the WRMSDs in the industrial workplace. Chapters 9 and 10 provide specific applications to hand tools and computer workstations, with which most of the upper limb WRMSDs have been associated. Thus, one chapter can be covered roughly every one and a half weeks in a typical semester-long course.

This textbook also attempts to assist the educator by providing numerous examples and problems with each chapter. A Web site (http://www.ie.psu.edu/courses/ie552) is available for on-line notes, background material, solutions, and sample exams. Comments and suggestions for improvement from users of this textbook are greatly appreciated. This is especially important if any outright errors are detected. Please simply respond to the *OOPS!* button on the Web site or contact the author directly by e-mail: axf@psu.edu. As with any Web site, this one will evolve continually.

Andris Freivalds

The Author

Andris Freivalds, Ph.D., is Professor in the Department of Industrial and Manufacturing Engineering and the Director of the Center for Cumulative Trauma Disorders at the Pennsylvania State University. He obtained his Ph.D. in Bioengineering in 1979 from the University of Michigan while assisting with the development of its 3D Static Strength Prediction Model. He later held a Faculty Summer Research Fellowship at the Bioengineering and Biodynamics Division of Aerospace Medical Research Laboratory at Wright Patterson Air Force Base in Ohio, during which time he became proficient with and developed a neuromusculature for the Articulated Total Body Model.

More recently, Dr. Freivalds has been concerned with the reduction of cumulative trauma disorders (CTDs) in U.S. industries through ergonomic tool and workplace design. This effort led to the founding of the Center for Cumulative Trauma Disorders with the cooperation of the Ben Franklin Partnership of the Commonwealth of Pennsylvania. This center has served as the source of ergonomic services for over 60 small- and medium-sized Pennsylvania companies in controlling their workplace hazards. As part of the services to better quantify and predict the stresses of workers employed in hazardous jobs, a CTD Risk Index and the "touch" glove, which measures hand movements and grip pressure, have been developed. In addition, with the cooperation of the Hershey Medical Center on a retrospective epidemiological study, Dr. Freivalds has been modeling individual attributes that may contribute to an individual's likelihood for developing CTDs.

Acknowledgments

The author wishes to acknowledge Professor Don B. Chaffin for providing him with the training and tools, as well as a model, to proceed with this endeavor. He thanks his graduate students — Neil Davidoff, Lynn Donges, Gerald Fellows, Carol Heffernan, Hyunkook Jang, Dongjoon Kong, Yongku Kong, Kentaro Kotani, Cheol Lee, Brian Lowe, Glenn Miller, Seikwon Park, Vishal Seth, Roberta Weston, Heecheon You, and Myunghwan Yun — for working long hours collecting the research data on which much of this book was based. Last, but not least, he expresses sincere gratitude to his wife, Dace Freivalds, for her patience, support, and valued assistance during the production of this textbook.

Contents

1

Introduction to Biomechanics

1.1 What Is Biomechanics?

Biomechanics is mechanics, the science that deals with forces and their effects, applied to biological systems. Traditionally, this has meant the human body at a relatively macro level. However, there need not be any such limitations, as any life-form can be studied at any level. More recently, perhaps because of the interest in the development of new drugs and measuring their effects on the body, biomechanical studies have progressed down to the level of a single cell. This book, however, focuses exclusively on the human body and the upper limbs.

Although biomechanics is based solidly on the principles of physics and mathematics developed in the 1600s and 1700s by Galileo, Newton, Descartes, Euler, and others, the first biomechanical observations as related to the function of the muscle and bones of the human body had already been made in the early 1500s by Leonardo da Vinci. Borelli, a student of Galileo, published the first treatise on biomechanics, *De Motu Animalium*, in 1680. Later in the 1700s, Ramazzini, whom many consider the first occupational physician, described in detail the forceful and extreme motions in butchering and other jobs leading to the development of musculoskeletal disorders and other diseases.

More recent advances that laid much of the groundwork for later human modeling include W. Braune and O. Fischer's *The Center of Gravity of the Human Body* in 1889, O. Fischer's *Theoretical Fundamentals for a Mechanics of Living Bodies* in 1906, and A.V. Hill's 50 years of detailed studies on muscle mechanics, ultimately culminating in a Nobel prize in 1922. The crossover of biomechanics into ergonomics, the science that deals with fitting work to the human operator, probably started with E.R. Tichauer using biomechanical principles to redesign tools for the workplace in the early 1970s. In the 1980s, the National Institute for Occupational Safety and Health (NIOSH) began specifically focusing on workplace-related musculoskeletal disorders (WRMSDs) as part of its Year 2000 Objectives to reduce workplace injuries.

1.2 Basic Concepts

Biomechanical principles can be applied to a system of bodies at rest, termed *statics*, or to a system of bodies in motion, termed *dynamics*. In such systems, bodies may be pushed or pulled by actions termed *forces*. Such forces always act in unison; i.e., if one body is pushing on another body, the second one is pushing back on the first body equally hard. This is Newton's third law, the *law of reaction*: for every action there is an equal and opposite reaction. Thus, if an operator is pinching or applying a force to a tool or a part, that tool or part is pushing back equally hard, as evidenced by the compression of the skin and underlying tissues.

Newton's first law is the *law of inertia*: a body remains at rest or in constant-velocity motion until acted upon by an external unbalanced force. Newton's second law is the *law of acceleration*: the acceleration of a body is proportional to the unbalanced force acting upon it and inversely proportional to the mass of the body. Mathematically this law is expressed as

$$F = ma \qquad (1.1)$$

where
F = force
m = mass
a = acceleration

A force can be characterized by three factors: magnitude, direction, and point of application. The *magnitude* is a scalar quantity that indicates the size of the push or pull action; e.g., a force of 10 N is twice as large as a force of 5 N. The *direction* of the force indicates the line of action of the force; i.e., a force applied perpendicular or normal to surface of a body will have an effect different from a force applied parallel to the surface, or in a shear direction. Note, the direction can range a full 360° in two dimensions, so that a normal force could be either pushing or pulling the body, depending on the angle defined. Typically for simplicity in modeling and calculations, the magnitude and direction are combined into one quantity termed a *vector*. Finally, the *point of application* of a force on a body is self-evident; i.e., the effect on an arm will be quite different if a force (such as a weight) is applied to the hand as opposed as to the elbow.

In this example, the weight acts as an *external force* to the arm, as it acts outside the body, while the muscular forces in the arm are *internal forces*, as they act inside the body. Note also that weight is not the same as mass; the weight is determined by the effect of gravity on the mass of the object and is measured in newtons (N, named after the English physicist and mathematician Sir Isaac Newton, 1642–1728) while the mass is measured in kilograms (kg). In some situations, a force will be distributed over an area rather than a single point of application. In that case, it is termed *pressure* and defined as

$$P = F/A \qquad (1.2)$$

where
P = pressure
A = area

If the force is newtons and area in meters squared, then the units of pressure are measured in pascals (Pa, named after French mathematician Blaise Pascal, 1623–1662).

Another important concept is the *moment* of a force or *torque*. A moment is the tendency of a force to cause rotation about a point or axis (depending on whether one is considering a two-dimensional or three-dimensional system). It is defined as the application of a force at a perpendicular distance from the point of rotation or the perpendicular component of a force to a lever arm. Mathematically, the moment equals force times distance or

$$M = r \times F \qquad (1.3)$$

where
M = moment
r = distance

1.3 Coordinate Systems

To define a vector or the direction of a force, a reference coordinate system needs to be defined. In a two-dimensional system, this can be done by dividing the plane into four quadrants using two perpendicular lines as axes (Figure 1.1A). The horizontal axis is defined as the x axis or *abscissa*, and the vertical axis is defined as the y axis or the *ordinate*. The point of intersection of the two axes is known as the *origin* of the system from which all point of applications are defined. Measurements are made in common units along the axes; positive values to the right of the origin on the x axis and above the origin for the y axis. Any point of application then can be defined using these coordinates; (0,0) is the origin and point A in Figure 1.1A is (3,4). Such a coordinate system is termed the *rectangular* or *Cartesian coordinate system* (named after the French mathematician René Descartes, 1596–1650). A third dimension can be easily added by placing the z axis perpendicular to both the x- and y-axes (Figure 1.1B).

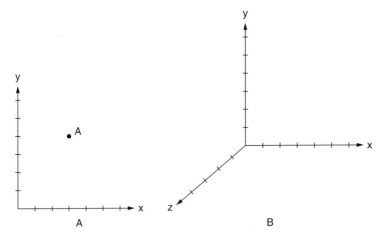

FIGURE 1.1
Rectangular or Cartesian coordinate system: (A) two dimensional; (B) three dimensional.

An alternate coordinate system is the *polar coordinate system* shown in Figure 1.2A. In this system all coordinates are measured with an angle θ, starting with 0° at the Cartesian *x* axis, moving full circle or 360° counterclockwise, and ending back at the same axis, and a distance *r* defined from the origin of the Cartesian coordinate system. The same point can be converted between the two coordinate systems with the following equations. From the polar to Cartesian system, use the equations:

$$x = r\cos\theta \tag{1.4}$$

$$y = r\sin\theta \tag{1.5}$$

From the Cartesian to the polar system, use the equations:

$$r = \left(x^2 + y^2\right)^{1/2} \tag{1.6}$$

$$\theta = \tan^{-1} y/x \tag{1.7}$$

For three dimensions, the *spherical coordinate system* with a distance *r* and two angles θ and φ can be used (Figure 1.2B). The same point can again be converted between the two coordinate systems. From the spherical to Cartesian system, use the equations:

$$x = r\sin\theta\cos\phi \tag{1.8}$$

$$y = r\sin\theta\sin\phi \tag{1.9}$$

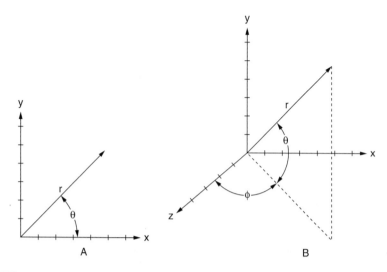

FIGURE 1.2
(A) Polar coordinate system (two dimensional); (B) spherical coordinate system (three dimensional).

$$z = r \cos \theta \tag{1.10}$$

From the Cartesian to the spherical system, use the equations:

$$r = \left(x^2 + y^2 + z^2\right)^{1/2} \tag{1.11}$$

$$\phi = \tan^{-1} y/x \tag{1.12}$$

$$\theta = \cos^{-1} z/r \tag{1.13}$$

1.4 Force Vector Algebra

The force *vector* shown in Figure 1.3 on a two-dimensional Cartesian coordinate system has a direction defined by the line originating at the origin (0,0) and ending at the point of application of (3,4). In vector notation, the direction can be also defined as $3i + 4j$, where i and j are termed the unit coordinate vectors for the x- and y-axes, respectively (k is used for the z axes). This vector is thus broken down into its x,y components, with a value of 3

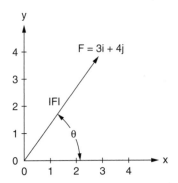

FIGURE 1.3
Cartesian coordinate system with vector $3i + 4j$.

for the x component and a value of 4 for its y component. The magnitude of a vector, based on Equation 1.6, is defined as

$$|F| = \left[F_x^2 + F_y^2\right]^{1/2} \tag{1.14}$$

where
F_x = the x component of the force vector F
F_y = the y component of the force vector F

For the above case, the magnitude has a specific value of

$$|F| = \left[3^2 + 4^2\right]^{1/2} = 5 \tag{1.15}$$

The directional angle θ (sometimes termed phase angle) can also be found from the components of the force vector from Equation 1.7 or

$$\theta = \tan^{-1}\left(F_y / F_x\right) \tag{1.16}$$

For the above case, the directional angle has a specific value of

$$\theta = \tan^{-1}\left(4/3\right) = 53.13° \tag{1.17}$$

These two values now define the force vector F in polar coordinates as $(5, 53.13°)$ and demonstrate the interchangeability of the notation between the two coordinate systems.

In the generic form, the force vector would be defined in the polar coordinate system as

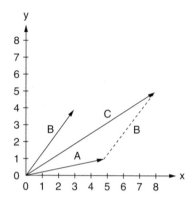

FIGURE 1.4
Addition of vectors A ($5i + j$) and B ($3i + 4j$) to create vector C ($8i + 5j$).

$$F = (r, \theta)$$ (1.18)

where the r is the magnitude $|F|$ and θ is the angle. The components along the x- and y-axes are defined as

$$F_x = F \cos \theta$$ (1.19)

$$F_y = F \sin \theta$$ (1.20)

For the specific force vector shown in Figure 1.3, the x,y components become

$$F_x = F \cos \theta = 5 \cos(53.13°) = 5(0.6) = 3$$ (1.21)

$$F_y = F \sin \theta = 5 \sin(53.13°) = 5(0.8) = 4$$ (1.22)

Two force vectors A and B can be added together to create a resultant force vector **C** by adding the x and y components (Figure 1.4). Since A is $5i + j$ and B is $3i + 4j$, then C is simply

$$C = 5i + j + 3i + 4j = 8i + 5j$$ (1.23)

This same resultant force vector can also be found graphically by placing the tail of force vector B to the tip of force vector A with the line between the tail of A and the tip of B creating the new resultant force vector C (see Figure 1.4). The same result can also be obtained by adding the tail of A to the tip of B.

One important manipulation of vectors is the vector *cross product*, which is used to calculate the moment of the force (from Equation 1.3), which is also a vector, but perpendicular to both the force and distance vectors. The sense of this resultant vector is determined by the *right-hand rule*, in which the fingers of the right hand pointing in the direction of the first vector are curled toward the second vector so as to cover the included angle between the two vectors. The extended thumb will then point in the resultant cross-product vector direction, which will be perpendicular to both of the original vectors. Mathematically, this can be expressed as

$$i \times j = k \quad \left(j \times i = -k\right)$$
$$j \times k = i \quad \left(k \times j = -i\right) \tag{1.24}$$
$$k \times i = j \quad \left(i \times k = -j\right)$$

Note, that this cross product also applies to the definition of a three-dimensional Cartesian coordinate system (see Figure 1.2B). Also, any vector crossed on itself (e.g., $i \times i$) is equal to zero, i.e., there is no unique perpendicular vector. There is also the *dot product* of vectors with both requiring the same direction (i.e., $i \cdot i$) and resulting in a purely scalar value.

1.5   Static Equilibrium

One result of Newton's first law is that bodies are typically studied in *static equilibrium*, which allows for several useful conditions. First, for the body to be in static equilibrium, it must be in *translational equilibrium*. Mathematically, this means that the net forces on the body must be zero or

$$\Sigma F = 0 \tag{1.25}$$

More practically, the forces are broken down into components by axes and result in

$$\Sigma F_x = 0 \quad \Sigma F_y = 0 \quad \Sigma F_z = 0 \tag{1.26}$$

Second, the body must also be in *rotational equilibrium*, which means that the net moments about any point in the body due to the external forces must also be zero. This can be expressed as

$$\Sigma M = 0 \tag{1.27}$$

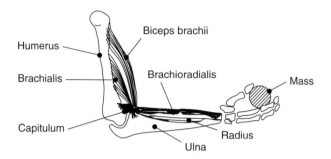

FIGURE 1.5
Musculature of the upper limb while holding a weight.

To study these conditions in detail, the body or the part of the body of interest is isolated and drawn as a *free-body diagram*. All the known forces are drawn accurately with respect to the magnitude, direction, and point of application. If a force is unknown, a representative arrow is included with an arbitrary direction. If a part of a body is isolated from another or more complete body, arbitrary reactive forces are included at that point of separation. Also, all moments are included.

Example 1.1: Static Equilibrium of the Upper Limb Holding a Weight

Consider the musculature of the upper limb as shown in Figure 1.5. There are three primary muscles involved in elbow flexion: the biceps brachii, the brachioradialis, and the brachialis, and one for elbow extension: the triceps brachii (see Section 2.1 for definitions of these terms). The hand holds a weight at the center of gravity of the hand. It would be of interest to find the muscle forces needed to hold this load at an elbow flexion of 90°. If the weight is merely being held, then this is a simpler case of statics, with no need to consider the dynamic effects from accelerations or initial velocities. Because the triceps is active only during elbow extension, it can be disregarded for elbow flexion. Also, including all three elbow flexors would result in a statically indeterminate situation; i.e., there are too many variables for the given amount of data or no one unique muscle force can be attributed to each muscle. The two smaller muscles are disregarded, leaving only the biceps brachii and the simpler case shown in Figure 1.6A.

Next, the forearm is isolated with all relevant reactive forces as shown in Figure 1.6B. The elbow joint is represented with two unknown reactive force F_{ex} and F_{ey}. The weight of the forearm is represented by a weight or force of 13 N acting downward through the forearm center of gravity, 12 cm distal of the elbow joint. The weight itself and the weight of the hand are represented by a force of 90 N acting downward at a distance of 31 cm from the elbow joint. The biceps brachii is represented by an

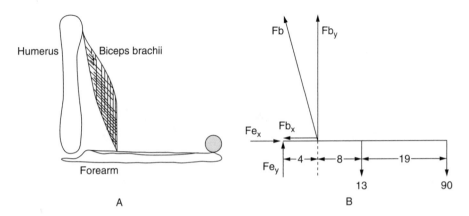

FIGURE 1.6
(A) Simplified upper limb while holding a weight; (B) free-body diagram of upper limb holding a weight.

unknown force F_b acting upward (i.e., lifting the forearm and weight up) at a point 4 cm distally of the elbow joint center of rotation. Because it is acting at an angle, the force is best represented in the vector form with x and y components of the form of Equations 1.19 and 1.20. The angle θ is found from Equation 1.16, where the distance of the origin of the biceps muscle is 30 cm from the elbow:

$$\theta = \tan^{-1}(30/4) = 82.4° \tag{1.28}$$

From Equations 1.19 and 1.20, the unknown x and y components of F_b are

$$F_{bx} = F_b \cos\theta = F_b \cos(82.4°) = 0.132 F_b \tag{1.29}$$

$$F_{by} = F_b \sin\theta = F_b \sin(82.4°) = 0.991 F_b \tag{1.30}$$

Then the unknown biceps muscle force can be represented by

$$F_b = 0.132 F_b i + 0.991 F_b j \tag{1.31}$$

The translational equilibrium of Equation 1.26 yields

$$\Sigma F_x = 0 = F_{ex} - F_{bx} = 0 \tag{1.32}$$

$$\Sigma F_y = 0 = F_{ey} - 0.991 F_b - 13 - 90 = 0 \tag{1.33}$$

Simplification of Equations 1.32 and 1.33 yields

$$F_{ex} = 0.132\,F_b \tag{1.34}$$

$$F_{ey} = 103 - 0.991\,F_b \tag{1.35}$$

The rotational equilibrium of Equation 1.27 can be established at any point, but is most convenient around the elbow joint center of rotation, as this eliminates both reactive components of the elbow joint, neither of which creates a moment around the point through which it passes. Using distances in meters yields

$$\Sigma M_e = 0$$
$$= (0.04i) \times (0.132\,F_b i + 0.991\,F_b j) + (0.12\,i) \times (-13\,j) + (0.31i) \times (-90\,j) \tag{1.36}$$

The accepted practice is to follow the right-hand rule as the force vector pushes down on its respective lever arm, with clockwise torques considered negative and counterclockwise torques considered positive. (However, as long as one is consistent, the opposite implementation can be used just as well.) Thus, in the above case, the weight- or gravity-induced torques are negative, while the muscle force–induced torque is positive. Of course, using the vector notation and cross products of Equation 1.24 automatically creates the proper moment, with $i \times i$ terms dropping out, $i \times j$ becoming k, and $i \times -j$ becoming $-k$. Simplifying Equation 1.36 yields

$$0.03964\,F_b k = 29.46\,k \tag{1.37}$$

$$F_b = 743.2\,\mathrm{N} \tag{1.38}$$

Substituting Equation 1.38 back into Equations 1.34 and 1.35 yields

$$F_{ex} = 0.132(743.2) = 98.1\,\mathrm{N} \tag{1.39}$$

$$F_{ey} = 103 - 0.991\,F_b = 103 - 0.991(743.2) = -633.5\,\mathrm{N} \tag{1.40}$$

In summary, the biceps brachii muscle (in reality, a combination of all three elbow flexor muscles) must exert an internal force of over eight times ($743.2/90 = 8.3$) the external force to maintain equilibrium. To find the individual contributions of each of the three elbow flexor muscles is an indeterminate situation and requires assumptions about the relative forces, typically determined from relative muscle cross-sectional areas. Also, there are considerable internal forces sustained in the elbow, especially because it acts as the pivot point for joint rotation.

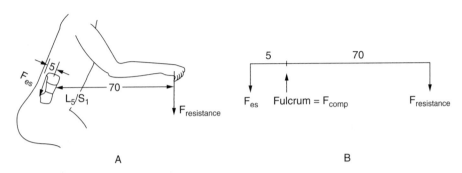

FIGURE 1.7
(A) The lower back modeled as a first-class lever. (B) Free-body diagram of the lower back.

The combination of forces acting around a pivot point or *fulcrum* (as in Example 1.1) is termed a *lever system*. The external weights or resistive forces are counterbalanced by an effort force, in this case the biceps brachii muscle force. Each acts through a respective moment or lever arm. The ratio of these forces, or of these moment arms, forms a quantity termed the *mechanical advantage* (ma):

$$\text{ma} = r_e / r_r = F_r / F_e \tag{1.41}$$

where
r_e = lever arm for the effort force
r_r = lever arm for the resistive force
F_e = the resistive force
F_r = the effort force

There are three different types of lever systems with different values for the mechanical advantage. In a *first-class lever* the fulcrum is located between the effort and resistance as in a playground teeter-totter or the erector spinae (F_{es}) muscles acting on the L_5/S_1 vertebra as a fulcrum to maintain an erect trunk position or while lifting a load ($F_{resistance}$ in Figure 1.7A). Note that in an approximate calculation using the free-body diagram of Figure 1.7B, disregarding alignment angles, and assuming an effort moment arm of 5 cm and a resistance moment arm of 70 cm, the mechanical advantage is

$$\text{ma} = r_e / r_r = 5/70 = 0.0714 \tag{1.42}$$

This, in reality, is a mechanical disadvantage and may be one of the factors in the high incidence of low back problems.

The versatility of the first-class lever system is demonstrated by changing the length of the moment arms to have a mechanical advantage that can be either greater or less than one. Thus, unequally heavy children can still use the teeter-totter by repositioning the fulcrum such that they are in relative equilibrium. Most extensor muscles act as first-class levers.

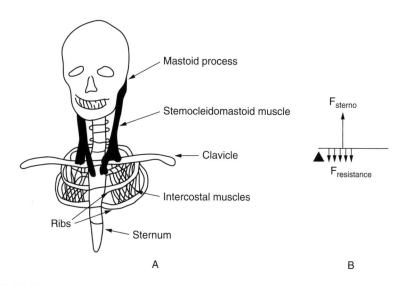

FIGURE 1.8
(A) The sternocleidomastoid muscle and clavicle modeled as a second-class lever. (B) Free-body diagram of the sternocleidomastoid muscle and clavicle.

In a *second-class lever*, the resistance is located between the effort and fulcrum and always results in a mechanical advantage greater than one; i.e., the effort is always less than the resistance. Examples include the wheelbarrow, a nutcracker, or a pry bar pulled upward. However, in the human body, it is difficult to find a true second-class lever. One possibility is the action of the sternocleidomastoid muscle during forceful inspiration (Figure 1.8A). The sternocleidomastoid muscle originates on the mastoid process of the skull and inserts on both the sternum and clavicle. The clavicle and sternum are tied into the ribcage through the attachments of the various intercostal muscles. Although, the sternocleidomastoid has a relatively direct insertion to the clavicle, which can be represented as a simple effort force F_{stern}, the resistance force is distributed over the length of the clavicle (Figure 1.8B). Therefore, for some part of the clavicle, the resultant pry bar action through the fulcrum at the sternum is a second-class level. (The point of application for a uniform distributed force is simply the midpoint of the distribution. For nonuniform distributions, the center of mass approach of Section 1.6 must be used.)

In a *third-class lever*, the effort is located between the fulcrum and the resistance and always results in a mechanical advantage less than one, or a mechanical disadvantage. The elbow flexion of Figure 1.6 and most other flexor muscles are good examples of third-class levers. The mechanical advantage of the biceps brachii from Example 1.1 is

$$\mathrm{ma} = F_r / F_e = 90 / 743.2 = 0.12 \qquad (1.43)$$

It would seem odd that there is again a mechanical disadvantage in the human body. This is typically the case for the upper and lower limbs, with the effort greater than the resistance. However, there is a trade-off. With the very short effort moment arms, small changes in muscle length will be amplified into large movements of the ends of the limbs. Thus, the human musculature is designed for speed and movement as opposed to strength.

1.6   Anthropometry and Center of Mass Determination

For the above static equilibrium analyses (Figure 1.5) and later biomechanical models, several key properties need to be known. Since, typically, the upper limb will be divided into its component segments, the segment link lengths, segment weights, and the location of the *center of mass* (cm, but often termed *center of gravity*, cg; both terms will be used interchangeably here) are needed. For specific cases, the segment link lengths can be measured directly using specialized calipers termed *anthropometers* or indirectly through stereo photography or laser or other optical surface scanning techniques while the segment weights can be determined directly by water displacement techniques (Miller and Nelson, 1976). Note, however, that the volume must be multiplied by a density factor, which is not always specifically known and can vary between individuals:

$$\text{Mass}(g) = \text{volume}(cm^3) \times \text{density}(g/cm^3) \qquad (1.44)$$

Specific density factors and segment properties have been compiled for the upper limbs in Table 1.1. The center of mass values in Table 1.1 has typically been found by the suspension technique of balancing a frozen cadaver segment along each of the three axes (Dempster, 1955). A pin is systematically moved along one axis until the balance point is found. The intersection of the three axial lines through each point determined the center of mass.

For a live person, the center of mass for a given segment, for example, the arm, can be found through a technique reported by LeVeau (1977). The person lies on a board, supported by a knife edge at one end and a force scale at the other, assuming two different positions relative to that segment, in this case the arm (Figure 1.9). As the upper limb is allowed to hang naturally, the center of mass for the body moves toward the head, decreasing the reading on the scale. With a few calculations based on simple mechanical principles, the weight of the upper limb can be determined. The full analysis is given in Example 1.2.

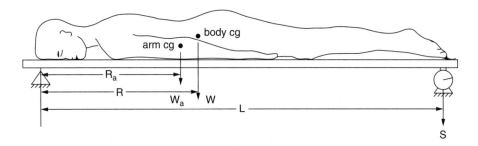

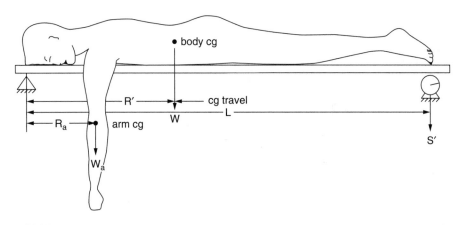

FIGURE 1.9
Method for determining the weight of the arm. (Redrawn from LeVeau, B., 1977. *Williams and Lissner Biomechanics of Human Motion*, 2nd ed., Philadelphia: W.B. Saunders, 214.)

Example 1.2: Determining the Weight of the Arm

In the fully prone posture, the body mass W is acting at a distance R from the left support. When the arm is hanging down, the whole body cg will have moved toward the head, with a shorter moment arm of R', and the scale will show a lower value of S' than in the first posture with S. Taking moments about the left support for each posture yields

$$SL - WR = 0 \tag{1.45}$$

$$S'L - WR' = 0 \tag{1.46}$$

where L is the distance between the scale and the left support. The corresponding moment arms are then

$$R = SL/W \tag{1.47}$$

$$R' = S'L/W \tag{1.48}$$

TABLE 1.1

Gross Anthropometric Data for the Upper Limbs

	Upper Arm	Forearm	Hand
Link definition[a]	Line between glenohumeral and elbow joint centers	Line between the elbow and wrist joint centers	Line between the wrist joint center and hand center of gravity
Proximal joint[a]	Glenohumeral	Elbow	Wrist
Joint center location[a]	Midregion of the palpable bone mass of the head and tuberosities of the humerus; with the arm abducted 45°, a line dropped perpendicular to the long axis from the acromion bisects the joint	Midpoint on a line between the lowest palpable point on the medial epicondyle of the humerus and a point above the radiale	Midpoint of a line between the radial styloid and the center of the pisiform, in line with the metacarpal III bone
Segment definition[a]	Acromion to radiale	Tip of elbow to styloid process	Base of hand to end of middle finger
Link to segment ratio[b]	0.89	1.07	0.506
Segment density[b,c] (g/cm³)	1.075	1.125	1.15
Segment length to stature ratio[c]	0.186	0.146	0.108
Segment mass to body mass ratio[c]	0.029	0.018	0.008
Segment cg to segment length ratio (from proximal end)[c]	0.452	0.424	0.397
Moment of inertia (I_{cm}) (10^{-4} kg m²)[b]	141	55	5
Moment of inertia (I_0) from proximal end (10^{-4} kg m²)[b]	407	182	19
Radius of gyration to segment length ratio (from proximal end)[d]	0.542	0.526	0.587

	Male			Female			Male			Female			Male			Female		
	5th	50th	95th	5th	50th	95th	5th	50th	95th	5th	50th	95th	5th	50th	95th	5th	50th	95th
Segment link length (cm)[e]	28.6	30.4	32.3	26.1	27.8	29.5	25.6	27.1	28.7	22.7	24.1	25.5	—	—	—	—	—	—
Segment length (cm)[a]	30.3	33.0	35.6	28.3	31.0	33.6	24.6	26.9	29.3	21.2	23.4	25.7	17.8	19.1	20.5	16.9	18.3	20.1
Segment mass (kg)[b]	1.6	2.1	2.8	1.3	1.7	2.5	0.9	1.2	1.6	0.7	1.0	1.4	0.4	0.4	0.6	0.3	0.4	0.5
Distance to cg from proximal end (cm)[b]	12.5	13.2	14.0	11.6	12.1	12.5	11.0	11.7	12.3	9.9	10.4	11.0	6.7	7.0	7.4	6.1	6.4	6.7

Note: See Figure 1.9 for landmarks; detailed data for the fingers are found in Tables 5.5 and 5.6.

a Webb Associates (1978).
b Dempster (1955).
c Roebuck et al. (1975).
d Plagenhoef (1966).
e Chaffin et al. (1999).

Note that in the second case, the whole body center of mass has moved anteriorly due to the movement of the arm.

A useful property for finding the center of mass of individual body segments is the *principle of moments:* the moments of the components must be equal to the moment of the whole. For each posture, this yields

$$WR = R_a W_a + R_b W_b \tag{1.49}$$

$$WR' = R_s W_a + R_b W_b \tag{1.50}$$

where

R_a = distance to the arm cg
W_a = weight of the arm
R_b = distance to the body minus the arm cg
W_b = body weight minus the arm weight
R_s = distance to the arm cg when hanging down, roughly the distance
        to the shoulder joint

By subtracting Equation 1.50 from Equation 1.49, the unknown value of R_b can be eliminated:

$$R_a - R_s = W(R - R')/W_a \tag{1.51}$$

Substituting Equations 1.47 and 1.48 into Equation 1.51 yields the final expression for the location of the arm cg from the shoulder joint:

$$R_a - R_s = L(S - S')/W_a \tag{1.52}$$

Alternatively, Equation 1.52 can be rearranged to yield the weight of the arm:

$$W_a = L(S - S')/(R_a - R_s) \tag{1.53}$$

The center of mass for a given body segment can also be calculated mathematically by extending the principle of moments. Assume that the truncated cylinder shown in Figure 1.10 represents a forearm. This shape can be cut into thin segments of thickness dr, each with a small force vector F representing the segment's weight and each acting a given distance r from the left-hand origin to create many small moments. Adding all the moments together should equal the total weight acting through a lever arm corresponding to the distance to the center of mass. Extending this concept to thinner and thinner segments and using integration to sum these moments, the center of mass can be found mathematically from

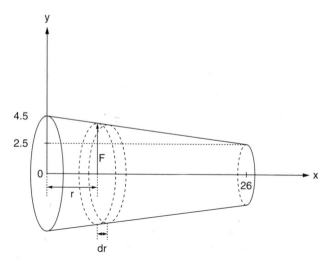

FIGURE 1.10
Method for determining the center of mass of the upper arm.

$$cm = \frac{\int rF\,dr}{\int F\,dr} \qquad (1.54)$$

The full details of the analysis are shown in Example 1.3.

Example 1.3: Determining the Center of Mass of the Upper Arm

For the stylized upper arm of Figure 1.10, the weight of each segment is the volume times a density factor. The volume is simply a disc of area $2F$ with thickness of dr. Assume a constant density factor of 1. (In reality, the density factor may vary with segment length, and then an actual value may need to be used.) The relationship of F with respect to r can be expressed as a line with the equation

$$F = -r/13 + 4.5 \qquad (1.55)$$

Then substituting Equation 1.55 into Equation 1.54 and integrating from 0 to 26 yield

$$cg = \frac{\int rF\,dr}{\int F\,dr} = \frac{\int \left(-r^2/13 + 4.5r\right)dr}{\int \left(-r/13 + 4.5\right)dr} = \left.\frac{\left(-r^3/39 + 2.25r^2\right)}{\left(-r^2/26 + 4.5r\right)}\right|_0^{26} = 11.76 \qquad (1.56)$$

Note that a distance of 11.76 cm from the left-hand origin or elbow is roughly 43.3% of the segment length of 26 cm, which corresponds closely to the relative cm locations given in Table 1.1 for a 5th percentile female.

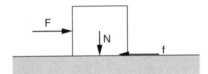

FIGURE 1.11
Frictional forces.

1.7 Friction

Friction is the interaction between two surfaces when coming into contact as one slides over the other (Figure 1.11). The resulting force in the lateral direction is termed the frictional force and depends on how tightly the surfaces are in contact and the material properties of the two surfaces, such as the roughness, which can be defined as the *coefficient of friction*. Mathematically, the frictional force can be expressed as

$$f = \mu N \tag{1.57}$$

where
f = frictional force
N = normal force
μ = coefficient of friction

Theoretically, the coefficient of friction should range from a lower limit of 0 to an upper limit of 1; i.e., the frictional force cannot exceed the normal force applied. However, under certain conditions, such as grasping with the grooved ridges found in the fingertips, frictional coefficients may exceed 1 and perhaps even reach values of 2 (Bobjer et al., 1993). Practically, it ranges from values as high as 0.75 for rubber on rough wood (LeVeau, 1977) to values as low as 0.08 for oiled steel on steel and 0.04 for high-molecular-weight polyethylene on steel (Weast, 1969). The latter properties are used in the designs used in low-friction artificial joints with coefficients of friction approaching 0.02 (Kitano et al., 2001). However, these still do not approach the coefficient of friction values of 0.003 to 0.005 found in real synovial joints (Unsworth et al., 1975), which most likely are attributable to the special hydrodynamic properties of synovial fluid described in Section 2.5.2.

The coefficient of friction also depends on movement. It is normally measured at the point one surface begins to slide with respect to the other, at which point it achieves the maximum value. It then decreases in value as the surfaces begin sliding more quickly. This leads to the classic physics example of static equilibrium: determining the steepest angle at which the

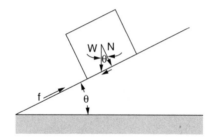

FIGURE 1.12
Determination of the coefficient of friction on an inclined plane.

block remains stationary without sliding down an inclined plane (see Example 1.4).

Example 1.4: Determination of the Coefficient of Friction on an Inclined Plane

The block of weight W (Figure 1.12) exerts a normal force N on a surface inclined at an angle of θ. This is also the component of the weight perpendicular to the inclined plane:

$$N = W\cos\theta \qquad (1.58)$$

The frictional force is the component of the weight parallel to the incline:

$$f = W\sin\theta \qquad (1.59)$$

Substituting Equations 1.58 and 1.59 into the definition of friction in Equation 1.57 and rearranging yield the coefficient of friction as a function of critical angle of the inclined plane:

$$\mu = f/N = \sin\theta/\cos\theta = \tan\theta \qquad (1.60)$$

This is one practical method for finding the maximum coefficient of friction between two surfaces.

Friction can also occur in pulley systems. A fixed pulley changes the direction of a force but not the magnitude of the force (Figure 1.13A). This principle allows for the reduction of forces in a free pulley, with each strand supporting one half of the weight (Figure 1.13B). A larger combination of n free pulleys with one fixed pulley (Figure 1.13C) reduces the force needed to lift the weight to

$$F = W/2^n \qquad (1.61)$$

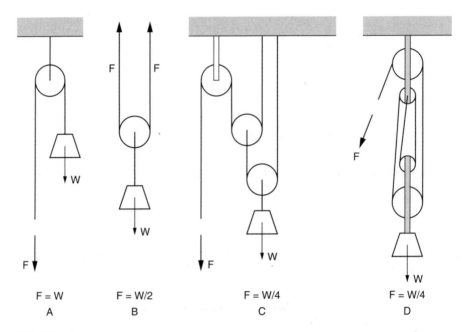

FIGURE 1.13
Pulley systems: (A) one fixed pulley; (B) one free pulley; (C) two free pulleys and one fixed pulley; (D) block and tackle.

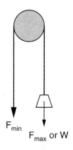

FIGURE 1.14
Crude pulley with friction.

Such a pulley system is more typically set up as a block and tackle with n free pulleys and n fixed pulleys (Figure 1.13D).

Although pulleys are assumed to be frictionless, this does not need to be the case. This is especially true for a crude pulley such as simply passing a rope around a pole (Figure 1.14), where the friction can assist in controlling the lowering of a heavy weight. The relationship between the two forces can be expressed as

$$F_{max} = F_{min}e^{\mu\theta} \qquad (1.62)$$

where
F_{max} = the larger of the two forces determined by movement in that direction
F_{min} = the smaller of the two forces
θ = the angle of contact between the rope and pole (radians)

Example 1.5: Friction on a Crude Pulley

Assuming that the coefficient of friction for a rough rope on a rough pole is approximately 0.5 and the angle of contact is 180° or π radians, then the force needed to lower a weight of 100 kg (equivalent to 980.7 N) is

$$F_{min} = \frac{980.7}{e^{0.5\pi}} = 980.7/4.81 = 203.9\,\text{N} \tag{1.63}$$

This force is only one fifth of that created by the weight itself. On the other hand, this setup would be very disadvantageous to lifting the weight as it would require

$$F_{max} = 980.7\,e^{0.5\pi} = 980.7\left(4.81\right) = 4{,}717.2\,\text{N} \tag{1.64}$$

or almost five times as much force as created by the weight itself.

1.8   Dynamics

Dynamics can be subdivided into *kinematics*, which is the study of pure motion, displacement, velocities, and acceleration, and into *kinetics*, which in addition studies the forces that produce that motion. Pure motion can either be rectilinear or circular. In the rectilinear case, the displacement vector of a body can be defined along the three axes of the Cartesian coordinate system as

$$s = xi + yj + zk \tag{1.65}$$

The velocity of that body is the change in displacement with respect to change in time and can be defined as an instantaneous velocity:

$$v = ds/dt \tag{1.66}$$

or as an average velocity:

$$\bar{v} = \Delta s/\Delta t \tag{1.67}$$

and is measured in meters per second. Similarly, the acceleration of that body can be defined as the change in velocity with respect to change in time in an instantaneous sense:

$$a = dv/dt \qquad (1.68)$$

or in an average sense:

$$\bar{a} = \Delta v/\Delta t \qquad (1.69)$$

and is measured in meters per second squared. The velocity and displacement vectors can be calculated for a given acceleration by integrating once for velocity:

$$v = at + v_0 \qquad (1.70)$$

where v_0 is the initial velocity, and integrating twice for displacement:

$$s = 1/2\, at^2 + vt + s_0 \qquad (1.71)$$

where s_0 is the initial displacement.

For circular motion, it is easier to use polar coordinates, in which case the angular displacement is defined as

$$s = r\theta \qquad (1.72)$$

The angular velocity and angular acceleration are defined as

$$\omega = d\theta/dt \qquad (1.73)$$

$$\alpha = d\omega/dt \qquad (1.74)$$

and measured in radians per second and radians per second squared, respectively. For a constant radius r, linear and angular quantities are related as follows:

$$v = r\omega \qquad (1.75)$$

$$a = r\alpha \qquad (1.76)$$

For studying kinetics, force effects on the body are also included. These forces follow Newton's second law defined previously in Equation 1.1. For circular motion, substituting Equation 1.76 into Equation 1.1 yields

$$F_t = mr\alpha \qquad (1.77)$$

where F_t is the *tangential force* acting at the center of mass of the body, α is the instantaneous angular acceleration of the body, and r is the distance of the body center of mass from the point of rotation. A second force acting on the body is the *centrifugal force* F_c acting along the radius of the rotation:

$$F_c = mr\omega^2 \qquad (1.78)$$

In terms of calculation moments and the rotational equilibrium analysis of Section 1.4, there is the moment created by the weight of the body acting a distance r, there is the tangential force acting a distance r, and a force component due to the mass of the body resisting change in angular velocity known as the *moment of inertia*:

$$M = I_{cm}\alpha \qquad (1.79)$$

where I_{cm}, the moment of inertia at the center of mass, is defined as the integral over the volume of the body:

$$I_{cm} = \int r^2 dm \qquad (1.80)$$

For a point mass, Equation 1.78 results in

$$I_{cm} = r^2 m \qquad (1.81)$$

Experimentally, moments of inertia for body segments are found by suspending frozen cadaver parts and swinging them as a pendulum (Lephart, 1984). The resulting period of oscillation yields an estimate of the moment of inertia:

$$I_0 = \frac{WL}{4\pi^2 f^2} \qquad (1.82)$$

where
I_0 = moment of inertia at the axis of suspension
W = weight of segment or mg
L = distance of center of mass to axis of suspension
f = period of oscillation

The moment of inertia at the center of mass located a distance L from the axis of suspension is found, by the parallel-axis theorem, to be

$$I_{cm} = I_0 - mL^2 \tag{1.83}$$

More practically, mean values for key body segments determined experimentally are given in Table 1.1.

Another useful parameter relating to moments of inertia is the *radius of gyration, K*. It is the effective distance from the axis of rotation, K, for which a point mass of Equation 1.82 yields an equivalent moment of inertia to the body segment:

$$K = \sqrt{\frac{I_{cm}}{m}} \tag{1.84}$$

The final rotational equilibrium equation for angular motion of a body can now be defined as the sum of three components:

$$\Sigma M = r \times mg + r \times F_t + I\alpha \tag{1.85}$$

Note that, since the centrifugal force acts through the point of rotation, it does not create a moment around the point of rotation.

For certain situations when the forces are not constant, it may be useful to apply concepts of work and energy to solving equations of motion. *Work* is the result of force acting on a body to produce motion and is measured as the product of the magnitude of the force vector times the amount of displacement of the body:

$$W = F \cdot s \tag{1.86}$$

Note that both vectors need to have the same direction and the dot product results in a purely scalar value. If the force is in newtons and the displacement in meters, the resulting unit is joules (J, named after the English physicist James Prescott Joule, 1818–1889).

Energy is the capacity of a system to do work and thus has the same units as work. It can be *potential energy* associated with position in the gravitational field or *kinetic energy* associated with linear displacement of a body. In the first case, it is defined as

$$E_p = mgh \tag{1.87}$$

where
E_p = potential energy
h = change in height with respect to gravity

In the second case, it is defined as

$$E_p = 1/2\, k s^2 \tag{1.88}$$

where
k = spring constant of an elastic body
s = linear displacement

Kinetic energy is associated with the energy released during motion of a body and is defined as

$$E_k = 1/2\, mv^2 \tag{1.89}$$

where
E_k = kinetic energy
m = mass of the body
v = rectilinear velocity of the body

The key principle in using work and energy for motion analyses is that work done on a body by a conservative force can be converted to kinetic and potential energies, the sum of which will always be constant for any position of the system; i.e., energy cannot be created or destroyed, but can only be transformed. This is known as the *law of the conservation of mechanical energy.*

Example 1.6: Potential Energy of a Falling Object

The average energy required for skull fracture is approximately 70 Nm. Consider a construction site or steel mill with an overhead crane carrying scrap metal. It would be of interest to determine the minimum height a 2-kg piece of metal would need to fall to cause skull fracture. Equation 1.87, with g = 9.807 m/s², yields

$$70 = 2 \times 9.807 \times h \tag{1.90}$$

Solving for h yields

$$h = 70/2/9.807 = 3.57\,\text{m} \tag{1.91}$$

This is not a very high height and demonstrates the need for wearing hard hats on industrial sites.

A similar analysis could be applied to the wrist, for an individual trying to break a fall with an outstretched arm after tripping. Considering a large body weight of 70 kg, the height would very minimal. However, the analysis is quite a bit more complicated because the weight is distributed along the length of the body and other parts of the body may come in contact with the ground first, absorbing some of the impact. Still, it is not an uncommon occurrence for an individual in a fall to fracture some of the bones in the wrist or the forearm.

Example 1.7: Kinetic Energy from a Flying Object

Again assume that the average energy required for skull fracture is approximately 70 Nm. Consider a powered lawnmower that picks up a stone weighing 0.01 kg and, through the action of the revolving blades, ejects it from the discharge chute of the mower. It would be of interest to determine the minimum velocity that would cause skull fracture. Equation 1.89 yields

$$70 = 1/2 \times 0.01 v^2 \tag{1.92}$$

Solving for velocity yields

$$v = \left(2 \times 70 / 0.01\right)^{1/2} = 118.3 \, \text{m/s} \tag{1.93}$$

Considering that the peripheral velocity of the blades for some mowers can achieve speeds of up to 100 m/s, it would not be unusual for a sufficiently large stone to cause major injury.

For further background material on biomechanics principles, useful examples, and practical applications to the human body, the reader is referred to LeVeau (1977) and Özkaya and Nordin (1991).

Questions

1. What is biomechanics?
2. Who are some of the historical figures that helped develop biomechanics as a science?
3. What factors characterize a force?
4. What characteristics are found in static equilibrium?
5. Compare and contrast the three different classes of levers. Give an example from the human body for each class.
6. What is the principle of moments? Why is it useful in biomechanics?
7. Define the coefficient of friction. How is it possible for it to exceed the value of one?
8. What is the difference between kinematics and kinetics?
9. Describe a method for determining the center of mass for a body segment.
10. Describe a method for determining the moment of inertia for a body segment.

11. What is the law of the conservation of mechanical energy? Give an example of where this may be applied.

12. How is the moment of inertia related to the radius of gyration for a body segment?

Problems

1.1. Consider Example 1.1, except that the included angle is now 135° instead of 90°. How would that change the force required of the biceps brachii and the mechanical advantage? Repeat for 45°. Relate these results to the development of certain types of strength-training equipment.

1.2. Consider the upper limb bent at 90°. The weight of the upper arm, forearm, and hand are represented by a forces of 21, 13, and 4 N, acting through the respective center of gravities as shown below. Find the center of gravity for the combined upper limb system.

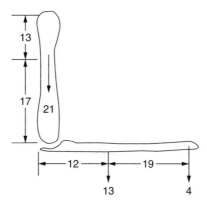

1.3. Consider the sternocleidomastoid muscle shown in Figure 1.8. Discuss the two different lever systems involved and the relative mechanical advantages for the respective ranges on the clavicle for which each type of lever system is applicable.

1.4. Consider a pilot using night vision goggles (force of 9 N), which are attached to the front of the helmet (force of 18 N). To counteract the resulting large downward torque of the head and consequent fatigue of the neck muscles, the pilot attaches a lead weight to the back of the helmet. Helmet cg is 2 cm in front of neck pivot point; goggle cg is 20 cm anterior of neck pivot point; lead weight cg is 10 cm behind neck pivot point; the head is of uniform density and exerts a force of 40 N. Find the appropriate lead weight that would best balance the head and eliminate neck fatigue. What critical assumption must be made before this problem can be started? Why is this assumption valid? What class of lever system is involved?

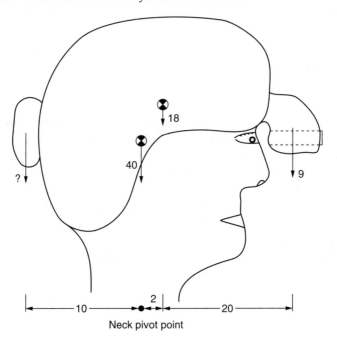

Neck pivot point

1.5. Traction is applied in line to the arm with a 15-kg weight suspended via three pulleys as shown below. Assuming frictionless pulleys, how much traction is applied to the arm?

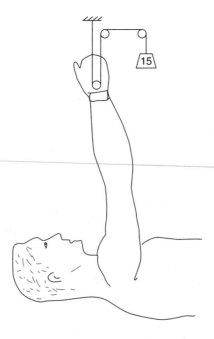

1.6. A patient is being lowered in a frictionless wheelchair down a 30° ramp. The total weight of the patient and wheelchair is 100 kg. A rope tied to a wheelchair takes a half turn around a pipe at the top of the ramp with μ = 0.2. What force must be applied to the rope to control the motion of the chair and patient?

1.7. A Russell traction (shown below) is used for immobilizing femoral fractures. Assuming μ = 0.05 and neglecting the weight of the leg, what weight is needed to produce a 30-kg traction force on the femur? What important features have been forgotten and usually must be done to the patient in these cases? Measure the angles needed directly from the drawing.

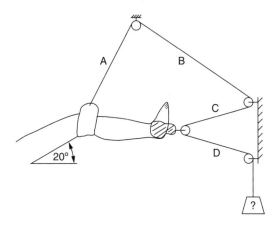

1.8. Assume that the energy level needed for shoulder fracture is approximately 70 J. What is the minimum weight needed for an object falling from a 10-m height to cause fracture? What is its velocity at impact?

References

Bobjer, O., Johansson, S.E., and Piguet, S., 1993. Friction between hand and handle. Effects of oil and lard on textured and non-textured surfaces; perception of discomfort, *Applied Ergonomics*, 24:190–202.

Chaffin, D.B., Andersson, G.B.J., and Martin, B.J., 1999. *Occupational Biomechanics*, 3rd ed., New York: John Wiley & Sons.

Dempster, W.T., 1955. *Space Requirements of the Seated Operator*, WADC-TR–55-159, Dayton, OH: Aerospace Medical Research Laboratories.

Kitano, T., Ateshian, G.A., Mow, V.C., Kadoya, Y., and Yamano, Y., 2001. Constituents and pH changes in protein rich hyaluronan solution affect the biotribological properties of artificial articular joints, *Journal of Biomechanics*, 34:1031–1037.

Lephart, S.A., 1984. Measuring the inertial properties of cadaver segments, *Journal of Biomechanics*, 17:537–543.

LeVeau, B., 1977. *Williams and Lissner Biomechanics of Human Motion*, 2nd ed., Philadelphia: W.B. Saunders.

Miller, D.I. and Nelson, R.C., 1976. *Biomechanics of Sport*, Philadelphia: Lea & Febiger.

Özkaya, N. and Nordin, M., 1991. *Fundamentals of Biomechanics*, New York: Van Nostrand Reinhold.

Plagenhoef, J.A., 1966. Methods for obtaining kinetic data to analyze human motions, *The Research Quarterly of the American Association for Health, Physical Education, and Recreation*, 37:103–112.

Roebuck, J.A., Kroemer, K.H.E., and Thomson, W.G., 1975. *Engineering Anthropometry Methods*, New York: Wiley-Interscience.

Unsworth, A., Dowson, D., and Wright, V., 1975. The frictional behavior of human synovial joints — Part I. Natural joints, *Transactions of the American Society of Mechanical Engineers, Series F, Journal of Lubrication Technology*, 97:369–376.

Weast, R.C., Ed., 1969. *Handbook of Chemistry and Physics*, Cleveland, OH: The Chemical Rubber Co., p. F15.

Webb Associates, Ed., 1978. *Anthropometric Source Book*, NASA 1024, Washington, D.C.: National Aeronautics and Space Administration.

2

Structure of the Musculoskeletal System

2.1 Gross Overview of Movements

The musculoskeletal system is a complex system of muscles, bones, and soft connective tissue that produces movement in the human body. The movements are three dimensional, centered around joints, but are typically defined in two dimensions along the three major planes (Figure 2.1): *sagittal,* observing the body from the side, *transverse,* observing the body from directly above the head, and *frontal,* observing the body from the front, i.e., face to face. These movements are defined with the human body in a *standard anatomical position,* as shown in Figure 2.1, with palms facing forward.

Movements of the trunk and neck in the sagittal plane include *flexion,* bending the trunk or neck forward, and *extension,* bending the trunk or neck backward. In the frontal plane, bending the trunk sideways results in lateral flexion, with the *lateral* direction farther away from the midline of the body, as opposed to the *medial* direction, which is closer to the midline. In the transverse plane, rotation of the trunk along the vertical long axis of the body (roughly the spinal column) results in *axial rotation.*

Movements of the shoulder girdle (as opposed to the *glenohumeral joint* or strictly the shoulder joint) in the sagittal or frontal plane include shoulder elevation, i.e., the raising the shoulders, and shoulder depression, i.e., the lowering of the shoulders. In the sagittal plane, drawing the shoulder forward results in *protraction,* while drawing the shoulders backward results in *retraction.*

Movements of the glenohumeral joint and hip joint in the sagittal plane include flexion, raising the arm or moving the thigh forward, and extension, pushing the arm or thigh backward of the midline. In the frontal plane, *abduction* is the raising the arm or thigh to the side, while *adduction* is lowering the arm or bringing the thigh closer to the midline. In transverse plane, rotation of the arm or leg along its long axis outward results in lateral or outward rotation, while rotation of the arm or leg along its long axis inward results in medial or inward rotation. Note that both the glenohumeral and hip joints are ball-and-socket type of joints, allowing for three degrees of rotational freedom.

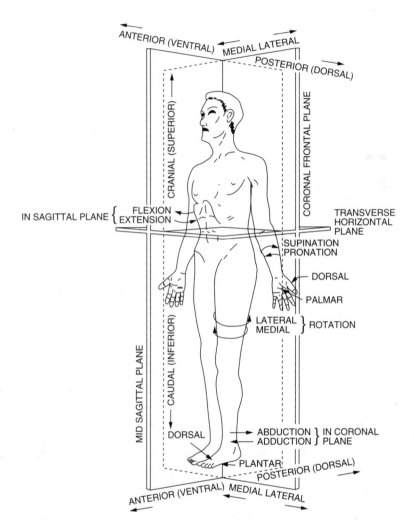

FIGURE 2.1

Standard anatomical posture with major movements shown. (From Chaffin, D.B. et al., 1999. *Occupational Biomechanics*, 3rd ed., New York: John Wiley & Sons. With permission.)

Movements of the elbow and knee joints in the sagittal plane include flexion, the bending from a fully straightened position or a decrease in the internal angle, and extension, an increase of the internal angle back toward the fully straightened position. Note that the elbow and knee joints are basically hinge or pin joints allowing only one degree of rotational freedom.

Movement of the wrist joint including the eight *carpal* bones in the wrist can be defined as follows. In the sagittal plane, flexion is bending the palm upward or closer to the forearm, while extension is bending the palm back or away from the forearm. In the frontal plane, *radial deviation* is moving the hand away from the trunk and closer to radius bone in the forearm, while *ulnar deviation* is moving the hand closer to the trunk and closer to the ulna in the forearm.

Movement of the ankle in the sagittal plane includes flexion or, more specifically, *dorsiflexion*, the raising of the dorsum or the top part of the foot, and extension or *plantar flexion*, moving the sole or the plantar part of the foot downward. If the *tarsal* bones of the foot are also involved, then *inversion* is bringing the sole of the foot inward and *eversion* is moving the sole of the foot outward.

Because of the large number of bones in the hand (Figure 2.2 and Figure 5.1), there are a correspondingly large number of joints and types of movement possible of the hand. The fingers are termed the *phalanges* and the palm is formed by the *metacarpals*. This is one reason the hand is such a good manipulative device that is difficult to replicate even with the finest robotic controls currently available. The thumb is the first digit, the index finger is the second, the middle finger is the third, the ring finger is the fourth, and the small finger is digit 5. MP refers to the metacarpophalangeal joint and IP refers to interphalangeal joints. MP and IP flexion is movement of the fingers closer to the palm, i.e., curling the fingers, while MP and IP extension is movement of the fingers away from the palm. Movement of the thumb perpendicularly away from the palm is abduction, with adduction closer to the palm. Movement of the thumb to oppose other digits pulpy surface to pulpy surface is *opposition*. The hand is considered to have a long axis defined by digit 3. Therefore, movements of digits 2, 4, and 5 away from this axis in the plane of the palm is abduction, and adduction is the return of the digits to their normal position.

Movement of the forearm can also be considered a joint action, because the two forearm bones, the *radius* and the *ulna*, rotate with respect to one another along the long axis. Rotation of the forearm to the palm-up position is *supination*, while to the palm-down position is *pronation*. Note that in all of these gross movements, there typically will be two opposing motions for each joint, each of which is controlled by a separate set of muscles.

2.2 The Skeletal System

The purpose of the skeletal system (see Figure 2.2) is both (1) to provide a rigid system of links, the bones, for the attachment of muscles and the basis of movement and (2) to protect the internal organs. There are more than 200 bones in the human body of various sizes, shapes, and mechanical properties. Interestingly, these characteristics can change dramatically in response to external stressors and, thus, living bones can be very dynamic systems.

Bones can be roughly categorized as either *long bones*, found in the extremities, i.e., the femur, the humerus, etc., or as *axial bones*, such as the skull, vertebrae, pelvis, etc. The long bones are characterized by a tubular shaft

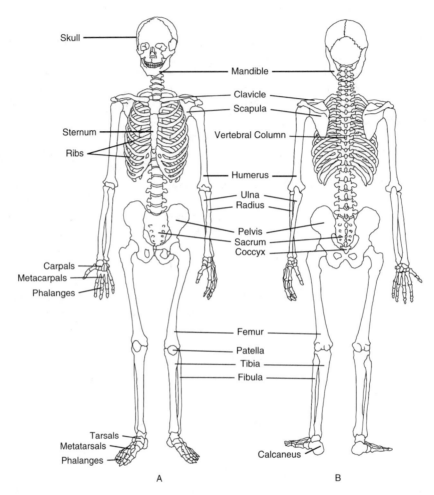

FIGURE 2.2
Major bones and in the human skeleton. (A) Anterior; (B) posterior.

termed the *diaphysis* and two enlarged rounded ends termed the *epiphyses* (Figure 2.3). The outer edge of the diaphysis is composed of higher mineral content and, thus, denser bone material, *cortical or compact bone*, while the center and epiphyses contain spongy, less dense bone material termed *cancellous* or *spongy bone*. To better distribute stress in this less dense region, a three-dimensional lattice-like structure of fibers, the *trabeculae*, has evolved. Interestingly, this is one of the very dynamic aspects of bone, with the trabeculae structure adapting to external stress in very visible patterns. This was first characterized by Wolff (1892) as "form follows function," now known as *Wolff's law*. The center of the diaphysis also contains bone marrow that produces red blood cells and blood vessels carrying away cells and bringing nutrients to the bone. This red blood cell production decreases

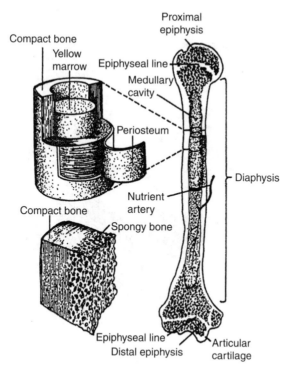

FIGURE 2.3

Diagram of a long bone, shown in longitudinal cross. (From Chaffin, D.B. et al., 1999. *Occupational Biomechanics*, 3rd ed., New York: John Wiley & Sons. With permission.)

dramatically by late adolescence with a concurrent increase in fatty deposits in the marrow.

Bone material is composed of cells and an extracellular matrix of fibers and a ground substance. The cells produce the extracellular matrix, which determines the mechanical properties of bone. The combined effect of the fibers and ground substance provides an additive effect for strength. An apt analogy is reinforced concrete with the concrete producing compressive strength and the rebars providing structural support. These cells are initially called *osteoblasts*, but gradually transform themselves into *osteocytes*, which become mineralized and isolated in the matrix. A third type of cells, the *osteoclasts*, performs a reverse process of gradually reabsorbing the bone structure. This again shows the very dynamic processes occurring in bone, with bone formation and resorption occurring simultaneously, especially in adaptive responses to external stressors and forces. This, however, is very different from the soft connective tissue, which, once formed, can only deteriorate, and is a partial explanation for the seriousness of repetitive motion injuries, which are slow to heal in connective tissue. On the other hand, bone, when injured, can actually heal to a stronger state than found initially.

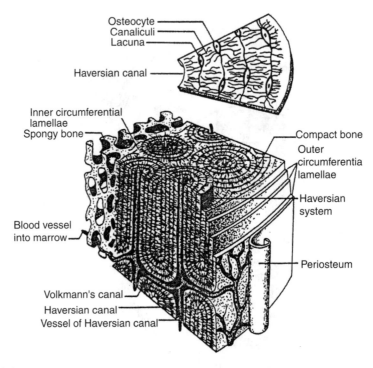

FIGURE 2.4
Diagram of the Haversian system within compact bone. (From Chaffin, D.B. et al., 1999. *Occupational Biomechanics*, 3rd ed., New York: John Wiley & Sons. With permission.)

The ground substance is *hydroxyapatite*, a crystalline structure of calcium while the fibers are primarily collagen fibers. During bone formation or *ossification*, the first bone called *woven bone* is laid down at outer edges of the *Haversian canal system* (Figure 2.4), or points of injury or fracture. Gradually, through the parallel arrangement of the collagen fibers and hydroxyapatite crystals, the woven bone becomes a more sheet-like *lamellar bone*. With repeated deposits of circumferential lamellae, cortical bone is formed and the overall bone gains strength. Note, this could be considered similar to production of plywood, which increases the overall strength of wood, or the laying down of steel strands in belted tires. Note, also, that this process follows mechanics principles of obtaining optimum strength. Bending strength is increased with increased moments of inertial, i.e., increasing cross-sectional areas and increasing the area farther from the point of rotation. That is, for the same amount or mass of material, a hollow tube is stronger than a solid tube (see Example 2.1).

Example 2.1: Bending Moments of Hollow Tubes

The elastic deflection of a support beam can be defined as the radius of curvature resulting from a bending moment applied to the beam:

$$\rho = EI/M \tag{2.1}$$

where
ρ = radius of curvature
E = the modulus of elasticity for the given material
I = moment of inertia of the cross section of the beam with reference to its axis
M = bending moment on the beam.

When there is a small bending moment or a very large moment of inertia, the radius of curvature approaches infinity, yielding a straight beam.

The moment of inertia of a solid beam with a circular cross section is

$$I = \pi r^4/4 \tag{2.2}$$

where r = radius of the circular cross section.
The moment of inertia of a tube is

$$I = \pi\left(r_1^4 - r_2^4\right)/4 \tag{2.3}$$

where r_1 = outer radius, r_2 = inner radius. For a solid tube, r_1 is zero and Equation 2.3 becomes equivalent to Equation 2.2.

The objective is to maximize the moment of inertia for a given amount of material defined as the area, which for the solid beam is

$$A = \pi r^2 \tag{2.4}$$

and for the tube is

$$A = \pi\left(r_1^2 - r_2^2\right) \tag{2.5}$$

For example, comparing a solid beam with a 1 cm radius and a tube with an outer radius of 3 cm and an inner radius of 2.828 (i.e., wall thickness of 0.172 cm) yields the same amount of material:

$$\pi 1^2 = \pi\left(3^2 - 2.828^2\right) = \pi \tag{2.6}$$

However, the moment of inertia for the solid beam is

$$I = \pi/4 \tag{2.7}$$

while the moment of inertia for the tube is

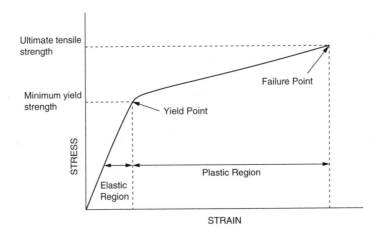

FIGURE 2.5
A typical stress–strain curve for a material in tension.

$$I = \pi\left(3^4 - 2.828^4\right)\big/4 = 17\pi\big/4 \qquad (2.8)$$

Thus, the moment of inertia for the hollow tube is 17 times larger than for a solid beam of the same amount of material resulting in a 17 times greater resistance to deflection for a given bending moment. This principle is used in the construction of pylons and products where weight is important, such as bicycles. Of course, carrying the principle to extremes would result in walls so thin that they would be easily damaged from direct pressure or impacts. Similarly, bones have evolved with a greater amount of solid material being deposited on the outer edge for greater strength.

2.3 Mechanical Properties of Bone

Stiffness and strength are important mechanical properties of bone. These are typically established through a *stress–strain curve* (Figure 2.5) obtained from a bone specimen placed in a testing jig. The load applied per unit area of the specimen is termed *stress*, while the deformation normalized to the initial length is termed *strain*. Initially, in a region termed the *elastic region*, the relationship between stress and strain is linear and repeatable during release of the loading. The slope of this region is the modulus of elasticity and represents the stiffness of the material:

$$\sigma = E\varepsilon \qquad (2.9)$$

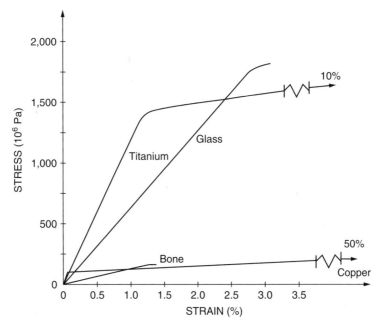

FIGURE 2.6
Stress–strain curves for bone and other materials in tension. Bone = compact bone from human femur (Reilly and Burstein, 1975); copper = 99.9% pure copper (Weast, 1969); glass = 6 mm strand, SiO_2 with 20% Na_2O (Weast, 1969); titanium = 6Al-4V alloy (Weast, 1969).

where
σ = stress (in Pa)
E = Young's modulus of elasticity (in Pa)
ε = strain (unitless)

Once loading exceeds the *yield point*, the material enters the *plastic deformation region* and will not return to its original shape when unloaded. At a certain point after considerable plastic flow, the material will eventually fail at the *failure point*. The relative material strengths at these points are termed the *minimum yield strength* and *ultimate tensile strength*.

Overall bone strength and properties are compared to those of other materials in Figure 2.6. Metals vary in ductility and show a definite plastic region while glass is very brittle and has no plastic region, failing at the end of the elastic region. A stiff metal, such as titanium, has an elongation range of less than 10% before failure, while a ductile metal, such as copper, may elongate up to 50% before failure. Bone has a less definite elastic region, perhaps up to 1% strain, and flows another 2% before failure.

When loaded in *tension* (Figure 2.7), the ultimate strength of bone is relatively comparable to copper. Not surprisingly, because of daily loading, bone is stronger in *compression* but relatively weak in shear loading (Figure 2.8). Also, because bone is *anisotropic*, its properties are very different depending

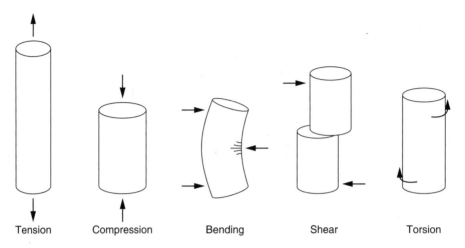

FIGURE 2.7
Schematic representation of various loading modes.

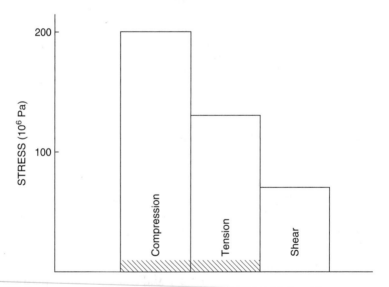

FIGURE 2.8
Ultimate strength at failure for human cortical bone specimens test in compression, tension, and shear. Shaded area indicates stresses experienced during running (Carter, 1978). (Adapted from Frankel and Nordin, 1980.)

on the direction of the applied forces as compared to the directional qualities of bone (Figure 2.9). This would seem quite logical considering the overlapping layers of lamellar patterns. Note, also, that the above properties apply to cortical bone having quite a dense structure (70 to 95%) as compared to cancellous bone, which with a 10 to 70% dense structure, is much weaker.

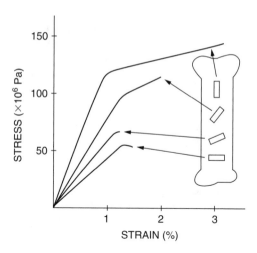

FIGURE 2.9

Stress–strain curves for cortical bone tested in tension in four different orientations. (Adapted from Reilly and Burstein, 1975.)

Typical daily loading of bone is compressive by nature and relatively low, around 4 MPa and rarely exceeding 12 MPa, measured during jogging (Carter, 1978). More extreme compressive loadings, as in impacts from falls, can result in fractures, typically found in vertebrae. *Shear* loading is applied parallel to the surface of the structure resulting in deformation of the internal cancellous bone (see Figure 2.4). A relatively typical shear fracture occurs to the femoral condyle during falls especially for older females with weaker bones. Bending fractures can occur when a load is applied at one end of the limb, with the other end relatively fixed, creating bending moment, and causing the limb to bend about the longitudinal axis. One outer surface of the bone is being lengthened through tensile loading, while the opposite outer surface is being compressed. Failure will tend to occur on the surface subjected to tension, because ultimate tensile strength is lower than ultimate compressive strength in cortical bone. For example, such bending moments may occur during skiing accidents, as the upper body falls forward over the top of a relatively immobile ski and ski boot, resulting in boot-top tibial fractures from falls (Frankel and Nordin, 1980). Torsional fractures may also occur in the same skiing accident, if the long ski tends to twist the tibia and fibula about the long axis.

Bone is very dynamic, changing size, shape, and structure as a result of the mechanical stresses placed upon it. As mentioned earlier, this was first observed by Wolff (1892) who characterized it in his "form follows function" law. Correspondingly, bone mass is deposited or reabsorbed as necessary at the critical locations, which is crucial, especially for those immobilized after injuries or in elderly individuals, most notably women. A 60-day immobilization of rhesus monkeys resulted in more than a 50% loss in compressive strength (Kazarian and Von Gierke, 1969). Full skeletal bone maturity is reached roughly at the age of 30. After age 30, bone loss, exemplified by a decrease in calcium, a decrease in cortical bone thickness and diameter, and a decrease in trabeculae in cancellous bone, occurs steadily, accelerating with increasing age.

Interestingly, a similar bone loss is found in astronauts returning from extended periods in space. The hypothesis is that the lack of mechanical strain in the bone from the lack of gravity leads to bone reabsorption. To prevent such bone loss, researchers have recommended exercise that maintains stress on bone for astronauts, specifically impact types of exercises that increase the strain rate in bone (Cavanagh et al., 1992). This has resulted in the development and deployment of specialized treadmills in which the astronaut is tethered to the treadmill with an elastic cord to maintain contact in the zero-*g* environment (McCrory et al., 1999).

2.4   Soft Connective Tissue

The soft connective tissue of the body — ligaments, tendons, fascia, and cartilage — provides support and structural integrity to the musculoskeletal system and transmits forces between components. All connective tissue, similar to bone, is composed of cells, an extracellular matrix of fibers, and a ground substance. The cells produce the extracellular matrix, which determines the mechanical properties of the connective tissue. The ground substance is typically a *proteoglycan*, a polysaccharide with a protein core, some lipids, and the ubiquitous water.

There are three main types of fibers: *collagen, elastin,* and *reticulin*. Collagen fibers provide strength and stiffness to the tissue, elastin fibers provide elasticity, while reticulin merely provides bulk. A stress–strain diagram for collagen (Figure 2.10) indicates a small toe region (up to 1% strain) in which the kinky strands are straightened, a relatively linear elastic region up to roughly 7% strain, and a plastic deformation region until ultimate failure at roughly 10% strain. The stress–strain diagram (Figure 2.11) for elastin is very different with almost pure elasticity (under minimal stress) up to roughly 200%, at which point the fibers have lost their elasticity, become stiff under increasing stress, and eventually fail without plastic deformation.

Ligaments connect bone to bone and provide stability at joints. They are typically 90% collagen with relatively straight arrangement of fibers with minimal elasticity (Figure 2.12). *Tendons* connect muscle to bone, transmitting the muscle force. They are composed almost completely of parallel bundles of collagen fibers with no elasticity. Tendons are often surrounded by a *synovial* lining sheath, which produces a very low friction synovial fluid to facilitate the gliding of tendons. The parallel arrangement is ideal for axial transmission of force. However, as a consequence the transverse properties are very much reduced. *Fascia* is connective tissue covering organs and

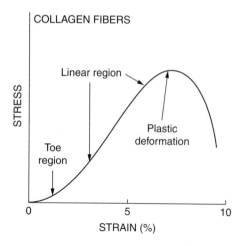

FIGURE 2.10
Stress–strain curve for collagen fibers in tension. (From Chaffin, D.B. et al., 1999. *Occupational Biomechanics*, 3rd ed., New York: John Wiley & Sons. With permission.)

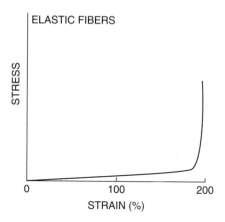

FIGURE 2.11
Stress–strain curve for elastin fibers in tension. (From Chaffin, D.B. et al., 1999. *Occupational Biomechanics*, 3rd ed., New York: John Wiley & Sons. With permission.)

muscles. It is very elastic (high percentage of elastin) with a very irregular arrangement of fibers, allowing elasticity in all direction. *Cartilage* covers articular bony surfaces and is found also in the ear, nose, and intervertebral discs. Of the three main types of cartilage, *hyaline cartilage* is found on the epiphysial areas of bone (see Section 2.5) and is a relatively homogeneous matrix of collagen fibers. *Fibrocartilage* is present in the intervertebral discs and is composed of collagen and elastin. *Elastic cartilage* is found in the ear and epiglottis of the throat.

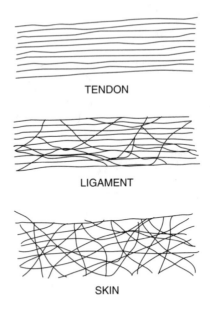

TENDON

LIGAMENT

SKIN

FIGURE 2.12
Schematic diagram of the structural orientation of tendon, ligament, and skin fibers. (From Chaffin, D.B. et al., 1999. *Occupational Biomechanics*, 3rd ed., New York: John Wiley & Sons. With permission.)

2.5   Joints

A joint is the interaction point between two or more bones. There are three types of joints, the most common of which is the articulating or freely moving joint. A layer of synovial fluid (the same as found in tendon sheaths) is found between the two articulating surfaces of the bones. Thus, these joints are sometimes also called synovial joints. If there is tissue connecting the two bones and it is fibrous such as in the skull, then these are termed fibrous joints. If the tissue is cartilage such as in the intervertebral discs, then these are termed cartilaginous joints.

2.5.1   Articular Joints

In an articular joint (Figure 2.13), the articulating ends of the bones are covered with a 1- to 5-mm-thick layer of connective tissue, the articular cartilage, and are surrounded by a synovial membrane (to contain the synovial fluid) and a joint capsule of ligaments. Many joints (such as the knee) have a disc of fibrocartilage (cartilage with higher collagen content) called a *meniscus* to better distribute forces and protect the bones. In fact, the main

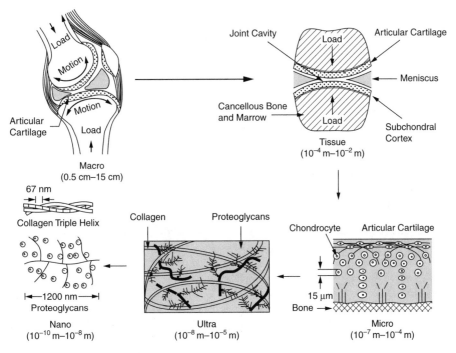

FIGURE 2.13

Important structural features of a typical articular joint. (From Mow, V.C. and Ratcliffe, A., 1997. In V.C. Mow and W.C. Hayes, Eds., *Basic Orthopaedic Biomechanics*, 2nd ed., Philadelphia: Lippincott-Raven, 113–178. With permission.)

purpose of articular cartilage is to spread loads over a larger area and to allow relative movements of the opposing surface with minimum friction and wear. Physiologically, articular cartilage is virtually devoid of both blood and lymph vessels, as well as nerves. This has important implications in terms of wear and potential regenerative capabilities.

Hyaline cartilage is primarily composed of the extracellular matrix with relatively few cells. The extracellular matrix is quite high in water content (60 to 80%), leaving only 20 to 40% solid material widely distributed. Of the solid part, 60% is collagen fibers and 40% is the proteoglycan gel, the ground substance composed of hyaluronic acid protein. The *chondrocyte* cells comprise less than 2% of the material and are arranged in a layered zone within the proteoglycan gel (see Figure 2.13). In the superficial tangential zone, the chondrocytes are oblong with their long axes aligned parallel to the articular surface. In the middle zone, the chondrocytes are round and randomly distributed, while in the deep zone the chondrocytes are columnar in arrangement and are perpendicular to the *tide mark*, which acts as a boundary to calcified cartilage and the bone. The collagen fibers are similarly distributed in the cartilage layer: densely packed parallel to the surface in the superficial tangential zone, randomly oriented in the middle zone, and perpendicular to the surface in the deep zone (Figure 2.14). This latter arrangement and zone

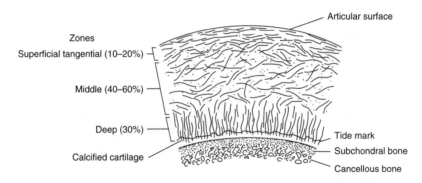

FIGURE 2.14
Layered structure of articular cartilage collagen network showing three distinct regions. (From Mow, V.C. and Ratcliffe, A., 1997. In V.C. Mow and W.C. Hayes, Eds., *Basic Orthopaedic Biomechanics*, 2nd ed., Philadelphia: Lippincott-Raven, 113–178. With permission.)

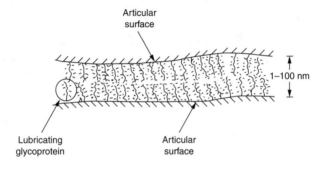

FIGURE 2.15
Schematic diagram of articular cartilage surface with a monolayer of lubricating proteoglycan. (From Mow, V.C. and Ateshian, G.A., 1997. In V.C. Mow and W.C. Hayes, Eds., *Basic Orthopaedic Biomechanics*, 2nd ed., Philadelphia: Lippincott-Raven, 275–316. With permission.)

are instrumental in anchoring the cartilage to the underlying bone (Mow and Ratcliffe, 1997).

The proteoglycan gel is composed of water and a brushlike polymeric macromolecule based on a hyaluronic acid core with many side units (Figure 2.14 and Figure 2.15). These molecules are strongly hydrophilic (because of regular fixed negative charges and a high concentration that attempts to dilute itself through osmosis) but are prevented from fully absorbing water and swelling by the collagen network. This constraint on swelling causes an increase in osmotic pressure and tensile stress on the collagen fibers when there is no external stress. When an external stress is applied to the cartilage surface, the internal pressure in the cartilage matrix increases, exceeding the osmotic pressure and causing water to be squeezed out of the cartilage, producing a natural lubricating system (see Section 2.5.2).

Mechanically, articular cartilage can be considered a biphasic material — a solid in terms of collagen and a liquid in terms of freely moving interstitial

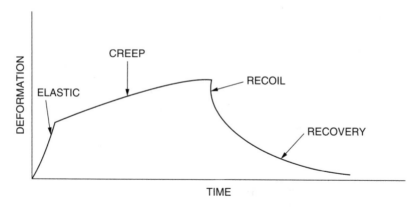

FIGURE 2.16
Stress–strain curve for articular cartilage. (From Chaffin, D.B. et al., 1999. *Occupational Biomechanics*, 3rd ed., New York: John Wiley & Sons. With permission.)

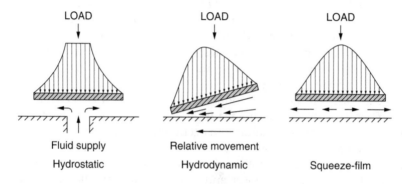

FIGURE 2.17
Diagrams illustrating three modes of joint lubrication: (A) hydrostatic, (B) hydrodynamic, (C) squeeze-film. (Adapted from Frankel and Nordin, 1980.)

water — perhaps, similar to a wet sponge. Correspondingly, it exhibits both elastic and viscoelastic properties under compression, with an initial elastic deformation, followed by a slow creep (Figure 2.16). Upon release of the load, an initial elastic recoil is followed by a slow recovery (Mow and Ratcliffe, 1997).

2.5.2 Joint Lubrication

As mentioned in Chapter 1, the articular surface has an extremely low coefficient of friction ($\mu = 0.003$ to 0.005; Linn, 1968; Unsworth et al., 1975), much lower than can be achieved with man-made materials and lubricants. This is due, it is thought, to the simultaneous application of three different lubrication mechanisms: hydrostatic, hydrodynamic, and squeeze film lubrication. In *hydrostatic lubrication*, loading of the joint forces the synovial fluid out of the pores of the cartilage and into the space between the articular surfaces (Figure 2.17A). As the joint is unloaded, the fluid is reabsorbed into the cartilage, similar to a sponge. In this case, the cartilage acts both as the pump and the reservoir for the lubricant.

In *hydrodynamic lubrication,* translational joint motion creates a wedge effect, further forcing synovial fluid between the articular surfaces (Figure 2.17B). In *squeeze-film lubrication,* even relatively normal pressures, the fluid is squeezed from the areas of high pressure to areas of lower pressure (Figure 2.17C). As the pressure in the first area decreases, fluid returns. Thus, there is continual movement of the synovial fluid between the articular surfaces just from the pressures due to normal walking or other activities (Mow and Ateshian, 1997).

2.5.3   Wear and Osteoarthritis

Wear is the removal of material from articulating surfaces, either by abrasion or adhesion of the interfacial surfaces or by fatigue through repetitive stressing and deformation of the contacting surfaces and repetitive exchange of the synovial fluid. Repetitive stressing of the extracellular matrix could cause (1) damage to the collagen fibers, (2) disruption of the proteoglycan gel network, or (3) impairment of the fiber/interfibrillar matrix interface. Repetitive exuding and imbibing of the interstitial fluid may cause a washing out of the proteoglycan molecules from the matrix or a reduction of the cartilage's self-lubricating ability.

Articular cartilage has been found to have a limited capacity for repair and regeneration, and if the stresses applied are large and sudden (excessive stress concentration), total failure can occur. Joints of people in certain occupations, such as football players' knees, ballet dancers' ankles, and miners' knees, are especially susceptible to high forces, fractures, damage to the load-spreading function of the menisci, and ligament ruptures allowing excessive movement of bone ends. It has been hypothesized that this progression of failure is related to (1) the magnitude of forces involved, (2) the total number of force peaks experienced, and (3) the rate of recovery, which is especially critical in some of the current repetitive motion disorders. Osteoarthritis occurs secondarily to the primary trauma in cartilage in the form of hemorrhages in the joint space, disorders of the collagen metabolism, and degradation of the proteolytic enzymes (Frankel and Nordin, 1980).

2.5.4   Cartilaginous Joints

Cartilaginous joints are primarily found in the intervertebral discs that separate the vertebral bones of the back. The disc consists of the *annulus fibrosus,* the outer onion-like fiber casings, and the *nucleus pulposus,* the gel-like center (Figure 2.18). As the disc is loaded the nucleus pulposus distributes the force uniformly to the outer annulus fibrosus, whose fibers can withstand the axial tensile stresses. A good analogy would be high-pressure tanks, whose fluid pressure is uniformly distributed to the walls, which are wrapped with glass fibers having very high tensile strength.

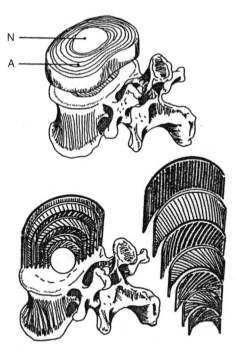

FIGURE 2.18
Structure of intervertebral disc: A = annulus fibrosus, N = nucleus pulposus. (From Chaffin, D.B. et al., 1999. *Occupational Biomechanics*, 3rd ed., New York: John Wiley & Sons. With permission.)

Both surfaces of the disc are covered by cartilage endplates, which are sufficiently porous to allow the diffusion of fluid across the end plate. Because the disc has no internal blood supply, this diffusion is its only means for receiving nutrients and eliminating wastes. This diffusion is accentuated by pressures created by loading of the vertebral column. Under high loading, fluid is forced out, while under decreased loading, fluid returns to the disc. As a result this can lead to a rather large shrinkage of the spin over the course of a day, 15 to 20 mm or roughly 1% of overall stature (DePukys, 1935). Anecdotally, astronauts returning from the zero-*g* space environment and minimal spinal loading have experienced spinal shrinkage two or three times that level. This phenomenon has been the basis for the development of *stadiometry*, measurement of spinal shrinkage as an indirect assessment of extended spinal loading (Eklund and Corlett, 1984).

Under repeated high loading, there is a tendency for the cartilage end plates to develop microfractures. These can lead to a greater net loss of fluid and an eventual drying of the nucleus pulposus and permanent shrinkage of the spine. More extreme fractures of the end plates or weakening of annulus fibrosus can lead to *disc herniation*, the bulging of the discs or even more catastrophic extrusion of the gel material. Further complications can result if the extruded material compresses nerve roots with consequent pain (sciatica) or even paralysis. Such events have typically been associated with high compressive forces combined with lateral bending or twisting actions on the spine and have led to extensive study and modeling of manual handling of loads.

Questions

1. Compare and contrast cortical and cancellous bone.
2. Describe the structural composition of bone. Give an example of a similar synthetic material.
3. Describe the stress–strain characteristics of bone. How do they compare to those of synthetic materials?
4. What is Wolff's law? Give several examples of where it may apply to bone.
5. Describe the basic structure of connective tissue.
6. What are the differences between ligaments, tendons, fascia, and cartilage?
7. Compare and contrast the three types of joints.
8. Describe the structure of an articular joint.
9. Describe the structure of hyaline cartilage. How does it compare to the basic structure of bone?
10. Explain why synovial joints have such low coefficients of friction, with respect to joint lubrication.
11. Describe the structure of intervertebral discs.

Problems

2.1. In addition to being hollow tubes, the long bones typically have larger diameters and thicker walls at the ends. Show the effect these characteristics have on bone strength (i.e., deflection). Note the comparable characteristic used in bicycle frame tubes is termed *double butted*.

2.2. Most support structures (bones, trees, etc.) seem to have a circular cross section. This would imply that a circular cross section is more resistant to bending than other shapes for a given amount of material. Compare the resistance to bending for a hollow square tube to a hollow circular tube of the same weight. The moment of inertia for a hollow square tube is given by

$$I = \left(w_1^4 - w_2^4\right)\big/4$$

where w_1 = outer width and w_2 = inner width.

2.3. The stress–strain curve for a material obeying Hooke's law is a line with a positive slope. Draw the experimentally determined stress–strain curve for a tendon. Explain the physiological basis for the differences this curve shows from that of the Hookean material.

References

Carter, D.R., 1978. Anisotropic analysis of strain rosette information from cortical bone, *Journal of Biomechanics*, 11:199–202.

Cavanagh, P.R., Davis, B.L., and Miller, T.A., 1992. A biomechanical perspective on exercise countermeasures for long term space flight, *Aviation, Space and Environmental Medicine*, 63:482–485.

Chaffin, D.B., Andersson, G.B.J., and Martin, B.J., 1999. *Occupational Biomechanics*, 3rd ed., New York: John Wiley & Sons.

DePukys, P., 1935. The physiological oscillation of the length of the body, *Acta Orthopaedica Scandinavica*, 6:338–347.

Eklund, J.A.E. and Corlett, E.N., 1984. Shrinkage as a measure of the effect of load on the spine, *Spine*, 9:189–194.

Frankel, V.H. and Nordin, M., 1980. *Basic Biomechanics of the Skeletal System*, Philadelphia: Lea & Febiger.

Kazarian, L.E. and Von Gierke, H.E., 1969. Bone loss as a result of immobilization and chelation: preliminary results in *Macaca mulatta*, *Clinical Orthopaedics*, 65:67–75.

Linn, F.C., 1968. Lubrication of animal joints: II The mechanism, *Journal of Biomechanics*, 1:193–205.

McCrory, J.L, Lemmon, D.R., Sommer, H.J., Prout, B., Smith, D., Korth, D.W., Lucero, J., Greenisen, M., Moore, J., Kozlovskaya, I., Pestov, I., Stepansov, V., Miyakinchenko, Y., and Cavanagh, P.R., 1999. Evaluation of a treadmill with vibration isolation and stabilization (TVIS) for use on the international space station, *Journal of Applied Biomechanics*, 15:292–302.

Mow, V.C. and Ateshian, G.A., 1997. Lubrication and wear of diarthrodial joints, in V.C. Mow and W.C. Hayes, Eds., *Basic Orthopaedic Biomechanics*, 2nd ed., Philadelphia: Lippincott-Raven, 275–316.

Mow, V.C. and Ratcliffe, A., 1997. Structure and function of articular cartilage and meniscus, in V.C. Mow and W.C. Hayes, Eds., *Basic Orthopaedic Biomechanics*, 2nd ed., Philadelphia: Lippincott-Raven, 113–178.

Reilly, D.T. and Burstein, A.H., 1975. The elastic and ultimate properties of compact bone tissue, *Journal of Biomechanics*, 8:393–405.

Unsworth, A., Dowson, D., and Wright, V., 1975. The frictional behavior of human synovial joints. Part I: Natural joints, *Transactions of the American Society of Mechanical Engineers, Series F, Journal of Lubrication Technology*, 97:369–376.

Weast, R.C., Ed., 1969. *Handbook of Chemistry and Physics*, Cleveland, OH: The Chemical Rubber Co., p. F15.

Wolff, J., 1892. *Das Gesetz der Transformation der Knochen* [*The Law of Bone Transformation*], Berlin: Hirschwald.

Woo, S.L.Y., Livesay, G.A., Runco, T.J., and Young, E.P., 1997. Structure and function of tendons and ligaments, in V.C. Mow and W.C. Hayes, Eds., *Basic Orthopaedic Biomechanics*, 2nd ed., Philadelphia: Lippincott-Raven, 113–178.

3

Neuromuscular Physiology and Motor Control

3.1 Introduction to Musculature

The more than 500 muscles in the body comprise close to 50% of the weight and 50% of the metabolic activity in the body. They are found as three different types of muscles: *skeletal muscles* attached to the bones, *cardiac muscle* found in the heart, and *smooth muscle* found in the internal organs and the walls of the blood vessels. Only skeletal muscles are discussed here in detail because of their relevance to motion. Skeletal muscles are attached to the bones on either side of a joint (Figure 3.1) by the tendons discussed previously and have the property of actively contracting and shortening, and in doing so, moving the bones. However, because muscle is soft tissue, the reverse action of active lengthening is not possible and a second set of muscle is required to return the limb to its original position. Thus, one or several muscles, termed *agonists* or prime movers, act as the primary activators of motion. An opposing set of muscles (typically on the opposite side of the joint), termed *antagonists*, counteracts the agonists and opposes the motion. Typically, one set of muscles is active, while the opposite set is relaxed. For example, during elbow flexion, the biceps or brachioradialis is the agonist (and also a flexor) while the triceps is the antagonist and also an extensor. However, during elbow extension, the triceps becomes the agonist (but is still an extensor), while the biceps becomes the antagonist. The muscle attachments to bones are also given specific names. The *origin* is the most *proximal* attachment, or the one nearest the trunk, while the *insertion* is the most *distal* or distant attachment from the trunk.

In terms of function, skeletal muscles can also be classified as spurt or shunt muscles. *Spurt* muscles originate far from the joint of rotation but are inserted close to the joint. Thus, they have short moment arms and can move the limb very rapidly but are relatively limited in the magnitude of effective strength. *Shunt* muscles are the opposite, with the origin close to the joint and the insertion point far from the joint. This creates a large moment arm and relative stabilizing effect on the joint. For example, in Figure 3.1 the biceps is the spurt muscle and the brachioradialis is the shunt muscle.

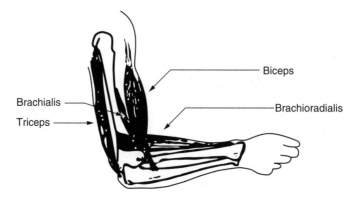

FIGURE 3.1
Muscles of the upper limb.

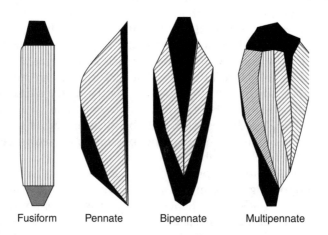

FIGURE 3.2
Patterns of muscle fiber arrangements.

Visually, skeletal muscles may have a variety of patterns with muscle fibers arranged either in parallel or obliquely to the long axis of the muscle (Figure 3.2). In *fusiform* muscles, the fibers lie parallel to the long axis, pull longitudinally, and allow for maximum velocity and range of motion, because of the relative length of the fibers. The biceps brachii is a good example of a fusiform muscle. In *pennate* or *unipennate* muscles, the fibers are arranged obliquely to the long axis, similar to the fibers in a bird feather cut in half. The extensor digitorum longus in the forearm is an example of a unipennate muscle. In bipennate muscles, the fibers are arranged obliquely on both sides of the long axis, as in a complete bird feather. Examples of bipennate muscles include the interosseous and typically the lumbricals in the hand. At the opposite extreme of parallel muscles are *multipennate* muscles, in which the fibers are relatively short and lie in several different oblique directions. Thus,

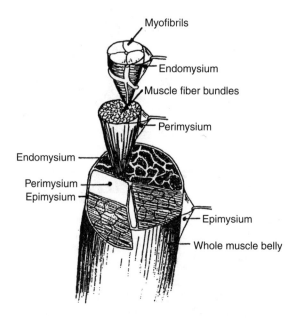

FIGURE 3.3
Transverse section of a muscle showing the various layers of fascia. (From Chaffin, D.B. et al., 1999. *Occupational Biomechanics*, 3rd ed., New York: John Wiley & Sons. With permission.)

they have a short range of motion, lower velocities, but can produce more power because of a larger cross-sectional area. The deltoid in the back of the shoulder is a good example of a multipennate muscle.

3.2 Structure of Muscle

The muscle consists of connective tissue in the form of fascia, muscle cells in the form of muscle fibers, and nerves. An outer layer of fascia, the *epimysium*, covers the muscle, inner layers of fascia, the *perimysium*, subdivide bundles of muscle fibers into *fasciculi*, and inner layers of fascia of *endomysium* covers individual muscle fibers (Figure 3.3). The fascia that binds fibers or groups of fibers extends to the end of the muscle and assists in firmly attaching the muscle and muscle fibers to the bone in the form of tendons. This gradual distribution of fascia throughout the muscle tissue is very important in the uniform transmission of force from the active contractile units to the tendon and bone. In addition, muscle tissue is penetrated by tiny blood vessels carrying oxygen and nutrients to the muscle fibers and by small nerve endings carrying electrical impulses from the spinal cord and brain.

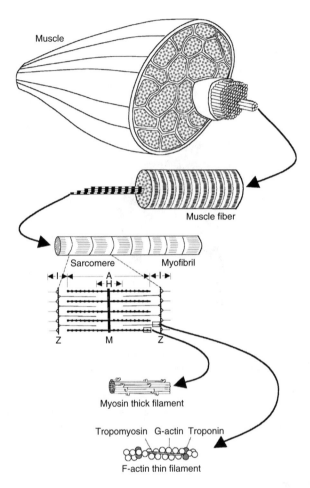

FIGURE 3.4
Organization of skeletal muscle from the muscle fibers to the protein filaments. (Adapted from McMahon, 1984.)

The muscle fibers or muscle cells are the smallest units in the muscle with independent action and may contain several nuclei. They are approximately 10 to 60 μm in diameter and range in length from 5 to 140 mm, depending on the size of the muscle. Each muscle fiber is further subdivided into smaller *myofibrils*, 1 μm in diameter, with roughly 1000 to 8000 of these per fiber. The myofibril contains the ultimate contractile mechanism in the form of protein filaments. There are two types of *myofilaments*: thick filaments, comprising long proteins with molecular heads, called *myosin*, and thin filaments comprising globular proteins, called *actin* (Figure 3.4).

The two types of filaments are interlaced with various amounts of overlap, giving rise to a striated appearance and the alternative name of *striated muscle*. These different bands are shown in Figure 3.4 with a gross division between A-bands (from anisotropic or different characteristics) of both thick

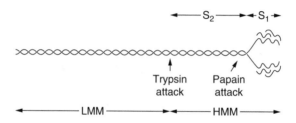

FIGURE 3.5

Schematic representation of the myosin molecule. (From Aidley, D.J., 1985. *The Physiology of Excitable Cells*, 2nd ed., Cambridge, U.K.: Cambridge University Press, 234. With permission.)

and thin filaments and I-bands (from *isotropic* or same characteristic) of just thin filaments. The thin filaments are held together by Z-discs (from the German *Zwischenscheibe* or inter disc), which also define one repeating unit within the myofibril, termed a *sarcomere*. The lighter band of non-overlapped thick filaments within the A-band is called the H-band (from the German *hell* for light or not as dark) and is bisected by the M-line (from the German *Mittelmembran* or middle membrane), a membrane that tends to hold the thick filaments together. The *sliding filament theory* of Huxley (1974) explains muscle contraction as a mechanism by which these filaments slide over one another rather than the filaments themselves shortening. This theory is supported by the observations that the I-bands and H-bands become narrower until they almost completely disappear. On the other hand, the A-band remains the same width throughout muscle contraction.

The thick filament is roughly 12 nm in diameter and composed of the long myosin molecules. Each myosin molecule (Figure 3.5) is roughly 150 nm long and consists of a tail composed of *light meromyosin* (LMM), which serves to bind the approximately 180 molecules together into a tight filament. The end of the myosin molecule has a head consisting of two subunits of *heavy meromyosin* (HMM), the S_1 and S_2 units. The S_1 unit provides the enzyme activity to cause the formation and breakage of cross bridges with the thin filament while the S_2 unit serves as the actual rotational bridge between the two types of filaments (Aidley, 1985).

The thin filament is a double helix of globular actin (G-actin) molecules 5 nm in diameter. Another protein, *tropomyosin*, serves to bring the globular actins together in chain, which is then sometimes termed fibrous actin (F-actin). At every seventh actin there is a third protein, *troponin*, which acts as an inhibitor of the cross-bridging to produce muscular contraction (Figure 3.6).

3.3 Basic Cell Physiology

A cell, including the muscle fiber, is composed primarily of *cytoplasm*, which is roughly 80% water but contains *mitochondria* used in the production of

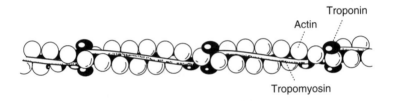

FIGURE 3.6
Schematic representation of the thin filament. (From Ebashi, S., Endo, M., and Ohtsuki, I., 1969. *Quarterly Reviews of Biophysics*, 2:351–384. With permission.)

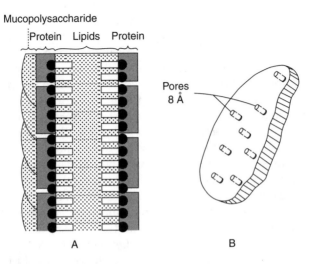

FIGURE 3.7
(A) Molecular organization of the cell membrane. (B) Pores in the cell membrane. (From Guyton, A.C., 1971. *Textbook of Medical Physiology*, Philadelphia: W.B. Saunders, 15. With permission from Elsevier Science.)

energy through metabolism and of a *nucleus* containing genetic material. The cell is surrounded by a *cell membrane,* which is a selective barrier for the passage of nutrients and wastes in and out of the cell. It also serves as the site for the action of hormones and the generation and transmission of electrical impulses. According to the *unit membrane theory* (Figure 3.7), the cell membrane is a bi-layer structure roughly 100 Å thick covered with a mucopolysaccharide surface. Below the surface is a protein layer followed by a phospholipid layer, which is then reversed for the inner layer. The polysaccharide and protein layers are *hydrophilic*, allowing water molecules to adhere to the surface, while the lipid layers prevent lipid-insoluble material to pass through. The thin mucopolysaccharide surface makes the outside different from the inside of the cell, allowing a differential charge buildup and a resulting cell potential. Materials can pass through this membrane in one of three different ways. Small charged molecules such as water pass

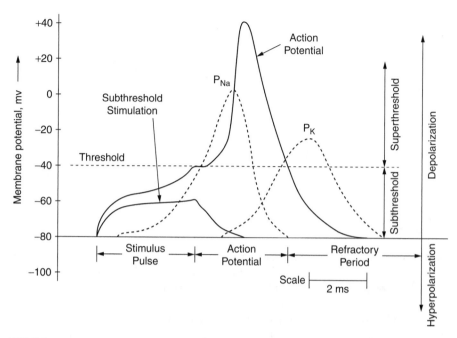

FIGURE 3.8
Formation of an action potential based on changes in Na$^+$ and K$^+$ ion flow.

through micropores. Larger molecules such as glucose pass through with the assistance of carrier molecules, while large lipids pass through easily because of their solubility in the lipid structure of the membrane.

The resting cell potential is created by an unequal concentration of ions; a high concentration of sodium (Na$^+$) and chloride (Cl$^-$) ions outside the cell and a high concentration of potassium (K$^+$) ions and negative proteins inside the cell. A relatively large potential of –70 mV is created by a very small (0.003%) excess amount of total ions. Also K$^+$ ions are much more permeable than Na$^+$ (about a 30:1 ratio) but because of the negative intracellular potential cannot easily diffuse out of the cell. Thus, in steady state, there is a continuous balance of concentration gradients vs. electrical gradients or potentials. However, there is still a continual leakage of K$^+$ ions out of the cell and Na$^+$ ions into the cell, which is rectified by an active sodium pump bringing the K$^+$ ions back in and the Na$^+$ ions back out.

An active disturbance of the membrane potential for the excitable cells (nerve and muscle cells), termed an *action potential*, creates the means for transmission of information for the activation of muscles and resulting movement. This disturbance can be in the form of hormones, electrical stimulation, chemical neurotransmitters, or even spontaneous changes such as in the smooth muscle of the gastrointestinal tract. In an action potential (Figure 3.8) there is an initial *depolarization* (a positive change in the membrane potential), which changes the permeability of the membrane allowing Na$^+$ ions to leak across the membrane down its concentration gradient. The

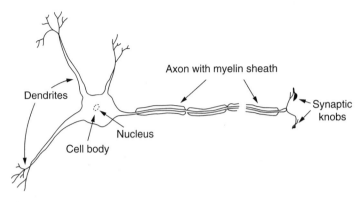

FIGURE 3.9
Schematic diagram of a neuron.

sodium pump cannot keep up and the inside of the cell becomes more positive. At a certain threshold point, around –40 mV, the membrane practically opens and the Na^+ ions (P_{Na} in Figure 3.8) flood across the membrane, dramatically changing the cell potential to positive values, reaching +30 to +40 mV. However, at the same time, because of the porosity of the membrane, K^+ ions (P_K in Figure 3.8) are also moving down their concentration gradient out of the cell, with the consequent reversal of cell polarity. Simultaneously, there is a sodium inactivation, shutting down Na^+ ion permeability with a reversal in the ratio of $Na^+:K^+$ permeability to a value of 1:20. The flow of K^+ ions out of the cell brings the cell potential back to –70 mV, sometimes with a brief hyperpolarization (more negative potential). The dramatic depolarization resulting in the action potential lasts for a brief time period, 1 to 2 ms. The return to normal steady state takes longer, anywhere from 1 to 15 ms. During this *refractory period*, the membrane cannot be easily stimulated again and the sodium pumps are working to return ionic balance to the cell. Note that once the initial disturbance reaches the threshold level, the process cannot be stopped. This is known as an *all-or-nothing response*. On the other hand, the depolarization process can reverse itself below threshold levels and will later be found to be one of the forms of control mechanisms within the neuromuscular reflex systems.

Note that, strictly speaking, no energy is required to produce an action potential. On the other hand, the sodium pump does require energy (in the form of ATP, discussed in Example 3.1). Also, the actual ion transfer is quite small and, in fact, should the sodium pumps be poisoned, up to 100,000 action potentials could still be generated before the ion concentrations would be sufficiently equilibrated to prevent further depolarizations.

Nerve cells, termed *neurons*, are carriers of electrical impulses that initiate muscle contraction (Figure 3.9). It also has a cell body with mitochondria for energy production and a nucleus with genetic material. More important is the *axon*, the long part of the neuron, which carries the action potential. Many axons are covered by *myelin*, a specialized fatty sheath that forces the action

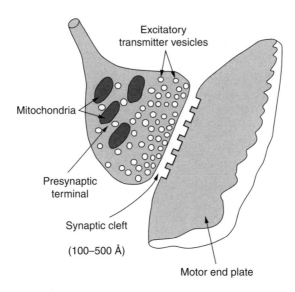

FIGURE 3.10

Anatomy of a synapse showing the synaptic knob and motor end plate. (From Guyton, A.C., 1971. *Textbook of Medical Physiology*, Philadelphia: W.B. Saunders, 15. With permission from Elsevier Science.)

potential to jump between gaps in the myelin, resulting in very high nerve conduction speeds. The *dendrites* are long and extensive branches off the cell body that serve to collect nerve impulses from other neurons. As with the invaginations in the brain, the dendrites greatly increase the surface area of the neuron with a much greater possibility for interconnections between neurons. The interconnection between a neuron and muscle cell is termed a *neuromuscular junction* and consists of a synaptic knob at the end of the neuron, a true gap termed the *synapse*, and the motor end plate, a specialized receptor, on the muscle fiber (Figure 3.10).

3.4 The Nervous System

Motor control of the muscles initiates in the *central nervous system* (CNS), which includes the brain, within and protected by the skull, and the spinal cord, passing through and protected by the vertebral column. The brain (Figure 3.11) can be subdivided into various areas, each containing a mass of nerve cells performing certain functions. To increase the motor control and other neural processing capability, the brain has developed deep invaginations, greatly increasing the surface area and thus space for more potential nerve cells, specifically their cell bodies. Among these areas, the *cerebral* or *sensorimotor* cortex covers the top surface of the brain and consists of both a

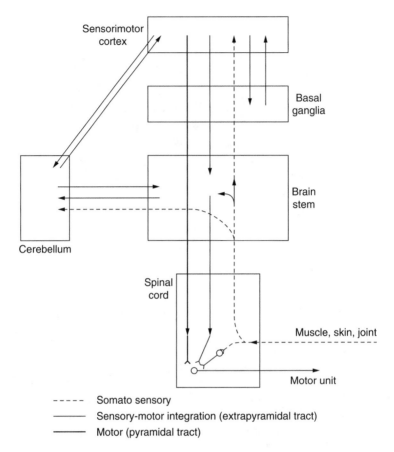

FIGURE 3.11
Schematic diagram of the central nervous system showing pyramidal and extrapyramidal tracts.
(Adapted from McMahon, 1984.)

motor part, from which the signals controlling muscle action originate, and
a sensory part, which receives feedback signals back from the muscles and
other parts of the body. The occipital lobe and the *cerebellum*, in the posterior
part, process visual information and feedback control for muscles, respectively. The frontal lobe is associated with emotion, the *basal ganglia* with
motor processing, and the *brain stem* with sensory processing.

The spinal cord carries various nerve pathways to the periphery of the body;
the main pathways are the *pyramidal tract*, involved in direct motor control, and
the *extrapyramidal tract*, also involved in motor control but through a more
circuitous pathway (see also Section 3.10). Once the nerves exit the spinal cord,
they become part of the peripheral nervous system. The peripheral nervous
system is subdivided into an *efferent* part, which carries information from the
CNS either to muscles, through the motor system, or to the heart and other
organs, through the autonomic system, and an *afferent* or sensory part, which
carries information back to the CNS, either from the muscles, through the

TABLE 3.1

Types of Neurons

Size	Group	Subgroup	Myelination	Size (µm)	Speed (m/s)	Function
Large	A	α (Ia)	Yes	12–20	72–100	Annulospiral
		α (Ib)	Yes	12–20	72–100	Golgi tendon organs
		β (II)	Yes	4–12	24–72	Flower spray
		γ (II)	Yes	1–4	6–24	Touch, somatic efferent
		δ (III)	No?	<1	0.6–2	Pain
Small	B		Yes	1–4	3–15	Visceral afferent/ efferent
Very small	C	(IV)	No	<1	0.6–2	Pain, temperature, visceral efferent

Source: Adapted from Matthews (1972).

somatic system, or from organs, through the visceral system. Each of the tracts or pathways in the CNS or nerves in the peripheral nervous system is composed of thousands of smaller neurons, which vary considerably in both size and function, as summarized in Table 3.1. These become more important in Section 3.10 regarding reflex pathways and motor control.

3.5 The Excitation–Contraction Sequence

The generalized excitation–contraction sequence of a nerve impulse traveling from the brain and causing a muscle contraction is as follows. An action potential originates in the motor cortex of the brain and travels down the pyramidal tract to the neuromuscular junction. There, a chemical neurotransmitter, acetylcholine (ACh), is released from vesicles in the synaptic knob. The ACh molecules diffuse across the synapse, to the motor end plate on the muscle fiber (Figure 3.10).

The ACh attaches to a receptor, causing a small potential at the motor end plate, termed a *miniature end plate potential* (MEPP). All of the MEPPs, from many ACh molecules, summate to create a motor end plate potential, which creates an action potential in the muscle fiber, in a one-to-one response. Eventually, an enzyme, cholinesterase, breaks down ACh into choline and acetic acid, which separately diffuse back to vesicles to be reformed into ACh.

Note that the neuromuscular junction is a very critical point in the neuromuscular system and a variety of poisons and drugs can have some very powerful effects here. Curare blocks the receptor sites, preventing muscle contraction (e.g., respiratory muscles) and eventually causing the individual to asphyxiate. Cocaine blocks the reuptake of choline and acetic acid, allowing continual stimulation, until the ACh is used up. Botulism blocks the release of ACh and thus prevents the excitation of muscle. The disease

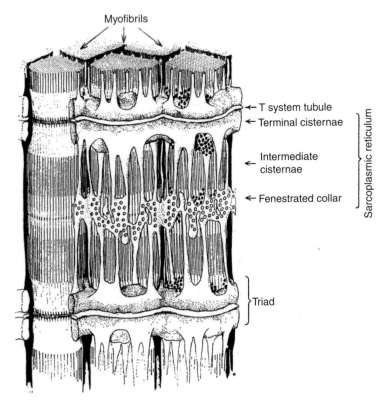

FIGURE 3.12
Schematic diagram of the sarcoplasmic reticulum surrounding myofibrils. (From Peachey, L.D., 1965. *Journal of Cell Biology,* 25(3, Pt. 2):209–232. With permission.)

myasthemia gravis causes a decrease in ACh receptor sites, reducing the motor end plate potential, and eventually reducing the strength of muscle contraction.

The muscle action potential changes the membrane permeability of a series of tubules and sacs surrounding the myofibrils, termed the *sarcoplasmic reticulum,* so as to release stored calcium ions (Ca^{++}) into the filaments (Figure 3.12). The calcium ions cause a change in the troponin-tropomyosin-actin complex on the thin filament removing an inhibition and allowing the further interaction between actin (A) and myosin (M) to occur. Troponin is a complex molecule with three subunits: troponin-T, which binds to tropomyosin; troponin-C, which binds with the calcium ions; and troponin-I, which is the actual inhibitory unit. Specifically, calcium ions cause the troponin complex to pull the tropomyosin out of the receptor site, which is occupied by the S_1 unit of myosin to for a bond.

At this point some energy is required and is provided by the most basic energy molecule, *adenosine triphosphate* (ATP). With the addition of some magnesium ions (Mg^{++}), the ATP begins to be split *(hydrolized)* by the S_1 unit of HMM:

$$ATP \cdot M \rightarrow ADP \cdot P_i \cdot M \tag{3.1}$$

A contortional change occurs in the S_1 head, allowing bonding to occur between the actin (A) and myosin (M):

$$ADP \cdot P_i \cdot M + A \rightarrow A\text{-}M \cdot ADP \cdot P_i \tag{3.2}$$

The ATP is completely hydrolized leaving a true bond in the form of a cross bridge between the thick and thin filaments:

$$A\text{-}M \cdot ADP \cdot P_i \rightarrow A\text{-}M + ADP + P_i \tag{3.3}$$

To break the actin–myosin bond, a fresh ATP molecule is needed:

$$A\text{-}M + ATP \rightarrow A + M \cdot ATP \tag{3.4}$$

Then, the myosin molecule is free to advance to the next G-actin molecule and repeat the previous steps in forming another cross bridge. For relaxation of the muscle, the Ca^{++} ions are released from troponin and are taken back up into sarcoplasmic reticulum. This last step again requires energy in the form of ATP.

Example 3.1: Metabolism, Energy, and ATP

ATP is created by the metabolism of the basic foods we eat: carbohydrates, fats, and proteins. This metabolism can occur in two different modes: *aerobic*, requiring oxygen, and *anaerobic*, not using oxygen. Aerobic metabolism uses a slow biochemical pathway, the citric acid or Krebs cycle, to generate 38 ATPs for each glucose molecule, the basic unit of carbohydrates:

$$C_6H_{12}O_6 + 6O_2 \rightarrow 6CO_2 + 6H_2O + 38\,ATP \tag{3.5}$$

On the other hand, anaerobic metabolism utilizes a fast glycolytic enzyme to break down the glucose molecule into two lactate molecules and produce two ATPs:

$$C_6H_{12}O_6 \rightarrow 2C_3H_6O_3 + 2\,ATP \tag{3.6}$$

The lactate molecule in the extracellular fluid of the body forms *lactic acid*, which is a direct correlate of fatigue. Thus, there is trade-off — aerobic metabolism is slow but very efficient, while anaerobic metabolism is very fast but inefficient and gives rise to fatigue.

Overall, there are several key steps in the excitation–contraction sequence. The calcium ions are key in inhibiting the troponin inhibitor. Energy, in the form of ATP, is needed for contraction, relaxation, and also Ca^{++} ion uptake. If somehow ATP production is completely stopped, the muscle cannot relax. This is the reason for rigor mortis in dead animals. The myosin molecule serves two functions. The S_2 unit bonds with actin to form the cross bridge while the S_1 unit acts as an enzyme to split ATP.

3.6   Motor Units

The *motor unit* is the functional unit of muscle, defined as one motor neuron (sometimes termed a *motoneuron*) and all of the muscle fibers innervated by the branches of the motor neuron axon. Motor units can vary in size considerably, from as low as 10 muscle fibers in the external rectus of the eye muscles, to as high as 2000 in the gastrocnemius in the calf. These muscle fibers are not clumped together but are distributed throughout the muscle, leading to a more distributed force production. Also, once an action potential is produced in the motor neuron, it travels down all of the branches of the motor neuron and activates all of the muscle fibers that it innervates in another type of all-or-nothing response. The ratio of muscle fibers to motor neuron is termed the *innervation ratio* and is important in determining muscle properties as discussed further in the next section

3.6.1   Types of Motor Units

There are three types of motor units, based on the functional characteristics of the component muscle fibers such as electrophysiological and biochemical properties. Typically. the slow twitch fibers (Type I or SO) are small with relatively low force but use aerobic metabolism and thus are good for sustained long-term effort without undue fatigue. On the opposite extreme, fast twitch fibers (Type IIB or FG) are large and respond quickly with high amounts of force, but fatigue quickly because of anaerobic metabolism. In between are fast but fatigue-resistant fibers (Type IIA or FOG) with moderate levels of force and moderate levels of fatigue due a reliance on both types of metabolism. The slow twitch fibers are typically small and found in smaller motor units; i.e., they have small innervation ratios. This leads to very precise control of force development and movement because each additional motor unit provides a small increase in force, i.e., ΔF_1 in Figure 3.13 (also a shallower slope). The fast twitch fibers are typically found in large motor units with large innervation ratios leading to larger jumps in force with each additional motor unit recruited and thus less precise control; i.e., compare ΔF_2 to ΔF_1 in Figure 3.13 (also a steeper slope).

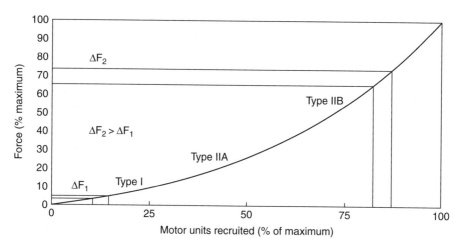

FIGURE 3.13
Motor unit recruitment demonstrating the size principle and precision in motor control.

The above process is a very specific orderly recruitment of motor units by the size of the neuron, with the smallest slow twitch, Type I fibers recruited first, followed by the intermediate fast, fatigue-resistant Type IIA fibers, and, finally, by the largest fast twitch, Type IIB fibers. This *size principle*, first postulated by Henneman et al. (1965), exists because the threshold for creating an action potential and firing the motor neuron is overcome more easily in the smallest neurons. For a given number of impulses from other neurons, the excitatory potentials summate most easily across the soma and the dendrites. In larger neurons, the same number of excitatory potentials is dispersed over a much larger surface area. Note that in terms of work design, it is inadvisable to perform precise activities immediately after heavy work. Some of the smaller motor units may have fatigued and larger ones will have been recruited with less precise control.

Typically a muscle will have all three types of fibers, but in varying quantities. Some muscles, such as the soleus in the calf, will have a preponderance of slow twitch fibers, while others, such as the brachioradialis, will have a preponderance of fast twitch fibers. To some degree, the characteristics of the fibers can be modified through specific training as in high-level sporting activities. However, to a large degree, the distribution of fibers is genetically determined. Thus, some individuals with a large proportion of slow twitch fibers will naturally be distance runners, while other individuals, with a large proportion of fast twitch fibers, will naturally be sprinters or power lifters. A general summary of motor unit characteristics is provided in Table 3.2.

3.6.2 Motor Unit Twitch

When the motor end plate of a muscle fiber is stimulated via the transfer of ACh, the MEPP causes an action potential to travel down the muscle fiber

TABLE 3.2

Motor Unit Characteristics

Characteristic	Type of Motor Unit		
	I/SO	IIA/FOG	IIB/FG
General label	Slow oxidative	Fast oxidative, glycolytic	Fast glycolytic
Contraction velocity	Slow	Fast	Fast
Tetanic frequency (Hz)	~30	~50–60	~100
Metabolism	Oxidative, aerobic	Fast oxidative + glycolytic, aerobic + anaerobic	Glycolytic, anaerobic
Fatigability	Fatigue resistant	Intermediate	Fast fatigable
Twitch force	Low	Medium	High
Twitch time (ms)	~120	~60–80	~20
Size of fibers/ motoneurons	Small	Intermediate	Large
Color	Red	Red	Pale
Proportion			
Brachioradialis	35%	—	65%
Biceps	40%	—	60%
Triceps	32%	—	68%
Soleus	80%	—	20%

releasing calcium ions from the sarcoplasmic reticulum and initiating the excitation–contraction sequence. The resulting contraction is called a twitch response and varies in size and duration depending on the type of muscle and muscle fibers involved, but not on the size of the stimulus, as for a motor unit the responses is an all-or-nothing response. There is always an initial *latency period* or a delay before a rise in tension is seen. This is due to the conduction time of the action potential down the muscle fiber and into the sarcoplasmic reticulum as well as the time for the calcium ions to be released from the sarcoplasmic reticulum.

Should the muscle fiber be stimulated again before the first twitch has died away, the second twitch reaches a higher force level. This is a potentiating effect because, during the relaxation period (and especially during the contraction period), there are still some calcium ions found in the myofibrils (termed the *active state*). Therefore, the protein filaments have not been completely inhibited and are easier to stimulate, resulting in a larger contraction. If the stimulation is repeated at higher frequency bursts (shorter interstimulation interval times), the resulting force output becomes even higher resulting in a steady force level termed unfused *tetanus*. Eventually with even higher frequencies, the ripples between successive twitches disappear, resulting in a fused tetanus with an even larger force output (Figure 3.14). However, this is the maximum force that can be produced by this motor unit at this given frequency, termed *tetanic frequency*. Higher frequencies will not yield any more increases in force. This tetanic frequency varies from a low of roughly 30 Hz in the soleus to over 300 Hz in the eye muscles. However, for the muscles in the upper limbs, the upper frequency is closer to 100 Hz.

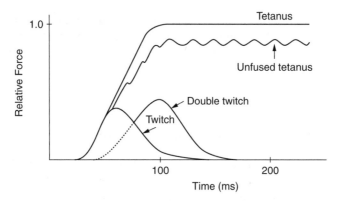

FIGURE 3.14
Twitch and tetanus. Sufficiently high frequency stimuli cause twitch forces to summate to yield a steady force termed tetanus.

The magnitude of muscle contraction, thus, depends to large extent on the frequency of stimulation, but also on the magnitude of stimulation, in which case, a greater number of motor units will be recruited. Note that two mechanisms for increasing muscular contraction are not completely independent. Based on the size principle and orderly recruitment of motor units, the smaller motor units have lower tetanic frequencies, while the larger motor units have higher tetanic frequencies.

Muscle contractions at a gross external level can be characterized in the following ways. Static or *isometric* contractions refer to force production without changes in muscle length. Dynamic contractions refer to conditions under which muscle length changes. If the muscle is shortening, then it is *concentric*. If the muscle is lengthening, then it is *eccentric*. Eccentric contractions are relatively uncommon is everyday life; walking or running downhill or trying to maintain control of a load too heavy to lift are a couple of examples. Dynamic contractions can be *isotonic*, in which the muscle force remains constant, or *isokinetic*, in which the muscle contracts at a constant velocity, or *isoinertial*, in which the muscle contracts at a constant acceleration. These constraints are imposed so as to have a controlled set of conditions in measuring or comparing dynamic muscle contractions.

Maximum muscle tension is determined by the number of muscle fibers involved. This, obviously, cannot be counted and is typically approximated by the cross-sectional area of the muscle, taken perpendicular to the fibers at the largest point of the muscle, called the belly. This tension or force factor ranges from 40 to 80 N/cm^2 depending on the researcher and the methods used to determine cross-sectional area. This is a relatively simple procedure for fusiform muscle in which the fibers are relatively parallel. However, for multipennate muscles the fiber arrangement varies considerably and no perpendicular cut can be easily achieved. Therefore, most researchers use the volume of the muscle (as determined by the weight of the muscle divided by the density) divided by length to obtain an average cross-sectional area.

Note that muscle cross section increases during muscle contraction as a result of the overlapping of filaments. However, muscle fibers also shorten during contraction causing the overall volume of the active muscle to remain constant.

3.7 Basic Muscle Properties (Mechanics)

Most of the basic muscle properties were determined by A.V. Hill and his colleagues at The University College, London, between 1910 and 1950 on isolated muscle preparations. These studies are summarized nicely in Hill's (1970) last treatise. Typically, a frog's sartorius muscle (having the ideal parallel or fusiform fiber arrangement) was mounted in an apparatus for stimulating the muscle and measuring muscle force As long as the muscle was kept in an oxygenated saline solution, the muscle fibers maintained their properties for several days. Because the preparation was typically in a glass container, it was termed *in vitro* as opposed to *in vivo*, or within a living body.

3.7.1 Active Length–Tension Relationship

The tension developed during muscle contraction is a nonlinear function that depends very specifically on muscle length. Maximum tension is found near the length that the muscle occupies in a relaxed state in the body, or *resting length*, and then drops off as the muscle either shortens or lengthens (Figure 3.15). At the resting length (position 3) there is maximum overlap between the thin filaments and all of the available cross-bridging zone of the thick filament, i.e., all myosin heads have a G-actin molecule to attach to. The plateau area between points 3 and 2 results because of the lack of myosin heads in the H-band, and as a result, even though the muscle fiber lengthens, no cross bridges are lost. However, at longer lengths, the tension drops off linearly because with each added increase in length fewer cross bridges are available. This drop off continue until roughly 170 to 180% of resting length, at which point, no overlap between the myosin heads and G-actin molecules is possible and no tension is produced.

When the muscle fiber shortens, on the other hand, the opposite thin filaments overlap and interfere with the bonding of myosin to actin, reducing tension (position 5). At position 6, or roughly 60% or resting length, there is complete interference of the thin filaments and no cross bridging is possible. Consequently, no force is produced. Also then thick filaments collide with the Z-disks, further complicating any possible cross bridging. This has been supported by electron micrographs, the complete disappearance of the I-bands and the narrowing of the A-bands.

This nonlinear length–tension relationship has been utilized in the development of various strength training devices (such as the Nautilus) to provide

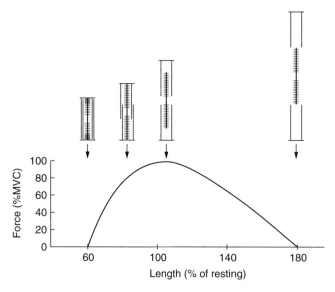

FIGURE 3.15
Active length–tension relationship in a muscle with corresponding sliding filament relationships. (Adapted from Gordon et al., 1966.)

the appropriate level of external resistance as the limb and muscles move through the range of motion.

3.7.2 Passive Length–Tension Relationship

The above property was a characteristic of stimulated muscle fibers, thus an active muscle property. However, muscle does not consist solely of the protein filaments, but also contains an extensive soft connective tissue network, primarily fascia composed of elastin. The passive properties of such tissue can be easily observed by recording the force as the passive (no electrical stimulation) muscle is stretched (Figure 3.16). The rate of tension increase is linear per applied stress:

$$d\sigma/d\ell = \alpha\sigma \qquad (3.7)$$

Integrating both sides yields

$$\sigma = ke^{\alpha\ell} \qquad (3.8)$$

When the muscle is stimulated, the tension changes dramatically because of the added effect of active contraction. The total muscle tension then becomes the combined effect of the active and passive force components (Figure 3.17) with a pronounced dip at 120 to 150% of resting length. This dip becomes more pronounced as the amount of fascia decreases in the muscle preparation. Thus, multipennate fibers, such as the deltoid, with

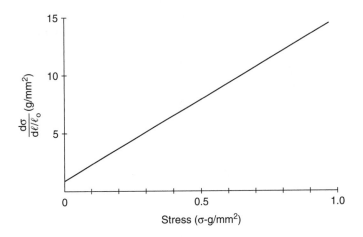

FIGURE 3.16
Passive length–tension relationship in a muscle. The stress-to-strain rate is a linearly increasing function of stress. (Adapted from Pinto and Fung, 1973.)

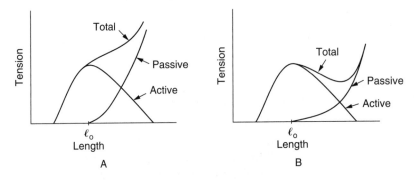

FIGURE 3.17
Combined active and passive length–tension relationships in (A) bipennate and (B) fusiform muscles. (Adapted from McMahon, 1984.)

short fibers and a relatively large amount of connective tissue will show almost a continual increase in muscle tension, while purely parallel-fibered muscle with relatively little connective tissue, such as the biceps, shows considerable dip. Note that a typical range of motion experienced by an *in vivo* muscle would be on the order of 80 to 120% resting length.

3.7.3 Velocity–Tension Relationship

It can be easily observed that during concentric motion, as the velocity of the movement increases, the amount of force developed by muscle decreases (Figure 3.18). Two factors contribute to this effect: (1) less efficient bonding in the cross bridges with more rapid sliding of the filaments past each other

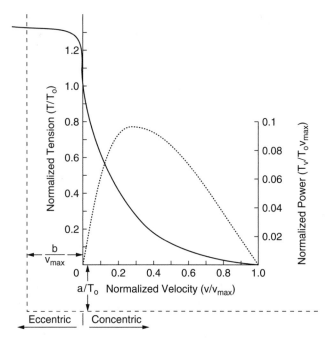

FIGURE 3.18

Hill's velocity–tension relationship. Note increase in force for concentric contractions and peak power at $0.3\ v_{max}$. (Adapted from McMahon, 1984.)

and (2) a damping effect of the fluid-filled muscle tissue. This relationship, also known as the force–velocity relationship, was first observed by Fenn and Marsh (1935) and later used by Hill (1938) to develop the first model of muscle. Interestingly, for eccentric motions, the tension developed by the muscle can increase to a higher value than observed in an isometric state (Katz, 1939). This is probably because breaking the protein cross bridges requires more force than holding them at their isometric limit. Also the external force must overcome latent viscous friction still present from the shortening stage (Winter, 1990). Eccentric contractions result in greater stress on and consequent microtrauma to the soft connective tissues within the muscle as evidenced by the greater soreness in eccentric exercise such as downhill running.

For the concentric part of the curve, Hill (1938) proposed an empirical quantitative formulation of the hyperbolic shape:

$$(T+a)(v+b) = (T_0 +a)b \qquad (3.9)$$

where
T = tension
T_0 = isometric tension
v = velocity

Note that the asymptotes of the hyperbola are not zero, but $T = -a$ and $v = -b$. A normalized form allows one to compare different muscles with one equation:

$$v' = (1 - T')/(1 + T'/k) \tag{3.10}$$

where
$v' = v/v_{max}$
$T'' = T/T_0$
$k = a/T_0 = b/v_{max}$

For most muscles, k ranges between 0.15 and 0.25.

The total mechanical power available from a muscle can be expressed as

$$\text{Power} = Tv = v(bT_0 - av)/(v + b) \tag{3.11}$$

and maximum power (depending on the value of k) occurs at roughly $0.3v_{max}$ and $0.3T_0$ and almost reaches a value of $0.1T_0v_{max}$. The advantage of maintaining an optimum velocity is demonstrated in bicycling, in which the rider will gear up or down depending on the external conditions of slope, wind, etc.

3.7.4 Active State Properties

The active state was originally meant to refer to the condition a contracting muscle is in as opposed to a resting state. More specifically, it refers to the residual tension in a muscle related to the amount of calcium remaining in the muscle filaments, at which time a greater force can be produced with a second stimulation. This was first demonstrated by Ritchie (1954) in a set of *quick release* experiments. The quick release of a stop mechanism (Figure 3.19) exposes the muscle to a constant load with a stimulation occurring at increasing times after the release. The muscle shortens against the load until the connection to the force transducer is taut, registering additional force on the transducer. After a sufficiently long period of time, the muscle has completed its contraction phase exhibiting minimal or no force on the transducer. The maximum point of the resulting set of curves defines the active state tension T_0 as function of time (and corresponds to the relaxation time for a twitch).

3.7.5 Developments Leading to Hill's Muscle Model

In a second set of quick release experiments, a load was attached to the muscle. The mechanism maintains the muscle in isometric tetanus appropriate for its length. After the release of the catch, the muscle is allowed to shorten (not held at constant length) but is regulated by the constant force of the load. The amount of shortening depends on the difference in force

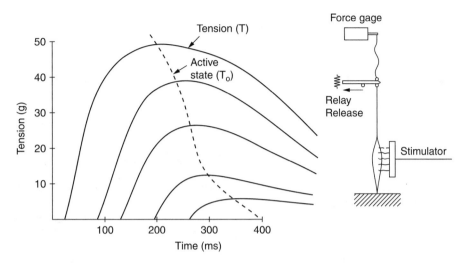

FIGURE 3.19
Quick release experiments defining the active state function. (From Ritchie, J.M., 1954. *Journal of Physiology*, 125:155–168. With permission.)

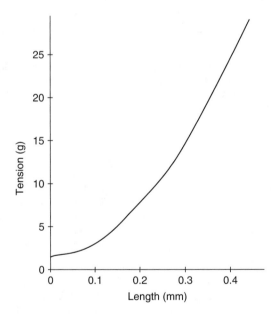

FIGURE 3.20
Length–tension relationship for the series elastic component. (Adapted from Jewell and Wilkie, 1958.)

generated before and after the release. Hill suggested that there is some sort of a spring or *series elastic element* in the muscle (Figure 3.20), which has a unique length for every tension level and is not dependent on velocity. This

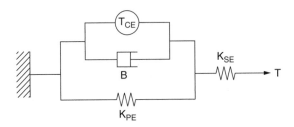

FIGURE 3.21
Hill's four-element model with a contractile component generating tension, T_{CE}.

element probably corresponds to the tendon structure and has a slope value of maximum tension over a 2% change in muscle resting length.

The passive tension curves suggest that there must also be a *parallel elastic element*, which resists passive stretching. This may represent the different types of fascia and membranes that are parallel to the filaments. The velocity–tension relationship (i.e., muscle force is greatest when velocity is zero) suggests that there is a dynamic resistance to movement or that force is dissipated while overcoming an inherent viscous resistance. Therefore, Hill proposed that the contractile element is a pure force generator with a parallel nonlinear *damping element* or dashpot. All of the proposed elements can be combined into a four-element muscle model frequently termed Hill's model (Figure 3.21). The model can also be expressed mathematically as a series of differential equations, which when solved will explain many of the basic mechanical properties of muscle. However, solution of these equations will be left until Chapter 4 when the introduction of Laplace transforms will allow for an easier solution of these equations.

3.7.6   Fatigue and Endurance

It can be easily shown that a maximum force (tetanic frequency, full motor unit recruitment) can only be maintained for a short period of time, 6 s, whereas a relatively low value of 15% of maximum can be maintained for extended periods of time, perhaps several hours. This corresponds exactly with the point at which the mechanical action of a contracting muscle becomes large enough to start compressing the weak (in compression) walls of arteries and occluding blood flow. As the muscle force increases, less blood reaches the working muscle with a corresponding decrease in oxygen availability. This means that the muscle must rely on a smaller amount of aerobic metabolism and a greater amount of glycolytic metabolism with concurrent fatigue. At roughly 70% max the blood flow is completely occluded and fatigue (as defined by the ability to maintain the given contraction level) occurs very quickly. This phenomenon (Figure 3.22) was first observed by Rohmert (1960) in the muscles of the upper limbs and can be quantified as a simple hyperbolic relationship with an asymptote at roughly 15% of maximum strength:

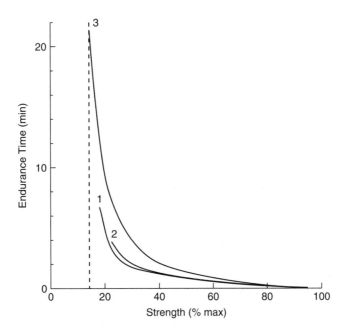

FIGURE 3.22
Endurance curves for various muscles. 1 = arm, leg, trunk (Rohmert, 1960). 2 = upper limbs pulling (Caldwell, 1963). 3 = biceps, triceps (Monod and Scherrer, 1965).

$$T_{end}(s) = \frac{1236.5}{(\%max - 15)^{0.618}} - 72.5 \qquad (3.12)$$

In addition to the depletion of nutrients in the muscle fibers, muscle fatigue may also occur in the neuromuscular junction due to a depletion of ACh in the nervous system with a depletion of ions to produce the action potentials, or perhaps in the protein filaments themselves with a decrease in contractility of the cross bridges. Note that full recovery from a maximum contraction of a 5 s duration may require a minimum of at least 2 min, if not more, and has led to standardized procedures to be used in properly assessing human strength (Chaffin, 1975). However, in terms of overall work efficiency, it is best to use short work–rest cycles. This does not allow the muscle to go into anaerobic metabolism and also utilizes the quick recovery of myoglobin stores as so aptly demonstrated by Åstrand et al. (1960b).

3.8 Energy, Metabolism, and Heat Production

Heat production in muscle was measured as early as 1848 by Helmholtz, but the real work was done by A. V. Hill and his colleagues from 1910 to

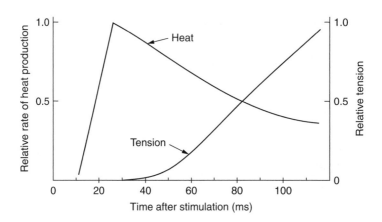

FIGURE 3.23
The activation heat rises quickly even before tension is developed. (Adapted from Hill, 1953.)

1950. To measure very small changes of heat production occurring in isolated muscle tissue samples, a very sensitive instrument such as the *thermocouple* was needed. A thermocouple works on the principle of two dissimilar metals (typically copper and nickel), which when connected create an electrical potential and current proportional to the surrounding temperature. Thus, when properly calibrated, the thermocouple becomes a very sensitive thermometer. Because the temperature changes for a single twitch in a muscle fiber are very small, on the order of 0.003°C, the sensitivity of the thermocouple needed to be improved. By connecting many thermocouples in series to yield a thermopile and using a sensitive galvanometer to measure very small currents, Hill was able to detect temperature changes as small as 0.000001°C.

Resting heat (H_{rest}) is a basic steady-state heat of muscle tissue, the simple consequence of the tissue being alive. This is a very small number, amounting to 0.0002 cal/g/min, and will be very much exceeded by the heat production occurring during active contraction. In both isometric and isotonic contractions, an *activation heat* (H_{act}), which appears 10 to 15 ms after the stimulus, begins to increase rapidly and reaches a maximum long before tension is fully developed (Figure 3.23). It coincides with the active state and, thus, is prolonged during tetanus. It also varies as a function of fiber length.

In an isotonic contraction, there is also additional heat termed the *heat of shortening* (H_{shor}). It was demonstrated by Fenn (1924) that a muscle that shortens produces more heat than when it contracts isometrically. Thus, it is sometimes called the *Fenn effect*, but the true relationship was refined by Hill (1938). In his experiments, a muscle was isometrically tetanized. It was then released and allowed to shorten against a load. With increasing loads, additional heat was produced with the extra heat (the difference between shortening and no shortening) due to true physical work being done. This physical work is the product of the force exerted and the distance the muscle moved.

The activation heat and heat of shortening are sometimes termed *initial heat* because they occur during muscle contraction as opposed to after the contraction, which is termed *relaxation* or *recovery heat* (H_{relax}). This relaxation heat can be liberated over a period of several minutes after contraction and corresponds to the muscle recovering oxygen and regenerating lactate to glucose and is as much as 50% greater than the initial heat.

There may be two other types of heat involved in muscle contraction. During eccentric contractions, the lengthening muscle also produces heat (H_{leng}), but it is much less than is produced in isotonic concentric-type work. This is evidenced by hikers sweating profusely while going uphill and putting on extra clothing while going downhill. Part of this difference may be explained by the larger tension created during eccentric contractions and part is due to energy being absorbed by bones and other connective tissues of the musculoskeletal system. This may explain the surprising soreness experienced after such downhill walking. Muscle may also show *thermoelastic heat* (H_{therm}). Most materials exhibit normal thermoelasticity, expanding when heated and cooling slightly when forcibly stretched. Rubber-like materials exhibit the opposite effect, heating when forcibly stretched. A muscle actually shows both effects; a resting muscle exhibits rubber thermoelasticity, while an active muscle exhibits normal thermoelasticity.

In summary, the various heats can be combined into the following total heat (H_{tot}) for an isotonic contraction:

$$H_{tot} = H_{rest} + H_{act} + H_{shor} + H_{relax} + H_{therm} \qquad (3.13)$$

with H_{shor} replaced by H_{leng} for eccentric contractions and H_{shor} eliminated for isometric contractions.

These heats correspond to chemical activity in the muscle, primarily the hydrolysis of ATP. ATP is regenerated from creatine phosphate (CP), an intermediary chemical compound:

$$ADP + CP \rightarrow ATP + Cr \qquad (3.14)$$

where Cr is the basic creatine molecule.

During work or exercise, the initial energy will come from ATP, which is regenerated by CP. Whereas the ATP stores in muscle fiber are used up almost instantly, CP can provide energy for 10 s or more (Figure 3.24). However, the ATP and CP has to be continually regenerated through the Krebs cycle. For high workloads, energy will be provided quickly through glycolysis, but this leads to higher concentrations of lactate and fairly quick fatigue. For lower workloads the aerobic contribution increases (Table 3.3) and keeps pace with the workload for extended periods of time. This was demonstrated very nicely by Åstrand et al. (1960b) in an experiment in which subjects exercised at a constant workload of 412 W (Figure 3.25). Those subjects that exercised for 10 s and took a 20-s rest were able to complete the full 30 min

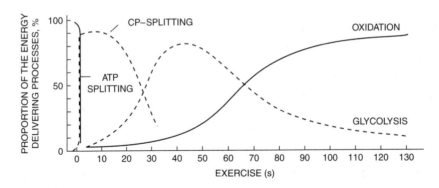

FIGURE 3.24
Schematic representation of energy sources during intense work. (From: Chaffin, D.B. et al., 1999. *Occupational Biomechanics*, 3rd ed., New York: John Wiley & Sons. With permission.)

TABLE 3.3

Percent Metabolic Energy Sources for Different Activities

Activity	Anaerobic		Aerobic (Oxidative)
	ATP + CP	Glycogen	
Weightlifting	98	2	0
Tennis	70	20	10
100 m run	95	5	0
1500 m run	20	60	20
Marathon run	0	5	95
Century bike ride	0	5	95

at low blood lactate levels, while those who exercised for 60 s and took 120-s breaks had extremely elevated blood lactate and could not even complete a 30-min bout of exercise.

During the shorter bouts of work, only ATP, CP, and some of the oxygen stored in muscle *(myoglobin)* was utilized. During the rest breaks, these sources were replenished with minimal penalty. For longer bouts of work, the muscle utilized the glycolytic process to produce energy quickly at the penalty of elevating blood lactate and incurring fatigue. Thus, the optimum arrangement of work is to have short, frequent work–rest cycles.

Note also the role of glycogen in the energy production process. By increasing the amount of carbohydrates in the diet *(carbohydrate loading)* 2 or 3 days prior to intense physical activity, the concentration of glycogen in the muscle can be increased from 1.5 g/100 g of muscle to 2.5 g (or even higher levels with more extreme dietary changes) with an associated increase in endurance for that sustained activity.

For more details on muscle physiology and mechanics, please refer to McMahon (1984), Aidley (1985), Jones et al. (1986), and Winter (1990).

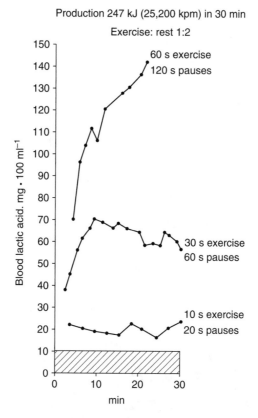

FIGURE 3.25

Blood lactate concentration in high intensity work performed in various work–rest cycles. (From Åstrand, P.O. and Rodahl, K., 1986. *Textbook of Work Physiology*, New York: McGraw-Hill. With permission.)

3.9 Receptors

Receptors are specialized nerve cells that provide the CNS information about external stimuli. Typically, they respond only to the specific stimuli they have evolved for, with increasing output in the form of higher-frequency action potentials with increasing magnitudes of stimulation. Thus, the photoreceptors in the retina respond only to light and the hair cells in the inner ear to sound pressure waves. They can be classified as *exteroreceptors*, those that respond to a conscious sensation such as above two examples, or as *proprioreceptors*, those that respond to unconscious sensations, such as those related to motor control, discussed below. Most receptors also have the basic property of *accommodation*, in which they adapt to a constant-level stimuli by decreasing the rate of firing (Figure 3.26).

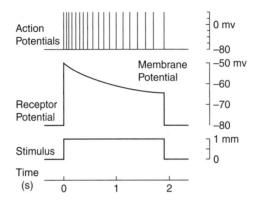

FIGURE 3.26
Receptor properties showing generation of action potentials and accommodation.

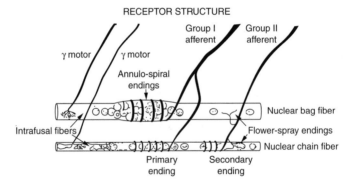

FIGURE 3.27
Schematic representation of nuclear bag and nuclear chain fibers and primary and secondary endings in a muscle spindle. (From Matthews, P.B.C., 1971. *Mammalian Muscle Receptors and Their Central Actions*, London: Edward Arnold. With permission.)

3.9.1 Muscle Spindles

Muscle spindles are modified muscle fibers that are thinner and shorter and have specialized neural receptor endings. They typically are located in parallel with the regular muscle fibers and respond to changes in fiber length and velocity changes. The muscle spindles have a connective tissue capsule giving rise to the name spindle or *fusiform* (Figure 3.27). The muscle fibers within the spindle are termed *intrafusal* fibers, while the regular muscle fibers outside the spindle are termed *extrafusal* fibers. Note that the extrafusal fibers are greater in number, larger in size (100 vs. 20 µm in diameter and 10 to 20 cm vs. 5 mm in length), and produce much more force. Also, the distribution of muscle spindles varies considerably according to the muscle; whereas the small muscles such as the interosseous of the fingers may have

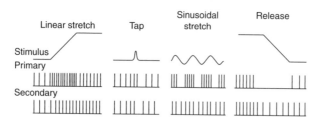

FIGURE 3.28

Typical response of primary and secondary endings to different types of stretch. (From Matthews, P.B.C., 1971. *Mammalian Muscle Receptors and Their Central Actions*, London: Edward Arnold. With permission.)

up to 120 spindles per gram of muscle, large muscle such as the gastrocnemius may have only 5 or fewer spindles per gram of muscle. This again has considerable implications for control, with the former allowing for very fine control and the latter for less fine control.

Muscle spindles have two types of receptors: *primary* and *secondary* endings. The primary endings, also known as the *annulospiral*, are found in the equatorial region of the spindle where there are few fibers (Figure 3.27). They generally are sensitive both to the displacement of the muscle and to the rate of displacement or velocity changes, and usually show a phasic response, with a 5-s transient peak and then a slower decay of about 1 min back to the baseline of no firing (Figure 3.28). They are innervated by Ia or α afferents and have a fairly low threshold.

The secondary endings, also known as *flower spray* endings, are found in the polar regions of the spindle, where there are many fibers (Figure 3.27). They are sensitive only to displacements, showing a tonic response, with a 5-s transient peak and then a fairly uniform firing rate proportional to the stretch (Figure 3.28). They are innervated by II or β nerve afferents and have a fairly high threshold. Both endings together are typically referred to as *stretch receptors*. A comparison of the two muscle receptors (as well as other receptors) is provided in Table 3.4.

The intrafusal muscle fibers are of two distinct types: *nuclear bag* and *nuclear chain* fibers (Figure 3.27). The nuclear bag fibers are about 8 mm long and have swollen equatorial regions, while the nuclear chain fibers are half as long with no central swelling. All nuclear bag and most nuclear chain fibers have primary endings, while all nuclear chain and some nuclear bag fibers have secondary endings. A typical muscle spindle will have two nuclear bag fibers and four to five nuclear chain fibers.

3.9.2 Golgi Tendon Organs

Golgi tendon organs are specialized encapsulated fascicles of dense collagen, which are offshoots from the primary tendon at the tendon–muscle junction. The fascicles, typically five, project into the muscle mass on the way to

TABLE 3.4

Summary of Receptor Characteristics

| | Muscle Spindles | | Golgi | | |
Characteristic	Primary Ending	Secondary Ending	Tendon Organs	Proprio-receptors	Pacinian Corpuscles
Afferent fiber	α (Ia)	β (II)	α (Ib)	γ?	γ?
Velocity (m/s)	80–125	50–80	80–125	6–20	6–20
Sensitivity	High	Low	High	—	—
Gain (#AP/s/unit)	100/mm	10/mm	20–180/kg	2/deg	—
Threshold, static	Low (~50 μm)	High (~500 μm)	20–200 g	Low	Medium
Threshold, dynamic	Low (~5 μm)	—	—	High (5°/ms)	Low (20 μm/2 ms)
Adaptation	1 min	4–5 h	3 s	Hours	6 ms

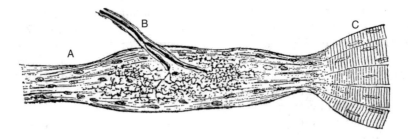

FIGURE 3.29

Schematic representation of a Golgi tendon organ: (A) tendon, (B) α afferent neuron, (C) muscle fibers. (From Matthews, P.B.C., 1971. *Mammalian Muscle Receptors and Their Central Actions*, London: Edward Arnold. With permission.)

becoming attached to a bundle of extrafusal muscle fibers (Figure 3.29). Branches of Ib or α sensory (afferent) nerves intertwine among the five bundles of collagen fibers, which in a relaxed Golgi tendon organ are spread open to reduce pressure on the nerve endings lying between them. During tension, these bundles straighten and crowd together, compressing the nerve endings and creating electrochemical changes in the nerve (Bridgman, 1968). Thus, the Golgi tendon organs respond to forces imposed on them by postural and locomotor activity, which could be in the form of passive forces developed by the muscle stretch and active forces resulting from muscle contraction. They have a surprisingly low threshold (Table 3.4) with the contraction of a single motor unit sometimes sufficient to excite the tendon organ. The response is a slowly adapting one (time constant = 3 s) with a threshold to active tension lower than that to passive tension. As opposed to muscle spindles, which are in parallel with extrafusal fibers and measure muscle length, Golgi tendon organs are in series with the extrafusal fibers and measure muscle tension.

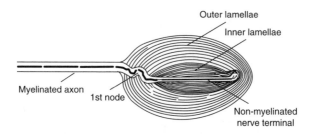

FIGURE 3.30
Schematic representation of a Pacinian corpuscle. (From Quilliam, T.A. and Sato, M., 1955. *Journal of Physiology*, 129:167–176. With permission.)

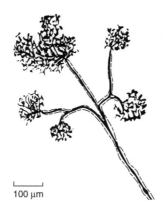

100 µm

FIGURE 3.31
Schematic representation of a Ruffini type ending found in joint capsules. (From Matthews, P.B.C., 1971. *Mammalian Muscle Receptors and Their Central Actions*, London: Edward Arnold. With permission.)

3.9.3   Other Receptors

Other receptors involved with motor control include Pacinian corpuscles and joint proprioreceptors, proprioreceptor referring to motor function. *Pacinian corpuscles* are pressure-sensitive receptors found on the fascia between muscles in the loose connective tissues near joints. Deformations of the outside covering are transmitted through the lamellae to the central nerve ending (Figure 3.30). The responses are very phasic, adapting in 6 ms or less.

Joint proprioreceptors are of two basic types: Ruffini type (Figure 3.31) and free nerve endings. The Ruffini type are of a tonic nature showing a 10-s transient and then maintaining a constant rate of firing proportional to the joint angle that lasts for hours. Furthermore, they show a long-term adaptation, such that it takes more than 10 min of baseline rest the same angular excursion will produce the same response. The response is bell shaped (Figure 3.32) with maximum sensitivity for a small range of specific angles. In

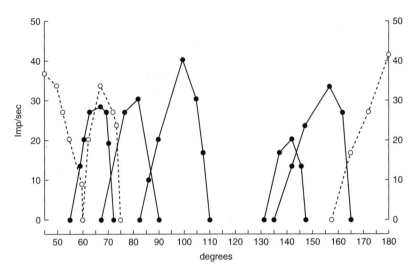

FIGURE 3.32
Bell-shaped response of joint proprioreceptors. Note the narrow range of angles to which the receptors respond. (From Matthews, P.B.C., 1972. *Mammalian Muscle Receptors and Their Central Actions*, London: Edward Arnold. With permission.)

addition, they are also sensitive to the angular velocity of movement, the discharge increasing for movements toward the specific angle and decreasing for movements away. For further information on muscle receptors, refer to Matthews (1972).

3.10   Reflexes and Motor Control

Axonal conduction of action potentials is a fundamental process in neural activity. Interconnections through synapses with other neurons or muscle fibers, as at the neuromuscular junction, form another component in this activity. For the motoneuron, at the neuromuscular junction, this was an excitation of the muscle fiber. At other locations, this process could be inhibitory. Furthermore, the motoneuron serves as an efferent pathway, away from the CNS, while other neurons serve as an afferent pathway, sending sensory information from receptors back to the CNS in the form of feedback. Thus, a set of neurons sending stimulus information to the CNS and receiving information back from the CNS, resulting in an appropriate response, can be considered as a system with a feedback loop. If this response is involuntary, i.e., does not require a conscious decision, then it is termed a *reflex*. A variety of such reflex pathways form the basis for motor control and they will be discussed in greater detail.

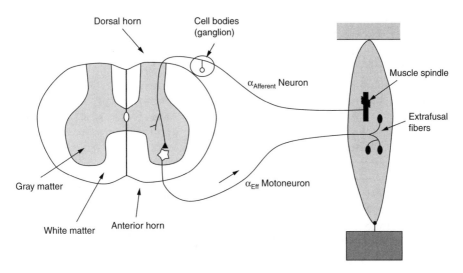

FIGURE 3.33
Schematic representation of a stretch reflex.

3.10.1 Stretch Reflex

The *stretch reflex* is the simplest reflex (Figure 3.33) consisting of five components. The first is the muscle spindle, the receptor that receives and processes the stimulus, in this case a stretch on the spindle. The second is an afferent neuron serving as the input pathway to the CNS. For the stretch reflex the afferent neuron is typically the largest neuron, the α or Ia type. The afferent neuron enters the spinal cord through the dorsal horn of the spinal cord and synapses on a motoneuron. Note that the synapse occurs in the central H-shaped darker region of the spinal cord termed *gray matter* as opposed to the *white matter* or lighter region are surrounding it. The gray matter receives its color from the motoneuron cell bodies while the white matter receives its color from the myelin sheaths of the descending pyramidal and extrapyramidal tracts. Note that the cell body for afferent sensory neuron is located outside of the spinal cord in a complex of numerous other such cell bodies, termed a *ganglion*.

The third component is the motoneuron cell body, which serves as an integrating center for information. In the simplest stretch reflex only one afferent input is required. However, in reality, the cell body is innervated with numerous other afferent inputs, some of which could also be inhibitory. The excitatory inputs depolarize that section of the motoneuron cell body in the form of *excitatory post-synaptic potentials* (EPSPs), similar to the MEPPs at the neuromuscular junction, except that a one-to-one response is not necessarily produced. Other innervating neurons, with a different neurotransmitter, may hyperpolarize the motoneuron cell body, creating *inhibitory post-synaptic potentials* (IPSPs), which then makes it more difficult for the neuron to be depolarize and fire an action potential. All of the EPSPs and IPSPs travel down the cell body membrane to the base of the axon, where all of the potentials summate and finally determine whether there is sufficient depolarization to create an action potential. Thus, the motoneuron cell body acts as a true integrating center or central processing unit.

The fourth component is the efferent path of the motoneuron. Again, this neuron is typically the largest α or Ia type so as to provide the fastest conduction velocity. The fifth component is the effector or the extrafusal fibers of the muscle, which contract upon stimulation. A typical stretch reflex is the *patellar reflex* tested by a physician tapping just below the knee of a free-hanging leg with a mallet. A vigorous tap stretches the tendon of the quadriceps muscle, which, after a brief delay, contracts the muscle, raising the leg slightly and relieving the stretch on the tendon. Failure to react indicates some problem in one of the components of the reflex arc, requiring further testing. This type of reflex is also sometimes termed a monosynaptic reflex because only one synapse is required.

Example 3.2: Timing Sequence of a Stretch Reflex

The timing sequence of a patellar tap reflex can be calculated as follows. The annulospiral, synapse, neuromuscular junction, and end plate all have approximately 1-ms delays. The large α neurons conduct action potentials at a minimum of 100 m/s. Assuming a knee tap and the neuron stretching 0.5 m to the L_5/S_1 level of the spinal cord, nerve conduction in either direction requires 5 ms (= 0.5/100). In addition the extrafusal fibers need a minimum of 20+ ms to generate enough force to contract and move the muscle. As a result there is a minimum of a 34-ms delay before any muscle contraction would be apparent.

Element	Time (ms)
Annulospiral	1.0
α_{aff}	5.0
Synapse	1.0
α_{eff}	5.0
Neuromuscular junction	1.0
End plate potential	1.0
Force buildup	20.0
Total	34.0 ms

3.10.2   γ-Loop Control

Muscle spindles consist of both stretch receptors and intrafusal contractile fibers. The latter serve as a means for controlling the gain of the stretch receptors. Contraction of the intrafusal fibers produces a stretch and excitation of the annulospiral comparable to that caused by an external mechanical stretch (Figure 3.34). A combination of both events would produce an even

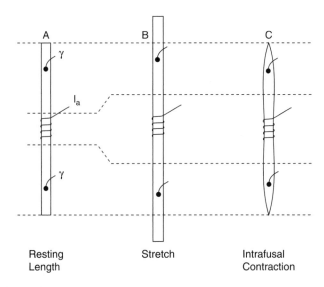

FIGURE 3.34
Activation of the annulospiral endings of a muscle spindle by (B) stretching the entire muscle
or by (C) intrafusal contraction. (A) Resting length. (Adapted from Schmidt, 1975.)

larger stimulation of the stretch receptors with a consequently more forceful
contraction of the extrafusal fibers.

The intrafusal fibers are innervated by smaller neurons of γ size (see Table
3.1), which emanate from the anterior horn of the spinal cord. Within the gray
matter area, collaterals of the α afferent neurons make synaptic connections
with γ neuron cell bodies in addition to α efferent motoneurons (Figure 3.35).
Should the initial stretch stimulus to the muscle spindle be weak, the resulting
stimulus through the stretch reflex of Figure 3.34 may not be sufficient to fully
contract the muscle and relieve the initial stretch. However, in the meantime,
the α afferent neuron have sent a signal through the γ efferent neuron to the
intrafusal fibers. Those fibers being much smaller in size would, according to
the Henneman et al. (1965) size principle, have a much greater likelihood of
being fired. The resulting contraction on the annulospiral would increase the
stretch stimulus sufficiently to eventually, after going around the stretch reflex
again, fire the extrafusal fibers. However, the resulting timing sequence of 87
ms (Example 3.3) would be considerably longer than the timing sequence of
34 ms (Example 3.2) for a pure stretch reflex. Note, also, that because several
synapses are involved the γ loop is one type of polysynaptic reflex.

Such γ control is a vital part of a length control system that the body uses
to maintain an upright position while under the influence of gravity. As a
result, many of the muscles, especially those in the neck, back, and lower
limbs, are continually in a state of lower or higher tension, which is referred
to as muscle tone. γ control also plays a part in *tremor*, the physiological
oscillation seen during sustained muscle contractions. For example, observe
the tremor at the end of a fingertip while holding the arm extended (this

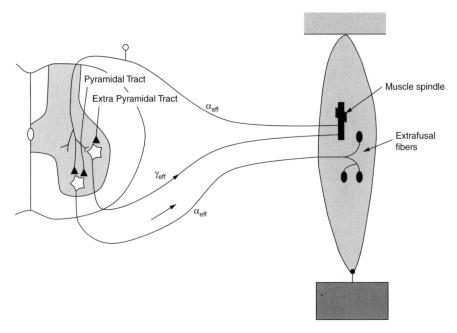

FIGURE 3.35
Schematic representation of a stretch reflex with the γ loop.

amplifies the tremor seen at the fingertip!). Eventually some of the motor units will fatigue, requiring the recruitment of additional motor units, typically larger ones. Much of this recruitment process proceeds through the γ loop. With larger and larger motor units being recruited, the increases in force will become more discrete and noticeable as tremor. The γ-loop time lag of 82 ms (Example 3.3) would yield physiological oscillations of approximately 12 Hz (= 1000/82). This compares very favorably to the values measured experimentally by Lippold (1970).

γ control is a factor in whiplash injuries from auto collisions. An unsupported head for a seat-belted occupant would have the tendency to swing forward violently, stretching the neck muscle spindles very quickly. This would result in a maximal stimulation of both the α efferent motoneurons and the γ efferents with a consequently maximal contraction of the neck muscles. The resultant sudden change in head acceleration from a positive to a negative value gives rise to the whiplash effect. The use of head restraints lessens the range motion of the head, thus reducing the magnitude of the acceleration change and the consequent injury.

Example 3.3: Timing Sequence of γ-Loop Control

The timing sequence of a stretch reflex with added γ-loop control can be calculated as follows. The annulospiral, synapse, neuromuscular junction, and end plate all have approximately 1-ms delays. The large α

neurons conduct action potentials at a minimum of 100 m/s. Assuming a knee tap and the neuron stretching 0.5 m to the L_5/S_1 level of the spinal cord, nerve conduction in either direction requires 5 ms (= 0.5/100 s). The γ neuron for the same length of 0.5 m but a slower speed of 25m/s requires 20 ms (= 0.5/25 s). The fastest muscle fibers need a minimum of 20+ ms to generate sufficient force to contract the muscle. As a result, there is a minimum of an 82-ms delay before any major muscle contraction would be apparent.

Element	Time (ms)
Annulospiral	1.0
α_{aff}	5.0
Synapse	1.0
γ_{eff}	20.0
Neuromuscular junction	1.0
Intrafusal force buildup	20.0
Annulospiral	1.0
α_{aff}	5.0
Synapse	1.0
α_{eff}	5.0
Neuromuscular junction	1.0
End plate potential	1.0
Extrafusal force buildup	20.0
Total	82.0 ms

3.10.3 α-γ Coactivation

Voluntary control of movement originates in the sensorimotor cortex with an action potential generated in the pyramidal neuron that stretches (in the case of leg movements) along the full length of the spinal cord through the pyramidal tract (see Figure 3.11). The pyramidal tract neurons then directly innervate the large α afferent motoneurons. Because these are large neurons with only one synapse involved, the result is a very quick time to initiate a movement. However, the trade-off is that there is a massive contraction of the extrafusal fibers resulting in a fairly ballistic type of movement with rather low precision.

Other neurons from the sensorimotor cortex will make various connections in the cerebellum and the basal ganglia, passing through the loosely defined extrapyramidal tract, and eventually reach the same level of the spinal cord as pyramidal neuron. There, the extrapyramidal neurons innervate γ efferents resulting in more controlled movements. Note that without the latter γ control, movements would be limited in magnitude because, with only α stimulation, the extrafusal fibers would contract, with corresponding contraction of the muscle spindles and removal of any further γ-loop activity. With simultaneous extrapyramidal tract activity, both α_{eff} and γ_{eff} are stimulated simultaneously, giving rise to a maximum extrafusal muscle contraction and maximum movement. This is known as α-γ coactivation (McMahon, 1984).

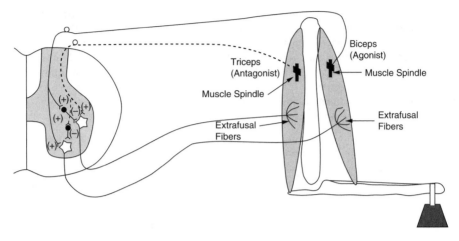

FIGURE 3.36
Schematic representation of a stretch reflex with reciprocal inhibition.

3.10.4   Reciprocal Inhibition

The stretch receptors also form an inhibitory reflex pathway, through an inter-neuron, to the antagonistic muscle (solid lines in Figure 3.36). Activity in the α afferent neuron results in both the excitation of the same side agonist extrafusal muscle fibers and the inhibition of the antagonistic extrafusal fibers. Termed *reciprocal inhibition*, this prevents the simultaneous activity of both sets of mus-cles, unless there is a conscious voluntary decision to override it. Should the muscular exertion be reversed (i.e., agonist becomes antagonist, and vice versa), then identical reciprocal inhibition pathways exist to again prevent simulta-neous activation of the muscles (dotted lines in Figure 3.36).

3.10.5   Clasp-Knife Reflex

The Golgi tendon organs also provide feedback in regulating motion and thus form another reflex pathway as well (Figure 3.37). The tendon organs are innervated by the largest α fibers, which also enter the dorsal horn of the spinal cord. However, instead of innervating directly on the α motor neuron, the action potentials are sent through an intermediary interneuron, which causes an inhibition on the α motor neuron. Upon a sudden force, such as jumping from a height with relatively stiff legs (with completely locked legs, bone and joint mechanics take over, resulting in potentially severe injuries), the Golgi tendon organs send a strong signal (high-fre-quency firing of action potentials) to the spinal cord, which through the interneuron becomes a strong inhibitory signal on the α_{eff} motor neuron. Consequently, extrafusal muscle contraction declines dramatically and the legs collapse as in a clasp knife. This is an example of a protective reflex, preventing the muscles from overproducing force. However, it is also

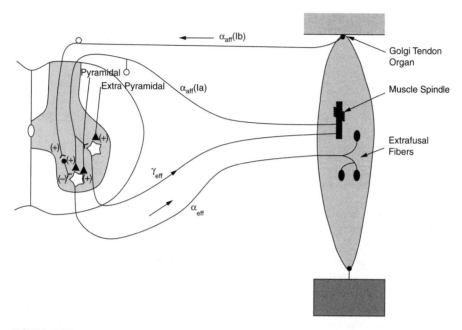

FIGURE 3.37
Schematic representation of the clasp-knife reflex with Golgi tendon organs.

thought that Golgi tendon organs play a broader, more complex role in regulating muscle tension through continuous feedback rather than a purely reactive role (Stuart et al., 1972).

3.10.6   Other Polysynaptic Reflexes

There are collaterals of the α efferent motor neuron that branch off within the gray matter of the spinal cord, synapse via interneurons called *Renshaw cells*, back to the parent cell body. With the signal passing through the inter-neuron, an inhibitory signal is provided, which acts to decrease the activity of the α efferent motor neuron. This is a form of negative feedback, guaran-teeing that weak motoneuron activity is transmitted undisturbed to the extrafusal muscle fibers, while excessive activity is dampened to prevent hyperactivity of the muscles.

In addition to reciprocal inhibition, which occurs to the antagonistic mus-cle, various other reflexes, known as *crossed* or *contralateral* reflexes, will occur to the other side of the body. For example, in Figure 3.38 a quick push on the underside of the right forearm will cause the extensors (triceps) to be stimulated causing elbow extension. This is a stretch reflex of the extensors (agonists) and reflex 1. Simultaneously, through reciprocal inhibition, the lateral antagonistic flexors (biceps brachii) are inhibited through reflex 2. In addition, the contralateral muscles of the left arm are also affected. The contralateral flexors (biceps brachii) are stimulated allowing the elbow to

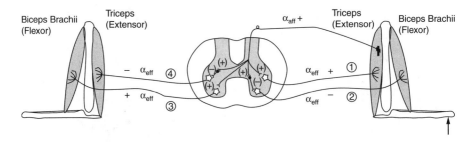

FIGURE 3.38
Schematic representation of polysynaptic and crossed reflexes: 1 = stretch reflex (monosynaptic);
2 = reciprocal inhibition; 3 = crossed flexor reflex; 4 = crossed extensor reflex.

flex in reflex 3. Simultaneously, through a more complex form of reciprocal
inhibition, the crossed extensors (triceps) are inhibited, allowing full elbow
flexion in reflex 4.

The existence of crossed reflexes, as discussed above, would seem to indicate
a superiority of alternating manipulations (180° out-of-phase) of the finger or
hand over parallel (completely in-phase) manipulations. In fact, such out-of-
phase motions, in which one finger flexes while the other extends, can be easily
maintained at low frequencies. However, as soon as the frequency increases to
a critical level, one finger abruptly shifts to an in-phase relationship, in which
both fingers flex in parallel (Kelso, 1981). This phenomenon has been explained
quite nicely in terms of nonlinear, coupled oscillators (Haken et al., 1985).
Similarly, Freivalds et al. (2000) found no significant differences between in-
phase and out-of-phase hand movements while performing various Purdue
Pegboard tasks. Apparently, training, practice, and voluntary factors determined at higher CNS levels can override the basic reflexes.

The full complexity of the reflex system can be difficult to ascertain. Matthews (1964) attempted a census on the cat soleus muscle to find the relative
number and distribution of various neuromuscular components. Within
roughly 25,000 extrafusal muscle fibers, he found 150 α motor neurons, 45
Golgi tendon organs, and 50 spindles within which were 50 primary (annulospiral) endings, 70 secondary (flower spray) endings, and 300 intrafusal
fibers with 100 γ neurons. Undoubtedly, all of the interconnections, directly
and indirectly through interneurons, at the spinal level, between all of these
components cannot be easily mapped. For further information on reflexes
and motor control, refer to Schmidt (1975) and McMahon (1984).

Questions

1. Discuss the trade-offs in the arrangement of muscle fibers.

2. Discuss the structure of muscle both at the gross and at the microscopic levels.

3. What is the sliding filament theory?

4. How is an action potential produced?

5. Compare and contrast pyramidal and extrapyramidal tracts in terms of motor control.

6. How is muscle contraction produced?

7. How is energy produced and utilized in the contractile process?

8. What is a motor unit?

9. What are the different types of motor units?

10. How is motor control affected by the size principle and orderly recruitment?

11. What is tetanus and how does it relate to the active state function?

12. What is an isometric muscle contraction? How can an isometric contraction lead to muscle force? That is, if the muscle does not move, cross bridging cannot occur. Explain.

13. What is an isotonic muscle contraction? Is it truly isotonic? Explain.

14. Explain the basis for an active length–tension relationship.

15. Explain the basis for the velocity–tension relationship.

16. What is the active state function? How was it first determined?

17. What is muscle fatigue and where does it occur? That is, what components of the musculoskeletal system may contribute to overall muscle fatigue?

18. What are the different components of heat production in muscle?

19. Describe the structure of a muscle spindle and relate it to the reception of sensory input.

20. What is a Golgi tendon organ?

21. What other proprioreceptors may be important in motor control?

22. Describe the pathway and components of a stretch reflex.

23. What effect does γ control have on motor control?

24. What is α-coactivation?

25. What is reciprocal inhibition?

26. What role does the Golgi tendon organ have in motor control?

27. What role does a Renshaw cell have in motor control?

28. What is a contralateral reflex?

29. Consider some of the various types of strength-training program or equipment that have been promoted over the years. What are the physiological bases for these? (For example, consider the Charles Atlas program of pressing on the opposite sides of a doorway!)

Problems

3.1. Quantitatively support Henneman's size principle. (*Hint:* Consider the surface area of a sphere.)

3.2. Using Hill's force–velocity and power curves shown in Figure 3.18:

   a. Derive the normalized form of Hill's force–velocity equation (Equation 3.10).

   b. Derive the power equation in its standard form (Equation 3.11).

   c. Show that the power curve peaks at approximately $0.3v_{max}$ and has an approximate value of $0.1T_0v_{max}$. (*Hint:* consider $0.15 < k < 0.25$, where $k = a/T_0 = b/v_{max}$.)

3.3. How does muscle endurance time change as the force level in a muscle contraction doubles from 20 to 40% of maximum force? What may explain this result?

References

Aidley, D.J., 1985. *The Physiology of Excitable Cells*, 2nd ed., Cambridge, U.K.: Cambridge University Press.

Åstrand, I., Åstrand, P.O., Christensen, E.H., and Hedman, R., 1960a. Intermittent muscular work, *Acta Physiologica Scandinavia*, 48:448–453.

Åstrand, I., Åstrand, P.O., Christensen, E.H., and Hedman, R., 1960b. Myohemoglobin as an oxygen store in man, *Acta Physiologica Scandinavia*, 48:454–460.

Åstrand, P.O. and Rodahl, K., 1986. *Textbook of Work Physiology*, New York: McGraw-Hill.

Bridgman, C.F., 1968. The structure of tendon organs in the cat: a proposed mechanism for responding to muscle tensions, *Anatomical Record*, 162:209–220.

Caldwell, L.S., 1963. Relative muscle loading and endurance, *Journal of Engineering Psychology*, 2:155–161.

Chaffin, D.B., 1975. Ergonomics guide for the assessment of human static strength, *Journal of the American Industrial Hygiene Association*, 35:201–206.

Chaffin, D.B., Andersson, G.B.J., and Martin, B.J., 1999. *Occupational Biomechanics*, 3rd ed., New York: John Wiley & Sons.

Ebashi, S., Endo, M., and Ohtsuki, I., 1969. Control of muscle contraction, *Quarterly Reviews of Biophysics*, 2:351–384.

Fenn, W.O., 1923. The relation between the work performed and the energy liberated in muscular contraction, *Journal of Physiology*, 58:373–395.

Fenn, W.O. and Marsh, B.S., 1935. Muscle force at different speeds of shortening, *Journal of Physiology*, 85:277–297.

Freivalds, A., Kong, D.J., and Murthy, S., 2000. Clarification of the "symmetrical use of both hands" principle of motion economy, *International Journal of Industrial Ergonomics*, 7:52–56.

Gordon, A.M., Huxley, A.F., and Julian, F.J., 1966. The variation in isometric tension with sarcomere length in vertebrate muscle fibres, *Journal of Physiology*, 184:170–192.

Guyton, A.C., 1971. *Textbook of Medical Physiology*, Philadelphia: W.B. Saunders.

Haken, H., Kelso, J.A.S., and Brinz, H., 1985. A theoretical model of phase transitions in human hand movements, *Biological Cybernetics*, 51:347–356.

Henneman, E., Somjen, G., and Carpenter, D., 1965. Excitability and inhibitability of motoneurons of different sizes, *Journal of Neurophysiology*, 28:599–620.

Hill, A.V., 1938. The heat of shortening and the dynamic constants of muscle, *Proceedings of the Royal Society*, 126B:136–195.

Hill, A.V., 1953. Chemical change and mechanical response in stimulated muscle, *Proceedings of the Royal Society*, 141:314–320.

Hill, A.V., 1970. *First and Last Experiments in Muscle Mechanics*, Cambridge, U.K: Cambridge University Press.

Huxley, A.F., 1974. Muscular contraction, *Journal of Physiology*, 243:1–43.

Jewell, B.R. and Wilkie, D.R., 1958. An analysis of the mechanical components in frog's striated muscle, *Journal of Physiology*, 143:515–540.

Jones, N.L., McCartney, N., and McComas, A.J., Eds., 1986. *Human Muscle Power*, Champaign, IL: Human Kinetics Publishers.

Katz, B., 1939. The relation between force and speed in muscular contraction, *Journal of Physiology*, 96:45–64.

Kelso, J.A.S., 1981. On the oscillatory basis of movement, *Bulletin of the Psychonomics Society*, 18:63–65.

Lippold, O.C.J., 1970. Oscillation in the stretch reflex arc and the origin of the rhythmical, 8–12 c/s component of physiological tremor, *Journal of Physiology*, 206:359–382.

Matthews, P.B.C., 1964. Muscle spindles and their motor control, *Physiological Reviews*, 44:219–288.

Matthews, P.B.C., 1972. *Mammalian Muscle Receptors and Their Central Actions*, London: Edward Arnold.

McMahon, T.A., 1984. *Muscles, Reflexes, and Locomotion*, Princeton, NJ: Princeton University Press.

Monod, H. and Scherrer, J., 1965. The work capacity of a synergic muscular group, *Ergonomics*, 8:329–338.

Peachey, L.D., 1965. The sarcoplasmic reticulum and transverse tubules of the frog's sartorius, *Journal of Cell Biology*, 25(3, Pt. 2):209–232.

Pinto, J.G. and Fung, Y.C., 1973. Mechanical properties of the heart muscle in the passive state, *Journal of Biomechanics*, 6:597–616.

Quilliam, T.A. and Sato, M., 1955. The distribution of myelin on nerve fibres from Pacinian corpuscles, *Journal of Physiology*, 129:167–176.

Ritchie, J.M., 1954. The effect of nitrate on the active state of muscle, *Journal of Physiology*, 125:155–168.

Rohmert, W., 1960. Ermittlung von Erholungspausen für statische Arbeit des Menschen [Determination of recovery times for human static work], *Internationale Zeitschrift für angewandte Physiologie einschliesslich Arbeitsphysiologie*, 18:123–164.

Schmidt, R.F., 1975. *Fundamentals of Neurophysiology*, Heidelberg: Springer-Verlag.

Stuart, D.G., Mosher, C.G., and Gerlach, R.L., 1972. Properties and central connections of Golgi tendon organs with special reference to locomotion, in Banker, B.Q., Przybylski, R.J., van der Meulen, J.P., and Victor, M., Eds., *Research in Muscle Development and the Muscle Spindle*, Amsterdam: Excerpta Medica, 437–464.

Winter, D.A., 1990. *Biomechanics and Motor Control of Human Movement*, 2nd ed., New York: John Wiley & Sons.

4

Modeling of Muscle Mechanics

4.1 Laplace Transforms and Transfer Functions

A transform is a means of converting a number or an expression into another form, a form that can be more easily manipulated and then inversely converted back to the original form of number or expression (see Figure 4.1). Consider that before the advent of computers, logarithms were commonly used to simplify multiplication and long division.

The Laplace transform (named after the French mathematician, Pierre Simon Laplace, 1749–1827) is a specific transformation for a function $f(t)$, defined as

$$\mathscr{L}\big[f(t)\big] = F(s) = \int_0^\infty f(t)e^{-st}dt \tag{4.1}$$

where $s = \sigma + j$, a complex number.

For $f(t)$ to be transformable it must meet the requirement that $\int_0^\infty |f(t)|e^{-\sigma t}\,dt < \infty$ for all real and positive σ. This is typically not a problem for most engineering functions, since $e^{-\sigma t}$ is a powerful reducing agent acting on the function $f(t)$.

As an example, perhaps the simplest Laplace transform is for a constant of value one. However, all functions being transformed using the Laplace operator should have a value of 0 for $t < 0$. Thus, the value of one should, technically, be defined as a *unit step function*, $u(t)$, which is equal to 0 for $t < 0$ and equal to 1 for $t \geq 0$. The resulting Laplace transform yields

$$\mathscr{L}\big[u(t)\big] = \int_0^\infty e^{-st}dt = \frac{-e^{-st}}{s}\bigg|_0^\infty = \frac{1}{s} \tag{4.2}$$

As a second example consider the exponential function $f(t) = e^{at}$. Note that this function is also only defined for values of $t \geq 0$; otherwise its value is zero.

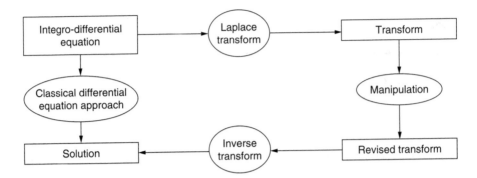

FIGURE 4.1
Algorithmic comparison of Laplace transforms with classical differential equation approach.

$$\mathcal{L}\left[e^{at}\right] = \int_0^\infty e^{at}e^{-st}dt = \int_0^\infty e^{-(s-a)t}dt = \left.\frac{-e^{-(s-a)t}}{s-a}\right|_0^\infty = \frac{1}{s-a} \tag{4.3}$$

With these two equations, a set of transform pairs has been established for two functions. This means that one does not need to perform the cumbersome integration repeatedly, but needs only to look up the appropriate transform. Thus, a table with similar transforms for other functions has already been established (see Table 4.1). However, not all functions will have the same exact form as in Table 4.1. In that case, several basic theorems listed in Table 4.2 will assist the user in the process of manipulating and calculating the transforms.

The inverse Laplace transform is defined as

$$f(t) = \frac{1}{2\pi j}\int_{\sigma-j\infty}^{\sigma+j\infty} F(s)e^{st}ds \tag{4.4}$$

but is generally not used, because of the uniqueness property, which states that there can not be two different functions having the same Laplace transform $F(s)$. Therefore, typically the Laplace transform table (Table 4.1) is used in reverse to determine the original function $f(t)$:

$$\mathcal{L}^{-1}\left\{\mathcal{L}\left[f(t)\right]\right\} = \mathcal{L}^{-1}\left[F(s)\right] = f(t) \tag{4.5}$$

4.1.1 Partial Fraction Expansion

Practically, to find the inverse Laplace transform, a *partial fraction expansion* of the polynomial function is performed through either the *algebraic approach*

TABLE 4.1

Table of Transforms

	$f(t)^a$	$F(s)$
1.	1 or $u(t)$	$\dfrac{1}{s}$
2.	t	$\dfrac{1}{s^2}$
3.	$\dfrac{t^{n-1}}{(n-1)!}$	$\dfrac{1}{s^n}$
4.	e^{at}	$\dfrac{1}{s-a}$
5.	te^{at}	$\dfrac{1}{(s-a)^2}$
6.	$\dfrac{1}{(n-1)!}t^{n-1}e^{at}$	$\dfrac{1}{(s-a)^n}$
7.	$\dfrac{1}{a-b}\left(e^{at}-e^{bt}\right)$	$\dfrac{1}{(s-a)(s-b)}$
8.	$1-e^{at}$	$\dfrac{-a}{s(s-a)}$
9.	$\dfrac{1}{\omega}\sin\omega t$	$\dfrac{1}{s^2+\omega^2}$
10.	$\cos\omega t$	$\dfrac{s}{s^2+\omega^2}$
11.	$1-\cos\omega t$	$\dfrac{\omega^2}{s\left(s^2+\omega^2\right)}$
12.	$\sin(\omega t+\theta)$	$\dfrac{s\sin\theta+\omega\cos\theta}{s^2+\omega^2}$
13.	$\cos(\omega t+\theta)$	$\dfrac{s\cos\theta-\omega\sin\theta}{s^2+\omega^2}$
14.	$e^{-\alpha t}\sin\omega t$	$\dfrac{\omega}{(s+\alpha)^2+\omega^2}$
15.	$e^{-\alpha t}\cos\omega t$	$\dfrac{s+\alpha}{(s+\alpha)^2+\omega^2}$
16.	$\sinh\alpha t$	$\dfrac{\alpha}{s^2+\alpha^2}$
17.	$\cosh\alpha t$	$\dfrac{s}{s^2-\alpha^2}$

Source: Van Valkenburg, M.E., 1964. *Network Analysis*, 2nd ed., Englewood Cliffs, NJ: Prentice-Hall. With permission.

TABLE 4.2

Basic Theorems for Laplace Transforms

1. Transform of linear combinations	$\mathcal{L}[af_1(t) + bf_2(t)] = aF_1(s) + bF_2(s)$
2. Transform of derivatives	$\mathcal{L}[d/dt(f(t))] = sF(s) - f(0^+)$
3. Transform of integrals	$\mathcal{L}[\int f(t)dt] = F(s)/s$
4. Transform for time shift	$\mathcal{L}[f(t-c)] = e^{-cs}\mathcal{L}[f(t)]$
5. Transform for s-shift	$\mathcal{L}[e^{bt}f(t)] = F(s-b)$
6. Transform for t-factor	$\mathcal{L}[t^n f(t)] = (-1)^n d^n/ds^n F(s)$

or the *residue approach* using differentiation. The first is conceptually very simple but may lead to computational difficulties for large functions. The second works well until repeated roots lead to complex differentiation. For most of our examples, the algebraic approach should suffice.

For the algebraic approach perform the following steps:

1. Express the transform as a ratio of polynomials (numerator over denominator) as $P(s)/Q(s)$.

2. Should the power of $P(s)$ be greater than the power of $Q(s)$, use long division to reduce the power of the numerator to less than the power of the denominator.

3. Manipulate the polynomial in the denominator $Q(s)$ as a product of factored polynomials in the form

$$Q(s) = s(s+s_1)(s+s_2)^2(s^2 + as + b)\ldots \tag{4.6}$$

where s_1, s_2 are termed roots and will yield the exponents for the inverse transform of Equation 4.3 (or Transform 4 in Table 4.1). Note that, through manipulation, the factor $s^2 + as + b$ can be expressed as $(s + \alpha)^2 + \beta^2$, where α and β represent real numbers in place of complex conjugate roots that may occur with a complete expansion of that factor.

4. Expand the factors as separate expressions with a polynomial in the numerator of a power lower than the denominator, with unknown constants. For factors that have a power, known as repeated roots, multiple fractions will have to be used, one for each power. Note that the numerator should include s terms up to one power less than found in the denominator.

5. The resulting expression will be of the form

$$\frac{P(s)}{Q(s)} = \frac{a_1}{s} + \frac{a_2}{(s+s_1)} + \ldots + \frac{a_3}{(s+s_2)} + \frac{a_4}{(s+s_2)^2} + \frac{a_5 s + a_6}{(s+\alpha)^2 + \beta^2} \tag{4.7}$$

6. Obtain a common denominator for the right-hand side of Equation 4.7, equate the numerators, and solve for the unknown coefficients a_i. Obviously, this will involve several equations with several unknowns. The more equations there are, the more difficult the process becomes.

For the residue approach, perform the following steps:

7. Multiply both sides of Equation 4.7 by the root term, i.e., $(s + s_1)$:

$$\frac{P(s)(s+s_1)}{Q(s)} = \frac{a_1(s+s_1)}{s} + a_2 + \frac{a_3(s+s_1)}{(s+s_2)} + \frac{a_4(s+s_1)}{(s+s_2)^2} + \frac{(a_5 s + a_6)(s+s_1)}{(s+\alpha)^2 + \beta^2} \quad (4.8)$$

8. Evaluate at $s = -s_1$. All right-hand terms, except for a_2, will become zero and

$$a_2 = \frac{P(s)(s+s_1)}{Q(s)}\bigg|_{s=-s1} \quad (4.9)$$

9. For repeated roots, multiply Equation 4.7 by the highest power of the root term, i.e., $(s + s_2)^2$:

$$\frac{P(s)(s+s_2)^2}{Q(s)} = \frac{a_1(s+s_2)^2}{s} + \frac{a_2(s+s_2)^2}{(s+s_1)} + a_3(s+s_2) + a_4 + \frac{(a_5 s + a_6)(s+s_2)^2}{(s+\alpha)^2 + \beta^2} \quad (4.10)$$

10. Evaluate at $s = s_2$. All terms, except for a_4, become zero.
11. Then differentiate both sides with respect to s and evaluate at $s = -s_2$, yielding the value for a_3. Obviously, there may be some difficulty in the differentiation. For higher powers, second and third derivatives are required. Note that, sometimes, a combination of the two methods can be used more effectively than each method separately.

Example 4.1: Complex Conjugate Roots by the Algebraic Method

The initial Laplace function is

$$\frac{P(s)}{Q(s)} = \frac{s+5}{(s+3)(s^2 + 4s + 5)} \quad (4.11)$$

Using Step 4, expand Equation 4.11 as partial fractions, reaching Step 5:

$$\frac{s+5}{(s+3)\left[(s+2)^2 + 1^2\right]} = \frac{a}{s+3} + \frac{bs+c}{\left[(s+2)^2 + 1^2\right]} \qquad (4.12)$$

Using Step 6 on Equation 4.12, obtain a common denominator and equate numerators yielding

$$s+5 = a\left[(s+2)^2 + 1^2\right] + (s+3)(bs+c) = (a+b)s^2 + (4a+3b+c)s + (5a+3c) \quad (4.13)$$

Solve for unknown coefficients in Equation 4.13 by equating terms with like powers of s:

$$0 = a+b$$
$$1 = 4a + 3b + c \qquad (4.14)$$
$$5 = 5a + 3c$$

Solving Equation 4.14 yields

$$a = 1, \; b = -1, \; c = 0 \qquad (4.15)$$

Substituting the coefficient values back into expanded partial fractions of Equation 4.12 yields

$$\frac{s+5}{(s+3)\left[(s+2)^2 + 1^2\right]} = \frac{1}{s+3} - \frac{s}{(s+2)^2 + 1^2} \qquad (4.16)$$

Take inverse Laplace transforms of the linear combination of terms in Equation 4.15 using Theorem 1 in Table 4.2. Using Transform 4 from Table 4.1 on the first term of Equation 4.16 yields

$$\mathcal{L}^{-1}\left(\frac{1}{s+3}\right) = e^{-3t} \qquad (4.17)$$

Expand the second term from Equation 4.16 appropriately so that the functions fit Transforms 15 and 16 from Table 4.1:

$$\frac{-s}{(s+2)^2 + 1^2} = \frac{-(s+2)}{(s+2)^2 + 1^2} + \frac{2}{(s+2)^2 + 1^2} \qquad (4.18)$$

The inverse Laplace transform of the first term in Equation 4.18 yields

$$\mathcal{L}^{-1}\left[\frac{-(s+2)}{(s+2)^2+1^2}\right]=-e^{-2t}\cos t \tag{4.19}$$

whereas the inverse Laplace transform of the second term in Equation 4.18 yields

$$\mathcal{L}^{-1}\left[\frac{2}{(s+2)^2+1^2}\right]=2e^{-2t}\sin t \tag{4.20}$$

Combining Equations 4.17, 4.19, and 4.20 yields the final expression:

$$f(t)=e^{-3t}-e^{-2t}\cos t+2e^{-2t}\sin t \tag{4.21}$$

Example 4.2: Repeated Roots by the Residue Method

The initial Laplace function is

$$\frac{P(s)}{Q(s)}=\frac{s+2}{(s+1)^2} \tag{4.22}$$

Using Step 4, expand Equation 4.22 as partial fractions, reaching Step 5:

$$\frac{s+2}{(s+1)^2}=\frac{a}{(s+1)}+\frac{b}{(s+1)^2} \tag{4.23}$$

Using Step 9, multiply both sides of Equation 4.23 by $(s + 1)^2$, yielding

$$s+2=a(s+1)+b \tag{4.24}$$

Then using Step 10, evaluate at $s = -1$, yielding $b = 1$. Next, using Step 11, take the derivative of Equation 4.24 with respect to s, which yields

$$\frac{d(s+2)}{ds}=1 \tag{4.25}$$

$$\frac{d[a(s+1)+b]}{ds}=a \tag{4.26}$$

Equating Equations. 4.25 and 4.26 yields $a = 1$. Then taking the inverse Laplace transform (Transforms 4 and 5 in Table 4.1) of Equation 4.23 yields the final transformed function:

$$\mathscr{L}^{-1}\left[\frac{1}{(s+1)} + \frac{1}{(s+1)^2}\right] = e^{-t} + te^{-t} = (t+1)e^{-t} \tag{4.27}$$

4.1.2 Transfer Functions

The concept of a *transfer function* is important in characterizing the properties of a system such as a muscle or a reflex. The transfer function can be considered a black box or operator that acts on an input function and transforms it into an output function. Thus, in a Laplace domain with all initial conditions set to zero, the ratio of the output, $y(s)$, to the input, $x(s)$, for that black box or system is defined as the transfer function, $H(s)$:

$$x(s) \rightarrow [H(s)] \rightarrow y(s) \quad \frac{y(s)}{x(s)} = H(s) \tag{4.28}$$

A special function, the *unit impulse* or *delta function*, $\delta(t)$, is used to better characterize system properties through the transfer function. The unit impulse could be considered a pulse whose magnitude approaches infinite height as the width of the pulse approaches zero with an area remaining constant and equal to one. The unit impulse has some very useful mathematical properties. Using Theorem 2 from Table 4.2, the derivative or change of slope for a unit step becomes infinite or the unit impulse, and the corresponding Laplace transform of a unit impulse is simply one:

$$\mathscr{L}[\delta(t)] = \mathscr{L}\left[\frac{d\,u(t)}{dt}\right] = sF(s) = s\left(\frac{1}{s}\right) = 1 \tag{4.29}$$

This property implies that by supplying a unit impulse forcing function to a system the output will simply be the transfer function of the system.

$$y(s) = H(s)x(s) = H(s) \tag{4.30}$$

Then by using an inverse transform, $H(t)$, the *impulse response* will describe system characteristics in a time domain. Obviously, such an input function cannot be realistically produced, although it is often used in an approximate mode to characterize some events occurring in mechanical systems. For example, the tendon tap in a patellar reflex could be considered a unit impulse for modeling purposes. More details on Laplace transforms can be

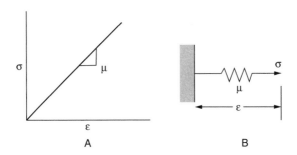

FIGURE 4.2
(A) Stress–strain characteristics of linear elastic spring. (B) Viscoelastic model of spring.

found in Kaplan (1962), Van Valkenburg (1964), or any other advanced calculus or network analysis textbook.

4.2 Viscoelastic Theory

Viscoelastic theory, introduced by Flügge (1975) and detailed by others including Christensen (1981), is the generalization of material or tissue elasticity and viscosity through the use of a variety of springs and dashpots. *Elasticity* is the property of a material that enables it to recover from a deformation produced in the material by an external force. In a perfectly elastic material such as a spring, all deformation is recovered upon release of the external forces and stress is proportional to strain (see Figure 4.2A). This can be represented by a linear spring model (Figure 4.2B) with a characteristic equation known as Hooke's law (named after the British physicist, Robert Hooke, 1635–1703):

$$\sigma = \mu\varepsilon \tag{4.31}$$

where
σ = stress or force per unit area
ε = strain or a change in length per original length, $(l - l_0)/l_0$
μ = spring constant

Note that in Section 2.3, when applied to materials, μ was termed Young's modulus of elasticity (named after the British physicist, Thomas Young, 1773–1829).

Viscosity is a property of a material or fluid that resists the force tending to make it flow. In a perfect fluid, the stress is proportional to the rate or velocity of flow (Figure 4.3A) and can be represented by a dashpot (Figure 4.3B) with its characteristic equation:

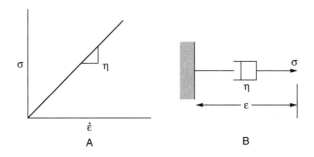

FIGURE 4.3
(A) Stress–strain rate characteristics of dashpot. (B) Viscoelastic model of dashpot.

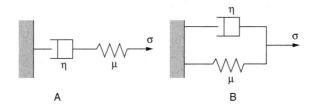

FIGURE 4.4
(A) Viscoelastic model of Maxwell fluid. (B) Viscoelastic model of Voigt solid.

$$\sigma = \eta \, d\varepsilon / dt \qquad\qquad (4.32)$$

where η = dashpot constant.

These basic viscoelastic elements can be used in various combinations to model material behavior. The two simplest mechanical models are the Maxwell fluid (named after the Scottish physicist James Maxwell, 1831–1879; Figure 4.4A) and the Voigt solid (named after the German physicist Woldemar Voigt, 1850–1919; Figure 4.4B).

In the Maxwell fluid under equilibrium conditions, the stress on the dashpot must equal the stress on the spring. Also, the total strain must be the sum of the individual strains for each component or element. We can express these relationships mathematically as

$$\varepsilon = \varepsilon_d + \varepsilon_s \qquad\qquad (4.33)$$

$$\sigma + \sigma_d = \sigma_s \qquad\qquad (4.34)$$

where
ε_d = strain in the dashpot
ε_s = strain in the spring
σ_d = stress in the dashpot and equal to the expression in Equation 4.32
σ_s = stress in the spring and equal to the expression in Equation 4.31

The overall goal is to express the stress–strain relationship for the full Maxwell fluid model. However, with more complicated models, combining the relationships expressed in Equations 4.33 and 4.34 could result in rather complex integro-differential equations for $\sigma(t)$ in the time domain. A much easier approach is to use Laplace transforms to express the equations in the Laplace domain and then to use algebraic manipulations to arrive at the desired expressions (note that $\sigma(s)$ and $\varepsilon(s)$ will typically be simply expressed as σ and ε):

$$\mathscr{L}\left[\sigma_d\left(t\right)\right] = \mathscr{L}\left[\eta\, d\varepsilon_d\left(t\right)/dt\right] = \eta s \varepsilon_d\left(s\right) \tag{4.35}$$

$$\mathscr{L}\left[\sigma\left(t\right)\right] = \mu\varepsilon_s\left(s\right) \tag{4.36}$$

Rearranging Equations 4.35 and 4.36 and using a constant σ yield

$$\varepsilon_d = \frac{\sigma}{\eta s} \tag{4.37}$$

$$\varepsilon_s = \frac{\sigma}{\mu} \tag{4.38}$$

Substituting Equations 4.37 and 4.38 in Equation 4.33 yields

$$\varepsilon = \frac{\sigma}{\eta s} + \frac{\sigma}{\mu} \tag{4.39}$$

Rearranging the expression yields either of two forms, depending on whether stress or strain is considered as the input:

$$\varepsilon = \frac{\mu + \eta s}{\mu \eta s}\sigma \tag{4.40}$$

$$\sigma = \frac{\mu \eta s}{\mu + \eta s}\varepsilon \tag{4.41}$$

In either case, the polynomial expression in s is the transfer function. The choice of expression is typically constrained by the experimental setup in applying a forcing function or by the desired modeling objective.

The transfer function can be similarly established for the Voigt body. If a strain is applied to the body, then each element, since they are in parallel, should be experiencing the same strain but different stresses. Therefore, the total stress is the sum of the stresses for each element:

$$\sigma = \sigma_d + \sigma_s \qquad (4.42)$$

$$\sigma = \eta s \varepsilon + \mu \varepsilon = \left(\eta s + \mu \right) \varepsilon \qquad (4.43)$$

The resulting transfer function is $\eta s + \mu$.

Note the development of an interesting relationship that can be used in simplifying the derivation of a transfer function. The two elements, the dashpot and the spring, can be considered to act similarly to a capacitor in the simplification of a network circuit; the values add directly to obtain an equivalent component when the individual components are found in a parallel arrangement:

$$\mu_{eq} = \mu_1 + \mu_2 \qquad (4.44)$$

where μ_{eq} = equivalent spring and μ_1, μ_2 = parallel spring elements.

When in series, the values are inverted, added and reinverted, i.e.:

$$\mu_{eq} = \left(\frac{1}{\mu_1} + \frac{1}{\mu_2} \right)^{-1} = \frac{\mu_1 \mu_2}{\mu_1 + \mu_2} \qquad (4.45)$$

where μ_{eq} = equivalent spring and μ_1, μ_2 = series spring elements.

This relationship can be used in easily developing the transfer function for a Kelvin body (named after the English physicist and mathematician William Kelvin, 1824–1907), which is the next more complicated viscoelastic model using three components (Figure 4.5A). Note that, excluding the contractile element, the Kelvin body is identical to the muscle model developed by Hill (1938, 1970) (see Figure 3.21). The dashpot and the spring element in series combine to yield the equivalent component shown in Figure 4.5B with a value of

$$\mu_{eq} = \frac{\mu_1 \eta s}{\mu_1 + \eta s} \qquad (4.46)$$

The equivalent component of Equation 4.46 and the spring element in parallel combine to yield the transfer function:

$$H(s) = \frac{\mu_1 \eta s}{\mu_1 + \eta s} + \mu_2 \qquad (4.47)$$

which, rearranged, results in the final transfer function (Figure 4.5C):

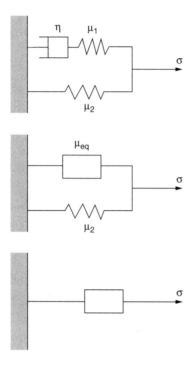

FIGURE 4.5
Derivation of the transfer function for the Kelvin model.

$$H(s) = \frac{(\mu_1 + \mu_2)\eta s + \mu_1 \mu_2}{\eta s + \mu_1} \tag{4.48}$$

The next step is to use the transfer function on a specific input to determine the resulting output. This will allow the experimenter to compare actual material properties with model responses, with the two most common properties stress relaxation and strain retardation. *Stress relaxation* is the resulting stress-over-time curve for a unit step input of strain. *Strain retardation* is the resulting strains-over-time curve for a unit step input of stress, sometimes also termed *creep*. This can be demonstrated quite nicely with the Voigt body and Equation 4.43 rearranged so that the input is stress and the output is strain:

$$\varepsilon(s) = \frac{\sigma(s)}{(\eta s + \mu)} \tag{4.49}$$

Using a unit step input of $\sigma(t) = u(t)$ and its Laplace transform of $\sigma(s) = 1/s$ yields the expression:

$$\varepsilon(s) = \frac{1}{(\eta s + \mu)s} \tag{4.50}$$

Using the algebraic approach to the partial fraction expansion of Equation 4.50 yields

$$\frac{1}{\eta(s + \mu/\eta)s} = \frac{1}{\eta}\left[\frac{a}{s} + \frac{b}{(s + \mu/\eta)}\right] \tag{4.51}$$

Obtaining a common denominator for the right side of Equation 4.51 and equating numerators yields

$$1 = as + a\mu/\eta + bs \tag{4.52}$$

Equating common powers of s terms in Equation 4.52 yields two equations in two unknowns:

$$a + b = 0 \tag{4.53}$$

$$a\mu/\eta = 1 \tag{4.54}$$

Solving Equations 4.53 and 4.54 yields

$$a = \eta/\mu \quad b = -\eta/\mu \tag{4.55}$$

Substituting the above values into Equation 4.51 and taking the inverse Laplace transform yields

$$\varepsilon(t) = 1/\mu \mathscr{L}^{-1}\left[\frac{1}{s} + \frac{1}{(s + \mu/\eta)}\right] \tag{4.56}$$

$$\varepsilon(t) = 1/\mu\left(1 - e^{\frac{-\mu t}{\eta}}\right) \tag{4.57}$$

A plot of Equation 4.57 (Figure 4.6) shows the characteristic creep that would be expected with a viscous damping element. As a constant stress is being continually applied to the Voigt material, the dashpot is continually yielding. However, with time the resulting increase in strain in the spring element has increased the internal stress, which ultimately will reach a value that resists the externally applied stress, stopping the creep process.

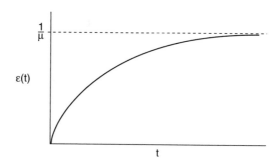

FIGURE 4.6
Stress retardation or creep in the Voigt solid.

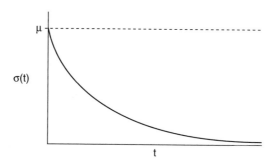

FIGURE 4.7
Stress relaxation in the Maxwell fluid.

Similarly, we can examine the properties of a Maxwell fluid. Using Equation 4.41 and a unit step strain input, the resulting stress becomes

$$\sigma(s) = \frac{\mu \eta s}{(\mu + \eta s)s} \tag{4.58}$$

Canceling out one s term in the denominator and numerator, factoring out a μ, and taking the inverse Laplace transform yields

$$\sigma(t) = \mathcal{L}^{-1}[\sigma(s)] = \mathcal{L}^{-1} \mu \left\{ \frac{1}{(s + \mu/\eta)} \right\} = \mu e^{\frac{-\mu t}{\eta}} \tag{4.59}$$

and the resulting stress relaxation curve in Figure 4.7.

Note that the calculation of a stress relaxation function for the Voigt body (Equation 4.43) results in an impulse function, which, although acceptable mathematically, is not realistic mechanically.

$$\mathscr{L}^{-1}\left[\sigma(s)\right] = \mathscr{L}^{-1}\left(\frac{\eta s + \mu}{s}\right) = \mathscr{L}^{-1}\left(\eta + \frac{\mu}{s}\right) = \eta\delta(t) + \mu u(t) \qquad (4.60)$$

Example 4.3: Initial and Final Value Theorems

As the transfer functions become more complicated, the corresponding functions in time become more complicated to plot. In such cases, either the initial value theorem or the final value theorem will provide the critical and initial and final values of the time plot. The *initial value theorem* is defined as

$$\lim_{t \to 0+} f(t) = \lim_{s \to \infty} sF(s) \qquad (4.61)$$

while the *final value theorem* is defined as

$$\lim_{t \to \infty} f(t) = \lim_{s \to 0} sF(s) \qquad (4.62)$$

Thus, the initial and final values, respectively, for the Voigt body creep function (Equation 4.57) can be found very simply from

$$\lim_{s \to \infty} sF(s) = \lim_{s \to \infty} \frac{s}{(\eta s + \mu)s} = 0 \qquad (4.63)$$

$$\lim_{s \to 0} sF(s) = \lim_{s \to 0} \frac{s}{(\eta s + \mu)s} = \frac{1}{\mu} \qquad (4.64)$$

4.3   Hill's Muscle Models

The basic mechanical properties, such as creep and stress relaxation, of Hill's three-element model (i.e., passive muscle with the contractile element removed, Figure 4.8A) can be determined as follows. The isotonic after-loaded experiments of Fenn and Marsh (1935) led to the velocity-tension relationship developed in Section 3.7.3 and shown in Figure 3.18. In terms of Hill's viscoelastic model, one can assume that initially the force on the parallel elastic element is negligible because the dashpot cannot move instantaneously. Obviously, with increasing time, the dashpot slowly yields and strain increases. However, for low to moderate strains, Hill's model can be simplified to the model shown in Figure 4.8B.

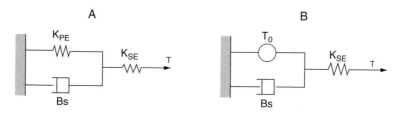

FIGURE 4.8
(A) Hill's three-element muscle model. (B) Simplified Hills muscle model.

In this simplified model, the force on the dashpot is

$$T_0 - T = Bv \tag{4.65}$$

where
T = tension
T_0 = isometric or maximum tension
v = velocity

This relationship can then be used to approximate the initial slope (i.e., velocities close to zero or minimal strain) of the velocity–tension relationship. Or more importantly, this initial slope provides an approximate value for the dashpot parameter B.

One can reach the same result starting with Hill's equation for the velocity–tension relationship:

$$(T + a)(v + b) = (T_0 + a)b \tag{4.66}$$

Multiplying the factors and subtracting common terms yield

$$Tv + av + Tb = T_0 b \tag{4.67}$$

Rearranging the terms yields and adding/subtracting the term $T_0 v$ yield

$$T(v + b) = T_0 b - av + T_0 v - T_0 v \tag{4.68}$$

Rearranging terms again yields

$$T(v + b) = T_0(v + b) - (a + T_0)v \tag{4.69}$$

Now dividing both sides by $(v + b)$ yields

$$T_0 - T = \frac{(a + T_0)}{(v + b)} v = Bv \tag{4.70}$$

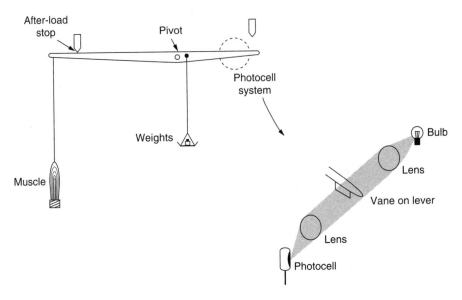

FIGURE 4.9
Quick stretch experiment for determining series elastic element. (From Aidley, D.J., 1985. *The Physiology of Excitable Cells*, 2nd ed., Cambridge, U.K.: Cambridge University Press, 265. With permission.)

where the term $(a + T_0)/(v + b)$ can be considered to be the initial slope of the velocity–tension relationship and an estimate of the dashpot parameter B.

From Hill's (1938) experiments on vertebrate muscles, the unknown constants a and b were found to be $T_0/4$ and $v_{max}/4$, respectively. Substituting these values into the expression for B from Equation 4.70 yields

$$B = \frac{a + T_0}{v + b} = \frac{1.25\,T_0}{v + v_{max}/4} \tag{4.71}$$

For values of velocity much less than $v_{max}/4$, B remains constant. Thus, again the initial slope of the velocity–tension curve can be used to estimate B. Data from Bawa et al. (1976) on the cat plantaris muscle have yielded values on the order of 4.6 g-s/mm.

K_{SE} can be determined from quick stretch experiments, in which a sudden pull is applied to a passive muscle at its resting length (Figure 4.9). On a quick pull the dashpot will not respond and all the strain will be absorbed in the series elastic element. Data from Jewell and Wilkie (1958) on the frog sartorius muscle yield values for K_{SE} on the order of 85 g/mm (Figure 4.10). Higher values of 380 g/mm for a cat plantaris muscle have been reported by Bawa et al. (1976). This large variation is due to a variety of factors: the experimental procedures, masses and elasticities in the equipment, the type of muscle, and from which animal it was taken. In addition, the stress–strain

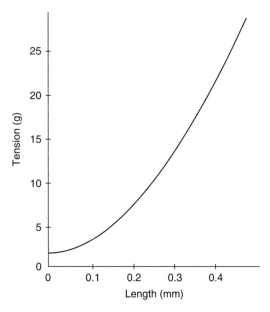

FIGURE 4.10
Length–tension relationship for a series elastic element. (Adapted from Jewell and Wilkie, 1958.)

relationship is not linear and can result in differing values for K_{SE} depending on the region of strain utilized.

K_{PE} is more difficult to determine and is typically done by looking at the second-order response to vibrations or other forcing functions. Bawa et al. (1976) indicate a value of 103 g/mm for a cat plantaris muscle. Note that K_{SE} is much stiffer than K_{PE}, which would seem reasonable considering that K_{SE} represents the tendon interface to the muscle, while K_{PE} represents the more elastic fascia separating bundles of muscle fibers.

4.3.1 Active Muscle Response

The active muscle response based on Hill's four-element model (Figure 4.11) can be found most easily by developing the transfer function for muscle model. First, the equilibrium equations need to be determined as follows. The internally developed muscle force T_{CE} is modified by the viscous damping element and parallel elastic element to become the externally measured tension, T. In the process, it is also transferred through the series elastic element, resulting in two equilibrium equations:

$$T = T_{CE} + Bs\varepsilon_i + K_{PE}\varepsilon_i \tag{4.72}$$

$$T = K_{SE}\left(\varepsilon - \varepsilon_i\right) \tag{4.73}$$

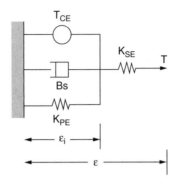

FIGURE 4.11
Hill's four-element active muscle model.

Equating Equations 4.72 and 4.73 and rearranging result in

$$T_{CE} = K_{SE}\,\varepsilon - \left(Bs + K_{PE} + K_{SE}\right)\varepsilon_i \qquad (4.74)$$

Solving Equation 4.73 for ε_i and substituting for ε_i into Equation 4.74 yield

$$\varepsilon_i = \varepsilon - T/K_{SE} \qquad (4.75)$$

$$T_{CE} = K_{SE}\,\varepsilon - \left(Bs + K_{PE} + K_{SE}\right)\varepsilon + \left(\frac{Bs + K_{PE} + K_{SE}}{K_{SE}}\right)T \qquad (4.76)$$

Rearrangement yields

$$T_{CE} = -\left(Bs + K_{PE}\right)\varepsilon + \left(Bs + K_{PE} + K_{SE}\right)/K_{SE}\,T \qquad (4.77)$$

Equation 4.77 can now be rearranged into two alternate forms: external muscle tension, T, as function of the active muscle contractile element tension, T_{CE}:

$$T = \frac{K_{SE}T_{CE}}{Bs + K_{PE} + K_{SE}} + \frac{K_{SE}\left(Bs + K_{PE}\right)}{Bs + K_{PE} + K_{SE}}\varepsilon \qquad (4.78)$$

or strain, ε, in terms of the active muscle contractile element tension and external tension:

$$\varepsilon = \frac{\left(Bs + K_{PE} + K_{SE}\right)T}{\left(Bs + K_{PE}\right)K_{SE}} - \frac{T_{CE}}{Bs + K_{PE}} \qquad (4.79)$$

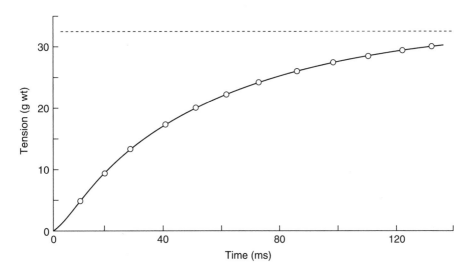

FIGURE 4.12
Tension buildup during isometric tetanus. (Adapted from Jewell and Wilkie, 1958.)

Note that both equations consist of two transfer functions, one for an external forcing function, either mechanical stress or strain, and the other for an internal forcing function from the contractile element.

4.3.2 Tension Buildup

Consider an *isometric experiment*, in which both ends of a muscle are rigidly fixed so that it cannot shorten. Then, when stimulated it contracts isometrically and the resulting external tension can be measured with a force gauge (Figure 4.12). This case can be examined using Equation 4.80, but with the second term in ε eliminated, since the muscle is stimulated isometrically and no strain (at least externally) is possible. Assuming a maximum tetanic stimulation, the input can be represented with a step function with magnitude T_{CE}. Using the Laplace transform of the step function, Equation 4.80 becomes

$$T = \frac{K_{SE} T_{CE}}{\left(Bs + K_{PE} + K_{SE}\right)s} \tag{4.80}$$

Factoring constants and rearrangement yield

$$T = \frac{K_{SE} T_{CE}}{B}\left\{\frac{1}{s+\left(K_{PE}+K_{SE}\right)/B}\right\}\frac{1}{s} \tag{4.81}$$

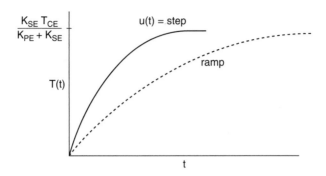

FIGURE 4.13
Calculated tension buildup using Hill's four-element model.

A partial fraction expansion yields

$$T = \frac{K_{SE}\,T_{CE}}{B}\left\{\frac{a}{s+\left(K_{PE}+K_{SE}\right)/B}+\frac{b}{s}\right\} \tag{4.82}$$

Using residues to solve for a and b yields

$$a = \left.1/s\right|_{s=-\left(K_{PE}+K_{SE}\right)/B} = -B\Big/\left(K_{PE}+K_{SE}\right) \tag{4.83}$$

$$b = \left.\frac{1}{s+\left(K_{PE}+K_{SE}\right)/B}\right|_{s=0} = B\Big/\left(K_{PE}+K_{SE}\right) \tag{4.84}$$

Substituting the coefficients a and b back into Equation 4.82 yields

$$T = \frac{K_{SE}T_{CE}}{B}\left\{\frac{-B\Big/\left(K_{PE}+K_{SE}\right)}{s+\left(K_{PE}+K_{SE}\right)/B}\right\}+\frac{B\Big/\left(K_{PE}+K_{SE}\right)}{s} \tag{4.85}$$

Taking the inverse Laplace transform and simplifying yield

$$T(t) = \frac{K_{SE}T_{CE}}{K_{PE}+K_{SE}}\left\{1-e^{-\left(K_{PE}+K_{SE}\right)t/B}\right\} \tag{4.86}$$

The plot of Equation 4.86 (Figure 4.13) corresponds nicely to the buildup of tension measured in the isometric experiment (Figure 4.12). Note that active muscle contractile tension, T_{CE}, is not directly transferred to the force gauge. Instead, it is modified by the combination of the parallel and series elastic elements as a reduced value. Should the values of K_{PE} and K_{SE} be relatively equal, the tension reduction is almost 50%. If the values are quite unequal, as in the actual muscle, then the reduction is relatively small. Also, note that the tetanic stimulation is not truly a unit step. It is more likely to be a steady increase in tension until maximum tension is achieved, which is best simulated by a *ramp function*, $f(t) = t$. In that case, the resulting tension function would have an additional term in t and a slight modification in the slope or rise of tension.

4.3.3 Stress Relaxation

Consider a quick stretch experiment, in which the passive muscle undergoes a step strain input of magnitude ε_0. In such case T_{CE} is zero and the first term can be eliminated and the Laplace transform of a unit step is ε_0/s:

$$T = \frac{K_{SE}\left(Bs + K_{PE}\right)}{Bs + K_{PE} + K_{SE}} \frac{\varepsilon_0}{s} \tag{4.87}$$

Rearrangement yields

$$T = K_{SE}\varepsilon_0 \frac{s + K_{PE}/B}{s\left[s + \left(K_{PE} + K_{SE}\right)/B\right]} \tag{4.88}$$

A partial fraction expansion yields

$$T = K_{SE}\varepsilon_0 \left\{\frac{a}{s + \left(K_{PE} + K_{SE}\right)/B} + \frac{b}{s}\right\} \tag{4.89}$$

Using residues to solve for a and b yields

$$a = \left.\frac{s + K_{PE}/B}{s}\right|_{s = -\left(K_{PE} + K_{SE}\right)/B} = \frac{K_{SE}}{K_{PE} + K_{SE}} \tag{4.90}$$

$$b = \left.\frac{s + K_{PE}/B}{s + \left(K_{PE} + K_{SE}\right)/B}\right|_{s=0} = \frac{K_{PE}}{K_{PE} + K_{SE}} \tag{4.91}$$

Substituting the coefficients a and b back into Equation 4.89 yields

$$T = \frac{K_{SE}\,\varepsilon_0}{K_{PE} + K_{SE}} \left\{\frac{K_{SE}}{s + \left(K_{PE} + K_{SE}\right)/B} + \frac{K_{PE}}{s}\right\} \tag{4.92}$$

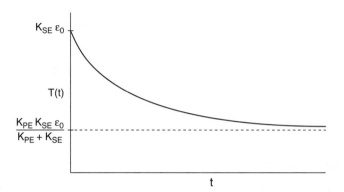

FIGURE 4.14
Calculated stress relaxation in Hill's four-element model.

Taking the inverse Laplace transform and simplifying yield the plot in Figure 4.14 and the function

$$T(t) = \frac{K_{SE}\,\varepsilon_0}{K_{PE} + K_{SE}} \left\{ K_{PE} + K_{SE}\, e^{-\left(K_{PE} + K_{SE}\right)t/B} \right\} \tag{4.93}$$

In this situation, the initial strain is all taken up in the series elastic element. However, the viscous damping element slowly yields, allowing the tension in the series elastic element to decrease to a point in which the tension between the two elastic elements is balanced. This phenomenon is termed stress relaxation and is observed in many tissues as well as engineering materials (Haddad, 1995).

4.3.4 Creep

The strain retardation or creep function for passive muscle can be generated in a similar manner to the stress relaxation of Section 4.3.3. Eliminate the active contractile component of T_{CE} from Equation 4.79, yielding

$$\varepsilon = \frac{\left(Bs + K_{PE} + K_{SE}\right)T}{\left(Bs + K_{PE}\right)K_{SE}} \tag{4.94}$$

Using a unit step input of external tension and dividing the numerator and denominator by B yield

$$\varepsilon = \frac{s + \left(K_{PE} + K_{SE}\right)\big/B}{K_{SE}\left(s + K_{PE}\big/B\right)s} \tag{4.95}$$

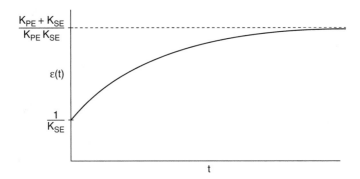

FIGURE 4.15
Calculated creep in Hill's four-element model.

Using the partial fraction expansion yields

$$\varepsilon = \frac{1}{K_{SE}}\left\{ \frac{a}{s + K_{PE}/B} + \frac{b}{s} \right\}$$ (4.96)

Solving for *a* and *b* using residues yields

$$a = \left.\frac{s + \left(K_{PE} + K_{SE}\right)/B}{s}\right|_{s=-K_{PE}/B} = \frac{-K_{SE}}{K_{PE}}$$ (4.97)

$$b = \left.\frac{s + \left(K_{PE} + K_{SE}\right)/B}{s + K_{PE}/B}\right|_{s=0} = \frac{K_{PE} + K_{SE}}{K_{PE}}$$ (4.98)

Taking the inverse Laplace transform and rearranging yield the creep function plotted in Figure 4.15 and the equation:

$$\varepsilon\left(t\right) = \frac{K_{PE} + K_{SE}}{K_{PE}K_{SE}} - \frac{e^{-\left(K_{PE}t/B\right)}}{K_{PE}}$$ (4.99)

Note that in this situation, with the initial application of a unit stress, the damping element does not respond. However, the series elastic spring yields to the stress with a step jump of movement. Then under continued loading the damping element begins to yield and allows the material to creep until the two elastic springs balance out the stress and the creep stops.

4.3.5 Time Constant

The creep rise (Equation 4.99) or stress relaxation (Equation 4.93) times are determined by the exponent in the exponential term. This exponential term can also be formulated as $e^{-t/\tau}$, where τ is the termed the *time constant* and, in the case of active force buildup (Equation 4.86) and stress relaxation (Equation 4.93), is equal to

$$\tau = B/\left(K_{PE} + K_{SE}\right) \qquad (4.100)$$

The exponential function drops from $e^0 = 1.0$ to $e^{-1} = 0.37$ in one time constant and to $e^{-2} = 0.14$ in two time constants, etc. For active force buildup, the rise becomes 0.63 in one time constant and 0.86 in two time constants.

For Hill's muscle model, substituting experimentally determined values for the viscoelastic elements yields a time constant of

$$B/\left(K_{PE} + K_{SE}\right) = 5/\left(103 + 380\right) = 0.0103\,\text{s} \qquad (4.101)$$

where from Bawa et al. (1976), $B = 5$ g-s/mm, $K_{PE} = 103$ g/mm, and $K_{SE} = 380$ g/mm. Using a smaller value from Jewell and Wilkie (1958) of $K_{SE} = 85$ g/mm with a correspondingly weaker $K_{PE} = 20$ g/mm yields

$$B/\left(K_{PE} + K_{SE}\right) = 5/\left(20 + 85\right) = 0.0476\,\text{s} \qquad (4.102)$$

This means that the rise time for twitch tension ranges from 10.3 to 47.6 ms to reach 63% of the final value and 20.6 to 95.2 ms to reach 86% of the final value. Note that these times correspond relatively closely to the twitch times for fast and slow twitch muscle fibers given in Table 3.2.

Note also the relative relationship between the time constant for stress relaxation (or force buildup) and for the creep function. Taking the ratio of the two yields

$$\frac{\tau_{relax}}{\tau_{creep}} = \frac{B/\left(K_{PE} + K_{SE}\right)}{B/K_{PE}} = \frac{K_{PE}}{K_{PE} + K_{SE}} \qquad (4.103)$$

Given that K_{SE} is much stiffer than K_{PE}, the time constant for stress relaxation is much smaller than the time constant for creep. This means that the muscle will relax much more quickly for stress than for strain changes.

4.4 Frequency Analysis

An alternative approach for muscle modeling and examining muscle properties is to consider the effects of a sinusoidal forcing function. Consider again the passive muscle from Equation 4.78, with T_{CE} set equal to zero:

$$T = \frac{K_{SE}\left(Bs + K_{PE}\right)\varepsilon}{Bs + K_{PE} + K_{SE}} \qquad (4.104)$$

From Table 4.1, a sinusoidal strain function:

$$\varepsilon(t) = \sin \omega t \qquad (4.105)$$

would be transformed to the Laplace domain as

$$\varepsilon(s) = \frac{\omega}{\left(s^2 + \omega^2\right)} \qquad (4.106)$$

Applying the transfer function of Equation 4.104 to a sinusoidal strain function of Equation 4.106 yields the muscle tension response in the Laplace domain:

$$T(s) = \frac{\omega K_{SE}\left(Bs + K_{PE}\right)}{\left(Bs + K_{PE} + K_{SE}\right)\left(s^2 + \omega^2\right)} \qquad (4.107)$$

A partial fraction expansion yields

$$T(s) = \frac{a}{\left(Bs + K_{PE} + K_{SE}\right)} + \frac{b}{\left(s^2 + \omega^2\right)} \qquad (4.108)$$

Without further calculations, it can be seen from Equation 4.108 that the sinusoidal strain forcing function results in a transient response in stress of the form e^{-at}, which dies down to zero as time becomes large, and a sinusoidal steady-state response, which continues for large times. To examine Equation 4.108 for various times or various frequencies of sinusoids requires considerable effort. Therefore, a simpler approach is needed to examine the frequency response characteristics for muscle through a formalized frequency analysis.

4.4.1 Generalized Approach

It can be shown that for a system with transfer function $H(t)$, a sinusoidal input of

$$x(t) = \sin \omega t \qquad (4.109)$$

will result in a sinusoidal output that is similar to the sinusoidal input in that it has the same frequency, but the magnitude may be altered and the two sinusoidal functions may be out of phase. Consider the output represented as

$$y(t) = H(t) x(t) = M(\omega) \sin(\omega t + \phi(\omega)) \tag{4.110}$$

where $M(\omega)$ = magnitude and $\phi(\omega)$ = phase angle.

The magnitude $M(\omega)$ can be represented quite simply in the Laplace domain as the magnitude of the transfer function:

$$M(\omega) = |H(s)|_{s=j\omega} = |H(j\omega)| \tag{4.111}$$

while the phase angle $\phi(\omega)$ can be represented as the phase angle of the transfer function or the argument of a complex variable, abbreviated as arg:

$$\phi(\omega) = \arg H(s)|_{s=j\omega} = \arg H(j\omega) \tag{4.112}$$

For any complex variable $X(\omega) + jY(\omega)$ (where $X(\omega)$ is the real part, $Y(\omega)$ is the imaginary part, and $j = \sqrt{-1}$ or $j^2 = -1$), the magnitude then can be expressed as

$$M(\omega) = \left[X(\omega)^2 + Y(\omega)^2 \right]^{1/2} \tag{4.113}$$

and the argument or phase angle as

$$\phi(\omega) = \tan^{-1} \left[Y(\omega) / X(\omega) \right] \tag{4.114}$$

For a complete frequency response analysis, the magnitude response of Equation 4.111 and phase angles of Equation 4.112 are plotted over the range of frequencies of interest.

4.4.2 Magnitude and Phase Angle in the Frequency Domain

Taking the Laplace transforms of Equations 4.109 and 4.110 yields Equation 4.111 with complex conjugate roots:

$$y(s) = \frac{H(s)\omega}{s^2 + \omega^2} = \frac{H(s)\omega}{(s+j\omega)(s-j\omega)} \tag{4.115}$$

Performing a partial fraction expansion yields the complex conjugate roots and other roots depending on the transfer function $H(s)$:

$$y(s) = \frac{a}{(s+j\omega)} + \frac{b}{(s-j\omega)} \tag{4.116}$$

The constants a and b can be found using the residue method:

$$a = \left.\frac{H(s)\omega}{(s-j\omega)}\right|_{s=-j\omega} = \frac{H(-j\omega)\omega}{-2j\omega} \tag{4.117}$$

$$b = \left.\frac{H(s)\omega}{(s+j\omega)}\right|_{s=j\omega} = \frac{H(j\omega)\omega}{2j\omega} \tag{4.118}$$

Substituting the constants into Equation 4.116 and taking the inverse Laplace transform yield the solution in the time domain:

$$y(t) = \frac{H(-j\omega)\omega e^{-j\omega t}}{-2j\omega} + \frac{H(j\omega)\omega e^{j\omega t}}{2j\omega} \tag{4.119}$$

Canceling the ω's and expanding $H(j\omega)$ into its complex conjugate form yield

$$y(t) = \frac{[X(\omega) - jY(\omega)]e^{-j\omega t}}{-2j} + \frac{[X(\omega) + jY(\omega)]e^{j\omega t}}{2j} \tag{4.120}$$

Rearranging terms yields

$$y(t) = X(\omega)\frac{e^{j\omega t} - e^{-j\omega t}}{2j} + Y(\omega)\frac{e^{j\omega t} + e^{-j\omega t}}{2} \tag{4.121}$$

From the Euler identities:

$$e^{j\omega} = \cos\omega + j\sin\omega \tag{4.122}$$

and

$$e^{-j\omega} = \cos\omega - j\sin\omega \tag{4.123}$$

sin *t* can be expressed as

$$\sin \omega t = \frac{e^{j\omega t} - e^{-j\omega t}}{2j} \qquad (4.124)$$

and cos *t* as

$$\cos \omega t = \frac{e^{j\omega t} - e^{-j\omega t}}{2} \qquad (4.125)$$

Substituting Equations 4.124 and 4.125 into Equation 4.121 yields the final solution in the time domain as

$$y(t) = X(\omega)\sin \omega t + Y(\omega)\cos \omega t \qquad (4.126)$$

To find the magnitude and phase, Equation 4.126 needs to be manipulated into an alternative form. Multiply and divide Equation 4.126 by the same term $(X(\omega)^2 + Y(\omega)^2)^{1/2}$ yielding

$$y(t) = \left(X(\omega)^2 + Y(\omega)^2\right)^{1/2} \left\{ \frac{X(\omega)\sin \omega t}{\left[\left(X(\omega)^2 + Y(\omega)^2\right)^{1/2}\right]^{1/2}} + \frac{Y(\omega)\cos \omega t}{\left(X(\omega)^2 + Y(\omega)^2\right)^{1/2}} \right\} \qquad (4.127)$$

Note that based on a right triangle with sides *X* and *Y*:

$$\cos \phi = \frac{X}{\left(X^2 + Y^2\right)^{1/2}} \qquad \sin \phi = \frac{Y}{\left(X^2 + Y^2\right)^{1/2}} \qquad (4.128)$$

Substituting Equation 4.128 into 4.127 yields

$$y(t) = M(\omega)\left\{\sin \omega t \cos \phi + \cos \omega t \sin \phi\right\} \qquad (4.129)$$

By trigonometric substitution, the alternative form of the solution in the time domain is

$$y(t) = M(\omega)\sin\left(\omega t + \phi(\omega)\right) \qquad (4.130)$$

where the magnitude, as indicated previously in Equation 4.113, is

$$M(\omega) = \left(X(\omega)^2 + Y(\omega)^2 \right)^{1/2}$$

(4.131)

and the phase angle, as indicated in Equation 4.114, is

$$\phi(\omega) = \tan^{-1} \frac{Y(\omega)}{X(\omega)}$$

(4.132)

Example 4.4: Calculation of Magnitude and Phase

Consider the simple transfer function:

$$H(s) = \frac{1}{s+1}$$

(4.133)

To find the magnitude and phase angle of $H(s)$, substitute $s = j\omega$ and multiply the numerator and denominator by the complex conjugate to form a complex variable of the form $X + jY$:

$$H(j\omega) = \frac{1}{1+j\omega} \frac{(1-j\omega)}{(1-j\omega)} = \frac{1-j\omega}{1+\omega^2} = \frac{1}{1+\omega^2} - \frac{j\omega}{1+\omega^2}$$

(4.134)

Note that only a pure imaginary component is used because of the Euler representation of sine and cosine functions in Equations 4.124 and 4.125. The magnitude is then

$$M = \left\{ \frac{1^2}{\left(1+\omega^2\right)^2} + \frac{\omega^2}{\left(1+\omega^2\right)^2} \right\}^{1/2} = \left\{ \frac{1}{1+\omega^2} \right\}^{1/2}$$

(4.135)

and the phase is

$$\phi = \tan^{-1} \frac{-\omega / \left(1+\omega^2\right)}{1 / \left(1+\omega^2\right)} = -\tan^{-1} \omega$$

(4.136)

Typically these frequency responses are plotted on log-log scales (Figure 4.16), so as to show the full range of possible frequencies. Also, on a log-

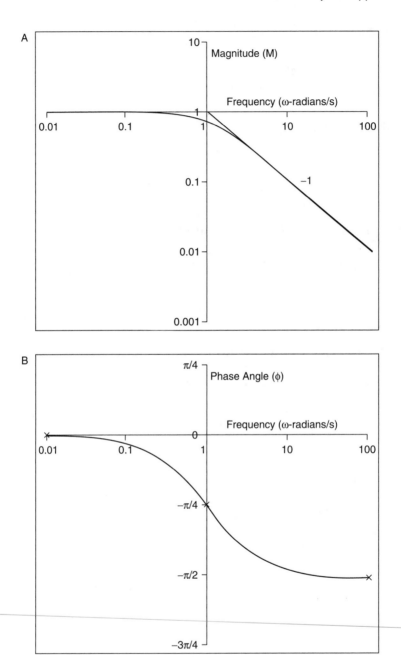

FIGURE 4.16
Magnitude (A) and phase angle (B) plots for $H(s) = 1/(s + 1)$.

log scale, several aspects of typical relationships are very much simplified. For very small ω, $\omega \ll 1$, the magnitude in Equation 4.135 is simply the value of 1 or a flat line for frequencies approaching $\omega = 1$ from the left-hand side. For very large ω, $\omega \gg 1$, the magnitude is essentially $1/\omega$, with the constant 1 in the denominator having little effect. On a log-log scale, $1/\omega$ is simply represented as line with a slope of −1. A critical point occurs at $\omega = 1$, which is known as a *break frequency*. There the two lines theoretically intersect, but the actual plot forms a curved connection. The actual magnitude at $\omega = 1$ is $1/\sqrt{2}$ or 0.707.

The phase angle is plotted in a similar manner although the ordinate for angles remains a linear scale. For very small angles, $\omega \ll 1$, $\tan^{-1} \omega = \omega$ and the phase angle is close to 0, but gradually decreasing (because of the minus sign) as ω becomes larger. For very large angles, as ω approaches ∞, $-\tan^{-1} \omega$ slowly approaches $-\pi/2$. At the break frequency of $\omega = 1$, the phase angle is $-\tan^{-1} 1$, which is equal to $-\pi/4$.

4.4.3 Magnitude and Phase Angle in the Laplace Domain

Frequency analysis can also be done in the Laplace or s-domain, in a more straightforward manner, as follows. The transfer function, $H(s)$ is put in a time constant format, i.e., the coefficient of s in each factor is put in the form of a time constant, $(1 + s\tau)$, where $\tau = 1/\omega_i$, and ω_i is the break frequency.

The magnitude plot is examined in terms of frequency ranges. Wherever ω (or s notation as used in the Laplace domain) is less than ω_i, the slope of the plot will be zero for factors in the denominator. If the ω is larger than ω_i, then the slope is equal to −1. If there are two s factors and ω is larger than both break frequencies, the slope becomes −2, etc. If there is an s factor in the numerator, similar rules apply, but the slopes are +1 or +2. This linearized approach for the magnitude is termed a *Bode plot* in electronics applications. In such cases the magnitude is typically expressed in terms of power with units of decibels.

The phase angle is determined by the simple relationship:

$$\phi = \alpha \pi / 2 \qquad (4.137)$$

where α = the average of the slopes of the magnitude plot for the immediately preceding and immediately following decade on either side of the frequency of interest. Further information on frequency plots and Bode plots can be obtained from Schneck (1992), Van Valkenburg (1964), or any other electrical engineering textbook.

Example 4.5: Calculation of Magnitude and Phase in the s-Domain

Consider the transfer function:

$$H(s) = \frac{5\left(1 + s/1\right)\left(1 + s/10\right)}{\left(1 + s/0.1\right)\left(1 + s/100\right)} \qquad (4.138)$$

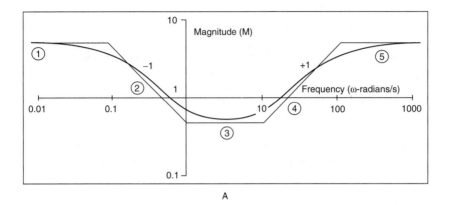

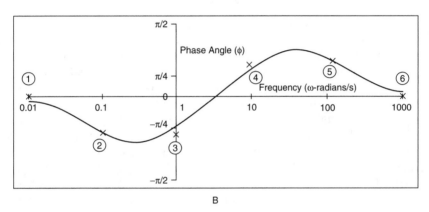

FIGURE 4.17
Magnitude (A) and phase angle (B) plots for $H(s) = [5(1 + s/1)(1 + s/10)]/[(1 + s/0.1)(1 + s/100)]$.

and the logical reasoning as follows, with the corresponding points marked on the curves in Figure 4.17. First consider the magnitude plot of Figure 4.17A.

1. The first or smallest break frequency is 0.1. For $\omega \ll 0.1$, $H(s)$ is approximately

$$H(s) = \frac{5(1)(1)}{(1)(1)} = 5 \tag{4.139}$$

with slope 0.

2. The next largest break frequency is 1. For $0.1 < \omega < 1$, $H(s)$ can be approximated as

$$H(s) = \frac{5(1)(1)}{(s/0.1)(1)} = \frac{0.5}{s} \tag{4.140}$$

or a downward sloping line with a slope of –1. Note that the +1 term has relatively little effect as compared to the s term.
3. The next break frequency is 10. For $1 < \omega < 10$, $H(s)$ can be approximated as

$$H(s) = \frac{5(s/1)(1)}{(s/0.1)(1)} = \frac{0.5s}{s} = 0.5 \tag{4.141}$$

or simply a flat line with slope 0.
4. The last break frequency is 100. For $10 < \omega < 100$, $H(s)$ can be approximated as

$$H(s) = \frac{5(s/1)(s/10)}{(s/0.1)(1)} = \frac{0.05s^2}{s} = 0.05s \tag{4.142}$$

or an upward sloping line with a slope of +1.
5. For $\omega \gg 100$, $H(s)$ can be approximated as

$$H(s) = \frac{5(s/1)(s/10)}{(s/0.1)(s/100)} = \frac{5s^2}{s^2} = 5 \tag{4.143}$$

or simply a flat line again at a value of 5. Finally, the corners at the break frequencies are rounded to obtain a smooth curve.

The phase angle plot will simply use the above slopes input into Equation 4.137.

1. For $\omega \ll 0.1$, the adjacent slopes are 0 on the magnitude plot, yielding $\phi = 0$.
2. At $\omega = 0.1$, the adjacent slopes are 0 and –1. The average value is –½, yielding $\phi = -\pi/4$.
3. For $\omega = 1$, the adjacent slopes are –1 and 0. The average value is –½, yielding $\phi = -\pi/4$.
4. For $\omega = 10$, the adjacent slopes are 0 and +1. The average value is +½, yielding $\phi = +\pi/4$.
5. For $\omega = 100$, the adjacent slopes are +1 and 0. The average value is +½, yielding $\phi = +\pi/4$.
6. For $\omega \gg 100$, the adjacent slopes are 0 and 0, yielding $\phi = 0$.

Again, a smooth curve is drawn through all of the points, yielding the plot shown in Figure 4.17B.

4.5   Frequency Analysis of Passive Muscle

Consider a passive muscle subject to a sinusoidal forcing strain function. Setting the tension of the contractile element to zero in Equation 4.78 yields the transfer function:

$$H(s) = \frac{K_{SE}(Bs + K_{PE})}{Bs + K_{PE} + K_{SE}}$$

(4.144)

Rearranging the expression to obtain an $(s + a)$ format, multiplying by the complex conjugate of the denominator term, and substituting $s = j$ yield

$$H(j\omega) = \frac{K_{SE}(K_{PE}/B + j\omega)\left[(K_{PE} + K_{SE})/B - j\omega\right]}{\left[(K_{PE} + K_{SE})/B + j\omega\right]\left[(K_{PE} + K_{SE})/B - j\omega\right]}$$

(4.145)

Simplification yields the real and imaginary parts:

$$H(j\omega) = \frac{K_{SE}\left[\omega^2 + K_{PE}(K_{PE} + K_{SE})/B^2 + j\omega K_{SE}/B\right]}{\omega^2 + \left[(K_{PE} + K_{SE})^2/B^2\right]}$$

(4.146)

To simplify calculations and plots, assume a very stiff series elastic element with a ratio of $K_{SE}/K_{PE} = 10$ and a ratio of $K_{PE}/B = 1$. Correspondingly, K_{SE}/B becomes equal to 10. Then, Equation 4.146 becomes

$$H(j\omega) = \frac{K_{SE}(\omega^2 + 11 + j10\omega)}{\omega^2 + 121}$$

(4.147)

The magnitude of $H(j)$ then becomes

$$M = K_{SE}\frac{\left[(\omega^2 + 11)^2 + 100\omega^2\right]^{1/2}}{\omega^2 + 121} = K_{SE}\frac{\left[\omega^4 + 122\omega^2 + 121\right]^{1/2}}{\omega^2 + 121}$$

$$= K_{SE}\frac{(\omega^2 + 1)^{1/2}}{(\omega^2 + 121)^{1/2}}$$

(4.148)

while the phase angle is

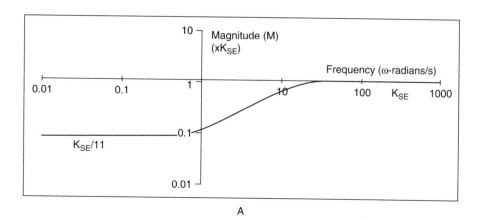

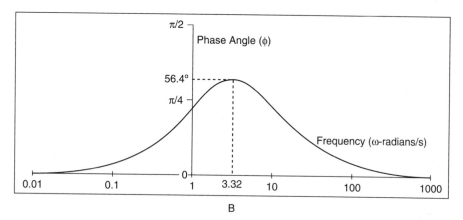

FIGURE 4.18
Magnitude (A) and phase angle (B) plots for $H(j) = [K_{SE}(\omega^2 + 11 + j10\ \omega)]/(\omega^2 + 121)$.

$$\phi = \tan^{-1}\frac{10\omega}{\omega^2 + 11} \tag{4.149}$$

To plot the magnitude, examine Equation 4.148 at small and large ω. For small ω, i.e., $\omega << 11$, the magnitude stays constant with a value of $K_{SE}/11$. For large ω, i.e., $\omega >> 11$, the magnitude also remains constant at a value of K_{SE}. For values of ω around 11 the values change smoothly as an ogive curve from $K_{SE}/11$ to K_{SE}. The complete magnitude plot is shown in Figure 4.18.

The phase angle plot is similarly constructed from Equation 4.149. For small ω, the phase angle is roughly equal to $\tan^{-1} \omega$ or zero and increases very gradually for increasing values of ω. For large ω, the phase angle is roughly equal to $\tan^{-1} 1/\omega$ or also zero for large values of ω. For values of ω around the break frequency, the values of the phase angle first increase and then decrease. The critical break frequency can be inferred from the denominator as $\omega = \sqrt{11}$ or can be calculated directly by finding the frequency at which point the phase angle reaches a maximum. This can be done by taking the derivative of Equation 4.149 with respect to ω and setting the resulting equation equal to zero:

$$\frac{d\phi}{d\omega} = \frac{d}{d\omega}\left\{ \tan^{-1}\frac{10\omega}{\omega^2+11} \right\} = 0 \qquad (4.150)$$

Using the following identity with $u = 10\,\omega/(\omega^2 + 11)$ yields

$$\frac{d\tan^{-1}u}{d\omega} = \frac{du/d\omega}{1+u^2} \qquad (4.151)$$

Only du/d is critical and is set equal to zero:

$$\frac{du}{d\omega} = \frac{10}{\omega^2+11} - \frac{20\omega^2}{\left(\omega^2+11\right)^2} = 0 \qquad (4.152)$$

yielding

$$\left(\omega^2+11\right)10 - 20\omega^2 = 10\omega^2 - 110 = \omega^2 - 11 = 0 \qquad (4.153)$$

The critical break frequency is then $\sqrt{11}$ = 3.32 and the maximum phase is $\tan^{-1}$ (1.51) or 56.4°. The complete phase angle plot is shown in Figure 4.18.

In terms of passive muscle, this means that at very low or high frequencies the forcing function and muscle response are practically in phase and elastically dominated by either the series elastic element (K_{SE}) for very high frequencies (i.e., the dashpot cannot respond sufficiently quickly, eliminating the parallel elastic element from the model) or by a combination of both elastic elements $K_{SE}/(K_{SE} + K_{PE})$ for very low frequencies (i.e., the dashpot responds, stretching the parallel elastic element with it). Around the critical break frequency the muscle is fully viscoelastic with the dashpot involved.

4.6   Hatze's Multielement Model

Hatze (1981) developed a muscle model considerably more complicated then Hill's four-element model (Figure 4.19). It is termed a *distributed model* because it starts at the sarcomere level, modeling all the individual structures rather than treating the complete muscle in a *lumped model* as done by Hill (1938). As with Hill's model, the purely contractile elements of the protein filaments are represented by CE_i. The parallel elastic elements of each sarcomere (PS_i) represent the surrounding fascia within muscle fibers such as

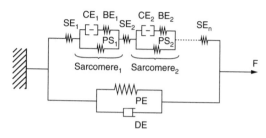

FIGURE 4.19
Distributed model of skeletal muscle. (Adapted from Hatze, 1981.)

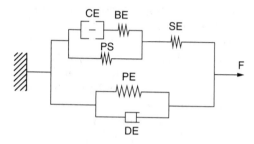

FIGURE 4.20
Lumped model of skeletal muscle.

the sarcolemna or endomysium, but do not individually include a damping component, as the sarcolemna are firmly attached to the Z-disks and do not allow appreciable movement. The damping element (DE) is contained in the fiber external structure and is thus placed parallel to the entire fiber. Similarly, the parallel elastic elements representing fascia are also placed parallel to the entire fiber. The series element is broken down into several components: a bridge element (BE_i) representing the elastic structures within the cross bridges and a series elastic element for the Z-disc (SE_1). Finally, at both ends of each muscle fiber are lightly damped series elastic elements (SE_2) representing the tendinous parts of the fiber.

Obviously, with hundreds and thousands of sarcomeres, such a distributed model for a complete muscle would be impossible to work with. Thus, a transition to a simple lumped model must be made. One justifiable assumption is that all the sarcomeres in a fiber are more or less identical and activated at approximately the same time. It follows then that all the SE_i for one fiber can be replaced by an equivalent single element SE. The same rationale can be applied to the elements CE_i, BE_i, and PS_i, resulting in the equivalent lumped elements of Figure 4.20.

A similar rationale can be used in lumping hundreds of muscle fibers into motor units and hundreds of motor units into a complete muscle. In general, although the motor units fibers are distributed randomly over a certain

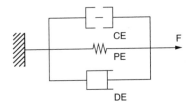

FIGURE 4.21
Simplified model of skeletal muscle.

volume of the muscle, all have a similar morphological contractile and his-
tochemical profiles. The motor units, however, vary in properties, and should
perhaps be represented by separate models.

Certain assumptions allow a further reduction of the lumped model to a
simpler lumped model yet. The series elastic element SE and bridge element
BE can be considered very stiff springs and eliminated completely. This
contention is supported by Bawa et al. (1976), who found $K_{SE} = 380$ g/mm
to be much larger than $K_{PE} = 103$ g/mm. K_{BE} can be considered to be in a
similar range with K_{SE}. Eliminating SE and BE results in a model with four
parallel elements, two of which are elastic and can be combined into one
parallel elastic element. The final simplified model is given in Figure 4.21.

The total force developed by the simplified model of Figure 4.21 can now
be expressed as

$$F = \left(f_{PE} + f_{CE} + f_{DE}\right)F_{MAX} \tag{4.154}$$

Note that each of the component elements is expressed as a fractional or
relative force, which is the final fraction to be scaled by the maximum force
developed by the muscle F_{MAX}.

Each element within the model needs further specification. Hill's model
assumed simple linear properties, which is not correct. For example, for the
parallel elastic element (PE), extensive tests on the tensile properties of
resting human sartorius muscle carried out by Yamada (1970) indicate an
exponential force–strain function (Figure 4.22):

$$f_{PE} = 0.00163\left(e^{7.66\varepsilon} - 1\right) \tag{4.155}$$

The velocity dependence of the damping element (DE) was expressed
previously as a simple dashpot. Alexander and Johnson (1965) separated the
damping properties into a passive coefficient and the active force–velocity
relationship, with the active component 6.4 times larger than the passive
component. Therefore, the Bawa et al. (1976) damping value for a cat plantaris muscle becomes 1.0 g-s/mm, which when normalized to the plantaris
resting length of 50 mm and maximum isometric tension of 245 g yields a

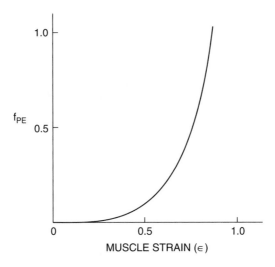

FIGURE 4.22
Force–strain function for the parallel elastic element of passive muscle.

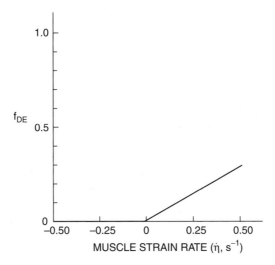

FIGURE 4.23
Viscous characteristics for the damping element of passive muscle.

normalized slope of $0.2F_{MAX}$ s/length. With maximum velocity for slow twitch fibers reaching 2.9 muscle lengths/s, fairly significant viscous damping forces ($0.6F_{MAX}$ at maximum velocity) can be obtained (Figure 4.23).

The contractile component can be modeled along its basic functions: the length–tension, velocity–tension, and active-state relationships. The first, as discussed previously, is determined by the number of active cross-links and

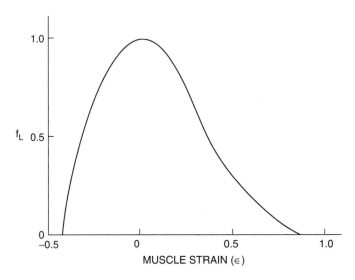

FIGURE 4.24
Length–tension relationship for active muscle.

overlap of the thick and thin filaments and can be represented from the data
of Gordon et al. (1966) by the function suggested by Hatze (1981):

$$f(\xi) = 0.32 + 0.71e^{-1.112(\xi-1)} \sin 3.722(\xi - 0.656) \tag{4.156}$$

where $f(\xi)$ is the normalized tension generation due to the length–tension
relationship and ξ is ℓ/ℓ_0 with $0.58 \le \ell \le 1.8$. This relationship (Figure 4.24)
shows a fairly peaked response with more than a 20% reduction in force for
less than ±20% changes in resting length.

The velocity–tension relationship is determined by the rate of breaking
and reforming of cross bridges with higher rates producing less effective
bonds. To account for the whole range of negative velocities (shortening or
concentric contractions) as well as positive velocities (lengthening or eccentric contractions) Hatze (1981) has defined the following expression:

$$f(\dot{\eta}) = \frac{0.1433}{0.1074 + e^{-1.409\sinh(3.2\dot{\eta}+1.6)}} \tag{4.157}$$

where
$f(\dot{\eta}) =$ normalized tension due to the velocity–tension relationship
$\dot{\eta} \quad = \dot{\epsilon}/\dot{\epsilon}_{MAX}$ or strain rate normalized to the maximum strain rate

This relationship shows a rapid increase in force up to an asymptotic value
34% greater than the maximum isometric contraction level and a very rapid

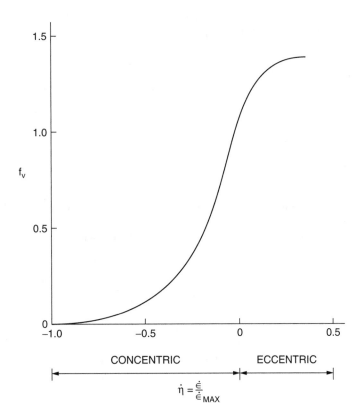

FIGURE 4.25
Velocity–tension relationship for active muscle.

decrease in force down to zero for maximum concentric contractions (Figure 4.25).

The active properties of the contractile element are also determined by the active state function $q(t)$. The relative force or tension due to the active state, f_q, is defined by the relative amount of calcium (Ca^{++}) bound to troponin, the inhibitor of bonding between the myosin heads on the thick filament and globular actin on the thin filament. If the maximum number of potential interactive sites on the thin filament are exposed by the action of Ca^{++}, then $q = 1$, while in a resting state q is very low, say, q_0. Thus, the isometric tension developed by a muscle fiber at a given length l_q is directly proportional to $q(t)$ (Hatze, 1981, p. 33). The tension developed as a consequence of the active state function can be defined as

$$f_q\left(t\right) = \frac{0.005 + 82.63\,v^2\left(1 - e^{-mt}\right)^2}{1 + 82.63\,v^2\left(1 - e^{-mt}\right)^2} \tag{4.158}$$

with the value of m to be determined later. For the complete details that led to development of this function, please refer to Example 4.6.

Example 4.6: Determination of the Active State Tension Function

To find the active state function $q(t)$, define γ to be the difference between the free Ca^{++} concentration γ_f and the free Ca^{++} concentration γ_0 in the resting fiber. However, for practical purposes, since $\gamma_0 << \gamma_f$, γ and γ_f basically identical. Let $\partial q / \partial \gamma$ denote the rate of change of the Ca^{++} concentration during the active state $q(t)$. The process of binding Ca^{++} ions to the troponin sites is hypothesized by Hatze (1981) and supported by the experimental studies of Ebashi and Eno (1968) to be a function of the length ℓ of the contractile element and of the difference between the maximum and present value of q and is controlled by a negative feedback loop:

$$\partial p / \partial \gamma = \rho_1^2(\varepsilon)(1-q) - 2\rho_2(\varepsilon)\rho_1(\varepsilon)p \qquad (4.159)$$

where p is defined as $\partial q / \partial \gamma$ and ρ_1 and ρ_2 are unknown functions to be determined. Note that Hatze's (1981) format has been changed by the substitution of standard strain ε for ξ, where

$$\xi = \varepsilon + 1 \qquad (4.160)$$

Solving the system of differential equations with initial conditions $p(0) = 0$ and $q(0) = q_0 = 0.005$ yields the normalized solution:

$$q(\varepsilon,\gamma) = 1 - \frac{(1-q_0)}{(m_1 - m_2)}\left\{m_1 e^{m_2\rho_1(\varepsilon)\gamma} - m_2 e^{m_1\rho_1(\varepsilon)\gamma}\right\} \qquad (4.161)$$

where

$$m_{1,2} = -\rho_2(\varepsilon) \pm \left[\rho_2^2(\varepsilon) - 1\right]^{1/2} \text{ for } \rho_2 > 1 \qquad (4.162)$$

Substituting experimentally found values, Hatze (1981) found

$$\rho_1^2(\varepsilon) = 2.34 \times 10^{14}\left\{\frac{\varepsilon + 0.44}{\varepsilon + 1.0}\right\}^{1/2} \text{ for } -0.44 < \varepsilon < 0.8 \qquad (4.163)$$

$$\rho_2(\varepsilon) = 1.05 \qquad (4.164)$$

With appropriate simplification for mammalian muscle provided by Hatze (1981, p. 40) and substituting Equations 4.162, 4.163, and 4.164 into Equation 4.161 we find

$$q(\xi, \gamma) = \frac{q_0 + \rho^2(\varepsilon)\gamma^2}{1 + \rho^2(\varepsilon)\gamma^2} \tag{4.165}$$

where

$$\rho(\varepsilon) = 125{,}780 \frac{(\varepsilon + 1)}{(1.9 - \varepsilon)} \tag{4.166}$$

The function γ, the free Ca^{++} ion concentration, can be represented as a function of time t and the relative stimulation rate v by a trend function, which represents the average behavior of γ in successive time intervals and which approaches a maximum value asymptotically and has the rate of increase proportional to the stimulation rate (Hatze, 1981, p. 39):

$$\partial\gamma/\partial t = m(1.373 \times 10^{-4} v - \gamma) \tag{4.167}$$

where v is the relative stimulation rate ranging between 0 and 1 and m is a constant to be determined later.

The rate of stimulation of motor units during voluntary contraction has been controversial. Several studies have found a fairly constant discharge frequency over a wide range of tension for individual motor units (Bigland and Lippold, 1954; Clamann, 1970), while others maintain that an increase in muscle tension is achieved in part by an increase in the stimulation rate and in part by an increase in the recruitment of motor units (Marsden et al., 1971; Person and Kudina, 1972; Milner-Brown et al., 1973b). However, the rise in frequency with a rise in tension is associated with a high frequency close to the maximum stimulation rate (Tanji and Kato, 1973). Thus, it is fairly reasonable to assume a constant stimulation rate and, therefore, a constant relative stimulation rate.

Now, solving Equation 4.167 with v constant yields

$$\gamma(t) = [\gamma(0) - 1.373 \times 10^{-4} v] e^{-mt} + 1.373 \times 10^{-4} v \tag{4.168}$$

where m is a unknown constant to be determined later. With $\gamma(0)$ much smaller than $1.373 \times 10^{-4} v$, Equation 4.168 reduces to

$$\gamma(t) = 1.373 \times 10^{-4} v [1 - e^{-mt}] \tag{4.169}$$

Substituting Equation 4.169 and Equation 4.166 with $\varepsilon = 0$ into Equation 4.165 yields the final active state function and its resultant relative force or tension:

$$f_q(t) = \frac{0.005 + 82.63\,v^2 \left(1 - e^{-mt}\right)^2}{1 + 82.63\,v^2 \left(1 - e^{-mt}\right)^2} \qquad (4.170)$$

Finally, f_{CE} can be redefined as a combination of the three different component relationships:

$$f_{CE} = f_q(t)\, f_\ell(\varepsilon)\, f_v(\dot{\eta}) \qquad (4.171)$$

An additional factor to consider is that the active state function will vary depending on the type of motor units and relative stimulation rate. Although the motor unit properties such as the stimulation rate will vary continuously from very slow twitch to very fast twitch fibers, for modeling simplicity, the motor units can be considered as grouped into two distinct populations, Type I or slow twitch and Type II or fast twitch units. The total muscle tension output (Equation 4.154) now becomes the sum of the force output from N_I type I motor units and from N_{II} type II motor units:

$$F = \left(f_{PE} + f_{CE_I} + f_{CE_{II}} + f_{DE}\right) F_{MAX} \qquad (4.172)$$

Also, the same total population of motor units can be subdivided into two other dynamically different populations: the N number of active motor units and the $\overline{N} - N$ number of inactive or fatigued motor units, where $\overline{N}$ is the total number of motor units in the muscle.

As mentioned previously, the motor units are recruited in a sequential order according to their size and twitch times. From Hatze (1981), the cumulative relative cross-sectional area u occupied by the recruited motor units increases by

$$u = u_0 e^{c(N-1)/\tilde{N}} \qquad (4.173)$$

where u_0 is the relative cross-sectional area of the smallest motor unit and ranges from 0 to 1 and c is a constant expressed as

$$c = -\ln u_0 \qquad (4.174)$$

For N large, Equation 4.173 reduces to

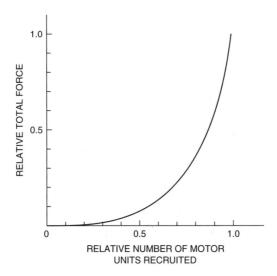

FIGURE 4.26
Muscle tension developed by orderly recruitment of motor units.

$$u_n = u_0 e^{cN/\tilde{N}} = u_0^{\left(1-N/\tilde{N}\right)} = u_0^{\left(1-n\right)} \qquad (4.175)$$

where n is the fraction of recruited or active motor units or $N/\overline{N}$. Examining the ratios of the smallest to the largest motor cross-sectional areas measured in muscle allows estimates of u_0 to be made. Experimental values of u_0 range from 0.005 for the rectus femorus to 0.009 for the biceps (Hatze, 1979), with an average value of 0.00673. Because the cross-sectional area increases exponentially, the total muscle tension also increases exponentially (Figure 4.26).

Combining the two sets of overlapping population distributions of motor units yields two distinct cases:

1. $N < N_I$, only parts of type I motor units are recruited and none of the type II is recruited because of the orderly recruitment pattern.
2. $N > N_I$, all type I motor units are recruited and some of the type II motor units are recruited, but none of the type I is inactive.

Additional appropriate motor unit properties are obtained from Henneman and Olson (1965). The contraction time t_c of a motor unit is a decreasing function of the fraction n of recruited motor units:

$$t_c = a - bn \qquad (4.176)$$

For type I motor units, Equation 4.176 becomes

$$t_{cI} = a_I - b_I n \quad \text{for } 0 \le n \le n_I \tag{4.177}$$

and, for type II motor units, Equation 4.176 becomes

$$t_{cII} = a_{II} - b_{II} n \quad \text{for } n_I \le n \le 1 \tag{4.178}$$

The constants can be determined from experimental data. For $n = 0$, the value of t_c corresponds to the contraction time of the slowest type I motor unit in the muscle or approximately equal to 0.1 s; for $n = n_I$, the value of t_c corresponds to the fastest type I motor unit (and slowest type II unit) or approximately 0.045 s; and for $n = 1$, the value of t_c corresponds to the fastest type II motor unit or approximately 0.01 s (Grimby and Hannerz, 1977). Substituting these values into Equations 4.172 and 4.173 and solving for the unknowns yield

$$a_I = 0.1 \tag{4.179}$$

$$b_I = 0.055/n_I \tag{4.180}$$

$$a_{II} = 0.01 + 0.035/(1 - n_I) \tag{4.181}$$

$$b_{II} = 0.035/(1 - n_I) \tag{4.182}$$

Equations 4.177 and 4.178 can now be expressed as

$$t_{cI} = 0.1 - 0.055 n/n_I \tag{4.183}$$

$$t_{cII} = 0.01 + 0.035(1 - n)/(1 - n_I) \tag{4.184}$$

Close (1965) showed that for mammalian skeletal muscle, the maximum normalized speed of shortening is related to the contraction time of a muscle, consisting predominantly of one fiber type, by

$$\dot{\varepsilon}_{MAX} = 0.297/t_c \tag{4.185}$$

This then indicates that the first or slowest motor unit at $n = 0$ has a relative contraction velocity of 2.97 lengths/s, while the last or fastest motor unit at $n = 1$ has a relative contraction velocity of 29.7 lengths/s. The value of $\dot{\varepsilon}_{MAX}$ is necessary for Equation 4.157.

The rate constant m in Equation 4.158 also depends on the contraction time:

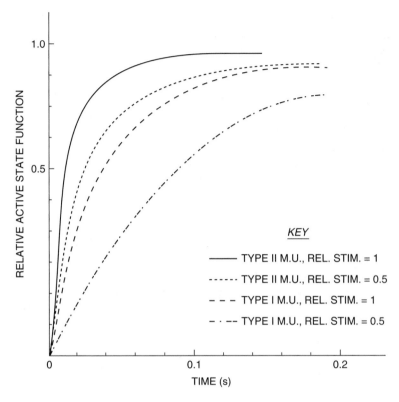

FIGURE 4.27
Muscle tension developed by the active state function for various conditions.

$$m = 0.372/t_c \qquad (4.186)$$

For the slowest motor unit ($n = 0$), $m = 3.72$, while for the fastest motor unit ($n = 1$), $m = 37.2$. The relative force or tension, $f_q(t)$, developed during the active state is plotted in Figure 4.27 for pure type I and type II motor units, as well as for different relative stimulation rates. Now, finally, Equation 4.158 is completely determined. Further details on the simplified Hatze muscle model can be found in Freivalds and Kaleps (1984) and Freivalds (1985).

4.7 Applications of the Hatze Muscle Model

One important factor affecting the accuracy in modeling the neuromusculature for dynamic simulation such as the Articulated Total Body Model (Freivalds and Kaleps, 1984) is the accuracy of the placement of the musculature, i.e., the origins and insertions of the muscle being simulated. Specific data, in many cases, are obtained by measuring directly from anatomical scaled photographs (McMinn and Hutchings, 1977). Obviously, some human error is involved, especially in using two-dimensional photographs of three-dimensional structures. Thus, it was decided to simulate errors in muscle placement and compare the muscle forces developed through while "stimulating" the muscle.

The simulation consisted of elbow flexion against a load with the three major elbow flexors: the biceps brachii, the brachialis, and the brachioradialis (see Figure 3.1). Using cross-sectional areas of 4.58, 4.63, and 1.37 cm² from Schumacher and Wolff (1966) and the maximum muscle force per area of 100 N/cm² from Hatze (1981) yielded maximum isometric tension values of 458, 463, and 137 N, respectively. Five different conditions were simulated. In Conditions 0 and 1, the origin of each muscle was displaced by ±10% of the insertion distance, respectively. In Condition 2, both the origin and insertion were shifted by 10%. In Condition 3, both the origin and insertion were shifted by 20%. Condition 4 was the control case with "true" origins and insertions. The simulation started with the hand holding a 270 N weight with the upper limb bent at 90° and the muscles stimulated for maximal contraction simultaneously. Since this weight exceeded the maximum weight that could be maintained by the elbow flexors, the muscles would necessarily be forced into eccentric contraction. This simulation corresponded closely in terms of muscle strength capabilities to the data of Wilkie (1950) who found his subjects could maintain a maximum of 196 N at the wrist.

The general pattern of the results shown in Figure 4.28 can be explained by the forces produced by the various components of the muscle model. Initially, since the weight exceeded the resting tonus of the muscles, the muscles were forcibly extended in an eccentric contraction, as exhibited by the rather sharp increase in force. As the arm is extended, the length–tension relationship contributes significantly in reducing the muscle force. The brachioradialis is affected the most because of its length, the biceps the least. However, for all four test conditions, there was a small deviation (average 3%, maximum 9%) from the control condition, indicating relatively low sensitivity for the location of the origins and insertions. Concentric contractions with smaller weights showed rapid decreases in muscle force due to the velocity–tension relationship. However, both simulations assumed maximal stimulation and recruitment to maximum force as in a ballistic movement. More commonly, movements are more controlled through the various feedback loops as well as voluntary control.

4.8 Control Theory and Motor Control

4.8.1 Basic Concepts

The musculoskeletal system, as any complex system, is composed of inputs, outputs, and either known or unknown (black box) components, which act

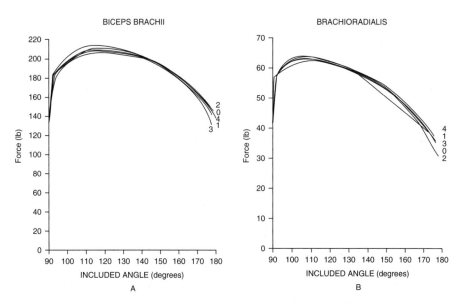

FIGURE 4.28
Force developed by the biceps brachii (A) and brachioradialis (B) while holding a load of 270 N under five different conditions: 0 = muscle origin displaced +10%; 1 = muscle origin displaced –10%; 2 = both origin and insertion displaced +10%; 3 = both origin and insertion displaced +20%; 4 = control case.

as transfer functions to modify the input to create the output. The action of the transfer function was discussed at length in Section 4.1.2. It might be valuable at this time to distinguish between open-loop and closed-loop systems. A *closed-loop system* performs some action that requires continuous control in the form of some comparison between the system output and the command input. This means there is continual feedback of information about any error that should be taken into account for successful operation. Thus, these types of systems are often referred to as *feedback systems*.

At the physiological level the muscle spindle system is a feedback system for muscle length and the Golgi tendon organs act as a feedback system for muscular tension. At a gross level, the tracking of a cursor on a computer screen with a pointer is a feedback system that requires a variety of information, including agonist muscle tension and length, antagonist muscle tension and length, to be fed back and compared to the input.

An *open-loop system* is one in which the command input is independent of the system output. This type of system, once activated, cannot be controlled any further, i.e., once the die is cast, fate is determined. Where as a guided missile is an example of a closed-loop system, a bullet from a rifle is an open-loop system. Such a system is sometimes termed a *feed-forward system*. At the physiological level, for example, when lifting a load, basic recruitment of α-efferent motor units at the cell body is an open-loop system. Either there is enough excitatory stimulation from the central nervous system or there is not. However, in the more complex sense, the muscle spindles will sense whether there is a stretching (i.e., the load is depressing the limb) and send feedback via the α-afferent pathway to provide further excitatory stimulation. At a gross level, a ballistic movement, such as throwing a ball, is theoretically an open-loop system, because once released the ball cannot be further controlled. However, there will be a variety of control actions and feedback loops occurring during the recruitment of appropriate muscle to provide the appropriate limb movement.

Open-loop tasks performed by a human operator will have the following characteristics:

1. The task performance is automatic. The operator utilizes previous experience and training to provide the best command input for the best output.
2. Since there is no feedback, the final outcome (whether the ball hits the target) may or may not be acceptable depending on system disturbances (such as wind) that cannot be directly controlled by the operator. Obviously, the operator will alter the motion on a second throw to better hit the target.
3. The degree of accuracy in performing such an open-loop task is dependent on both the operator's skill level and the presence of outside disturbances.

Closed-loop tasks performed by a human operator will have the following characteristics (as compared to an open-loop task):

1. The task performance requires continuous feedback of system output. For example, in the above tracking task, the location of the pointer with respect to the cursor must be continually observed for best performance.
2. Task performance increases with an increased ability to more precisely reproduce or control the command input, i.e., the pointer location.
3. System performance is less sensitive to external disturbances, since corrections can be or are made continually.
4. There is an increased tendency toward system oscillation and instability as described in more detail later.

4.8.2 First-Order System

Using Hill's four-element model, the external muscle tension was developed in Equation 4.78 as a function of the internal tension from the contractile element and the external strain:

$$T = \frac{K_{SE}T_{CE}}{Bs + K_{PE} + K_{SE}} + \frac{K_{SE}\left(Bs + K_{PE}\right)\varepsilon}{Bs + K_{PE} + K_{SE}} \qquad (4.187)$$

Typically, such linear lumped models give rise to transfer functions that have polynomials in s both in the numerator and denominator, where the power of s in the numerator should typically be lower than the power of s in the denominator for system stability (e.g., an impulse response would not be feasible). The *roots* of these polynomials are those values that make the polynomial equal to zero.

The roots of the denominator have a special significance because they characterize the exponential and/or sinusoidal terms of the impulse response. It is called the *characteristic function* of the system and its roots are called the *poles* of the system. The roots of the numerator affect the magnitude and phase of the response, but not its basic nature. They are called the *zeros* of the system.

Assuming an isometric contraction for the characteristic muscle function in Equation 4.187 yields the simpler form:

$$T = \frac{K_{SE}T_{CE}}{Bs + K_{PE} + K_{SE}} + \frac{K_{SE}T_{CE}/B}{s + 1/\tau} \qquad (4.188)$$

where $1/\tau$ is the pole of the system and $\tau = B/(K_{PE} + K_{SE})$ is the time constant of the system. In a frequency analysis, the critical break frequency is $\omega = 1/\tau$. This basic system is known as a *first-order system* because there is only one pole or the power of s in the denominator is one. The step response and frequency analysis are shown in Figure 4.29.

4.8.3 Second-Order System

A *second-order system* has two poles or the power of s in the denominator (or the characteristic function) is two. This is probably the most common and most intuitive model of physical systems and is used to represent the mass-spring-dashpot system of Figure 4.30:

$$\frac{\varepsilon\left(s\right)}{\sigma\left(s\right)} = \frac{1}{Ms^2 + Bs + K} \qquad (4.189)$$

where
M = mass of the object
B = damping constant
K = spring constant

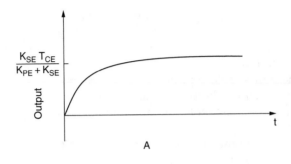

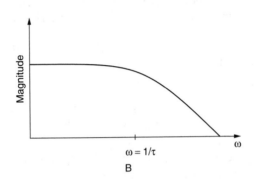

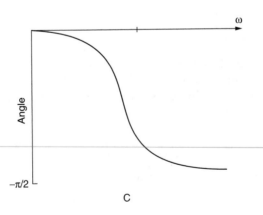

FIGURE 4.29
Step response (A), magnitude plot (B), and phase angle plot (C) for a first-order system. $T = (K_{SE}T_{CE})/(Bs + K_{PE} + K_{SE})$.

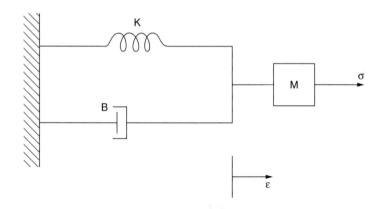

FIGURE 4.30
Simple mass–spring–dashpot system giving rise to second-order dynamics.

Reorganizing Equation 4.189 yields the characteristic form of a second-order system:

$$\frac{\varepsilon(s)}{\sigma(s)} = \frac{\omega_n^2/K}{s^2 + 2\omega_n \zeta s + \omega_n^2} \tag{4.190}$$

where ω_n is termed the undamped *natural frequency* and is the frequency at which the system would oscillate if the damping, B, were zero. It is defined as

$$\omega_n = \left(K/M\right)^{1/2} \tag{4.191}$$

ζ is termed the *damping ratio* and is defined as

$$\zeta = \frac{B}{2\omega_n} \tag{4.192}$$

The frequency response of such a second-order system is obtained by replacing s with $j\omega$ in Equation 4.190, yielding

$$H(\omega) = \frac{\omega_n^2/K}{-\omega^2 + 2j\omega_n \zeta\omega + \omega_n^2} = \frac{\omega_n^2}{K} \frac{1}{\left(\omega_n^2 - \omega^2\right) + 2j\zeta\omega_n\omega} \tag{4.193}$$

Multiplying the numerator and denominator the complex conjugate yields

$$H(\omega) = \frac{\omega_n^2}{K} \frac{\left(\omega_n^2 - \omega^2\right) - 2j\zeta\omega_n\omega}{\left(\omega_n^2 - \omega^2\right)^2 + 4\zeta^2\omega_n^2\omega^2} \tag{4.194}$$

The magnitude, as defined from Equation 4.113, is

$$M(\omega) = \left[X(\omega)^2 + Y(\omega)^2\right]^{1/2} = \frac{\omega_n^2}{K}\left[\left(\omega_n^2 - \omega^2\right)^2 + 4\zeta^2\omega_n^2\omega^2\right]^{-1/2} \tag{4.195}$$

For small ω, $\omega \ll \omega_n$, the magnitude is

$$M(\omega) = 1/K \tag{4.196}$$

with a slope of zero on the magnitude plot. For large ω, $\omega \gg \omega_n$, the magnitude becomes

$$M(\omega) = \frac{1}{K}\frac{\omega_n^2}{\omega^2} \tag{4.197}$$

with a slope of –2 on the magnitude plot.
 The phase angle, from Equation 4.114, is defined as

$$\phi(\omega) = \tan^{-1}\left[Y(\omega)/X(\omega)\right] = \tan^{-1}\frac{2\zeta\omega_n\omega}{\left(\omega_n^2 - \omega^2\right)} \tag{4.198}$$

For small ω, $\omega \ll \omega_n$, the phase angle is

$$\phi(\omega) = \tan^{-1}2\zeta\omega/\omega_n \approx 0 \tag{4.199}$$

For large ω, $\omega \gg \omega_n$, the phase angle is

$$\phi(\omega) = -\tan^{-1}2\zeta\omega_n/\omega \approx -\tan^{-1}\infty = -180° \tag{4.200}$$

The resulting magnitude and phase plots, for various values of ζ, are shown in Figure 4.31.
 For a larger range of values of ζ, the second-order system exhibits four distinct types of behavior. Figure 4.32 summarizes these responses in a *pole-zero diagram*. For $\zeta = 0$, the system is termed *undamped* and the impulse response will be a steady-state sinusoid of frequency ω_n. For $\zeta < 1$, the system

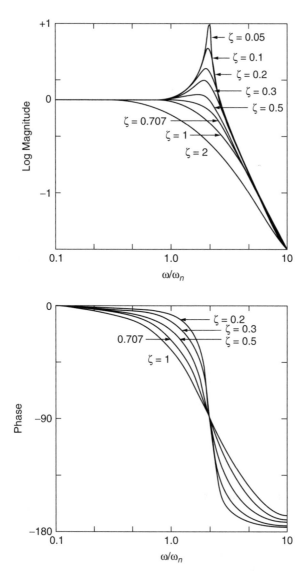

FIGURE 4.31

Magnitude and phase plots for a second-order system for various values of ζ. (From Milsum, J.H., 1966. *Biological Control Systems*, New York: McGraw-Hill. With permission.)

is termed *underdamped* and sinusoids of ω_n will die out over time. For $\zeta = 1$, the system is termed *critically damped* and the impulse response rises and then dies out. Note that in this case the pole is repeated. For $\zeta > 1$, the system is termed *overdamped* and the impulse response dies out more quickly than for the critically damped case. Note that for poles on the positive side of the pole-zero diagram, the resulting exponential envelope for the sinusoids explodes. This is termed an unstable system and is discussed later. The

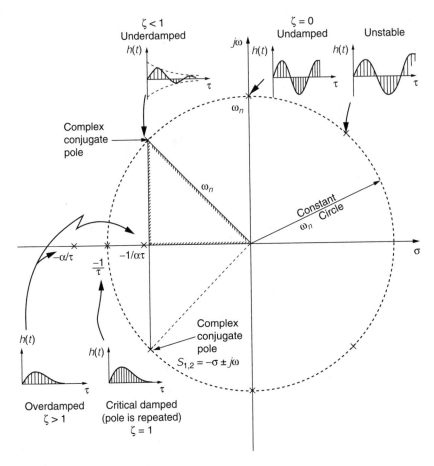

FIGURE 4.32
Impulse responses for a second-order system for various pole locations. (From Milsum, J.H., 1966. *Biological Control Systems*, New York: McGraw-Hill. With permission.)

transfer functions and step responses for these four cases are given in Table 4.3. Further details on such systems and responses can be found in Milsum (1966), Melsa and Schultz (1969), and Stark (1968).

Example 4.7: Step Response of a Second-Order System

Assume a critically damped ($\varsigma = 1$) second-order system similar to the mass-spring-dashpot system of Equation 4.189, with a step stress (e.g., muscle force) input. The resulting strain output (i.e., movement) is

$$\varepsilon\left(s\right) = \frac{\omega_n^2/K}{\left(s^2 + 2\omega_n s + \omega_n^2\right)s} = \frac{\omega_n^2}{K}\frac{1}{\left(s+\omega_n\right)^2} \qquad (4.201)$$

TABLE 4.3

Transfer Functions and Step Responses of Second-Order Systems

Damping Ratio	Type of Damping	Transfer Function	Frequency Domain Step Response	Time Domain Step Response
$\zeta = 0$	Undamped	$\dfrac{\omega_n^2}{s^2+\omega_n^2}$	$\dfrac{\omega_n^2}{s\left(s^2+\omega_n^2\right)}$	$1-\cos\omega_n t$
$0 < \zeta < 1$	Underdamped	$\dfrac{\omega_n^2}{s^2+2\zeta\omega_n s+\omega_n^2}$	$\dfrac{\omega_n^2}{s\left(s^2+2\zeta\omega_n s+\omega_n^2\right)}$	$1-\dfrac{e^{-\zeta\omega_n t}}{\sqrt{1-\zeta^2}}\sin\left(\omega_n\sqrt{1-\zeta^2}\,t+\tan^{-1}\sqrt{\left(1-\zeta^2\right)}/\zeta\right)$
$\zeta = 1$	Critically damped	$\dfrac{\omega_n^2}{\left(s+\omega_n\right)^2}$	$\dfrac{\omega_n^2}{s\left(s+\omega_n\right)^2}$	$1-\left(1+\omega_n t\right)e^{-\omega_n t}$
$\zeta > 1$	Overdamped	$\dfrac{\omega_n^2}{\left(s+\omega_n/\alpha\right)\left(s+\alpha\omega_n\right)}$	$\dfrac{\omega_n^2}{s\left(s+\omega_n/\alpha\right)\left(s+\alpha\omega_n\right)}$	$1-\dfrac{\left(e^{-\alpha\omega_n t}-a^2 e^{-\omega_n t/\alpha}\right)}{\alpha^2-1}$

Source: Milsum, J.H., 1966. *Biological Control Systems*, New York: McGraw-Hill. With permission.

A partial fraction expansion of Equation 4.201 yields

$$\varepsilon(s) = \frac{a}{s} + \frac{b}{s+\omega_n} + \frac{c}{(s+\omega_n)^2} \tag{4.202}$$

Using the residue method the following solutions are obtained:

$$a = \left. \frac{\omega_n^2}{K(s+\omega_n)^2} \right|_{s=0} = \frac{1}{K} \tag{4.203}$$

$$c = \left. \frac{\omega_n^2}{Ks} \right|_{s=-\omega_n} = \frac{-\omega_n}{K} \tag{4.204}$$

$$b = \left. \frac{\omega_n^2}{K} \frac{d(1/s)}{ds} \right|_{s=-\omega_n} = \left. \frac{-\omega_n}{Ks^2} \right|_{s=-\omega_n} = \frac{-1}{K} \tag{4.205}$$

Substituting Equations 4.203, 4.204, and 4.205 into Equation 4.202 yields

$$\varepsilon(s) = \frac{1}{K}\left\{ \frac{1}{s} - \frac{1}{s+\omega_n} - \frac{\omega_n}{(s+\omega_n)^2} \right\} \tag{4.206}$$

Taking the inverse Laplace transform yields the final solution as shown in Table 4.3:

$$\varepsilon(t) = \frac{1}{K}\left\{ 1 - \left(1 + \omega_n t\right)e^{-\omega_n t} \right\} \tag{4.207}$$

4.8.4 Human Information Processing and Control of Movements

One approach to modeling and understanding movement is to use information theory. *Information theory* measures information in bits, where a *bit* is the amount of information of information required to decide between two equally likely alternatives. The term *bit* came from the first and last part of the words *bi*nary dig*it* used in the computer and communication theory to express the on/off state of a chip or the polarized/reverse polarized position of small pieces of ferromagnetic core used in archaic computer memory. Mathematically, this can be expressed as

$$H = \log_2 n \tag{4.208}$$

where H = the amount of information and n = the number of equally likely alternatives.

With only two alternatives, such as the on/off state of a chip or the toss of an unweighted coin, there is 1 bit of information presented. With ten equally likely alternatives, such as the numbers from 0 to 9, 3.322 bits of information can be conveyed ($\log_2 10 = 3.322$). An easy way of calculating $\log_2$ is to use the following formula:

$$\log_2 n = 1.4427 \times \ln n \tag{4.209}$$

When the alternatives are not equally likely, the information conveyed is determined by

$$H = \Sigma p_i \times \log_2 \left(1/p_i\right) \tag{4.210}$$

where p_i = the probability of the ith event and i = alternatives from 1 to n.

As an example, consider a weighted coin such that heads come up 90% of the time and tails only 10% of time. The amount of information conveyed in a coin toss becomes

$$H = 0.9 \times \log_2 \left(1/0.9\right) + 0.1 \times \log_2 \left(1/0.1\right)$$
$$= 0.9 \times 0.152 + 0.1 \times 3.32 = 0.469 \text{ bits} \tag{4.211}$$

The amount of information that a human processes can be quantified through a *choice-reaction time* experiment, in which the operator responds to several stimuli with several appropriate responses. This can be considered simple decision making and, and based on the human information processing system, the response time should increase as the number of alternative stimuli increases. The response is nonlinear (Figure 4.33A) but, when decision complexity is quantified in terms of the amount of information conveyed in bits, then the response becomes linear (Figure 4.33B) and is referred to as the *Hick–Hyman law* (Hick, 1952; Hyman, 1953):

$$RT = a + bH \tag{4.212}$$

where
RT = response time (s)
H = amount of information (bits)
a = intercept
b = slope, sometimes referred to as the information processing rate

Note that when there is only one choice (e.g., when the light appears, press the button), H equals zero and the response time is equal to the intercept.

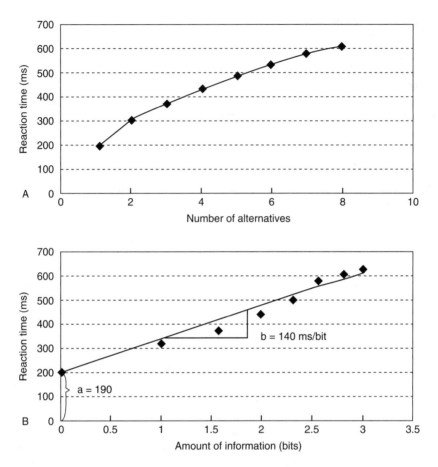

FIGURE 4.33
Hick–Hyman law illustrated with raw data (A) and information expressed in bits (B).

This is known as *simple reaction time*. It can vary depending on the type of stimulus (auditory reaction times are about 40 ms faster than visual reaction times), the intensity of the stimulus, and preparedness for the signal.

Information theory was applied to the modeling of human movement by Fitts (1954) who developed the *index of difficulty* to predict movement time. The index of difficulty was defined as a function of the distance of movement and target size in a series of positioning movements to and from identical targets:

$$ID = \log_2\left(2D/W\right) \tag{4.213}$$

where
ID = index of difficulty (bits)
D = distance between target centers
W = target width

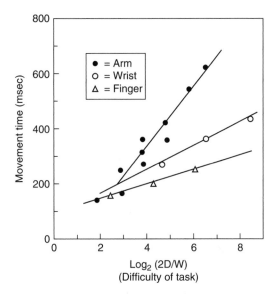

FIGURE 4.34

Fitts' law illustrating arms, wrist, and finger movements. (From Sanders, M.S. and McCormick, E.J., 1993. *Human Factors in Engineering and Design*, 7th ed., New York: McGraw-Hill. With permission.)

Movement time was found to follow the Hick–Hyman law, now termed *Fitts' law*:

$$MT = a + b \text{ ID} \tag{4.214}$$

where
MT = movement time (s)
a = intercept
b = slope

In a particularly successful application of Fitts' law, Langolf et al. (1976) modeled human movement by different limbs across a wide range of distances, including very small targets visible only with the assistance of a microscope. Their results (Figure 4.34) yielded slopes of 105 ms/bit for the arm, 45 ms/bit for the wrist, and 26 ms/bit for the finger. The inverse of the slope is interpreted, according to information theory, as the motor system *bandwidth*. In this case, the bandwidths were 38 bits/s for the finger, 23 bits/s for the wrist, and 10 bits/s for the arm. This decrease in information processing rates was explained as the result of added processing for the additional joints, muscles, motor units, receptors, etc.

Interestingly, Langolf et al. (1976) also showed that the typical human movement response to a unit-step input follows a second-order response. The desired input is a step change in displacement of the hand from a starting

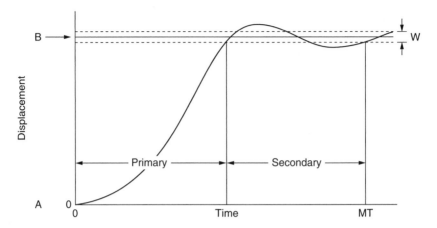

FIGURE 4.35
Typical movement response in target acquisition showing second-order control. (Adapted from Langolf et al., 1976.)

point *A* to a target or an ending point *B* with an arbitrary width *W*. The response shows the actual displacement of the hand plotted against time with two distinct phases (Figure 4.35). The first or primary phase consists of acceleration and deceleration of the hand resulting in a relatively overall constant velocity. The second or secondary phase consists of homing into the target, with one or more overshoots and undershoots, thus showing the characteristic oscillation of an underdamped second-order control system. This is in contrast to rapid, almost, ballistic type motions produced in a boxing punch or jab, which operates in an open-loop fashion with minimal or no feedback.

4.9   Root Locus Approach to Muscle Modeling

4.9.1   The Root Locus Method

An open-loop system with no feedback can be simply represented as a black box for the plant with function *G*(*s*) (Figure 4.36A). The *plant* can be considered a simple transfer function or element that exerts control over the input, to transform it into the output. A closed-loop system has a feedback path, which may also have a transfer function element to it represented as *H*(*s*) (Figure 4.36B). With more elements, the representation, termed a *block diagram*, may become more complicated. Therefore, there are several identities that may be useful for manipulating such block diagrams (Figure 4.37). The most useful is Identity 6, which will typically be used to convert a feedback system to a simple transfer function for further manipulation or inverse transform calculation.

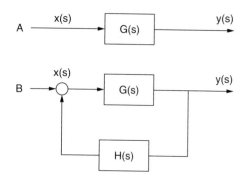

FIGURE 4.36
(A) Open-loop system. (B) Closed-loop system with feedback path.

Example 4.8: Derivation of Identity 6

The difference between the input $x(s)$ and the feedback path can be defined as an error function, $e(s)$, which is then operated on by the plant $G(s)$ to yield the output:

$$y(s) = G(s)e(s) \tag{4.215}$$

This error function can be formally defined as

$$e(s) = x(s) - H(s)\,y(s) \tag{4.216}$$

Substituting Equation 4.215 into Equation 4.216 then yields

$$y(s) = G(s)\big[x(s) - H(s)\,y(s)\big] = G(s)\,x(s) - G(s)\,H(s)\,y(s) \tag{4.217}$$

Collating $y(s)$ terms and dividing both sides by $x(s)$ yield the final expression:

$$\frac{y(s)}{x(s)} = \frac{G(s)}{1 + G(s)\,H(s)} \tag{4.218}$$

Note that if it were a positive feedback system, then the plus sign in Equation 4.218 would become a minus sign.

For a real system to function properly it must also be a stable system. There are several definitions of stability; however, they all apply to the steady-state response (i.e., as $t \to \infty$) rather than the transient response. The classic definition of stability is that $G(t)$ is finite as defined by

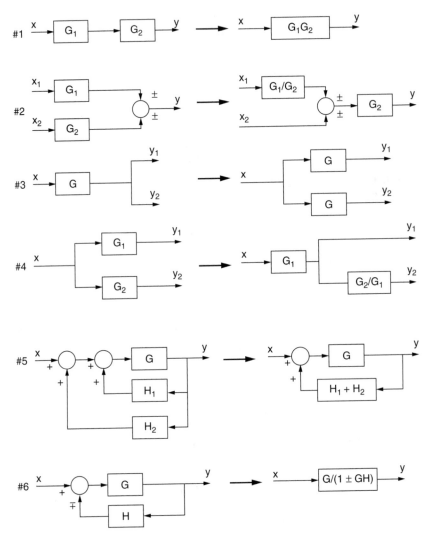

FIGURE 4.37
Block diagram identities.

$$\int_0^\infty \left| G(t) \right| dt < \infty \qquad\qquad (4.219)$$

However, as shown previously, working in the time domain can be difficult. Therefore, in practice, the Laplace domain and an alternate definition of stability are used: the poles of the closed-loop transfer function, $y(s)/x(s)$, lie in the left half of the s-plane.

In the generalized representation of a control loop (Figure 4.36B), $G(s)$ is typically referred to as the *plant*, with an internal gain control K, and $H(s)$ is the feedback element. One of the easiest aspects of controlling the stability of the system is to adjust the gain K of the controller as needed. The overall system transfer function (according to Identity 6) is

$$\frac{y(s)}{x(s)} = \frac{KG(s)}{1 + KG(s)H(s)} \tag{4.220}$$

This representation is referred to as the *closed-loop transfer function*. The characteristic function of this transfer function is determined by the denominator and, effectively, by $KG(s)H(s)$. Consequently, the term $KG(s)H(s)$, referred to as the *open-loop transfer function*, can be used to determine system stability.

There is a graphical analytical procedure for determining the location of the poles (and zeros) of this open-loop transfer function as a function of certain systems parameters, most typically the controller gain K. This *root locus* plots the poles or roots of the open-loop transfer function as a function of K using a structured procedure given as a set of 12 rules in Table 4.4. These are explained below in relation to the relatively simple open-loop transfer function:

$$KG(s)H(s) = \frac{K(s+2)}{s(s+6)} \tag{4.221}$$

Rule 1. Number of branches. The number of branches of the root-locus plot is equal to the number of poles of the open-loop transfer function. In Equation 4.221, there are two poles, $s = 0$ and $s = -6$, yielding two branches.

Rule 2. Starting points. The branches of the root locus start at the poles of the open-loop transfer function. In Equation 4.221, the branches start at $s = 0$ and $s = -6$. Note that, for the system identified by Equation 4.221 to be stable, as s approaches the poles (in which case the denominator goes to zero and the transfer function goes to infinity), K must approach zero. Thus, $K = 0$ at the poles.

Rule 3. End points. The branches of the root locus terminate at the zeros of the open-loop transfer function. For the example in Equation 4.221, the branches terminate at $s = -2$. Another zero needs to be identified and will eventually be found somewhere at infinity. Note that the system identified by Equation 4.221 can be stable as s approaches the zero (in which case the numerator goes to zero) even if K approaches infinity. Thus, $K = \infty$ at the zeros.

Rule 4. Behavior on the real axis. A point on the real axis is part of the root locus if an odd number of poles and/or zeros lie to the right of this

TABLE 4.4

Summary of Root Locus Construction Rules

Rule 1:	Number of branches	There is one branch for each pole of the open-loop transfer function $KG(s)H_{eq}(s)$.
Rule 2:	Starting points ($K = 0$)	The branches of the root locus start at the poles of $KG(s)H_{eq}(s)$.
Rule 3:	End points ($K = \infty$)	The branches of the root locus end at the zeros of $KG(s)H_{eq}(s)$.
Rule 4:	Behavior along the real axis	The root locus exists on the real axis at every point for which an odd number of poles and/or zeros lie to the right.
Rule 5:	Gain determination	At a point s_1 on the root locus, the gain is given by: $$K = \frac{1}{\left| G(s)H_{eq}(s) \right|}\Bigg|_{s = s_1}$$
Rule 6:	Symmetry of locus	The root locus is always symmetric with respect to the real axis.
Rule 7:	Breakaway or reentry points	The root locus breaks away from the real axis at a point of relative maximum gain and returns to the real axis at a point of relative minimum gain.
Rule 8:	Breakaway or reentry angles	At points of breakaway or reentry, the branches of the root locus are separated by an angle of $\pm 180°/\alpha$. where α is the number of branches that intersect.
Rule 9:	Asymptotic behavior for large K	The asymptote angles are given by $$\phi = \frac{180° + k360°}{p - z} \quad k = 0, 1, 2, \ldots, p - z - 1$$ and the origin of the asymptotes is $$OA = \frac{\sum (\text{Pole Locations}) - \sum (\text{Zero Locations})}{p - z}$$
Rule 10:	Imaginary-axis crossing	The branches of the root locus across the imaginary axis at points where the phase shift is 180°.
Rule 11:	Sum of the closed-loop poles	If $p - z \geq 2$, the sum of the closed-loop pole is a constant.
Rule 12:	Angles of departure and arrival	The angles of departure and arrival at complex conjugate poles and zeroes are determined by satisfying the angle criterion near the pole or zero in question.

Source: Melsa, J.L. and Schultz, D.G., 1969. *Linear Control Systems,* New York: McGraw-Hill. With permission.

point. This means that for the system of Equation 4.221 the root locus exists between 0 and –2 and from –6 leftward, as shown in Figure 4.38A.

Rule 5. Value of gain. The value of the gain, K, can be determined at a given point, $s = s'$, on the root locus by evaluating the characteristic function of the closed loop transfer function:

$$1 + KG(s)H(s) = 0 \tag{4.222}$$

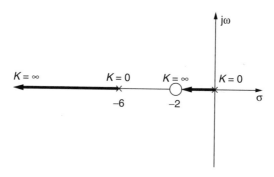

FIGURE 4.38
Root locus plot for [K(s + 2)]/[s(s + 6)].

or, in an alternate form,

$$KG(s)H(s) = |1|$$ (4.223)

at a phase angle of 180°. Consequently, the value of gain *K* is

$$K = \frac{1}{\left| G(s)H(s) \right|_{s=s'}} = \frac{s(s+6)}{(s+2)} \bigg|_{s=s'}$$ (4.224)

For the system of Equation 4.221, the following values of gains can be calculated:

s	−0.1	−1.0	−1.5	−1.9
K	0.31	5.0	13.5	77.9

Rule 6. Symmetry. The root locus is symmetric with respect to the real or x-axis. If the poles of the open-loop transfer function happen to be complex conjugate roots, then these roots will lie equidistant above and below the real axis. This means that the root locus will necessarily deviate from the x-axis and may have breakaway and reentry points and angles to the real axis. However, for Equation 4.221, the root locus lies completely on the x-axis as shown in Figure 4.38.

For the rest of the rules a slightly more elaborate root locus will be utilized. Its open-loop transfer functions is defined as

$$KG(s)H(s) = \frac{K(s+6)}{s(s+2)}$$ (4.225)

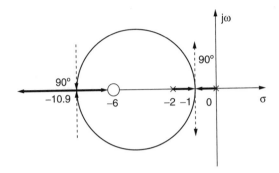

FIGURE 4.39
Root-locus plot for $[K(s + 6)]/[s(s + 2)]$.

The first six rules yield the following characteristics for the root locus. From Rule 1, there are two poles and, thus, two branches. From Rule 2, the starting points are the poles, $s = 0$ and $s = -2$. From Rule 3, the ending points are the one direct zero of $s = -2$ and another zero, implied at $s = -6$. From Rule 4, the two branches of the root locus would start on the real axis at 0 and –2, head toward each other, then breakaway somewhere from the real axis and finally reenter the real axis beyond –6. Based on these rules and Rule 6 of symmetry, an approximate root locus for Equation 4.225 is given by Figure 4.39A.

Rule 7. Breakaway or reentry points. The root locus breaks away from the real axis at a point of relative maximum gain and reenters the real axis at a point of relative minimum gain. The relative maximum and minimum points for a continuous function can be determined by taking the derivative of the function, setting it equal to zero, and solving for the roots, i.e.,

$$d\left[G(s)H(s)\right]\big/ds = 0 \tag{4.226}$$

or

$$\frac{d}{ds}\left\{\frac{1}{G(s)H(s)}\right\} = 0 \tag{4.227}$$

depending on whichever form is easier to differentiate. In terms of the final solution, the form does not matter since one is the expression for K and the maximum, while the other is the expression for $1/K$ or the minimum. Differentiation of Equation 4.225 yields

$$\frac{d}{ds}\left\{\frac{s(s+2)}{s+6}\right\} = \frac{2s+2}{s+6} - \frac{\left(s^2 + 2s\right)}{\left(s+6\right)^2} = 0 \tag{4.228}$$

Simplification of Equation 4.228 yields

$$s^2 + 12s + 12 = 0 \qquad (4.229)$$

Based on the quadratic formula, the roots for Equation 4.229 are

$$s = \frac{-b \pm \sqrt{b^2 - 4ac}}{2a} = \frac{-12 \pm \sqrt{12^2 - 4 \times 12}}{2} = -1.1 \text{ and } -10.9 \qquad (4.230)$$

Therefore, without even calculating the exact value of gain, the root locus breaks away from the real axis at –1.1 and reenters at –10.9.

Rule 8. Breakaway and reentry angles. At the breakaway and reentry points, the angle of breakaway and reentry is determined by $180°/\alpha$, where α is the number of branches intersecting at that point. For Equation 4.225, $\alpha = 2$ and the breakaway and reentry angles are $\pm 180°/2 = \pm 90°$.

Rule 9. Asymptotic behavior. For cases in which the number of poles p exceeds the number of zeros z, there will an indirect zero at infinity with the root locus showing asymptotic behavior as it moves toward that indirect zero. Note that in such situations the gain K will also be increasing in value. There will $p - z$ number of asymptotes with the angle of the asymptote with respect to the real axis given by

$$\text{Angle} = \pm\pi/(p-z), \pm 3\pi/(p-z), \ldots \qquad (4.231)$$

Also, the origin of the asymptotes is given by the centroid equal to

$$\text{Origin} = \frac{\Sigma \text{ poles} - \Sigma \text{ zeros}}{p - z} \qquad (4.232)$$

For Equation 4.225, $p = 2$, $z = 1$, and $p - z = 1$. Therefore, there is one asymptote with angle of $-\pi$. The origin of the asymptote is not critical in the case of just one asymptote, but will be in the case of two or more asymptotes.

The final root locus for the system as represented by Equation 4.225 is shown in Figure 4.39B. Note that, although the transfer function appears to be quite similar to the transfer function of the system as represented by Equation 4.221, the resulting root loci are quite different.

Rule 10. Imaginary axis crossing. The branches of the root locus cross the imaginary axis at points where the phase shift is 180°. Consider a system represented by the following open-loop transfer function:

$$KG(s)H(s) = \frac{K(s+2)}{s(s-1)(s+6)} \qquad (4.233)$$

From Rule 1, there are three poles and, thus, three branches of the root locus. From Rule 2, the starting points are the poles 0, +1, and –6. From Rule 3, the end points are the direct zero at –2 and two indirect zeros at infinity. From Rule 4, the root locus will exist on the real axis between 0 and +1 and between –6 and –2. From Rule 6, the root locus will be symmetrical. From Rule 7, the breakaway point can be determined from maximum relative gain. Rather than performing a difficult differentiation, it could be approximated as midway between 0 and +1. Substituting several values of s around +0.5 yields the following values of gain K and a maximum at +0.45, where K is

$$K = \left| \frac{s(s-1)(s+6)}{(s+2)} \right|$$

(4.234)

s	0.40	0.45	0.50	0.55
K	0.640	0.652	0.650	0.636

From Rule 8, there are two diverting branches and the breakaway angle is $180°/2 = 90°$. From Rule 9, $p = 3$ and $z = 1$, and $p - z = 2$. The asymptote angles are given by $180°/2 = 90°$ and the centroid origin for the asymptotes is $[0 - 6 + 1 - (-2)]/2 = -1.5$.

Now, using Rule 10, one can find the imaginary axis crossing point by finding the phase angle of the transfer function and setting it equal to zero (i.e., $\tan 180° = 0$):

$$G(j\omega)H(j\omega) = \frac{2 + j\omega}{-5\omega^2 - j(\omega^3 + 6\omega)}$$

(4.235)

Multiplying the numerator and denominator by the complex conjugate of the denominator yields

$$G(j\omega)H(j\omega) = \frac{2 + j\omega}{\left[-5\omega^2 - j(\omega^3 + 6\omega)\right]} \frac{\left[-5\omega^2 + j(\omega^3 + 6\omega)\right]}{\left[-5\omega^2 + j(\omega^3 + 6\omega)\right]}$$

(4.236)

This expression simplifies to

$$G(j\omega)H(j\omega) = \frac{-(\omega^4 + 16\omega^2) + j(-3\omega^3 + 12\omega)}{-25\omega^4 - \omega^2(6 + \omega^2)^2}$$

(4.237)

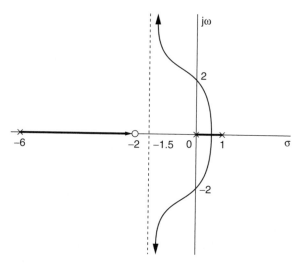

FIGURE 4.40
Root locus plot for $[K(s + 2)]/[s(s - 1)(s + 6)]$.

The phase angle is determined by the arc tangent of the imaginary part over the real part, which is equal to 180°. This also means that the ratio of the imaginary part over the real part equals zero, as the arc tangent of zero is 180°. Consequently, the imaginary part alone must also equal zero:

$$-3\omega^3 + 12\omega = 0 \tag{4.238}$$

The solution to the equation is ω equals either 0 or ± 2. Substituting in $\omega = 2$ into the expression for magnitude based on Equation 4.223 yields a value of $K = 10$ at the critical crossing point and the complete root locus is shown in Figure 4.40.

$$\left| G(j\omega)H(j\omega) \right| = \frac{\left[\left(\omega^4 + 16\omega^2\right)^2 + \left(-3\omega^3 + 12\omega\right)^2 \right]^{1/2}}{25\omega^4 + \omega^2 \left(6 + \omega^2\right)^2} \tag{4.239}$$

$$\left| G(j\omega)H(j\omega) \right| = \frac{\left[\left(2^4 + 16 \times 4\right)^2 + \left(-3 \times 2^3 + 12 \times 2\right)^2 \right]^{1/2}}{25 \times 2^4 + 2^2 \left(6 + 2^2\right)^2} = \frac{80}{800} = \frac{1}{K} \tag{4.240}$$

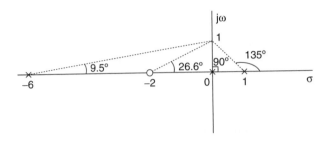

FIGURE 4.41
Graphical approach to finding imaginary axis crossing point.

Thus, for all values of gain, K, ranging from the starting point with $K = 0$ up to $K = 10$, the roots will likely be on the right half of the s plane and the system will be unstable. Note that the exact crossing point, $\omega = \pm 2$, yields a pure sinusoidal response in the time domain. Because the function does not expand to infinity, but also does not approach zero, it could be considered a form of limited stability.

There is also a graphical approach that can be much simpler for complicated expressions of s. It is based on the characteristic equation of Equation 4.222 exhibiting a phase angle relationship of 180° (Equation 4.223 or 4.224). Although this relationship applies to any point on the root locus, it is very tedious to take random points on the s plane and determine whether the phase angle criterion is true. However, there are a relatively limited number of points available for which the crossing of the imaginary axis will satisfy this criterion. At the critical crossing point the total phase-angle contributions from each of the poles and zeros of the open-loop control system should add up to 180°. In the format of Rule 9, the angles from each pole and zero to the critical crossing point summate to 180°:

$$\Sigma \text{ pole angles} - \Sigma \text{ zero angles} = 180° \qquad (4.241)$$

For the system defined by Equation 4.234 and whose root locus is shown in Figure 4.40, the phase angle relationship works as follows. Because the breakaway point on the right half of the s plane is 0.45 and the asymptote line is −1.5, a rough estimate for the crossing point is relatively small ω, perhaps $\omega = 1$ (Figure 4.41). Starting with the pole at −6, the phase angle at the crossing point is

$$\tan^{-1} 1/6 = 9.5° \qquad (4.242)$$

For the zero at −2, the phase angle at the crossing point is

$$\tan^{-1} \tfrac{1}{2} = 26.6° \qquad (4.243)$$

The pole at the origin creates a 90° phase angle. The pole at +1 yields a phase angle of:

$$180° - \tan^{-1}1 = 180° - 45° = 135° \tag{4.244}$$

The sum of all these phase angles according to Equation 4.241 is

$$9.5° + 90° + 135° - 26.6° = 207.9° \tag{4.245}$$

This sum is close to but a bit larger than the required 180° angle. By increasing ω, the angle to the zero at –2 increases and the angle to the pole at +1 decreases, bringing the sum closer to 180°. At $\omega = 2$, the respective angles in Equation 4.241 become

$$18.4° + 90° + 116.6° - 45° = 180° \tag{4.246}$$

Note that the origin also satisfies the 180° phase angle relationship and, in a limited sense, is a crossing point. In this particular case, it is the pole at zero and a starting point for the root locus.

A third and final approach may also be used. For this, Rule 11 is used.

Rule 11. Sum of the poles. If $p - z \geq 2$, the sum of the poles remains a constant independent of K. For the system defined by Equation 4.233, there are three poles and one zero, allowing Rule 11 to be used. The sum of the poles (with $K = 0$) is $-6 + 0 + 1 = -5$. Therefore, at $s = -5$, the sum of the other two poles must be zero, indicating that they are complex conjugates on the imaginary axis. The value of K must be the same for whichever pole is used to calculate it. Thus, instead of using the complex conjugate roots, K can be calculated much more quickly using the root or pole at $s = -5$.

$$K = \left| \frac{s(s-1)(s+6)}{(s+2)} \right|_{s=-5} = \left| \frac{(-5)(-6)(1)}{(-3)} \right| = 10 \tag{4.247}$$

Rule 12. Complex poles and zeros. The angles of departure from complex poles and the angle of arrival at complex zeros are determined by the 180° phase angle criterion. Consider a system represented by the following open-loop transfer function:

$$KG(s)H(s) = \frac{K}{s^2 + 2s + 2} \tag{4.248}$$

The denominator is partitioned into two complex conjugate roots:

$$KG(s)H(s) = \frac{K}{(s+1+j)(s+1-j)} \tag{4.249}$$

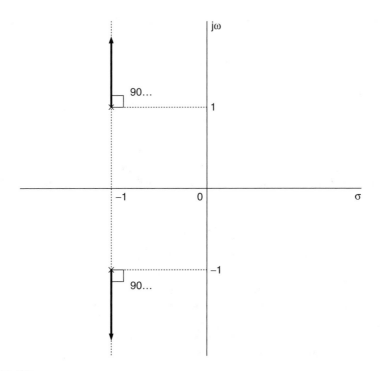

FIGURE 4.42
Root locus plot for $K/(s^2 + 2s + 2)$ showing complex poles.

From Rule 1, there are two poles and, thus, two branches of the root locus. From Rule 2, the starting points are the poles $-1 - j$ and $-1 + j$. From Rule 3, the end points are two indirect zeros at infinity. From Rule 4, the root locus cannot exist on the real axis because there can never be an odd number of roots. From Rule 5, the root locus will be symmetrical. From Rule 9, the asymptote angles are $\pm 180°/2 = \pm 90°$. From Rule 12, the angles of departure are determined as follows. For the top pole $(-1 + j)$, the angle of departure plus the angle to bottom pole $(90°)$ must sum to $180°$. Therefore, the departure angle is $90°$. From Rule 5 and symmetry, the angle of departure for the bottom pole is $-90°$ and the final complete root locus is shown in Figure 4.42.

The root locus plots and frequency analysis magnitude and phase angle plots for a variety of different simple transfer functions are given in Table 4.5. These will be useful in helping to identify the transfer functions and develop models based on experimentally observed data for different physiological entities. Further details on root locus plots can be found in Melsa and Schultz (1969) or other textbooks on linear control systems.

4.9.2 Muscle Spindle Model

Because the muscle spindle consists of intrafusal muscle fibers in the pole region and the elastic annulospiral element in the nuclear bag region, it

TABLE 4.5

Summary of Root Locus, Magnitude, and Phase Angle Plots for Several Simple Transfer Functions

Transfer Function	Root Locus	Frequency Analysis	
		Magnitude	Phase Angle (ϕ)
$\dfrac{1}{s}$ (a) Integrator			
$\dfrac{1}{s+1}$ (b) Single lag			
$\dfrac{s}{s+1}$ (c) Derivative with lag			
$\dfrac{1}{T} \times \dfrac{s+T}{s+1},\ T<1$ (d) Phase lead			
$\dfrac{1}{T} \times \dfrac{s+T}{s+1},\ T>1$ (e) Phase lag			

Transfer Function	Root Locus	Frequency Analysis	
		Magnitude	Phase Angle (ϕ)
$\dfrac{1}{s^2}$ (f) Inertial system			
$\dfrac{1}{s(s+1)}$ (g) Integrator with lag			
$\dfrac{1}{(s+1)(s+T)},\ T>1$ (h) Double lag			
$\dfrac{1}{s^2+2\zeta s+1},\ \zeta>1$ (i) Damped oscillator			

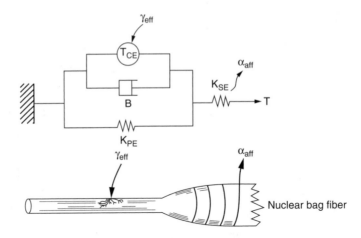

FIGURE 4.43
Schematic model of a muscle spindle. (Adapted from McMahon, 1984.)

would be reasonable to use Hill's four-element model to also represent the muscle spindle (Figure 4.43). The pole region would then be represented by a dashpot B in parallel with a parallel elastic element, K_{PE}, and the contractile element, T_{CE}. Input from the gamma neurons is assumed to control the force level generated by the contractile element. The series elastic element of the intrafusal fibers is combined with the elastic element of the annulospiral element for a combined K_{SE}. Obviously, the values of the muscle spindle parameters will be different from the values for Hill's muscle model.

In principle, the spindle provides information not only on length but also on the rate of change of length. Upon an instantaneous stretch, the dashpot element cannot change its length instantaneously. Therefore, all of the stretch is initially taken up by the series elastic element, K_{SE}, and there is a large increase in the firing rate of the α afferent neuron proportional to the stretch ε_0. If the amount of stretch is increased, the initial amount of firing is also increased (see Figure 3.28). After the initial stretch is over, the dashpot slowly extends, allowing K_{PE} to take up some of the increased length, so that the firing rate drops to a steady level substantially below the initial peak.

Should the gamma system not be activated, this drop in the firing rate can be modeled very similarly to passive muscle in a quick stretch experiment. Consider Equation 4.78 and the step stretch of the muscle spindle.

$$T = \frac{K_{SE}\left(Bs + K_{PE}\right)}{Bs + K_{PE} + K_{SE}} \frac{\varepsilon_0}{s} \tag{4.250}$$

A partial fraction expansion yields

$$T = \frac{K_{SE}\varepsilon_0}{K_{PE} + K_{SE}} \left\{ \frac{K_{SE}}{s + \left(K_{PE} + K_{SE}\right)/B} + \frac{K_{PE}}{s} \right\} \tag{4.251}$$

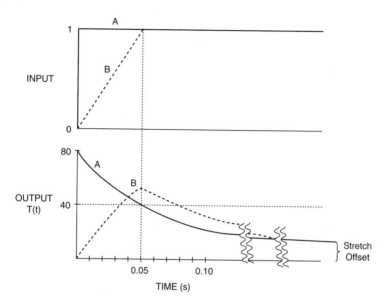

FIGURE 4.44
Calculated muscle spindle response to a step input (A) and ramp input (B).

Taking the inverse Laplace transform, simplifying, and using numerical data on muscle (not the spindle) from Bawa et al. (1976) of $B = 5$ g-s/mm, and from Jewell and Wilkie (1958) of $K_{SE} = 80$ g/mm and the weaker $K_{PE} = 20$ g/mm, yield $\tau = B/(K_{PE} + K_{SE}) = 5/(20 + 80) = 0.05$ s and the response in the time domain of

$$T(t) = \frac{K_{SE}\,\varepsilon_0}{K_{PE} + K_{SE}}\left\{K_{PE} + K_{SE}e^{-(K_{PE}+K_{SE})t/B}\right\} = 16\varepsilon_0\left(1 + 4e^{-t/0.05}\right) \quad (4.252)$$

Assuming $\varepsilon_0 = 1$, Equation 4.251 yields the resultant plot shown in Figure 4.44A.

Experimentally instantaneous stretches are not realistic. In practice, the application of the stretch becomes more of a steep ramp function, which can be also modeled using Laplace transforms. In this particular case, assume a ramp, $20t$, reaching the value of 1 in one time constant of 0.05 s. The response then becomes

$$T = \frac{K_{SE}\left(Bs + K_{PE}\right)}{Bs + K_{PE} + K_{SE}}\frac{20\varepsilon}{s^2}\,0 \quad (4.253)$$

Rearrangement and a partial fraction expansion yield

$$T = 20K_{SE}\varepsilon_0\left\{\frac{a}{s + \left(K_{PE} + K_{SE}\right)/B} + \frac{b}{s^2} + \frac{c}{s}\right\} \quad (4.254)$$

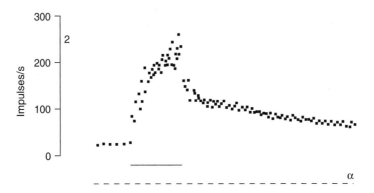

FIGURE 4.45
Muscle spindle response (afferent firing frequency) to a stretch of constant velocity (i.e., ramp function). (From Bessou, P., Emonet-Dénand, F., and Laporte, Y., 1965. *Journal of Physiology*, 180:649–672. With permission.)

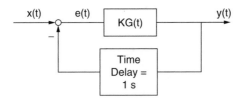

FIGURE 4.46
Closed-loop system with a time delay of 1 s in the feedback path.

Using residues to solve for a and b yields

$$a = \left.\frac{s + K_{PE}/B}{s^2}\right|_{s = -(K_{PE} + K_{SE})/B} = \frac{-K_{SE}B}{\left(K_{PE} + K_{SE}\right)^2} \tag{4.255}$$

$$b = \left.\frac{s + K_{PE}/B}{s + \left(K_{PE} + K_{SE}\right)/B}\right|_{s=0} = \frac{K_{PE}}{K_{PE} + K_{SE}} \tag{4.256}$$

$$c = \left.\frac{d}{ds}\left\{\frac{s + K_{PE}/B}{s + \left(K_{PE} + K_{SE}\right)/B}\right\}\right|_{s=0} = \frac{K_{SE}B}{\left(K_{PE} + K_{SE}\right)^2} \tag{4.257}$$

Substituting the coefficients a, b, and c back into Equation 4.254, taking the inverse Laplace transform, and simplifying yield

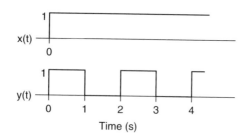

FIGURE 4.47
Output of a closed-loop system with a time delay of 1 s to a unit step input.

$$T(t) = \frac{20K_{SE}{}^2\varepsilon_0}{\left(K_{PE} + K_{SE}\right)^2}\left\{1 - e^{-\left(K_{PE}+K_{SE}\right)t/B} + \frac{K_{PE}\left(K_{PE} + K_{SE}\right)}{K_{SE}B}\,t\right\}$$

$$= 64\varepsilon_0\left(1 - e^{-t/0.05} + 5t\right)$$

(4.258)

The resulting plot (Figure 4.44B) for a sluggish stretch input (i.e., not a true step input, but a very steep ramp, reaching the value of 1 in one time constant of 0.05 s) shows a sluggish rise in the firing frequency, reaching a peak level lower than for a true step input, and then a fall to a steady-state firing rate. This plot also corresponds very nicely to data observed by Bessou et al. (1965), shown in Figure 4.45.

4.9.3 Time Delays

Time delays in a neuromuscular system can occur because of synaptic crossing times, neural conduction times, times for the calcium ions to release from the sarcoplasmic reticulum and diffuse into the surrounding muscle tissue. In an engineering control system, time delays in a negative feedback system can result in oscillatory behavior of the output even though the input is steady. This can obviously cause problems with stability.

An example of a pure time delay in a negative feedback loop is shown in Figure 4.46. The Laplace transform of a pure time delay corresponds to a time shift transform from Table 4.2:

$$\mathcal{L}\left[f\left(t - a\right)\right] = e^{-as}\,\mathcal{L}\left[f\left(t\right)\right] = e^{-as}$$

(4.259)

Using the Laplace transform of the closed-loop response from Equation 4.218 and assuming a simple plant with a gain of 1 yields the final closed-loop transfer function:

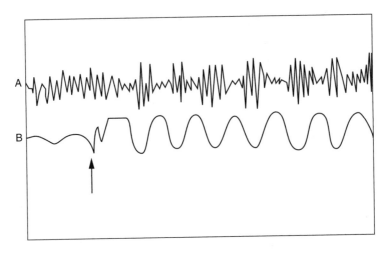

FIGURE 4.48
(A) Electromyograph (EMG) from extensor digitorum communis. (B) Self-sustained oscillations in the middle finger elicited from a small tap at the arrow (7 oscillations over 600 ms). (From Lippold, O.C.J., 1970. *Journal of Physiology*, 206:359–382. With permission.)

$$\frac{y(s)}{x(s)} = \frac{1}{1+e^{-as}} \tag{4.260}$$

Using a unit step input with Laplace transform of $1/s$ yields an output response of

$$y(s) = \frac{1}{s\left(1+e^{-as}\right)} \tag{4.261}$$

The inverse transform (from a detailed mathematics handbook such as Selby (1970) is

$$y(t) = \tfrac{1}{2}\left[1-\left(-1\right)^{n}\right] n-1 < t < n \tag{4.262}$$

The input step and output square wave responses are plotted in Figure 4.47. Although the output response is a stylized response, it still supports the principle of time delays in a negative feedback system causing oscillatory behavior. This phenomenon was particularly observed by Lippold (1970) who elicited tremor in an extended finger with a small initial mechanical perturbation. These oscillations were found to be in phase with groups of muscle action potentials recorded from the extensor digitorum communis muscle (Figure 4.48) and were thought to originate due to time delays in the neuromuscular loops as described in Chapter 3, particularly when the loop gain is greater than one.

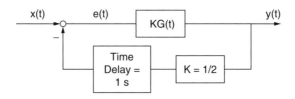

FIGURE 4.49
Closed-loop system with a time delay of 1 s and attenuator of ½ in the feedback path.

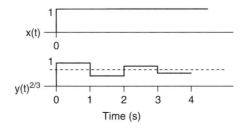

FIGURE 4.50
Output of a closed-loop system with a time delay of 1 s and attenuator of ½ in the feedback path.

An alternative approach is to examine the system in Figure 4.46 directly. The error, $e(t)$, is the difference between the input $x(t)$ and the feedback path, which is $y(t - 1)$, i.e., the output delayed by 1 s. Note, also, that in this case, $y(t) = e(t)$, since there is only a gain of one in the direct open-loop path. At $t = 0$, the input jumps to value of one, which is also the output for up to $t = 1$, as the feedback path is delaying the output signal for 1 s. At $t = 1$, the feedback passes its value of 1 to the junction and, as a negative feedback, is subtracted from one, yielding an output of 0 for the next second, up to $t = 2$. At $t = 2$, the previous value 0 is passed through the feedback loop which has no effect on the input, which passed through unchanged to the output which jumps to one. This square wave continues *ad infinitum* as a form of oscillatory behavior and a destabilizing factor in motor control.

In engineering systems, the system may be stabilized by introducing an attenuator into the feedback loop, such that the loop gain is less than one. Therefore, consider an attenuator of ½ in the feedback path (Figure 4.49). Now, reexamine the system flow directly. At $t = 0$, the input jumps to a value of one, which is also the output for up to $t = 1$, since the feedback path is delaying the output signal for 1 s. At $t = 1$, the feedback passes its attenuated value of ½ to the junction and, as a negative feedback, is subtracted from one, yielding an output of ½ for the next second, up to $t = 2$. At $t = 2$, the previous value of ½ is passed through the feedback loop, reduced to ¼ and subtracted from the input value of 1, yielding an output value of ¾. This value is reduced to ⅜ in the next cycle and subtracted from 1, yielding an output value of ⅝, etc. The oscillations are decreasing (Figure 4.50) and the final converging value can be calculated from the closed-loop transfer function:

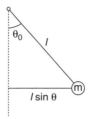

FIGURE 4.51
Undamped pendulum defined in terms of displacement.

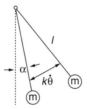

FIGURE 4.52
Undamped pendulum defined in terms of velocity control.

$$\frac{y(s)}{x(s)} = \frac{G(s)}{1+G(s)H(s)} = \frac{1}{1+1(\frac{1}{2})} = \frac{2}{3} \tag{4.263}$$

This is comparable to the experience of hearing the loud screech of public address systems, whose microphone happens to pick up sound from its own speaker and through the amplification creates oscillations. The screech goes away when the gain on the amplifier is decreased. Similarly, Lippold (1970) showed that tremor could be decreased by inflating a blood pressure cuff on the oscillating limb. This reduced the blood flow to the neuromuscular system and most likely decreased the gain in the feedback loop.

4.9.4 Velocity Control

Consider an undamped pendulum that is released from an angle θ_0 (Figure 4.51). With no damping the pendulum will swing past center, reach an identical angle θ_0 on the other side, and continue back and forth in a pure harmonic oscillation. The torque acting to restore the pendulum to the center position depends on the horizontal component of the angle θ and balances the moment of inertia for the pendulum:

$$ml^2 \ddot{\theta} = -mgl\sin\theta \tag{4.264}$$

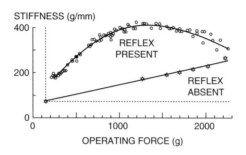

FIGURE 4.53

Muscle stiffness with and without reflexes present. (From Hoffer, J.A. and Andreassen, S., 1981. *Journal of Neurophysiology*, 45:267–285. With permission.)

which for small angles (when $\sin\theta \approx \theta$) becomes

$$\ddot{\theta} + g/l\ \theta = 0 \tag{4.265}$$

The solution to this is similar to the undamped mass–spring–dashpot system equation:

$$s^2 + \omega_n^2 = 0 \tag{4.266}$$

The future position of the pendulum can be predicted by an angle θ^+, which is defined by the present angle θ (Figure 4.52) and a change in position determined by the velocity of movement:

$$\theta^+ = \theta + k\ \dot{\theta} \tag{4.267}$$

Note that the velocity is negative, i.e., restoring the pendulum back to center. If the restoring force is proportional to α rather than θ, then substituting Equation 4.267 back into Equation 4.265, in the Laplace domain, yields

$$\ddot{\theta} + g/l\left(\theta + k\ \dot{\theta}\right) = \ddot{\theta} + gk/l\ \dot{\theta} + g/l\ \theta = \left(s^2 + gks/l + g/l\right)\theta = 0 \tag{4.268}$$

The pendulum can be considered analogous to muscle force in the stretch reflex. If muscle force is proportional to stretch only, one would get pure oscillations only. But when the stretch receptors are sensitive to both displacement and velocity, the velocity term contributes a damping and stabilizing effect to the reflex (McMahon, 1984).

4.9.5 Reflex Stiffness

Motor control and maintenance of muscle stiffness were generally thought to be solely due to muscle spindles, either directly through the α afferent

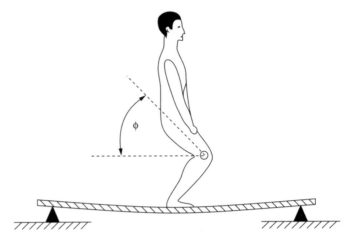

FIGURE 4.54
Measurement of *in vivo* reflex stiffness by natural frequency. (Adapted from Greene and McMahon, 1979.)

and α efferent pathways or through greater control of the γ efferent pathway. However, more recent studies have shown the influence of lower-level feedback also from Golgi tendon organs, which were once thought to respond only to excessive forces as in the clasp-knife reflex.

Detailed studies of a decerebrate cat soleus, using incremental applications of muscle stretch, show increases in muscle force from which the reflex stiffness of the muscle can be calculated (Hoffer and Andreassen, 1981). The effects for the initial small increases in force show a corresponding increase in muscle stiffness (Figure 4.53). However, as the muscle force levels increase, the stiffness plateaus. When the soleus nerve is cut, the response is very different with a continual increase in stiffness, indicating that the reflex maintenance of stiffness has been lost.

In human experiments (Greene and McMahon, 1979), male subjects stood on a beam with knees flexed at a constant angle (Figure 4.54). Slight vertical bouncing motions at appropriate frequencies (as determined by the natural frequency of a second-order damped system for the appropriate masses) produced resonant bouncing deflections in the beam. The range of frequencies for this resonance was very narrow, indicating a fine level of tuning. Using second-order system calculations the stiffness of the leg muscles could be calculated. Interestingly, a doubling of the body weight (by holding weights) caused less than 10% increase in muscle stiffness, indicating a reflex response in maintaining a constant muscle stiffness over a wide range of conditions.

Example 4.9: Development of Model for Parkinson Tremor

Frequency analysis data on normal and Parkinson's patients (Stark, 1968) was used to develop a transfer function model (Figure 4.55). Many pathological types of tremor are caused by lesions in the brain as opposed to

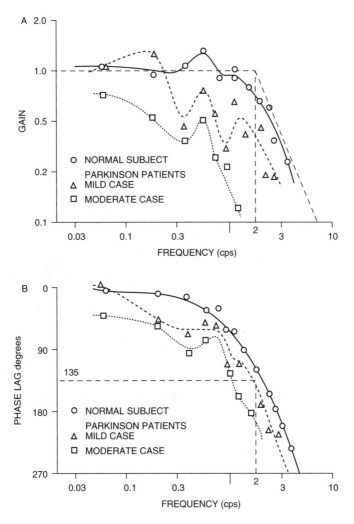

FIGURE 4.55
Magnitude (A) and phase angle (B) plots for normal subjects and for patients with Parkinson's. (From Stark, L., 1968. *Neurological Control Systems*, New York: Plenum Press. With permission.)

perturbations of the normal stretch reflex as performed by Lippold (1970). Parkinson's disease is one example in which arteriosclerotic changes in the basal ganglia, especially in elderly people, cause large-amplitude tremors of low frequency (2 to 3 Hz, much lower than the normal tremor of 10 to 11 Hz) and rigidity of movements. In this particular example, the transfer function for normal subjects will be derived. Based on the magnitude plot of Figure 4.55A, a breakpoint at approximately 2 Hz can be identified. This corresponds to a frequency of $2\pi \times 2$ or 12.5 radians. At this point the slope drops off at

$$\frac{\Delta y}{\Delta x} = \frac{\log(1) - \log(0.1)}{\log(2) - \log(6)} = -2 \tag{4.269}$$

From Table 4.5(f), this indicates a double pole and a transfer function of the form:

$$\frac{y(s)}{x(s)} = \frac{K}{(s + 12.5)^2} \tag{4.270}$$

A double pole should yield a –90° phase lag at the critical frequency (–180° at large frequencies) of 2 Hz on the phase plot (Figure 4.55B). However, the actual phase lag is –135°, which indicates that the additional –45° of phase lag must be due to a time lag. From the Laplace representation of a pure time delay in Equation 4.259 and the Euler identity in Equation 4.122, the phase lag of a time delay is found to be

$$\theta = \tan^{-1} \frac{-\sin a\omega}{\cos a\omega} = -a\omega \tag{4.271}$$

A 45° angle is equal to $2 \times 45°/360°$ or 0.78 radians. Substituting 0.78 radians into Equation 4.271 yields a time constant at the critical frequency of

$$a = 0.78/\omega = 0.78/12.5 = 0.06 \text{ s} \tag{4.272}$$

The revised form of the transfer function now becomes

$$\frac{y(s)}{x(s)} = \frac{Ke^{-0.06s}}{(s + 12.5)^2} \tag{4.273}$$

The value of gain K can be determined by finding the magnitude of the transfer function in Equation 4.273 and setting it equal to one. This is a fairly difficult process but can be simplified if one realizes that the gain of one also occurs as frequency approaches zero. Substituting $s = 0$ into Equation 4.273 yields a K of 156 and the final form of the transfer function:

$$\frac{y(s)}{x(s)} = \frac{156e^{-0.06s}}{(s + 12.5)^2} \tag{4.274}$$

The response for patients with Parkinson's is more difficult to model, deviating considerably from the normal second-order feedback system. It almost appears that the opposing agonist and antagonist feedback systems are permanently switched on, counteracting typical feedback and leading to permanent contraction of muscles and rigidity in the muscles. Much of this is due to the lesions in the basal ganglia and consequent interference in the normal functioning of the γ-loop feedback systems.

Questions

1. What is the purpose of using Laplace transforms in biomechanical modeling?
2. What are the trade-offs of using the algebraic and residue approaches in partial fraction expansions?
3. What is a transfer function?
4. Given that a unit impulse is not a realistic function, what purpose does an impulse response provide?
5. Compare and contrast the two basic elements in viscoelastic theory.
6. What is a stress relaxation function?
7. What is creep?
8. How do the time constants for the stress relaxation and creep functions compare in Hill's three-element model?
9. What are the frequency characteristics of passive muscle?
10. What is the difference between a distributed and a lumped model?
11. Compare and contrast open- and closed-loop systems.
12. What is the difference between a first- and second-order system?
13. What are poles and zeros?
14. What purpose do the roots of the characteristic function serve?
15. What is the natural frequency and how does it relate to motor control?
16. What is a bit?
17. Explain the Hick–Hyman law in terms of information processing.
18. What is the index of difficulty?
19. Explain Fitts' law in terms of motor control.
20. What is system bandwidth?
21. What is the difference between an open-loop and a closed-loop transfer function? What useful purpose does each provide?
22. What effect does a time lag in a feedback loop have on system performance? How can it be controlled?

Problems

4.1. Find entry 3 in the Laplace transform table (Table 4.1) from entry 1.

4.2. Find entry 4 from entry 1.

4.3. Find entry 10 from entry 9.

4.4. Find the Laplace transform of $\sin^2 t$.

4.5. Find the Laplace transform of $te^{2t}u(t-1)$.

4.6. Find the inverse Laplace transform of $3s/(s^2+1)(s^2+4)$.

4.7. Find the inverse Laplace transform of $(s+1)/(s^2+2s)$.

4.8. Find the inverse Laplace transform of $1/(s+1)(s+2)^2$.

4.9. Find the transfer function, $H(s)$, for this model.

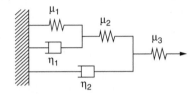

4.10. Compare these two viscoelastic models:

   a. Find the transfer function $H(s) = \varepsilon(s)/\sigma(s)$ for both models.

   b. Find the strain for an impulse and step stress input for Model 1.

   c. How are the parameters of the two models related? (*Hint:* They are alternate ways of representing the same Hill's passive three-element muscle model!)

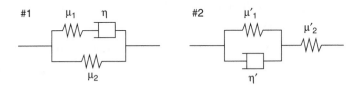

4.11. The ratio of peak twitch tension generated from a single stimulus to tetanic tension generated from tetanic stimulation is termed the twitch/tetanus ratio. Research shows that it is higher in fast twitch muscles than in slow twitch muscles. Use Hill's four-element active muscle model to calculate the twitch/tetanus ratio for fast and slow twitch muscles. Assume isometric tension.

4.12. Find the magnitude and phase plots for $10/s(10+s)$.

4.13. Find the magnitude and phase plots for $10(s+1)/s(s+10)^2$.

4.14. Consider a new viscoelastic element called a "slipshot," which can be represented in the Laplace domain as $1/(s + 2)$. A more complex gel-like element can be created by putting a dashpot (with coefficient of one) in series with the slipshot.

   a. Find the gel's transfer function $H(s) = \sigma(s)/\varepsilon(s)$.

   b. What are the gel's stress and strain retardation functions?

   c. What is the frequency response for the gel?

4.15. a. Simplify the following block diagram to a basic closed loop feedback system:

   b. Find the overall transfer function.

   c. Calculate a step response for $K = 1$.

   d. Find the root locus plot.

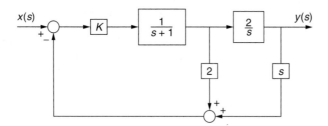

4.16. Find the root locus plot for $10K/(s^3 + 12s^2 + 20s)$. For what K is the system stable?

4.17. Find the root locus plot for $K(s + 2)/(s^2 + 2s + 2)$. For what K is the system stable?

References

Aidley, D.J., 1985. *The Physiology of Excitable Cells*, 2nd ed., Cambridge, U.K.: Cambridge University Press.

Alexander, R.S. and Johnson, P.D., 1965. Muscle stretch and theories of contraction, *American Journal of Physiology*, 208:412–416.

Bahler, A.S., 1967. Series elastic component of mammalian skeletal muscle, *American Journal of Physiology*, 213:1560–1564.

Bawa, P., Mannard, A., and Stein, R.B., 1976. Predictions and experimental tests of a viscoelastic muscle model using elastic and inertial loads, *Biological Cybernetics*, 22:139–145.

Bessou, P., Emonet-Dénand, F., and Laporte, Y., 1965. Motor fibres innervating extrafusal and intrafusal muscle fibres in the cat, *Journal of Physiology*, 180:649–672.

Bigland, B. and Lippold, O.C.J., 1954. Motor unit activity in the voluntary contraction of human muscle, *Journal of Physiology*, 125:322–225.

Christensen, R.M., 1981. *Theory of Viscoelasticity: An Introduction*, 2nd ed., New York: Academic Press.

Clamann, H.P., 1970. Activity of single motor units during isometric tension, *Neurology*, 20:254–260.

Close, R.I., 1965. The relation between intrinsic speed of shortening and duration of the active state of muscle, *Journal of Physiology*, 180:542–559.

Ebashi, S. and Endo, M., 1968. Calcium ion and muscular contraction, *Progress in Biophysics and Molecular Biology*, 18:125–183.

Fenn, W.O. and Marsh, B.S., 1935. Muscle force at different speeds of shortening, *Journal of Physiology*, 85:277–297.

Fitts, P., 1954. The information capacity of the human motor system in controlling the amplitude of movement, *Journal of Experimental Psychology*, 47:381–391.

Flügge, W., 1975. *Viscoelasticity*, 2nd ed., Berlin: Springer-Verlag.

Freivalds, A., 1985. Incorporation of Active Elements into the Articulated Total Body Model, AAMRL-TR-85-061, Wright-Patterson Air Force Base, OH: Armstrong Aerospace Medical Research Laboratory.

Freivalds, A. and Kaleps, I., 1984. Computer-aided strength prediction using the Articulated Total Body Model, *Computers & Industrial Engineering*, 8:107–118.

Gordon, A.M., Huxley, A.F., and Julian, F.J., 1966. The variation in isometric tension with sarcomere length in vertebrate muscle fibers, *Journal of Physiology*, 184:170–192.

Greene, P.R. and McMahon, T.A., 1979. Reflex stiffness of man's antigravity muscles during kneebends while carrying extra weights, *Journal of Biomechanics*, 12:881–891.

Grimby, L. and Hannerz, J., 1977. Firing rate and recruitment order of toe extensor motor units in different modes of voluntary contraction, *Journal of Physiology*, 264:864–879.

Haddad, Y.M., 1995. *Viscoelasticity of Engineering Materials*, New York: Chapman & Hall.

Hatze, H., 1979. A teleological explanation of Weber's law and the motor unit size law, *Bulletin of Mathematical Biology*, 41:407–425.

Hatze, H., 1981. *Myocybernetic Control Models of Skeletal Muscle*, Pretoria, South Africa: University of South Africa.

Henneman, E. and Olson, C.B., 1965. Relations between structure and function in the design of skeletal muscle, *Journal of Neurophysiology*, 28:581–598.

Hick, W.E., 1952. On the rate of gain of information, *Quarterly Journal of Experimental Psychology*, 4:11–26.

Hill, A.V., 1938. The heat of shortening and the dynamic constants of muscle, *Proceedings of the Royal Society*, 126B:136–195.

Hill, A.V., 1970. *First and Last Experiments in Muscle Mechanics*, Cambridge, U.K.: Cambridge University Press.

Hoffer, J.A. and Andreassen, S., 1981. Regulation of soleus muscle stiffness in premamillary cats: intrinsic and reflex components, *Journal of Neurophysiology*, 45:267–285.

Hyman, R., 1953. Stimulus information as a determinant of reaction time, *Journal of Experimental Psychology*, 45:423–432.

Jewell, B.R. and Wilkie, D.R., 1958. An analysis of the mechanical components in frogs striated muscle, *Journal of Physiology*, 143:515–540.

Kaplan, W., 1962. *Operational Methods for Linear Systems*, Reading, MA: Addison Wesley.

Langolf, G., Chaffin, D., and Foulke, J., 1976. An investigation of Fitts' law using a wide range of movement amplitudes, *Journal of Motor Behavior*, 8:113–128.

Lippold, O.C.J., 1970. Oscillation in the stretch reflex arc and the origin of the rhythmical, 8–12 c/s component of physiological tremor, *Journal of Physiology*, 206:359–382.

Marsden, C.D., Meadows, J.C., and Merton, P.A., 1971. Isolated single motor units in human muscle and their rate of discharge during maximal voluntary effort, *Journal of Physiology*, 217:12P–13P.

McMahon, T.A., 1984. *Muscles, Reflexes, and Locomotion*, Princeton, NJ: Princeton University Press.

McMinn, R.M.H. and Hutchings, R.T., 1977. *Color Atlas of Human Anatomy*, Chicago, IL: Yearbook Medical Publishers.

Melsa, J.L. and Schultz, D.G., 1969. *Linear Control Systems*, New York: McGraw-Hill.

Milner-Brown, H.S., Stein, R.B., and Yemm, R., 1973a. The orderly recruitment of human motor units during voluntary isometric contractions, *Journal of Physiology*, 230:359–370.

Milner-Brown, H.S., Stein, R.B., and Yemm, R., 1973b. Changes in firing rates of human motor units during linearly changing voluntary contractions, *Journal of Physiology*, 230:371–390.

Milsum, J.H., 1966. *Biological Control Systems*, New York: McGraw-Hill.

Person, R. and Kudina, L.P., 1972. Discharge frequency and discharge pattern of human motor units during voluntary contraction of muscle, *Electroencephalography and Clinical Neurophysiology*, 32:471–483.

Sanders, M.S. and McCormick, E.J., 1993. *Human Factors in Engineering and Design*. 7th ed., New York: McGraw-Hill.

Schneck, D., 1992. *Mechanics of Muscle*, 2nd ed., New York: New York University Press.

Schumacher, G.H. and Wolff, E., 1966. Trockengewicht und physiologischer Querschnitt der menschlichen Skelettmuskulatur, II. Physiologischer Querschnitte [Dry weight and physiological cross section of human skeletal muscle, II. Physiological cross section], *Anatomischer Anzeiger*, 119:259–269.

Selby, S.M., Ed., 1970. *CRC Standard Mathematical Tables*, 18th ed., Cleveland, OH: Chemical Rubber Company.

Stark, L., 1968. *Neurological Control Systems*, New York: Plenum Press.

Tanji, J. and Kato, M., 1973. Firing rate of individual motor units in voluntary contraction in abductor digital minimi muscle in man, *Experimental Neurology*, 40:771–783.

Van Valkenburg, M.E., 1964. *Network Analysis*, 2nd ed., Englewood Cliffs, NJ: Prentice-Hall.

Wilkie, D.R., 1950. Relation between force and velocity in human muscle, *Journal of Physiology*, 110:249–280.

Yamada, H., 1970. *Strength of Biological Materials*, Baltimore: Williams & Wilkins.

5

Models of the Upper Limbs

5.1 Anatomy of the Hand and Wrist

5.1.1 Bones of the Hand and Wrist

The human hand has 27 bones divided into three groups: 8 *carpal* bones in the wrist, 5 *metacarpal* bones, and 14 *phalanges* of the fingers. The *carpal* bones are arranged in two rows and have names reflecting their shapes (Figure 5.1). The bones of the distal row, from the lateral side to the medial side, include the *trapezium* (four sided with two parallel sides), *the trapezoid* (four sided), the *capitate* (the central bone), and the *hamate* (hook shaped). These four bones fit together tightly bound by interosseous ligaments to form a relatively immobile unit that articulates with the metacarpals to form the *carpometacarpal* (CMC) joint. The bones of the proximal row include the *scaphoid* (boat shaped), the *lunate* (half-moon shaped), *the triquetrum* (triangle shaped), and the *pisiform* (pea shaped). The proximal surfaces of the scaphoid, lunate, and triquetrum form a biconvex elliptical surface, which articulates with the biconcave surface of the distal extremity of the radius. The articulation between the proximal and distal rows is termed the mid-carpal joint while articulations between adjacent bones are called intercarpal joints.

The five metacarpal bones are cylindrical in shape and articulate proximally with the distal carpal bones and distally with the proximal phalanges of the digits. The bases of the metacarpal bones of the index and middle fingers are linked together tightly and articulate little with the trapezoid and the capitate bones in the CMC joint. On the other hand, the CMC joint for metacarpals of the ring and little fingers with the hamate allows up to 10 to 15° and 20 to 30° of flexion/extension, respectively. The arched shafts of the metacarpal bones form the palm and the distal ends are spherical in shape, allowing articulation with the base of the corresponding phalanges. Interosseous muscles and extensor tendons run along the concave side and the large and smooth dorsal surface of the shaft, respectively, while the distal ends have a grooved volar surface for the flexor tendons (Nordin and Frankel, 2001).

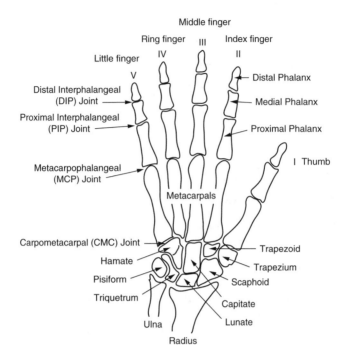

FIGURE 5.1
Bones and joints of the right hand (palmar view).

There are three phalanges for each digit and two for the thumb for a total of 14 bones. They are labeled proximal, middle, and distal phalanges (with the middle one missing in the thumb), according to their positions and become progressively smaller. The heads of the proximal and middle phalanges are bicondylar, facilitating flexion and extension and circumduction. The shafts are semicircular in cross section (the palmar surface is almost flat), as opposed to the cylindrical metacarpals. The axes of the distal phalanges of the index, ring, and little fingers are, respectively, deviated ulnarly, radially, and radially from the axes of the middle phalanges (Gigis and Kuczynski, 1982).

5.1.2   Joints of the Hand

There are four joints in each finger, in sequence from the proximal to distal: CMC, *metacarpophalangeal* (MCP), *proximal interphalangeal* (PIP), and *distal interphalangeal* (DIP) joints (see Figure 5.1). As mentioned in Section 5.1.1, the CMC joints are formed by the bases of the four metacarpals and the distal carpal bones and are stabilized by interosseous ligaments to form a relatively immobile joint. However, a major function of the CMC joint is to form the hollow of the palm and allow the hand and digits to conform to the shape of the object being handled (Norkin and Levangie, 1992).

The MCP joints are composed of the convex metacarpal head and the concave base of the proximal phalanx and stabilized by a joint capsule and ligaments. Flexion of 90° and extension of 20 to 30° from neutral take place in the sagittal plane. The range of flexion differs among fingers (and individuals) with the index finger having the smallest flexion angle of 70° and the little finger showing the largest angle of 95° (Batmanabane and Malathi, 1985). Radial and ulnar deviation of approximately 40 to 60° occurs in the frontal plane, with the index finger showing up to 60° abduction and adduction, the middle and ring fingers up to 45°, and the little finger about 50° of mostly abduction (Steindler, 1955). The range of motion at the MCP joint decreases as the flexion angle increases because of the bicondylar metacarpal structure (Youm et al., 1978; Schultz et al., 1987). There is also some axial rotation of the fingers from a pronated to a supinated position as the fingers are extended. In the reverse motion, the fingers crowd together as they enter flexion (Steindler, 1955).

The IP joints, as hinge joints, exhibit only flexion and extension. Each finger has two IP joints, the PIP and the DIP, except the thumb, which has only one. Volar and collateral ligaments, connected with expansion sheets of the extensor tendons, prevent any side-to-side motion. The largest flexion range of 100 to 110° is found in the PIP joints, while a smaller flexion range of 60 to 70° is found in the DIP joints. Hyperextension or extension beyond the neutral position, due to ligament laxity, can also be found in both DIP and PIP joints (Steindler, 1955).

5.1.3   Muscle of the Forearm, Wrist, and Hand

The muscles producing movement of the fingers are divided into two groups — extrinsic and intrinsic — based on the origin of the muscles. The *extrinsic* muscles originate primarily in the forearm, while the *intrinsic* muscles originate primarily in the hand. Therefore, the extrinsic muscles are large and provide strength, while the intrinsic muscles are small and provide precise coordination for the fingers. Each finger is innervated by both sets of muscles, requiring good coordination for hand movement.

The extrinsic muscles are divided into flexors found primarily on the anterior forearm (Figure 5.2) and extensors found primarily on the posterior forearm (Figure 5.3). Most of the flexors originate from the medial epicondyle of the humerus while most of extensors originate from the lateral epicondyle of the humerus. Both sets of muscles insert on the carpal bones, metacarpals, or phalanges. Each group can be further divided into superficial and deep groups of muscles as categorized in greater detail in Table 5.1.

The intrinsic muscles are divided into three groups: the thenar, the hypothenar, and the midpalmar muscle groups. The *thenar* group acts on the thumb and comprises the thenar eminence at the base of the thumb. The *hypothenar* group acts on the little finger and comprises the hypothenar eminence at the base of the medial palm. The midpalmar muscles act on all of

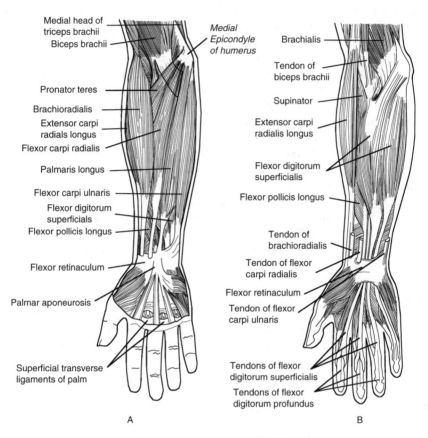

Medial head of
triceps brachii
Biceps brachii

Medial Epicondyle of humerus

Brachialis

Tendon of
biceps brachii

Pronator teres

Supinator

Brachioradialis

Extensor carpi
radials longus

Flexor carpi radialis

Extensor carpi
radialis longus

Palmaris longus

Flexor digitorum
superficialis

Flexor carpi ulnaris

Flexor pollicis longus

Flexor digitorum
superficials
Flexor pollicis longus

Tendon of
brachioradialis

Flexor retinaculum

Tendon of flexor
carpi radialis

Palmar aponeurosis

Flexor retinaculum

Tendon of flexor
carpi ulnaris

Superficial transverse
ligaments of palm

Tendons of flexor
digitorum superficialis

Tendons of flexor
digitorum profundus

A   B

FIGURE 5.2
Anterior muscles of the right hand: (A) superficial layer, (B) middle layer. (Adapted from Spence, 1990.)

the phalanges except the thumb. Primarily located on the palmar side, these intrinsic muscles allow for the independent flexion/extension and abduction/adduction of each of the phalanges, giving rise to precise finger movements. These muscles are shown in Figure 5.4 and categorized in Table 5.2.

5.1.4 Flexor Digitorum Profundus and Flexor Digitorum Superficialis

The *flexor digitorum profundus* (FDP) and flexor *digitorum superficialis* (FDS) are the main finger flexor muscles and are involved in most repetitive work. Using electromyography (EMG), Long et al. (1970) identified the FDP as the muscle performing most of the unloaded finger flexion, while the FDS comes into play when additional strength is needed, with the FDP comprising about 12% of the total muscle capability below the elbow. There is significant variation in force contributions of the FDS tendons for each finger (0.9 to 3.4%) while the FDP tendons provide a relatively constant force contribution

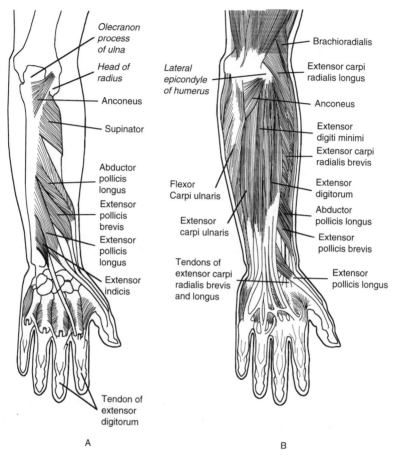

FIGURE 5.3
Posterior muscles of the right hand: (A) deep layer, (B) superficial layer. (Adapted from Spence, 1990.)

to each finger (2.7 to 3.4%). This results in a relatively large range of force ratios, from 1.5 to 3. Average FDP resting tendon fiber length is slightly shorter than for the average FDS tendon. Table 5.3 provides a summary of the general mechanical characteristics of the FDP and FDS tendons for each finger.

The FDP originates from the proximal anterior and medial surface of the ulna and inserts into the base of the distal phalanx (Figure 5.5). In the midforearm, the muscle divides into two bellies: the radial and the ulnar. The radial part inserts into the index finger, while the ulnar part inserts into middle, ring, and little fingers. Consequently, the latter three fingers tend to move together, while the index finger can function independently of the others. The FDP tendon passes along the finger through a series of pulleys, which maintain a reasonably constant moment arm for flexing or extending the finger. Before inserting into the distal phalanx, the FDP passes through a split in the FDS tendon (Fahrer, 1971; Steinberg, 1992; Brand and Hollister, 1993).

TABLE 5.1

Extrinsic Muscles of the Hand and Wrist

Group	Layer	Name	Nerve	Function
Anterior	Superficial	Flexor carpi radialis	Median	Flexes and adducts hand Aids in flexion/pronation of forearm
		Palmaris longus	Median	Flexes hand
		Flexor carpi ulnaris	Ulnar	Flexes and adducts hand
	Middle	Flexor digitorum superficialis	Median	Flexes phalanges and hand
	Deep	Flexor digitorum profundus	Median, ulnar	Flexes phalanges and hand
Posterior	Superficial	Extensor carpi radialis longus	Radial	Extends and abducts hand
		Extensor carpi radialis brevis	Radial	Extends hand
		Extensor digitorum	Radial	Extends little finger
		Extensor digiti minimi	Radial	Extends little finger
		Extensor carpi ulnaris	Radial	Extends and adducts hand
	Deep	Abductor pollicis longus	Radial	Abducts thumb and hand
		Extensor pollicis brevis	Radial	Extends thumb
		Extensor pollicis longus	Radial	Extends thumb
		Extensor indicis	Radial	Extends index finger

Source: Adapted from Spence (1990); Tubiana (1981).

5.1.5 Flexor Tendon Sheath Pulley Systems

The tendon sheath is a double-walled tube, surrounding the tendons and containing synovial fluid. The synovial sheath provides both a low-friction-gliding as well as a nutritional environment for the flexor tendon. The flexor tendon sheath, sometimes termed the fibrosseous tunnel, begins at the neck of the metacarpal phalanx, ends at the distal interphalangeal joint, and is held against the phalanges by pulleys. These pulleys primarily act to prevent tendon bowstringing across the joints during flexion but also maintain a relatively constant moment arm.

The pulleys can be divided into three types based on their locations: a palmar aponeurosis pulley, five *annular* (ring-shaped) pulleys (A1, A2, A3, A4, and A5), and three *cruciate* (cross-like) pulleys (C1, C2, and C3). The A2 and A4 pulleys are located on the proximal and middle phalanges, while the A1, A3, and A5 pulleys are located at the palmar surface of the MCP, PIP, and DIP joints (Figure 5.6) The A2 and A4 pulleys are most important for normal function and a stable joint, with the A3 and other pulleys coming into play when the A2 and A4 have been damaged (Manske and Lesker, 1977; Idler, 1985; Lin et al., 1990). Such damage to the pulleys can occur in extreme activities, in which much of the body weight is supported by the fingers, such as rock climbing. Although the A3 pulley is relatively weaker and closer to the PIP joint, it is more flexible and stretches, transferring the load to the A2 and A4 pulleys, which then fail first (Marco et al., 1998).

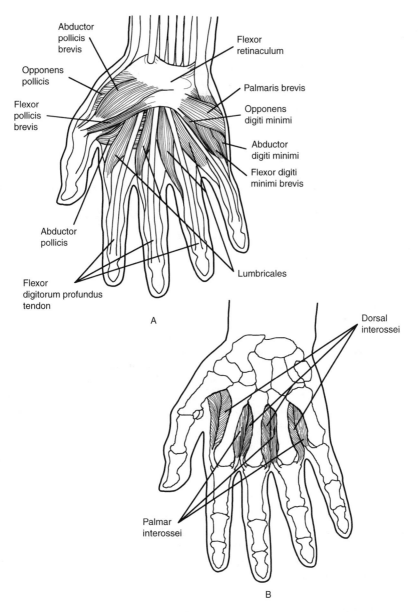

FIGURE 5.4
Intrinsic muscles of the hand: (A) palmar view, (B) dorsal view. (Adapted from Spence, 1990.)

5.1.6 Wrist Mechanics

The seven main muscles involved in wrist and hand motion are flexor carpi radialis (FCR), flexor carpi ulnaris (FCU), flexor digitorum profundus (FDP), flexor digitorum superficialis (FDS), extensor carpi radialis brevis (ECRB),

TABLE 5.2

Intrinsic Muscles of the Hand and Wrist

Group	Name	Nerve	Function
Thenar muscles	Abductor pollicis brevis	Median	Abducts thumb
	Opponens pollicis	Median	Pulls thumb toward little finger
	Flexor pollicis brevis	Median	Flexes thumb
	Adductor pollicis	Ulnar	Adducts thumb
Hypothenar	Palmaris brevis	Ulnar	Folds skin on ulnar side of palm
muscles	Abductor digiti minimi	Ulnar	Abducts little finger
	Flexor digiti minimi	Ulnar	Flexes little finger
	Opponens digiti minimi	Ulnar	Pulls little finger toward thumb
Midpalmar	Lumbricales	Median, ulnar	Flex proximal phalanges
muscles	Dorsal interossei	Ulnar	Abduct fingers
	Palmar inerossei	Ulnar	Adduct fingers

Source: Adapted from Spence (1990); Tubiana (1981).

TABLE 5.3

General Characteristics of the FDP and FDS Tendons

	Resting Fiber Length (cm)[a]		Moment Arm (cm)[b]						Relative Force of Finger Flexors (%)[c]		
			DIP Joint		PIP Joint		MCP Joint				
Finger	FDP	FDS	FDP	FDS	FDP	FDS	FDP	FDS	FDP	FDS	FDP/FDS
Index	6.6	7.2	0.65	—	0.98	0.83	1.01	1.21	2.7	2.0	1.35
Middle	6.6	7.0	0.70	—	1.07	0.87	1.16	1.40	3.4	3.4	1.00
Ring	6.8	7.3	0.68	—	1.04	0.85	1.04	1.30	3.0	2.0	1.50
Little	6.2	7.0	0.60	—	0.85	0.74	0.89	0.98	2.8	0.90	3.11

[a] Brand et al., 1981.
[b] Ketchum et al., 1978.
[c] Brand and Hollister, 1993.

extensor carpi radialis longus (ECRL), and extensor carpi radialis ulnaris (ECU) (Garcia-Elias et al., 1991). The primary function of the FCR, FCU, ECRB, ECRL, and ECU is to move the wrist, while the FDP and FDS are secondary wrist movers. The primary function of the FDP and FDS is to flex and extend the fingers and secondarily to rotate the wrist. The FDP and FDS pass through carpal tunnel. The primary muscles and tendons involved with wrist movements of flexion, extension, radial, and ulnar deviation planes are listed below (An et al., 1981):

Flexion: FCR and FCU

Extension: ECRB, ECRL, and ECU

Radial deviation: FCR, ECRB, and ECRL

Ulnar deviation: FCU and ECU

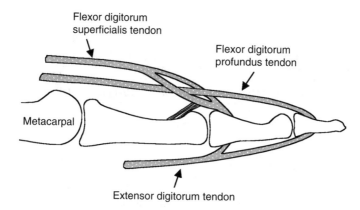

FIGURE 5.5
FDP and FDS tendons of a typical digit. (From Thompson, J.S., 1977. *Core Textbook of Anatomy,* Philadelphia: J.B. Lippincott. With permission.)

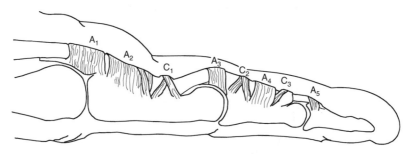

FIGURE 5.6
Pulley structure of the finger (A = annular, C = cruciate). (Adapted from Nordin and Frankel, 2001.)

The parameters that have been commonly used to describe the muscles are muscle fiber length (FL) and physiological cross-sectional area (PCSA). Muscle length is related to mechanical potential for tendon excursion, and the maximum tension of the muscle to its PCSA (An et al., 1991). In moving the wrist, each tendon across the wrist joint slides a certain distance to execute the movement, and the tendon excursion and moment arm at various wrist joint angles can be measured and derived through experiments (Armstrong and Chaffin, 1978; An et al., 1991). Muscle parameters, tendon excursions, and moment arms at wrist joint (An et al., 1981, 1991; Lieber et al., 1990) are summarized in Table 5.4. The magnitudes of tendon excursion were measured over a 100° range of motion in the flexion–extension plane and a 50° range of motion in the radial-ulnar deviation plane in forearm neutral position.

Table 5.4 reveals that the FCR, FCU, and ECRB provide larger tendon excursion during flexion and extension movement than ECRL and ECU, while ECRL and ECU have greater tendon excursion during radial and ulnar

TABLE 5.4

Physiological and Mechanical Properties of Wrist Joint Muscles and Tendons

Muscle and Tendon	Physiological Size		Tendon Excursion (mm)		Moment Arm (mm)[a]	
	Length (cm)	PCSA (cm²)	F/E plane	R/U plane	F/E plane	R/U plane
FCR	10.9–12.4	2.0	25 ± 4	7 ± 1	+15 ± 3	+8 ± 2
FCU	15.2–15.4	3.2–3.4	28 ± 4	12 ± 3	+16 ± 3	−14 ± 3
ECRB	13.8–15.8	2.7–2.9	20 ± 3	11 ± 1	−12 ± 2	+13 ± 2
ECRL	11.8–18.3	1.5–2.4	12 ± 3	17 ± 1	−7 ± 2	+19 ± 2
ECU	13.6–14.9	2.6–3.4	10 ± 2	16 ± 2	−6 ± 1	−17 ± 3

[a] + denotes flexion and radial deviation; − denotes extension and ulnar deviation.

Source: Adapted from An et al. (1981, 1991); Lieber et al. (1990).

TABLE 5.5

Phalange Lengths as Percent of Hand Length for Males and Females

Phalanx	Proximal	Medial	Distal
Thumb	17.1	—	12.1
Index	21.8	14.1	8.6
Middle	24.5	15.8	9.8
Ring	22.2	15.3	9.7
Little	17.7	10.8	8.6

Source: Davidoff (1990); Davidoff and Freivalds (1993).

deviation movement. The results also demonstrate that the FCR and FCU are prime muscles for flexion, ECRB for extension, ECRL for radial deviation, and ECU for ulnar deviation. In spite of the three-dimensional orientation of the wrist tendons to the rotation axes and the complexity of carpal bone motion, Table 5.5 indicates that the moment arms of wrist motion are maintained fairly consistently and correspond well with the anatomical location of the tendons. According to An et al. (1991), these findings are related to the anatomical considerations; the extensor retinaculum ensures a consistent relationship of the wrist extensors (ECRB, ECBL, and ECU) to the rotation axes, while the FCR is firmly fixed in the fibro-osseous groove, and the FCU infixed on the pisiform.

5.1.7   Select Finger Anthropometry Data

As discussed in Section 1.5, for any sort of biomechanical modeling using static equilibrium analyses, it is necessary to have a variety of key anthropometric properties, such as segment link lengths, segment weights, the location of the center of gravity, the location of the center of joint rotation,

TABLE 5.6

Interphalangeal Joint Dimensions — Mean and
(Standard Deviations) in mm

Joint	Breadth		Thickness	
	Male	Female	Male	Female
IP (I)	22.9 (3.8)	19.1 (1.3)	20.1 (1.5)	16.8 (1.0)
PIP (II)	21.3 (1.3)	18.3 (1.0)	19.6 (1.3)	16.3 (1.0)
DIP (II)	18.3 (1.3)	15.5 (1.0)	15.5 (1.3)	13.0 (1.0)
PIP (III)	21.8 (1.3)	18.3 (1.0)	20.1 (1.5)	16.8 (1.0)
DIP (III)	18.3 (1.3)	15.2 (1.0)	16.0 (1.3)	13.2 (1.0)
PIP (IV)	20.1 (1.3)	18.3 (1.0)	18.8 (1.3)	15.8 (1.0)
DIP (IV)	17.3 (1.0)	14.5 (0.8)	15.2 (1.3)	12.5 (0.8)
PIP (V)	17.8 (1.5)	14.5 (0.8)	16.8 (1.3)	14.0 (1.0)
DIP (V)	15.8 (1.3)	13.2 (0.8)	13.7 (1.3)	11.4 (0.8)

Note: I = thumb, II = index finger, III = middle, IV = ring,
V = little finger.

Source: Garrett (1970a,b).

TABLE 5.7

Location of Finger Joint Centers
from Distal End of Phalanx

Finger	DIP	PIP	MCP
Index	18	13	20
Middle	15	12	20
Ring	13	12	19
Little	17	14	24

Note: DIP distances as % of medial phalanx length, PIP and MCP distances
as % of proximal phalanx length.

Source: Adapted from An et al. (1979).

the range of motion for each joint, and muscle insertion points. Not all of
this information has been measured or documented at the level of individual
phalanges, but the following tables may provide some useful data: Table 5.5,
phalange lengths; Table 5.6, interphalangeal joint dimensions; Table 5.7,
interphalangeal joint flexion and extension ranges; Table 5.8, joint center
locations; and Table 5.9, tendon insertion points. The last two tables were
adapted from the data of An et al. (1979) based on three separate coordinate
systems located at the center of joint rotation for each phalanx, as shown in
Figure 5.7. Note the x-axis is in the axial direction of the phalanx, with the
positive direction pointing proximally. The y-axis is perpendicular with the
positive direction pointing dorsally. The positive z-axis points radially for
the right hand. However, any deviations in the z-direction were generally
minimal and were omitted for simplicity. The tendon insertion points of

TABLE 5.8

Interphalangeal Joint Flexion and Extension Ranges —
Means and (Standard Deviations) in Degrees

Joint	Flexion		Extension	
	Male	Female	Male	Female
MCP (I)	56.3 (21.8)	60.0 (14.5)	3.7 (7.4)	11.2 (13.2)
IP (I)	62.3 (22.2)	67.2 (16.9)	21.5 (22.8)	21.5 (23.6)
MCP (II)	85.2 (7.4)	84.7 (7.8)	15.1 (10.7)	20.9 (8.0)
PIP (II)	94.8 (13.7)	103.8 (5.0)	0.3 (1.3)	0.0
DIP (II)	77.5 (13.0)	81.0 (5.4)	1.3 (3.5)	0.9 (3.6)
MCP (III)	86.7 (6.7)	89.1 (7.6)	13.5 (10.0)	19.7 (7.2)
PIP (III)	88.8 (23.8)	102.2 (5.0)	0.0	0.3 (5.7)
DIP (III)	80.2 (12.0)	83.5 (7.0)	0.0	0.9 (3.6)
MCP (IV)	86.0 (5.1)	87.4 (6.4)	13.5 (10.0)	19.4 (8.3)
PIP (IV)	93.2 (13.4)	100.9 (6.4)	0.0	0.0
DIP (IV)	79.1 (12.8)	80.0 (8.5)	0.0	0.9 (3.6)
MCP (V)	83.7 (7.9)	86.5 (6.8)	14.1 (8.3)	21.5 (6.8)
PIP (V)	90.5 (13.4)	96.6 (6.9)	0.0	0.0
DIP (V)	77.8 (11.5)	78.5 (10.7)	0.7 (2.6)	1.2 (3.8)

Source: Davidoff and Freivalds (1993).

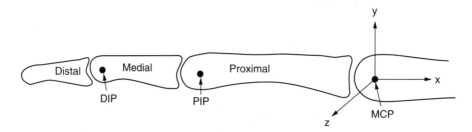

FIGURE 5.7
Finger coordinate system. (Adapted from An et al., 1979.)

Table 5.9 correspond approximately to the location of the five annular pulleys
described in Section 5.1.5. This still allows for adequate modeling of finger
flexion in the *x*–*y* plane. Other, more functional, data on the hand can be
found in Garrett (1971) and detailed data on muscle moment arms and
tendon excursions for the index finger can be found in An et al. (1983).

5.2   Static Tendon–Pulley Models

Landsmeer (1960, 1962) developed three biomechanical models for finger flexor
tendon displacements, in which the tendon–joint displacement relationships

TABLE 5.9

Representative Tendon Insertion Distances for Each Finger with Respect to That Joint's Center Coordinate System

| | | Index Finger | | | | Middle Finger | | | | Ring Finger | | | | Little Finger | | | |
| | | Distal | | Proximal | | Distal | | Proximal | | Distal | | Proximal | | Distal | | Proximal | |
Joint	Muscle	x	y	x	y	x	y	x	y	x	y	x	y	x	y	x	y
DIP	FDP	-18	-13	25	-22	-19	-12	26	-22	-19	-13	26	-22	-18	-15	2	-20
PIP	FDP	-22	-14	18	-17	-27	-15	22	-14	-28	-16	23	-16	-24	-15	20	-18
	FDS	-22	-11	18	-13	-27	-11	22	-12	-28	-13	23	-13	-24	-13	20	-15
MCP	FDP	-24	-17	13	-27	-30	-18	16	-26	-31	-16	17	-26	-27	-20	15	-28
	FDS	-24	-22	13	-31	-30	-18	16	-31	-31	-19	17	-29	-27	-24	15	-32

Note: See Figure 5.7. DIP distances as % of medial phalanx length, PIP and MCP distances as % of proximal phalanx length.

Source: Adapted from An et al. (1979).

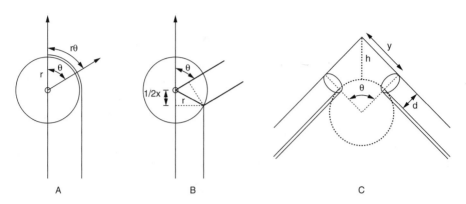

FIGURE 5.8
Landsmeer's tendon models: (A) Model I, (B) Model II, (C) Model III. (Adapted from Landsmeer, 1962.)

are determined by the spatial relationships between the tendons and joints. In Model I (Figure 5.8A), Landsmeer assumed that the tendon is held securely against the curved articular surface of the proximal bone of the joint, and the proximal articular surface can be described as a trochlea. Such a model is particularly useful in describing extensor muscles. The tendon displacement relationship is described by

$$x = r\theta \tag{5.1}$$

where
x = tendon displacement
r = distance from the joint center to the tendon
θ = joint rotation angle

However, if the tendon is not held securely, it may be displaced from the joint when the joint is flexed and will settle in a position along the bisection of the joint angle (Figure 5.8B). Model II is useful for describing tendon displacement in intrinsic muscles as

$$x = 2r\sin(\theta/2) \tag{5.2}$$

Landsmeer's (1960) Model III depicts a tendon running through a tendon sheath held securely against the bone, which allows the tendon to curve smoothly around the joint (Figure 5.8C). The tendon displacement is described by

$$x = 2\left[y + \tfrac{1}{2}\theta\left(d - y/\tan\tfrac{1}{2}\theta\right)\right] \tag{5.3}$$

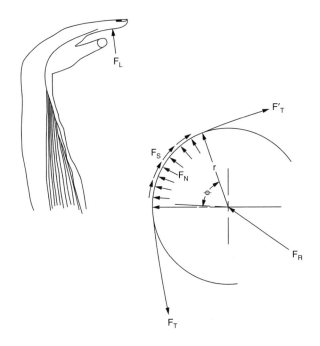

FIGURE 5.9
Armstrong tendon–pulley model for the wrist. (From Chaffin, D.B. et al., 1999. *Occupational Biomechanics*, 3rd ed., New York: John Wiley & Sons. With permission.)

where
y = tendon length to joint axis measured along long axis of bone
d = distance of tendon to the long axis of bone

For small angles of flexion (< 20°), tan θ is almost equal to θ, and Equation 5.3 simplifies to

$$x = d\theta \tag{5.4}$$

Armstrong and Chaffin (1979) proposed a static model for the wrist based on Landsmeer's (1962) tendon Model I and LeVeau's (1977) pulley-friction concepts (Figure 5.9). Armstrong and Chaffin (1978) found that, when the wrist is flexed, the flexor tendons are supported by *flexor retinaculum* on the volar side of the carpal tunnel. When the wrist is extended, the flexor tendons are supported by the carpal bones. Thus, deviation of the wrist from neutral position causes the tendons to be displaced against and past the adjacent walls of the carpal tunnel. They assumed that a tendon sliding over a curved surface is analogous to a belt incurring friction forces while wrapped around a pulley, as described in Section 1.7. The radial reaction force on the ligament or the carpal bones, F_R, can be characterized as follows:

$$F_R = 2F_T e^{\mu\Theta} \sin\left(\theta/2\right) \tag{5.5}$$

where
F_R = radial reaction force
F_T = tendon force or belt tension
μ = coefficient of friction between tendon and supporting tissues
θ = wrist deviation angle (in radians)

The resulting normal forces on the tendon exerted by the pulley surface can be expressed per unit arc length as

$$F_N = \frac{2F_T e^{\mu\theta} \sin(\theta/2)}{r\theta} \qquad (5.6)$$

where
F_N = normal forces exerted on tendon
r = radius of curvature around supporting tissues

For small coefficient of frictions, comparable to what is found in joints ($\mu <$ 0.04) and for small angles of θ, Equation 5.6 reduces to the simple expression:

$$F_N = F_T/r \qquad (5.7)$$

Thus, F_N is a function of only the tendon force and the radius of curvature. As the tendon force increases or the radius of curvature decreases (e.g., small wrists), the normal supporting force exerted on tendon increases. F_R, on the other hand, is independent of radius of curvature but is dependent on the wrist deviation angle.

This tendon–pulley model provides a relatively simple mechanism for calculating the normal supporting force exerted on tendons that are a major factor in work-related musculoskeletal disorders (WRMSDs). However, this model does not include the dynamic components of wrist movements such as angular velocity and acceleration, which might be risk factors in WRMSDs.

5.3 Dynamic Tendon–Pulley Models

Schoenmarklin and Marras' (1990) dynamic biomechanical model extended Armstrong and Chaffin's (1979) static model to include a dynamic component of angular acceleration (Figure 5.10). The dynamic model is two dimensional in that only the forces in flexion and extension plane are analyzed. This model investigates the effects of maximum angular acceleration on the resultant reaction force that the wrist ligaments and carpal bones exert on tendons and their sheaths.

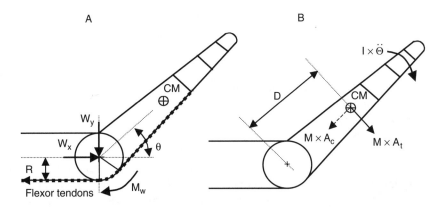

FIGURE 5.10
Dynamic tendon–pulley model for the wrist. (A) Free-body diagram; (B) mass × acceleration diagram. (Adapted from Schoenmarklin and Marras, 1990.)

Key forces and movements in the model include the reaction force at the center of the wrist (W_x and W_y), the couple or moment (M_w) required to flex and extend the wrist, and the inertial force ($M \times A_n$ and $M \times A_t$) and inertial moment ($I \times \ddot{\Theta}$) acting around the hand's center of mass. For equilibrium, the magnitude of moment around the wrist in the free-body diagram must equal the magnitude of moment acting around the hand's center of mass in the moment acceleration diagram:

$$F_T R = \left(MA_t + MA_c\right)D + I\ddot{\Theta} \tag{5.8}$$

where
M = mass
A_t = tangential acceleration
A_c = centripetal acceleration
F_T = tendon force
I = moment of inertia of the hand in flexion and extension
$\ddot{\Theta}$ = angular acceleration

Thus, the hand is assumed to accelerate from a stationary posture, so, the angular velocity is theoretically zero, resulting in zero centripetal force ($A_c = V^2/R = 0$). Then,

$$F_T R = MDA_t + I\ddot{\Theta} \tag{5.9}$$

$$F_T R = MD^2\ddot{\Theta} + I\ddot{\Theta} \tag{5.10}$$

$$F_T = \frac{\left(MD^2 + I\right)\ddot{\Theta}}{R} \tag{5.11}$$

$$F_R = 2\frac{\left(MD^2 + I\right)\ddot{\Theta}}{R}\sin\frac{\theta}{2} \qquad (5.12)$$

where
R = radius of curvature of the tendon
D = distance between the center of mass of hand and wrist
M = weight of hand
θ = wrist deviation angle

The above equations indicate that the resultant reaction force, F_R, is a function of angular acceleration, radius of curvature, and wrist deviation. Thus, exertion of wrist and hand with greatly angular acceleration and deviated wrist angle would result in greater total resultant reaction forces on the tendons and supporting tissues than exertions with small angular acceleration and neutral wrist position. According to Armstrong and Chaffin (1979), increases in resultant reaction force would increase the supporting force that the carpal bones and ligaments exert on the flexor tendons, therefore increasing the chance of inflammation and risk of carpal tunnel syndrome (CTS). Therefore, these results might provide theoretical support to why angular acceleration variable can be considered a risk factor of WRMSDs.

The advantage of Schoenmarklin and Marras' (1990) model is that it does include the dynamic variable of angular acceleration into assessment of resultant reaction force on the tendons. But the model is two dimensional, and it does not consider the coactivation of antagonistic muscles in wrist joint motions. This points to the need for further model developments to account for additional physiological factors.

5.4 Complex Tendon Models

Any model that incorporates more than the one muscle–tendon unit of the above models, all of sudden, becomes much more complicated, because the number of unknown muscle forces exceeds the number of equilibrium or constraint equations. This is known as the statically indeterminate problem. The two main approaches utilized in solving this problem are reduction methods and optimization methods.

5.4.1 Reduction Methods

The main objective of the reduction method is to reduce the number of excessive variables until the number of unknown forces is equal to the number of required equilibrium equations eliminating static indeterminacy.

Smith et al. (1964) initiated mathematical analyses of the finger tendon forces to find the effects of the flexor tendons acting on MCP joint deformed by rheumatoid arthritis. They used a two-dimensional model to analyze the MCP joint and muscle forces of the index finger during tip pinch. To reduce the number of unknown muscle forces, the following assumptions were applied: (1) the sum of the interosseous (I) forces is treated as a single force 2I; (2) half of the interosseous forces of I act at the PIP joint and the other half act at the DIP joint; (3) the lumbrical (L) is much smaller than the I, as much as I. They solved the three moment equations using these assumptions and anthropometrical data of the index finger obtained from a cadaver hand in a tip pinch position. They reported the tendon forces normalized to the external force F, as $3.8F$. $2.5F$, $0.9F$, and $0.3F$ for the FDP, FDS, I, and L, respectively. They also found a value of $7.5F$ for the MCP joint force. The results indicate that the flexor tendons are dominant and the forces are many times larger than the intrinsic muscle forces during tip pinch.

Chao et al. (1976) presented a comprehensive analysis of the three-dimensional tendon and joint forces of the fingers in pinch and power grip functions. Kirschner wires (K-wires) were drilled through the phalanges to fix the finger configuration in the desired position and different surgical wires were inserted into the tendon and muscles of hand specimens of the cadaver to identify different tendons on x-ray film. The exact orientations of finger digits and the locations of the tendons were defined by bi-planar x-ray analysis. Through a free-body analysis, 19 independent equations were obtained for 23 unknown joint and tendon forces. Using the permutation-combination principle of setting any four of the nine tendon forces equal to zero solved the indeterminate problem. The selection of these tendons was based primarily on EMG responses and physiological assessment. They found that high constraint forces and moments at the DIP and PIP joints were found during pinches, whereas large magnitudes of constraint forces at the MCP joint were found during power grips. The total of the intrinsic muscles (RI, UI, and LI) produced a greater force than the total of the flexor tendons (FDP and FDS) in both pinch and power grip actions.

5.4.2 Optimization Methods

An alternative method using a typical optimization technique was suggested by Seireg and Arvikar (1973) and Penrod et al. (1974). In this approach, force equilibrium equations and anatomical constraint relationships were used for the equality constraints and the physiological limits on the tendon; muscle and joint forces were applied as the inequality constraints. In addition, the most important factor in this method is optimal criteria that correspond to the objective function of the formulation. The possible solutions can vary based on the optimal criteria selected.

Chao and An (1978a) studied the middle finger during tip pinch and power grip actions, with an aid of three-dimensional analysis. They analyzed the same problem using the optimization and linear programming (LP) technique of Chao et al. (1976) instead of the previously described EMG and permutation-combination method. The predicted middle finger muscle and joint forces were very similar to those of the previous study (Penrod et al., 1976), except for the intrinsic muscle forces whose predicted values were considerably lower. They found that the highest joint contact forces for all three joints occurred for pinch grip rather than power grip. They also found that the main flexors (FDP and FDS) were most active in both pinch and power grip functions, whereas the intrinsic muscles were less active in power grip than in pinch.

An et al. (1985) also applied LP optimization techniques to solve the indeterminate problem of a three-dimensional analytic hand model. The ranges of muscle forces of the index finger under isometric hand functions, such as tip pinch, lateral key pinch, power grip, and other functional activities were analyzed. FDP and FDS carried high tendon forces compared with other muscles in most hand functions, although the predicted FDS force was zero in a pinch grip. The long extensors (LE) and two intrinsic muscles contributed large forces in the key pinch. The large force of these intrinsic muscles in pinch action can be explained by the role of these muscles in maintaining balance and stabilization of the MCP joint. The joint constraint forces for each finger were also studied. The Chao et al. (1976) study showed a trend for joint constraint forces in which the DIP joint had the lowest force and the force progressively increased for the PIP joint and was largest at the MCP joint. An et al. (1985) showed the same trend in lateral pinch functions.

5.4.3   Combined Approaches

Chao and An (1978b) used a graphical presentation with a combined permutation and optimization technique to solve the statically indeterminate tendon force problem. They analyzed the maximum tip pinch force of the index finger as a function of external force directions (0, 30, and 45°) and the DIP joint flexion angles (10 to 50°). The results showed that the pinch strength relied on the direction of applied external force, as well as the finger joint configuration. The tendon forces of the index finger were also studied with the same finger posture as that in the Chao et al. (1976) study, but only one angle (45°) of the external force was assumed. Also, the predicted extrinsic extensor tendon force was considerably larger than in their previous studies.

Weightman and Amis (1982) presented a good critical review for the previously published studies and applied their two-dimensional finger model to the analysis of resultant joint forces and muscle tensions in various pinch actions. To create a statically determinate problem, all joints were assumed to be pin joints with a fixed center of rotation during flexion. The relationships of the intrinsic muscle forces were assumed identical to those of Chao and An (1978a), except that the long extensor muscles forces dropped to zero. They also used the PCSA of the muscles to define the force distributions in the intrinsic muscles. Their results compared to other previously published studies with a good correlation of both muscle and joint force predictions. Based on these comparisons, they verified that a two-dimensional finger model could be valid for analyzing two-dimensional finger actions, even though realistically any finger motion is still three dimensional.

5.5 A Two-Dimensional Hand Model

From a biomechanical perspective, the extrinsic finger flexors, FDP and FDS, comprise the main sources of power for finger flexion in grasping type motions, especially the power grip. Also, because most of the tendon–pulley attachments are in line with the long axis (i.e., x-axis) of the phalanges (see Section 5.1.7) and there are small lateral force components (i.e., along the z-axis), only two axes, the x and y, need to be defined. Therefore, a simple two-dimensional model utilizing those two tendons should be sufficient for most applications.

To further define the model, several other assumptions need to be made. These are as follows:

1. The effects of intrinsic muscles and extensors on the finger flexion can be neglected because these muscles will typically be in a relaxed state during the normal range of motion for a power grip (Armstrong, 1976; Cailliet, 1994).

2. All of the interphalangeal and metacarpal joints (DIP, PIP, and MP joints) are assumed to be pure hinge joints, allowing only flexion and extension.

3. Anatomic analysis shows that the FDS is inserted by two slips to either side of the proximal end of the middle phalanx (Steinberg, 1992; Cailliet, 1994). It is assumed that each FDS tendon is inserted to the palmar side of the proximal end of the middle phalange, parallel to the long axis. In a two-dimensional biomechanical model, the effect of having two splits inserted along the sides of the bone is the same as having one tendon inserted on the palmar side of the proximal end of the middle phalange.

4. Tendons and tendon sheaths are modeled as a frictionless cable-and-pulley system. Therefore, a single tendon passing through several joints maintains the same tensile force (Chao et al., 1976).

5. The externally applied forces are assumed to be a single unit-force exerted at the midpoint pulp of a distal phalange for pinch or by three-unit forces applied normally at the midpoint of each phalange and metacarpal bone for grasp as shown in Figure 5.10. The direction

of the force is assumed to be perpendicular to the long axis of the bone.

6. The weight of the bones together with other soft tissues on the hand is assumed to be negligible.

7. Due to indeterminacy, the tendon force ratio of FDP to FDS at each phalange is assumed to be 3:1, i.e., $\alpha = 0.333$ (Marco et al., 1998).

8. FDP and FDS tendon moment arms (in millimeter) are estimated for DIP, PIP, and MCP joints of different thickness equations from the equations of Armstrong (1976):

$$PR_{ik} = 6.19 - 1.66X_1 - 4.03X_2 + 0.225X_3 \qquad (5.13)$$

$$SR_{ik} = 6.42 + 0.10X_1 - 4.03X_2 + 0.225X_3 \qquad (5.14)$$

where
PR_{ik} = FDP moment arm for the ith finger and kth joints
SR_{ik} = FDS moment arm for the ith finger and kth joints
X_1 = 1 for PIP and 0 for all others
X_2 = 1 for DIP and 0 for all others
X_3 = joint thickness (mm) from Table 5.6

Consequently, the pertinent equations are as follows:

$$PR_{DIP} = 2.16 + 0.225X_3 \qquad (5.15)$$

$$PR_{PIP} = 4.53 + 0.225X_3 \qquad (5.16)$$

$$SR_{PIP} = 6.52 + 0.225X_3 \qquad (5.17)$$

$$PR_{MCP} = 6.19 + 0.225X_3 \qquad (5.18)$$

$$SR_{MCP} = 6.42 + 0.225X_3 \qquad (5.19)$$

Four Cartesian coordinate systems are established to define the locations and orientations of the tendons and to describe the joint configuration (Figure 5.11). There are two coordinate systems for both the middle and proximal phalanges and only one system for the distal and metacarpal phalanges. The y-axis is defined along the long axis of the each phalanx, from the proximal end to the distal end. The x-axis is defined as perpendicular to the long axis of each phalanx and in the palmar-dorsal plane, from the palmar side to the dorsal side of the finger bone. Both x- and y-axes have their origins at the

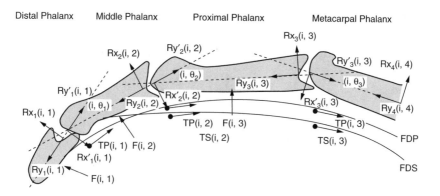

FIGURE 5.11
Free-body diagram for a two-dimensional hand model. For symbols and notation, see text. (From Kong, Y.K., 2001. Optimum Design of Handle Shape through Biomechanical Modeling of Hand Tendon Forces, Ph.D. dissertation, University Park, PA: Pennsylvania State University. With permission.)

center of the proximal end of phalanx. Note that these definitions are different from that used by An et al. (1979) in Figure 5.7 and Tables 5.8 and 5.9.

In terms of notation, subscript i refers to fingers, with 1 to 4 for the index, middle, ring, and little fingers, respectively, subscript j refers to joints, with 1 to 4 for the DIP, PIP, MP, and wrist joints, respectively, while subscript k refers to phalanges, with 1 to 4 for the distal, middle, proximal phalanges, and the metacarpal bone, respectively.

In terms of model input values, the external force on each phalange of each finger is indicated by $F(i,k)$. The finger joint flexion angles, measured with reference to straight fingers as the hand is lying flat, are indicated by (i,θ_j). The length of each phalanx for each finger is indicated by $L(i,k)$.

For the model output variables, the FDP tendon force for each phalanx of each finger is indicated by $TP(i,k)$. The FDS tendon force for each phalanx of each finger is indicated by $TS(i,k)$. Finally, joint constraint forces along the X_k- and Y_k-axes are indicated by $Rx_k(i,j)$ and $Ry_k(i,j)$, respectively.

To solve for the above unknown model output variables, a static equilibrium analyses (per Section 1.5) of each phalanx must be performed. Specifically the summation of forces acting on each phalanx in the x- and y-axes must be zero. Similarly, the summation of all moments acting on each phalanx must also be equal to zero. The resulting equations for the distal phalanx are

$$TP(i,1) = 0.5L(i,1)F(i,1)/PR(i,1) \tag{5.20}$$

$$Ry_1(i,1) = TP(i,1)\cos(i,\theta_1) \tag{5.21}$$

$$Rx_1(i,1) = TP(i,1)\sin(i,\theta_1) - F(i,1) \tag{5.22}$$

For the middle phalanx, they are

$$TP(i,2) = \frac{\left[0.5F(i,2) - Rx_1(i,1)\cos(i,\theta_1) + Ry_1(i,1)\sin(i,\theta_1)\right]L(i,2)}{\alpha SR(i,2) + PR(i,2)} \tag{5.23}$$

$$TS(i,2) = \alpha TP(i,2) \tag{5.24}$$

$$Ry_2(i,2) = Rx_1(i,1)\sin(i,\theta_1) + Ry_1(i,1)\cos(i,\theta_1) + (\alpha+1)TP(i,2)\cos(i,\theta_2) \tag{5.25}$$

$$Rx_2(i,2) = Rx_1(i,1)\cos(i,\theta_1) - Ry_1(i,1)\sin(i,\theta_1) + (\alpha+1)TP(i,2)\sin(i,\theta_2) \\ - F(i,2) \tag{5.26}$$

For the proximal phalanx, they are

$$TP(i,3) = \frac{\left[0.5F(i,3) - Rx_2(i,2)\cos(i,\theta_2) + Ry_2(i,2)\sin(i,\theta_2)\right]L(i,3)}{\alpha SR(i,3) + PR(i,3)} \tag{5.27}$$

$$TS(i,3) = \alpha TP(i,3) \tag{5.28}$$

$$Ry_3(i,3) = Rx_2(i,2)\sin(i,\theta_2) + Ry_2(i,2)\cos(i,\theta_2) + (\alpha+1)TP(i,3)\cos(i,\theta_3) \tag{5.29}$$

$$Rx_3(i,3) = Rx_2(i,2)\cos(i,\theta_2) - Ry_2(i,2)\sin(i,\theta_2) + (\alpha+1)TP(i,3)\sin(i,\theta_3) \\ - F(i,3) \tag{5.30}$$

One interesting application of such a biomechanical hand model is to identify the optimum handle size for gripping so as to minimize tendon forces. However, in a typical power grip, there are two alternative ways in which the geometry of a cylindrical handle surface and phalange contacts can be defined. In Grip I (Figure 5.12), the point of contact between the distal phalange (L_1) and a handle is assumed to be at the middle point of the distal phalange; i.e., the distal phalange is divided into two equal lengths ($L_1/2$). The bisector of the DIP angle establishes a right triangle with the distal phalanx as the base and the altitude passing through the contact point to the center of handle. Through trigonometry, the DIP joint angle then becomes

$$\theta_1' = 2\tan^{-1}\left[2(R+D_1)/L_1\right] \tag{5.31}$$

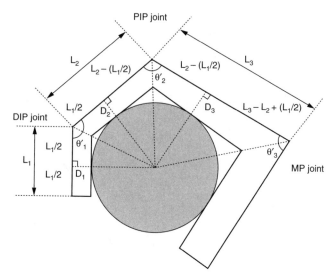

FIGURE 5.12

Schematic diagram of Grip I. (From Kong, Y.K., 2001. Optimum Design of Handle Shape through Biomechanical Modeling of Hand Tendon Forces, Ph.D. dissertation, University Park, PA: Pennsylvania State University. With permission.)

where
θ'_1 = DIP joint angle
R = radius of the cylindrical handle
D_1 = thickness of distal phalanx

The second contact point (between the middle phalange, L_2, and the handle) divides the middle phalange into two unequal lengths, one being $L_1/2$ (due to the DIP bisector) and the other being $L_2 - L_1/2$. The bisector of the PIP angle establishes a right triangle with the medial phalanx as the base and the altitude again passing through the contact point to the center of handle. Through trigonometry, the PIP joint angle then becomes

$$\theta'_2 = 2\tan^{-1}\frac{2(R+D_2)}{2L_2 - L_1} \tag{5.32}$$

where
θ'_2 = PIP joint angle
D_2 = thickness of medial phalanx

The third contact point with the handle also divides the proximal phalange (L_3) into two parts, one the same length as the proximal part of middle phalange ($L_2 - L_1/2$) and the other ($L_3 - L_2 + L_1/2$). The bisector of the MP angle established another right triangle as previously leading to

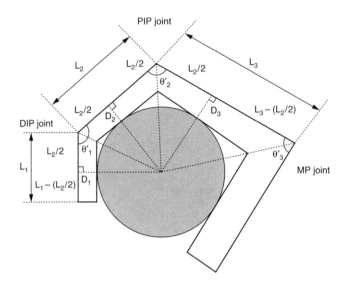

FIGURE 5.13
Schematic diagram of Grip II. (From Kong, Y.K., 2001. Optimum Design of Handle Shape through Biomechanical Modeling of Hand Tendon Forces, Ph.D. dissertation, University Park, PA: Pennsylvania State University. With permission.)

$$\theta'_3 = 2\tan^{-1}\frac{2(R+D_3)}{2L_3 - 2L_2 + L_1} \tag{5.33}$$

where θ'_3 = MP joint angle.

In the case of Grip II (Figure 5.13), the second contact point is assumed to divide the medial phalanx into two equal lengths ($L_2/2$). The perpendicular bisector of the medial phalanx forms two identical right triangles, yielding equal DIP and PIP joint angles (θ'_1 and θ'_2):

$$\theta'_1 = \theta'_2 = 2\tan^{-1}\left[2(R+D_2)/L_2\right] \tag{5.34}$$

The third contact point divides the proximal phalange into two unequal lengths. One is $L_2/2$ while the other is $L_3 - L_2/2$. The MP joint angle (θ'_3) can then be estimated as

$$\theta'_3 = 2\tan^{-1}\frac{2(R+D_3)}{2L_3 - L_2} \tag{5.35}$$

Based on this biomechanical hand model, tendon forces for each finger and in total were calculated for both types of grip and for 11 cylindrical handles with diameters ranging from 10 to 60 mm. For Grip I, tendon forces were minimized at 30 to 35 mm, 38 to 43 mm, 40 to 45 mm, and 25 to 30

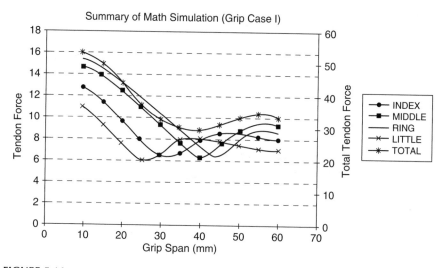

FIGURE 5.14

Finger tendon forces for Grip I. (From Kong, Y.K., 2001. Optimum Design of Handle Shape through Biomechanical Modeling of Hand Tendon Forces, Ph.D. dissertation, University Park, PA: Pennsylvania State University. With permission.)

mm for index, middle, ring, and little fingers, respectively. The total of tendon force for all fingers was minimized for an approximately 40-mm cylindrical handle (Figure 5.14). As the size of the handle deviated above or below 40 mm, the total tendon forces increased.

For Grip II, tendon forces were minimized at 23 to 28 mm, 28 to 33 mm, 28 to 33 mm, and 20 to 25 mm for index, middle, ring, and little fingers, respectively. The total of tendon force for all fingers was minimized for an approximately 28-mm cylindrical handle (Figure 5.15). The combined results for each type of grip are summarized in Table 5.10. As noted previously, as the size of the handle deviates from the optimum size, tendon forces increase. This is an important principle that should be utilized in the design of hand tools (see Section 9.3.2). Also, in either type of grip, the optimal handle sizes depends greatly on which finger is considered. Therefore, a purely traditional cylindrical handle cannot provide optimality for all fingers simultaneously and alternative handle shapes need to be considered (see Section 9.3.3). Further details can be found in Kong (2001) and Kong, Freivalds, and Kim (in press) with applications to meat hook handles in Kong and Freivalds (2003).

5.6 Direct Measurement Validation Studies

Directly measured tendon forces under isometric finger function were first reported by Bright and Urbaniak (1976). They developed a strain gauge to

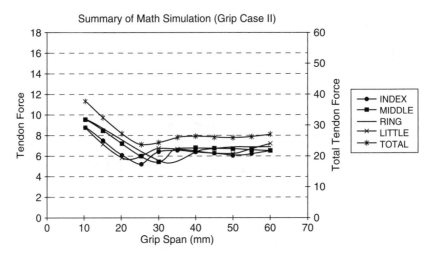

FIGURE 5.15
Finger tendon forces for Grip II. (From Kong, Y.K., 2001. Optimum Design of Handle Shape through Biomechanical Modeling of Hand Tendon Forces, Ph.D. dissertation, University Park, PA: Pennsylvania State University. With permission.)

TABLE 5.10

Summary of Optimal Cylindrical Handle Sizes

Finger	Grip I	Grip II	Combined Grip
Index	30	25	25–30
Middle	40	30	30–40
Ring	40	30	30–40
Little	25	20	20–25

measure the tendon forces in both tip pinch and power grip actions during operative procedures. Flexor tendon forces were found to be in the range of 40 to 200 N and 12.5 to 150 N for the FDP and FDS, respectively, in power grip action, while 25 to 125 N for the FDP and 10 to 75 N for the FDS in pinch action. Because they directly measured the tendon forces only, they did not report the actual applied pinch and power grip force and the ratio of tendon force to the externally applied force.

Schuind et al. (1992) directly measured the flexor tendons (FPL, FDP, and FDS) during various finger functions. They developed an S-shaped tendon force transducer and measured the flexor tendon forces in pinch and power grip functions. Also, a pinch dynamometer was used to record the applied loads in pinch action. The tendon forces showed proportionality to the externally applied forces. To compare their results with the previously published mathematical finger models, they normalized their tendon forces, as a ratio of the tendon force to the applied forces. In tip pinch, the ratios were 3.6*F,*

7.92F, and 1.73F, for the externally applied force F, for the FPL, FDP, and FDS, respectively. In lateral pinches, the ratios were 3.05F, 2.9F, and 0.71F for the FPL, FDP, and FDS, respectively. Although the FDP and FPL showed high forces during tip and lateral pinch, the maximal values recorded are probably on the lower side of the potential forces, which could be explained by the significantly weaker pinch and power grip forces during carpal tunnel surgery due to the denervation or partial anesthesia of the sensory area of the median nerve. However, the magnitude of tendon forces was similar to values reported by Bright and Urbaniak (1976), although direct comparison is not possible as the applied force was not recorded in their study.

In another *in vivo* tendon force measurement study, Dennerlein et al. (1998) measured only the FDS tendon forces of the middle finger at three finger postures, which ranged from extended to flexed pinch postures, using a gas-sterilized tendon force transducer (Dennerlein et al., 1997) and a single axis load cell. The investigation was centered on the average ratio of the FDS tendon tension to the externally applied force. The average ratio ranged from 1.7F to 5.8F, with a mean of 3.3F, in the study. Tip pinches with the DIP joint flexed were also studied with a tendon-to-tip force ratio of 2.4F. These ratios were compared with the results of their own three finger models as well as other contemporarily published isometric tendon force models. These ratios were larger than those of other studies. The average values were also slightly higher than that (1.73F) of Schuind et al.'s (1992) *in vivo* tendon force measurement study. It was found that the tendon force ratios and muscle strength varied substantially from individual to individual, although the ratio of force from tendon to tendon was relatively constant within the same limb for all studies (Ketchum et al., 1978; Brand et al., 1981; Dennerlein et al., 1998). A summary of these tendon force models is given in Table 5.11.

5.7   Critical Evaluation of Modeling Approaches

Although the intrinsic muscles are more active in pinch action than in power grip action, the relative magnitudes of the main flexor tendon forces (such as FDP and FDS) are usually high in both actions. These *in vivo* tendon forces of the flexors are presented in Table 5.12 based on the previous studies. In general, these averages and ranges of tendon forces are very similar, with a few exceptions. Schuind et al. (1992) showed lower FDS tendon forces in power grip action than those of other types of grips. The tendon force ranges of Brand et al. (1981) show similar magnitudes with Bright and Urbaniak (1976) power grips. Ketchum et al. (1978) and Bright et al. (1976) tip pinch actions also show the similar ranges of tendon forces. Schuind et al. (1992) represented the significant differences between FDP and FDS tendon forces in both pinch and power grip, whereas the others showed that the force of FDP tendon was only slightly larger than that of the FDS tendon. These

TABLE 5.11

Summary of Tendon Force Models

Model		Ref.	Key Features
Static		Landsmeer (1960, 1962)	Simplest tendon pulley model
		Armstrong and Chaffin (1978, 1979)	Pulley model with tendon force
Dynamic		Schoenmarklin and Marras (1990)	Pulley model with acceleration
Complex tendon forces	Reduction	Smith et al. (1964)	2D, scaled tendon forces
		Smith et al. (1964)	3D, some forces set equal to zero
	Optimization	Seireg and Arvikar (1973)	Objective function with constraints
		Penrod et al. (1974)	Objective function with constraints
		Chao and An (1978a)	3D, linear programming
		An et al. (1985)	3D, linear programming
	Combined	Chao and An (1978b)	Graphical, optimization
		Weightman and Amis (1982)	Some $F = 0$, some $F \propto$ muscle area
In vivo studies		Bright and Urbaniak (1976)	Strain gauge
		Schuind et al. (1992)	S-shape tendon force transducer
		Dennerlein et al. (1998)	Gas-sterilized tendon force transducer

TABLE 5.12

In Vivo FDP and FDS Tendon Forces (kg)

Study	Finger Configuration	FDP	FDS
Brand et al. (1981)	—	14.9* (13.5–17.0)	10.4* (4.5–17)
Ketchum et al. (1978)	MCP joint flexion	5.7* (5.27–6.18)	6.12* (3.73–7.63)
Bright and Urbaniak (1976)	Tip Pinch	2.5–12.5	1.0–7.5
	Power grip	4.0–20.0	1.25–15.0
Schuind et al. (1992)	Tip pinch	8.3 (2.0–12.0)	1.9 (0.3–3.5)
	Power grip	4.0 (1.9–6.4)	0.6 (0.0–0.9)

* Average tendon forces for all fingers.

discrepancies can be explained by the different finger postures utilized in each study, as each finger could have various functional muscle capacities depending on its joint configuration (Chao and An, 1978b).

In all these *in vivo* tendon force studies, the muscle and tendon forces were proportional to the externally applied forces. However, these predicted maximum tendon forces are probably lower than the true potential forces because these experiments were performed during carpal tunnel surgery under local anesthesia in the median nerve innervation area. In such case, the muscles are partially inactive and produce lower pinch and power grip forces. To normalize these tendon forces, the ratios of the tendon force to the applied force, FDP to FDS, and joint forces were studied for both pinch and power grip functions (Table 5.13 and Table 5.14).

TABLE 5.13

Tendon and Joint Forces during Pinch (normalized to external force)

Study	Pinch Type	Muscle Force				Joint Force		
		FDP	FDS	FDP/FDS	I	DIP	PIP	MCP
Bright and Urbaniak (1976)	Tip	2.50–12.5 kg*	1.0–7.5 kg*					
Schuind et al. (1992)	Tip	7.92	1.73	4.60				
	Lateral	2.90	0.71	4.08				
Dennerlein et al. (1998)	Tip	—	3.30 (1.7–5.8)					
Smith et al. (1964)	Tip	3.80	2.50	1.52	2.10			7.50
Chao et al. (1976)	Tip, Radial, Ulnar	4.32	0.73	5.90	7.05			8.80
Chao and An (1978)	Tip***	3.30	3.10	1.06	2.41	5.60	6.00	
Chao and An (1978)	Tip	3.97	0.82	4.84	3.11	4.68	8.29	8.51
Weightman and Amis (1982)	Tip	2.40**	1.85**	1.30				
An et al. (1985)	Tip	1.93–2.08	1.75–2.16		0–0.99	2.40	4.40	3.50

Note: * = tendon force; ** = average value for various finger configurations; *** = middle finger tip pinch.

TABLE 5.14

Tendon and Joint Forces in Power Grip (normalized to external force)

| Study | Finger | Tendon Force | | | | Joint Force | | |
		FDP	FDS	FDP/FDS	I	DIP	PIP	MCP
Bright and Urbaniak (1976)		4.0–20.0*	1.25–15.0*					
Schuind et al. (1992)		4.0**	0.6**	6.67				
Chao et al. (1976)	Index	2.77	2.53	1.09	15.76	3.09	4.35	12.70
	Middle	3.05	4.23	0.72	13.10	3.17	7.11	13.90
	Little	3.37	3.40	0.99	15.21	3.31	6.02	14.50
Chao and An (1978)	Middle	3.37	3.75	0.90	1.64	3.89	6.80	5.18
An et al. (1985)	Index	3.17–3.47	1.51–2.14		0.1–1.19	2.8–3.4	4.5–5.3	3.2–3.7

Note: * = tendon force, unit: kg; ** = mean tendon forces, unit: kg.

Average ratios of tendon forces to the applied forces in the tendon force prediction models were, for an external force of F, $3.5F$, $1.8F$, and $3.67F$ for the FDP, FDS, and I (intrinsic) tendons in pinch, while $3.14F$, $3.48F$, and $11.4F$ were for FDP, FDS, and I tendons in power grip, respectively. Generally, all data agreed with high contributions of flexor tendons (FDP and FDS) for both pinch and power grip actions, although intrinsic tendons showed high variations among those data. The average ratios of FDP to FDS were also obtained, 2.92:1 and 0.93:1 for pinch and power grip, respectively. These data showed the significant strength contribution of the FDP tendon to the pinch, as opposed to the fairly equal contributions of these two flexors to the overall power grips.

Although they did not measure the externally applied force with the tendon forces in a power grip, Schuind et al. (1992) attempted to validate these mathematical solutions experimentally. They used the pinch dynamometer only for measuring the amount of the applied force for pinch functions. Thus, the mean tendon forces were applied for validating power grip functions in this study.

In pinch studies, Schuind et al. (1992) reported the higher ratio of FDP to the applied force ($7.92F$) than the result ($3.5F$) of mathematical tendon force prediction models. The FDS ratio to the applied force ($1.73F$), however, was fairly similar to the average ratio ($1.8F$) in the finger model studies. Because of the large force measurement for the FDP tendon, a higher ratio of FDP/ FDS ($4.6F$) was presented in their study than that of finger model studies. Dennerlein et al. (1998) also found higher ratios of the FDS tendon to the applied force ($3.3F$) than those of mathematical finger model studies.

In power grip studies, there are few *in vivo* data on the ratio of tendon force to externally applied force. Thus, only the FDP:FDS ratio of direct measurement study can be used for the comparison with finger model studies. Schuind et al. (1992) presented a 6.67:1 ratio based on their mean tendon forces of FDP and FDS. The force of FDP was significantly larger than that of FDS in direct measurement studies (Table 5.12). DP and FDS showed similar contributions to power grip ($3.14F$ for FDP and $3.48F$ for FDS; Kong, 2001) and a FDP:FDS ratio of 0.93:1 was also calculated in finger force prediction models. The variability of these results may be expected because all researchers did not use the same finger characteristics: moment arms, finger configurations, and angles of the applied forces to the finger tip regarding the function of intrinsic vs. flexor muscles during pinch and power grips. Based on the solutions from the three moment equations, Smith et al. (1964) found that flexor tendons usually carry larger forces than other intrinsic muscles during tip pinch. Chao and An (1978b) also supported this result in their study. They showed the flexors were most active and produced high tendon forces in both pinch and power grip actions. However, Chao et al. (1976) and An et al. (1985) suggested contradictory results for the contributions of intrinsic muscles in finger actions. They presented higher contributions of intrinsic muscles than those of flexors did in pinch and power grip functions. In general, although the magnitude of the intrinsic muscle force was less than that of the flexors, the intrinsic muscles were more active in pinches than in power grip. An et al. (1985) also agreed with high intrinsic muscle forces in pinches and explained it by the need for these intrinsic muscles to balance and stabilize the large MCP joint forces.

Most of these studies showed similar trends for joint forces. Small constraint forces and moments were seen at both the DIP and PIP joints, while the constraint forces and moments were considerably higher at the MCP joint in both actions. DIP and PIP joint forces of the power grip actions were relatively lower than those of the pinch actions. It may explain why hands are more adaptable in performing powerful grip actions rather than with pinches since it is more difficult to maintain the proper stability requirements at the distal joints (Chao et al., 1976).

Questions

1. Describe the structural anatomy of the hand and wrist.
2. Describe the musculature needed to produce a gripping action.
3. What are the major differences between extrinsic and intrinsic muscles?
4. Compare and contrast the flexor digitorum profundus and flexor digitorum superficialis.
5. Describe the flexor tendon–pulley systems.
6. What is bowstringing?
7. Compare and contrast the three Landsmeer pulley models.
8. What is the reasoning behind the development of tendon strain and tendinitis in repeated manual exertions?

9. What is the reasoning behind the development of tendon strain and tendinitis in hand motions with extreme deviations?

10. Why is it thought that individuals with small wrists may be more susceptible to injuries than those with large wrists?

11. How do the effects of dynamics modify the static tendon–pulley models?

12. How can static indeterminancy problems be handled in hand/wrist models?

13. In a model of a power grip, what are the two major approaches or assumptions needed to begin the modeling process?

14. Compared to the external forces, what are the ranges of tendon forces predicted by modeling and reported by direct measurement? What are the differences between a power and pinch grip?

Problems

5.1. Complete the development of Landsmeer's Model III, that is, derive Equation 5.3.

5.2. Compare the differences in tendon forces predicted by the three Landsmeer models.

5.3. What is the relative difference in tendon forces resulting between the two different assumptions used in modeling a power grip (i.e., Kong's Grip I and Grip II)?

5.4. Using Kong's (2001) model, estimate the tendon forces (normalized to external force) required for pressing down with an extended finger (e.g., pressing a button).

References

An, K.N., Chao, E.Y., Cooney, W.P., and Linscheid, R.L., 1979. Normative model of human hand for biomechanical analysis, *Journal of Biomechanics*, 12:775–788.

An, K.N., Hui, F.C., Morrey, B.F., Linscheid, R.L., and Chao, E.Y.S., 1981. Muscle across the elbow joint: a biomechanical analysis, *Journal of Biomechanics*, 14:659–669.

An, K.N., Ueba, Y., Chao, E.Y., Cooney, W.P., and Linscheid, R.L., 1983. Tendon excursion and moment arm of index finger muscles, *Journal of Biomechanics*, 16:419–425.

An, K.N., Chao, E.Y., Cooney, W.P., and Linscheid, R.L., 1985. Forces in the normal and abnormal hand, *Journal of Orthopaedic Research*, 3:202–211.

An, K.N., Horii, E., and Ryu, J., 1991. Muscle function, in An, K.N., Berger, R.A., and Cooney, W.P. (Eds.), *Biomechanics of the Wrist Joint*, New York: Springer-Verlag, pp. 157–169.

Armstrong, T.J., 1976. Circulatory and Local Muscle Responses to Static Manual Work, Ph.D. dissertation, Ann Arbor, MI: University of Michigan.

Armstrong, T.J. and Chaffin, D.B., 1978. An investigation of the relationship between displacements of the finger and wrist joints and the extrinsic finger flexor tendons, *Journal of Biomechanics*, 11:119–128.

Armstrong, T.J. and Chaffin, D.B., 1979. Some biomechanical aspects of the carpal tunnel, *Journal of Biomechanics*, 12:567–570.

Batmanabane, M. and Malathi, S., 1985. Movements at the carpometacarpal and metacarpophalangeal joints of the hand and their effect on the dimensions of the articular ends of the metacarpal bones, *Anatomical Record*, 213:102–110.

Brand, P.W. and Hollister, A., 1993. *Clinical Mechanics of the Hand*, 2nd ed., St. Louis, MO: Mosby-Year Book.

Brand, P.W., Beach, R.B., and Thompson, D.E., 1981. Relative tension and potential excursion of muscles in the forearm and hand, *Journal of Hand Surgery*, 6:209–218.

Bright, D.S. and Urbaniak, J.S., 1976. Direct measurements of flexor tendon tension during active and passive digit motion and its application to flexor tendon surgery, *Transactions 22nd Annual Orthopedic Research Society*, 240.

Cailliet, R., 1994. *Hand Pain and Impairment*, 3rd ed., Philadelphia: Davis.

Chaffin, D.B., Andersson, G.B.J., and Martin, B.J., 1999. *Occupational Biomechanics*, 3rd ed., New York: John Wiley & Sons.

Chao, E.Y.S. and An, K.N., 1978a. Determination of internal forces in human hand, *Journal of Engineering Mechanics Division ASCE*, 104:255–272.

Chao, E.Y.S. and An, K.N., 1978b. Graphical interpretation of the solution to the redundant problem in biomechanics, *Journal of Biomechanics*, 11:159–167.

Chao, E.Y.S., Opgrande, J.D, and Axmear, F.E., 1976. Three-dimensional force analysis of finger joints in selected isometric hand functions, *Journal of Biomechanics*, 9:387–396.

Cooney, W.P and Chao, E.Y.S., 1977. Biomechanical analysis of static forces in the thumb during hand function, *Journal of Bone and Joint Surgery*, 59A:27–36.

Davidoff, N.A., 1990. The Development of a Graphic Model of a Human Hand, M.S. thesis, University Park, PA: Pennsylvania State University.

Davidoff, N.A. and Freivalds, A., 1993. A graphic model of the human hand using CATIA, *International Journal of Industrial Ergonomics*, 12:255–264.

Dennerlein, J.T, Miller, J., Mote, C.D., Jr., and Rempel, D.M., 1997. A low profile human tendon force transducer: the influence of tendon thickness on calibration, *Journal of Biomechanics*, 30:395–397.

Dennerlein, J.T, Diao, E., Mote, C.D., Jr., and Rempel, D.M., 1998. Tensions of the flexor digitorum superficialis are higher than a current model predicts, *Journal of Biomechanics*, 31:295–301.

Fahrer, M., 1971. Considerations on functional anatomy of the flexor digitorum profundus, *Annales de Chirurgie*, 25:945.

Garcia-Elias, M., Horii, E. and Berger, R.A., 1991. Individual carpal bone motion, in An, K.-N., Berger, R.A., and Cooney, W.P., Eds., *Biomechanics of the Wrist Joint*, New York: Springer-Verlag, 61–75.

Garrett, J.W., 1970a. Anthropometry of the Air Force Female Hand, AMRL-TR-69-26, Wright Patterson Air Force Base, OH: Aerospace Medical Research Laboratory.

Garrett, J.W., 1970b. Anthropometry of the Hands of Male Air Force Flight Personnel, AMRL-TR-69-42, Wright Patterson Air Force Base, OH: Aerospace Medical Research Laboratory.

Garrett, J.W., 1971. The adult human hand: some anthropometric and biomechanical considerations, *Human Factors*, 13:117–131.

Gigis, P.I. and Kuczynski, K., 1982. The distal interphalangeal joints of the human fingers, *Journal of Hand Surgery*, 7:176–182.

Idler, R.S., 1985. Anatomy and biomechanics of the digital flexor tendons, *Hand Clinic*, 1:3–12.

Ketchum, L.D., Thompson, D., Pocock, G., La, C., and Wallingford, D., 1978. A clinical study of forces generated by the intrinsic muscles of the index finger and the extrinsic flexor and extensor muscles of the hand, *Journal of Hand Surgery*, 3:571–578.

Kong, Y.K., 2001. Optimum Design of Handle Shape through Biomechanical Modeling of Hand Tendon Forces, Ph.D. dissertation, University Park, PA: Pennsylvania State University.

Kong, Y.K. and Freivalds, A., 2003. Evaluation of meat hook handle shapes, *International Journal of Industrial Ergonomics*, 32:13–23.

Kong, Y.K., Freivalds, A., and Kim, S.E., in press. Evaluation of handles in a maximum gripping task, *Ergonomics*.

Landsmeer, J.M.F., 1960. Studies in the anatomy of articulation, *Acta Morphologica Nederlands*, 3–4:287–303.

Landsmeer, J.M.F., 1962. Power grip and precision handling, *Annals of Rheumatoid Diseases*, 21:164–170.

LeVeau, B., 1977. *William and Lissner Biomechanics of Human Motion*, Philadelphia: W.B. Saunders.

Lieber, R.L., Fazeli, B.M., and Botte, M.J., 1990. Architecture of selected wrist flexor and extensor muscles, *Journal of Hand Surgery*, 15:244–250.

Lin, G.T., Cooney, W.P., Amadio, P.C., and An, K.N., 1990. Mechanical properties of human pulleys, *Journal of Hand Surgery*, 15B:429–434.

Long, C., Conrad, P.W., Hall, E.A., and Furler, S.L., 1970. Intrinsic-extrinsic muscle control of the hand in power grip and precision handling: an electromyographic study, *Journal of Bone and Joint Surgery*, 52A:853–867.

Manske, P.R. and Lesker, P.A., 1977. Strength of human pulleys, *Hand*, 9:147–152.

Marco, R.A.W., Sharkey, N.A., and Smith, T.S., 1998. Pathomechanics of closed rupture of the flexor tendon pulleys in rock climbers, *Journal of Bone and Joint Surgery*, 80A:1012–1019.

Nordin, M. and Frankel, V.H., 2001. *Basic Biomechanics of the Musculoskeletal System*, 3rd ed., Philadelphia: Lippincott/Williams & Wilkins.

Norkin, C.C. and Levangie, P.K., 1992. *Joint Structure & Function: A Comprehensive Analysis*, Philadelphia: Davis.

Penrod, D.D., Davy, D.T., and Singh, D.P., 1974. An optimization approach to tendon force analysis, *Journal of Biomechanics*, 7:123–129.

Schoenmarklin, R.W. and Marras, W.S., 1990. A dynamic biomechanical model of the wrist joint, *Proceedings of the Human Factors Society 34th Annual Meeting*, Santa Monica, CA: Human Factors Society, 805–809.

Schuind, F., Garcia-Elias, M., Cooney, W.P., III, and An, K.N., 1992. Flexor tendon forces: *in vivo* measurements, *Journal of Hand Surgery*, 17A:291–298.

Schultz, R.B., Stroave, A., and Krishnamurthy, S., 1987. Metacarpophalangeal joint motion and the role of the collateral ligaments, *International Orthopaedics*, 11:149–155.

Seireg, A. and Arvikar, R.B., 1973. A mathematical model for evaluation of forces in lower extremities of musculoskeletal system, *Journal of Biomechanics*, 6:313–326.

Smith, E.M., Juvenile, R.B., Bender, L.F., and Pearson, J.R., 1964. Role of the finger flexors in rheumatoid deformities of the metacarpophalangeal joints, *Arthritis and Rheumatism*, 7:467–480.

Spence, A.P., 1990. *Basic Human Anatomy*, 3rd ed., Redwood City, CA: Benjamin Cummings.

Steinberg, D.R., 1992. Acute flexor tendon injuries, *Orthopaedics Clinics of North America*, 23:125–140.

Steindler, A., 1955. *Kinesiology of the Human Body under Normal and Pathological Conditions*, Springfield, IL: Charles C Thomas.

Thompson, J.S., 1977. *Core Textbook of Anatomy*, Philadelphia: J.B. Lippincott.

Tubiana, R., Ed., 1981. *The Hand*, Vol. 1, Philadelphia, PA: Saunders.

Weightman, B. and Amis, A.A., 1982. Finger joint force predictions related to design of joint replacements, *Journal of Biomedical Engineering*, 4:197–205.

Youm, Y., McMurty, R.Y., Flatt, A.E., and Gillespie, T.E., 1978. Kinematics of the wrist, *Journal of Bone and Joint Surgery*, 60A:424–431.

6

Musculoskeletal Disorders and Risk Factors

6.1 The Extent of the Problem

There are six major surveys that have estimated the magnitude of musculoskeletal disorders (MSDs) in the general U.S. population: the National Health and Nutrition Examination Survey from 1976 to 1988, the National Ambulatory Medical Care Survey of 1989, the National Health Interview Surveys of 1988 and 1995, the Health and Retirement Survey from 1992 to 1994, and the Social Security Supplemental Security Income Survey of 1998. Unfortunately, all are based on individual self-reports and not on medical diagnosis, and none identifies the work-relatedness aspect, if any, of these disorders. Given that the vast majority of adults are in the active workforce, there would be difficulty in finding comprehensive data on an occupationally unexposed group, which, by definition, would be unrepresentative of the U.S. adult population.

In terms of overall MSDs, the 1988 National Health Interview Survey found a prevalence of almost 15% for the U.S. population (Lawrence et al., 1998), which stayed relatively constant at 13.9% for the 1995 survey (Praemer et al., 1999). However, Social Security Supplemental Security Income Survey of 1998 did indicate a noticeable increase in prevalence with age, 16.9% for those 50 to 59 and 23.9% for those 60 to 65. In terms of upper limb MSDs, the 1988 National Health Interview Survey found a prevalence of 9.4% in the hand or wrist, with 1.5% specifically carpal tunnel syndrome and 0.4% tendinitis (Tanaka et al. 1995). Interestingly, when based on reported symptoms, the prevalence for carpal tunnel syndrome can be as high as 14.4%, but when referred for a clinical diagnosis the prevalence drops to 2.7% (Atroshi et al., 1999).

Information about the work-related nature of MSDs is again difficult to obtain, as there is not one central comprehensive surveillance data system. Perhaps the best source of data is the Annual Survey of Occupational Injuries and Illnesses Survey, produced by the U.S. Department of Labor's Bureau of Labor Statistics (BLS). It covers private industry but excludes self-employed, small farms, and federal, state, and local government agencies, or about 25% of the total workforce, and is collected primarily from the injury and illness data reports required by the Occupational Safety and Health Administration (OSHA Form 200). One category subset is labeled "disorders associated with

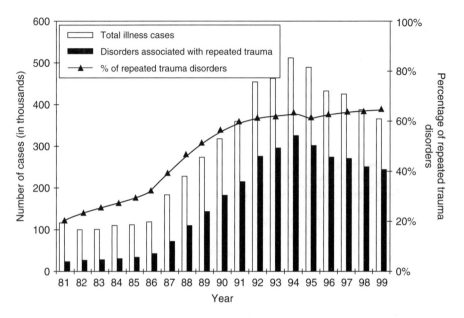

FIGURE 6.1

Incidence of disorders primarily associated with repeated trauma in private industry, 1982–1999. (Adapted from Bureau of Labor Statistics: http://www.bls.gov/iif/oshsum.htm.)

repeated trauma" and provides a historical trend in MSDs. The number of cases was relatively steady from 1976 to 1982 at around 22,000, then increased sharply to 332,100 by 1994, at which point there was a gradual reduction to 246,700 by 1999 (Figure 6.1). This recent decline was speculated to have occurred as a result of a better recognition of such MSDs and the implementation of industrial health and safety programs (Conway and Svenson, 1998).

Further evidence for the work-relatedness of these types of musculoskel-etal injuries can be found from the survey data of Tanaka et al. (1995, 1997). Of the 1.87 million reporting having symptoms of carpal tunnel syndrome, a third were diagnosed has having the condition by the health-care provider and more than one half believed these were work related. Of the nearly 600,000 reporting tendinitis symptoms, 28% were labeled as work related by a health-care provider. In summary, all of these surveys and studies indicate a large-scale work-related problem that had a rapid growth in the 1980s and early 1990s with a slight decline in recent years.

6.2   Common MSDs and Their Etiology

There are a large variety of MSDs that have some commonality both in the physiological or anatomical characteristics and in the general location of the

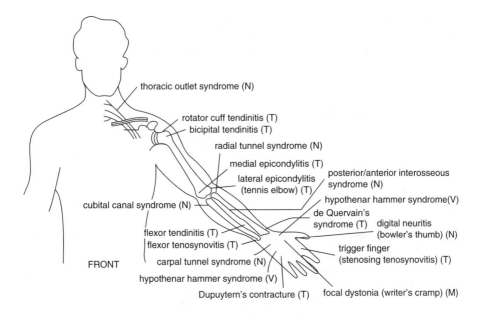

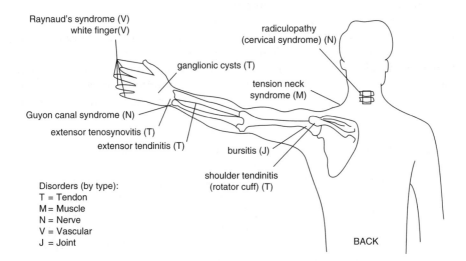

FIGURE 6.2

Examples of musculoskeletal disorders that may be work related. (From Kuorinka, I. and Forcier, L., 1995. *Work Related Musculoskeletal Disorders (WMSDs): A Reference Book for Prevention*, London: Taylor & Francis. With permission.)

problem (Figure 6.2). For introducing and describing common MSDs it is best to categorize them by the anatomical characteristics, while later, in providing more detailed scientific evidence for risk factors, it is best to categorize them by joint. It would not be unusual for a complaining worker or the medically untrained ergonomist to lump medically different disorders into one collective "shoulder" disorder, since, probably, neither can identify the disorder more specifically. From the anatomical viewpoint, MSDs can be classified into six basic types: tendon, muscle, nerve, vascular, bursa, and bone/cartilage.

6.2.1   Tendon Disorders

The tendon, as described previously in Chapter 2, is the part of the muscle and the surrounding fascia transmitting force from the muscle that attaches to the bone and produces joint motion. In places where there is a great deal of movement (e.g., fingers, wrist, shoulder) the tendon may pass through a sheath that protects and lubricates the tendon to reduce friction. When this sheath and the tendon within become inflamed, it is termed *tenosynovitis*. When a tendon without the sheath becomes inflamed, it is termed *tendinitis*. This inflammation can progress to the point of having microtrauma or even visible fraying of the tendon fibers. Sometimes, cases are further identified as to sublevel where found on the tendon. *Enthesopathy* or insertional tendinitis occurs at the tendon–bone interface with relatively little inflammation. A common one is enthesopathy of the extensor carpi radialis brevis from the lateral epicondyle, resulting from forceful, twisting motions, which then is referred to as *lateral epicondylitis*, or more commonly as *tennis elbow*. *Peritendinitis* refers to the inflammation of the tendon proper, where there is no tendon sheath, while the inflammation of the muscle–tendon interface is termed *myotendinitis*. Although technically they are all different disorders, they are often found together and exhibit similar symptoms of localized pain and tenderness and are typically collectively referred to as tendinitis. Two common examples of tendinitis are *bicipital tendinitis*, or inflammation of the long head of the biceps tendon as it passes over the head of the humerus through the bicipital groove caused by hyperabducting the elbow or forceful contractions of the biceps, and *rotator cuff tendinitis*, inflammation of tendons of various muscles around the shoulder (supraspinatus, infraspinatus, teres minor) caused from abducted arms or arms raised above the shoulders.

Acute cases of tenosynovitis may develop localized swelling, a narrowing or *stenosing* of the sheath, and even the formation of a nodule on the tendon, causing the tendon to be become temporarily entrapped or *triggered* as it attempts to slide through the sheath. If this occurs in the index finger, typically used in repeatedly and forcefully activating a power tool, it is colloquially termed *trigger finger*. Many times, upon attempting to straighten the finger and stretch the tendon, the tendon will crackle or crepitate leading to the more complete term of *stenosing tenosynovitis crepitans*. Other examples of tenosynovitis in the hand include *de Quervain's disease* with inflammation of the tendons of the abductor pollicis longus and extensor pollicis brevis of the thumb. Repetitive forceful motions of the thumb in a variety of tasks, even games, lead to such problems and also to names popularized in the media referring back to those tasks, e.g., *Atari or Nintendo thumb* (Reinstein, 1983). *Dupuytren's contracture* is formation of nodules in the palmar fascia, an extension of the tendon of the palmaris longus muscle, leading to triggering of the ring and little fingers. Tenosynovitis of the flexor tendons (carpi, digitorum profundus, and superficialis) within the wrist from repeated forceful wrist motion may lead to carpal tunnel syndrome. Similarly, repeated opening of scissors or other tools may lead to tenosynovitis in the extensor tendons in the fingers. A by-product of tenosynovitis is the excess release of synovial fluid, which may collect and form fluid-filled *ganglionic cysts* that appear as nodules under the skin on the surface of the hand.

The mechanism of injury for tendon disorders depends on a variety of factors, some of which have been investigated in animal studies. Exercise with controlled conditions can have positive long-term effects by increasing tendon cross-sectional area and strength. Remodeling of the tendon can occur with the laying down of additional fibrocartilaginous tissue (Woo et al., 1980). However, when the exercise becomes excessive (high rates of loading in rabbits), there are degenerative changes in the tendon with increased number of capillaries, inflammatory cells, edema, microtears, and separation of fibers consistent with pathology of tendinosis in humans. Elevated temperatures and hypoxia in the core of the tendon may play a role in these degenerative changes (Backman et al., 1990). When a tendon experiences compressive loading in addition to tension, e.g., curving around a bone or ligament as in the Armstrong and Chaffin (1978) tendon–pulley model, the tendon becomes transformed from linear bands of collagen fascicles into irregular patterned fibrocartilage with changes in the proteoglycans (Malaviya et al., 2000). Coincidentally, tendon strength, at least in rats, decreases with age (Simonsen et al., 1995).

6.2.2 Muscle Disorders

Muscle disorders start as simple muscle soreness or pain, termed *myalgia*, in workers, both old and especially new workers, performing unaccustomed strenuous or repetitive work. The affected area will be sore and tender to touch because of microstrain and inflammation of the tissue, termed *myositis*. If the work is soon stopped (e.g., a one-time job or a weekend activity), relief will occur in several days. If the work is continued a gradual manner (i.e., a break-in period), generally a conditioning process occurs, the muscle heals, becomes accustomed to task, and becomes more resistant to injury. However, if the work is continued in an excessive manner (i.e., few rest periods, frequent overtime), the muscle strain and myalgia become chronic and the disorder becomes *myofascial pain syndrome*. The muscle may spasm, dysfunction, and temporary disability may result. In chronic stages, the disorder is characterized by chronically painful spastic muscles, tingling sensations, nervousness, and sleeplessness and is termed *fibromyalgia* or *fibrositis*. It is aggravated by both repeated activities and also, paradoxically, by rest; it may be worse upon rising in the morning. Another characteristic of fibro-myalgia is the presence of *trigger points*, small areas of spastic muscle that are tender to touch surrounded by unaffected muscle. Pressure on these trigger points will often result in pain shooting up or down the extremity. Details on trigger points and treatments of these disorders can be found in Travell and Simons (1983).

One specific and rather common myofascial syndrome is the *tension-neck syndrome*, characterized by pain and tenderness in the shoulder and neck region for clerical workers and small-parts assemblers, who typically are slightly hunched forward for better visibility and have contracted the upper back (trapezius) and neck muscles (Kuorinka and Forcier, 1995). More active and excessive muscle contraction may lead to a *writer's cramp* or *focal dystonia*. It was first noticed in Victorian England in scriveners who were responsible for copying contracts by hand using quills gripped firmly. The resulting spasms were first described in detail by Wilks (1878) and later by others (Sheehy and Marsden, 1982) as resulting from the repetitive forceful contrac-tions of the hand with complications induced by co-contractions of the forearm flexors and extensors. The problem is that individuals tend to over-grip tools or other objects by as much as a factor of 5. The problem is further exacerbated by carpal tunnel syndrome or other neurological disorders that reduce sensory feedback and increase overgripping to a factor of 10 (Lowe and Freivalds, 1999).

The mechanism of injury for muscle disorders is quite different from tendon disorders. Typically, muscle injury occurs as the result of excessive external forces on the passive structures, mainly connective tissue, rather than from overuse. Excessive muscle use will result in muscle fatigue, lim-iting contractile capability before cellular damage can occur. This fatigue is due to intramuscular pressure exceeding capillary pressure (about 30 mmHg) causing ischemia and hypoxia to the active muscle fibers (Sjøgaard and Søgaard, 1998) which then may contribute to alterations in the intracel-lular pH, lactic acid, calcium and potassium concentrations, and may upset overall homeostasis (Sjøgaard and Jensen, 1997). Eccentric contractions, in which external loads cause the sarcomeres to lengthen during active cross-bridging, are also likely to cause structural damage, inflammation, hemor-rhaging, and loss of force-generating capacity (McCully and Faulkner, 1985; McComas, 1996). Based on an exponential relationship that exists between stress and the number of cycles, with greater stress requiring fewer cycles, there should be a theoretical stress limit, below which injury could be avoided (Warren et al., 1993). However, no such value has been derived for human muscle. There are also indications that passive stretch (Noonan et al., 1994) and vibration (Necking et al., 1966) contribute to muscle injury. As for tendons, there are age-related changes in skeletal muscle, with a gradual decrease in strength starting at age 40 and increasing more dramatically after age 65 (Faulkner et al., 1990). Although most of this is related to inactivity, some 20% of the decrease cannot be prevented with exercise (Faulkner and Brooks, 1995).

6.2.3 Nerve Disorders

Nerve entrapment occurs between two different tissues, muscles, bones, ligaments, or other structures, and may be due to a variety of diseases, such as hyperthyroidism or arthritis, vascular disorders or edema, in addition to chronic work-related trauma. During entrapment, pressure on the nerve will impair blood flow and oxygenation of the Schwann cells and the myelin sheath with consequent effects on the axonal transport system and production of action potentials. If the pressure is high enough, mechanical blocking of the depolarization process will occur (Lundborg, 1988). A complicating factor is that entrapment at one location of the nerve (which may be up to 1 m in length) increases the susceptibility to further injury at points either distal or proximal to the first location, due to impairment of the axonal flows of ions. This multiple entrapment, known as the *double crush syndrome*, makes it even more important that ergonomists consider the whole extremity when analyzing a job and diagnosing potential problems.

The most common nerve entrapment of the upper limbs is *carpal tunnel syndrome*. The *carpal tunnel* is formed by eight carpal bones on the dorsal side and the transverse carpal ligament (flexor retinaculum, which serves to prevent bowstringing) on the palmar side of the wrist (Figure 6.3). Through this tunnel, in a tight fit, pass various blood vessels, flexor tendons, and the median nerve, which innervates the index and middle fingers and parts of the thumb and ring finger. Any additional increase in the contents of the tunnel will increase the pressure on the median nerve with consequent disruption of nerve conduction. This may occur in pregnant females when additional water retention results in swelling of the contents of carpal tunnel (Punnett et al., 1985) or in clerical, assembly, garment, and food processing workers from forceful repetitive wrist flexions/extensions or ulnar/radial deviations. The resulting friction of the tendons when sliding through their sheaths wrapped around the carpal tunnel bones or ligaments in the Armstrong and Chaffin (1978) tendon–pulley model (presented in Section 5.2) is compensated for by additional secretions of synovial fluid. This causes swelling, increases resting carpal canal pressures by as much as a factor of three (Okutsu et al., 1989), and compresses the median nerve resulting in shooting pains, especially at night, tingling and numbness, and loss of fine motor control to the above-mentioned fingers.

Two other nerves, the ulnar and radial, pass through the wrist area, although not through the carpal tunnel. The ulnar nerve enters the hand at Guyon's canal on the medial (little finger) side, innervating the little finger and part of the ring finger. Sometimes the ulnar nerve is entrapped, leading to the *Guyon canal syndrome* with tingling and numbness of the associated fingers. The ulnar nerve may also be trapped farther back in either the ulnar groove or the cubital tunnel formed by the two heads of the flexor carpi ulnaris near the elbow in the *cubital tunnel syndrome* as a result of direct pressure on the area from resting the elbows on sharp table edges or twisting motions at the elbow. Symptoms include pain and soreness at the medial elbow and tingling and numbness in the associated fingers. An acute blow to the ulnar nerve at the ulnar groove results in the "funny bone" sensation.

The radial nerve also passes into the forearm just below the lateral epicondyle near the head of the radius. Compression of the nerve due to a contracted muscle or bones will result in localized pain and tenderness and tingling and numbness in the thumb, termed the *radial tunnel syndrome*. A similar effect will result from an entrapment of a deep branch of the radial nerve (interosseous) within the supinator muscles of the forearm in the arcade of Frohse in the *posterior interosseous syndrome*. This condition will also exhibit a weakness in extensor muscles for the wrist and little finger.

The median nerve can similarly be trapped both at the elbow, in the *pronator teres syndrome*, and in the forearm, in the *anterior interosseous syndrome*. In the first case, the median nerve is trapped beneath the two heads of the pronator teres muscle, as a result of inflammation and swelling of muscle from constant pronation as in the classic "clothes wringing" motion. Symptoms include spasm and tightness of the pronator teres muscle, resulting in pain on the palm side of forearm and symptoms distally that are similar to those of carpal tunnel syndrome and may result in misdiagnosis. The only difference is that the palmar cutaneous branch of median nerve branches off before the carpal tunnel. Therefore, it will produce impaired sensations in the palm in the pronator teres syndrome but not the carpal tunnel syndrome (Parker and Imbus, 1992). In the second case, the anterior interosseous branch of the median nerve can be compressed by the deep anterior forearm muscles from overuse. Because the nerve innervates muscles in the mid-forearm and the flexor pollicis longus, symptoms include pain in the front of the forearm and difficulty producing an O-shaped pattern in a thumb–index finger tip pinch (Parker and Imbus, 1992).

Farther back on the upper limb, the *thoracic outlet syndrome* is entrapment of the brachial plexus (and also the subclavian artery and vein) in one or more different sites: the scalenus muscles in the neck, between the clavicle and first rib, and between the chest wall and the pectoralis minor muscle (Figure 6.3). Symptoms include numbness or tingling and pain in the arm and hand, especially on the ulnar side. Even the spinal nerve roots that form the brachial plexus (cervical vertebrae C5, C6, C7, C8) may be compressed between the intervertebral openings in *cervical radiculopathy*. These openings may narrow due to degenerative disc disease or arthritis, which may be further exacerbated by repetitive neck motions. Symptoms include tingling and numbness and pain radiating to various locales determined by the innervation of the appropriate nerve root.

In a different type of nerve disorder, *digital neuritis*, direct pressure while grasping tools (e.g., scissors) or other items with sharp edges may result in inflammation and swelling of the underlying nerve and eventual numbness in the associated digit. Again, the aggravating task or item may lead to descriptive colloquial names such as *bowler's thumb* (Howell and Leach, 1970; Dunham et al., 1972) or *cherry pitter's thumb* (Viegas and Torres, 1989).

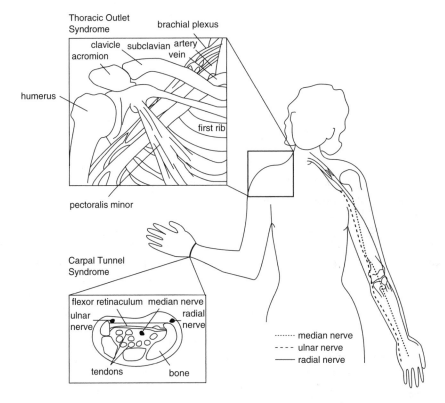

FIGURE 6.3

Carpal tunnel and thoracic outlet syndromes. (From Kuorinka, I. and Forcier, L., 1995. *Work Related Musculoskeletal Disorders (WMSDs): A Reference Book for Prevention*, London: Taylor & Francis. With permission.)

Extraneural compression pressures as low as 30 mmHg decrease intraneural flow and impair axonal transport within peripheral neurons. After several hours of compression, inflammation leads to fibrin deposits, proliferation of fibroblasts, which after several days leads growth of fibrous tissues. After a week, demyelination and axonal degeneration are observed, with the degree of injury correlated with the external pressure (Dyck et al., 1990). Chronic nerve compression in rats shows a similar etiologic pattern, ending in nerve fiber degeneration (Sommer et al., 1993; Mosconi and Kruger, 1996). Vibration exposure shows similar edema formation, demyelination, and ultimately nerve degeneration both experimentally induced in rats (Chang et al., 1994) and from occupational exposure in humans (Strömberg et al., 1997). Although experimental studies on spinal nerve root compression are much less common than for peripheral nerves, the injury mechanisms appear to be similar. Direct acute mechanical compression leads to intraneural edema and subsequent fibrosis (Rydevik et al., 1976). Chronic nerve compression may be less severe with changes evolving gradually allowing for adaptation of the axons and vasculature. On the other hand, the compression leads to an increase in neurotransmitters that stimulate pain transmission (Cornefjord et al., 1997).

6.2.4   Vascular Disorders

In vascular disorders, one or more of three different factors — vibration, cold temperatures, and direct pressure — cause ischemia of the blood supply to nerves and muscle resulting in hypoxia to the tissue with tingling, numbness, and loss of fine control. In the *hand/arm vibration syndrome* (HAVS), vibration (e.g., from power tools) activates the smooth muscle surrounding arterioles causing a clamping action and loss of blood flow (*ischemia*) to the hand resulting in a blanching or the colloquial *white finger syndrome*. This will also result in numbness and an inability to perform precision work. Cold temperatures have a very similar ischemic effect on the arterioles through a local vasoconstrictor reflex. However, some individuals, especially women in northern climates, have an especially pronounced response leading to painful sensations, termed *Raynaud's syndrome*. The prevalence of HAVS increases markedly when there is a combination of vibration from power tool usage in cold environments, e.g., railroad work (Yu et al., 1986), stone cutting (Taylor et al., 1984), mining (Hedlund, 1989), and forestry work (Olsen and Nielsen, 1988). Vibration also happens to be a major factor in carpal tunnel syndrome (see Section 6.2.3).

Direct pressure on the circulatory vessels can also cause ischemia and loss of fine motor control, effects similar to vibration or cold. This can occur in thoracic outlet syndrome, where the subclavian vessels are in close proximity to the brachial plexus and are similarly entrapped within the shoulder area, or in the *hypothenar hammer syndrome*, where the ulnar artery is compressed against the hypothenar eminence (muscle below the little and ring fingers) during hand hammering.

6.2.5   Bursa Disorders

Bursitis is inflammation of *bursae*, closed sacs filled with synovial fluid. Bursae are usually located in areas with potential for friction and help facilitate the motion of tendons and muscles over bone protuberances, especially around joints. Bursitis may be caused by friction, trauma, inflammatory diseases such as rheumatoid arthritis, and by bacteria. In the upper limbs, it is found at the elbow (olecranon bursa) and the shoulder (subacromial bursitis), the latter developing as part of the degeneration of the rotator cuff tendons. The most common occupationally induced bursitis, however, is in the knee (prepatellar bursitis) found in carpet layers due to the kneeling posture and use of the knee kicker (Thun et al., 1987).

6.2.6 Bone and Cartilage Disorders

Arthritis can be of two forms: *rheumatoid arthritis*, which is a generalized inflammatory process associated with diseases such as gout, and *osteoarthritis*, which is a degenerative process of joint cartilage. Despite an increase in cartilage water content and increased synthesis of proteoglycans, the cartilage decreases in thickness, with increased trauma to subchondral bone resulting in sclerosis. How the process begins is quite unclear. Many cases are idiopathic, having no clear predisposing factors, while other cases may occur as a result of specific trauma or injury to the joint. There is some evidence that repetitive work such as lifting may contribute to osteoarthritis severity in the shoulder joint (Stenlund et al., 1992).

The above MSDs, for convenience purposes, have been summarized in Table 6.1. Further details on specific types of MSDs can be found in Parker and Imbus (1992) and Kuorinka and Forcier (1995).

6.3 Medical Diagnosis and Treatment of MSDs

If a worker reports musculoskeletal pain, the physician will perform a physical examination with a series of steps to identify the disorder. The first is a general inspection of the patient, looking for asymmetry between the two sides of the body or for other visible irregularities like ganglionic cysts or swelling. The second part involves a series of range of motion (ROM) maneuvers. These include passive, resisted, and active motions. In a passive ROM, the patient is told to relax and the physician moves the patient's limb through a set of positions. Because the muscles and tendons surrounding the joint are generally relaxed, any pain or stress may be more a joint problem. However, if there is tightness or limited ROM there may be a case of tenosynovitis. In resisted ROM, the patient attempts to move the limb while the physician holds the limb steady (Figure 6.4). Because the muscles and tendons are contracting without the joint moving, problems in the muscles and tendons may be better identified. However, any muscle weakness may also be due to nerve entrapment. In active ROM tests, the patient moves the limb, and all aspects of the musculoskeletal system are examined.

In the third step, the physician may check for localized pain, tenderness, and trigger points by palpating or pressing with the fingers against various parts of the body. This will help identify the most inflamed parts of the body. However, pain can be generalized or even referred, with respect to nerves, and, therefore, one needs to be careful not to draw misleading conclusions.

In the fourth step, a series of specific diagnostic tests may be performed to isolate specific MSDs. In *Finkelstein's test* (Figure 6.5) the patient wraps the fingers around the thumb and deviates the wrist in the ulnar direction (Finkelstein, 1939). If pain occurs at the radial styloid at the wrist and along

TABLE 6.1

Common MSDs by Tissue Type and Their Associated Features

Tissue	General Injury	Common Specific Injuries (Colloquial Terms)	Occupational Risk Factors	Characteristic Features
Tendons	Tendinitis	Lateral epicondylitis (tennis elbow)	Repetitive forceful supination with wrist extension	Microtears in fibers, fraying of tendon, localized pain, tenderness, limited motion
		Medial epicondylitis (golfer's elbow)	Repetitive forceful pronation with wrist flexion	
		Bicipital tendinitis (shoulder pain)	Reaching overhead	
		Supraspinatus tendinitis (rotator cuff)	Outward shoulder rotations	
	Tenosynovitis	Flexor tenosynovitis in index finger (trigger finger)	Repetitive finger flexion	Thickening of synovial sheath, swelling, narrowing of space for tendon, resulting in localized pain and tenderness, triggering, and crackling sounds
		de Quervain's disease (Nintendo thumb)	Repetitive thumb flexion	
		Dupuytren's contracture (ring/little fingers)	Repetitive forceful gripping	
		Flexor tenosynovitis in wrist	Repetitive wrist motions (precursor to carpal tunnel syndrome)	
		Extensor tenosynovitis in fingers	Repetitive finger extension	
		Ganglionic cysts	Repetitive joint motions (by-product of tenosynovitis)	Fluid-filled sacs that may form bumps on skin
Muscles	Acute strain	Myalgia	Overuse of muscle	Muscle pain from microstrains
	Chronic strain	Myositis, myofascial syndromes, fibromyalgia, fibrositis, in various areas	Overuse of muscle	Chronic myalgia from inflammation of muscle and surrounding fibrous tissue, presence of trigger points or tender areas, commonly idiopathic
		Tension neck syndrome (stiff neck)	Static neck flexion	
	Cramping	Focal dystonia (in finger = writer's cramp)	Excessive gripping	Cramping, pain, limited motion
Nerve related	Nerve entrapment	Carpal tunnel syndrome	Repetitive forceful wrist motion	Median nerve entrapment at wrist, pain and tingling in index and middle fingers
		Guyon canal syndrome	Repetitive wrist flexion/extension, hand hammering, pressure on wrist	Ulnar nerve entrapment near wrist, pain/tingling in little finger

Category	Disorder	Risk factors	Description
	Cubital tunnel syndrome	Repetitive elbow flexion with wrist extension, pressure on elbow	Ulnar nerve entrapment in the ulnar groove or cubital tunnel at the elbow, pain and tingling in little finger
	Posterior interosseous syndrome	Repetitive wrist extension	Radial nerve entrapment in the forearm, pain in forearm and thumb
	Anterior interosseous syndrome	Repetitive wrist motions	Median nerve entrapment in the forearm, pain in midforearm
	Radial tunnel syndrome	Repetitive forearm rotation, wrist flexion with pronation, wrist extension with supination	Radial nerve entrapment at the elbow, pain on palm side of forearm
	Pronator teres syndrome	Repetitive pronation with finger flexion (gripping)	Median nerve entrapment at the elbow
	Thoracic outlet syndrome	Reaching above shoulders, repetitive use of shoulders	Entrapment of brachial plexus in shoulder area, pain in the arm, headaches
	Cervical syndrome or radiculopathy	Repetitive neck motions	Compression of spinal nerve roots in the neck, pain radiating down arm
Direct compression	Digital neuritis (bowler's thumb)	Gripping object with sharp edges	Pain, tingling, and loss of fine control in the fingers
Vascular / Ischemia	Hand/arm vibration syndrome (white fingers)	Vibration	Ischemia of ulnar artery, tingling, numbness, loss of fine control in hand
	Hypothenar hammer syndrome	Hand hammering	Ischemia of subclavian vessels, tingling, numbness in the arm
	Thoracic outlet syndrome	Reaching above shoulders, repetitive use of shoulders	Idiopathic ischemia of blood supply due to cold
	Raynaud's syndrome (white fingers)	Cold temperatures	
Joints / Bursitis	Subacromial bursitis, adhesive capsulitis(frozen shoulder)	Repetitive should motions, lifting	Thickening of bursa, pain, limited motion
Arthritis	Inflammatory, rheumatoid	Systemic disease, not work related	Inflammation and thickening of synovial tissues
	Osteoarthritis, degenerative	Repetitive joint motions	Thinning of cartilage, symptoms confused with other MSDs

Note: In many cases several types of disorders may occur simultaneously and the symptoms can be quite broad, nonspecific, and overlapping.

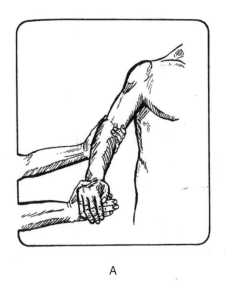
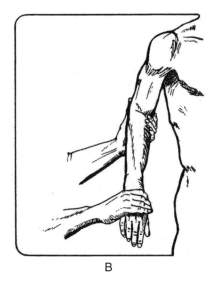

A   B

FIGURE 6.4
Resisted range of motion maneuvers as a diagnosis for MSDs. (A) Resisted flexion and extension; (B) resisted ulnar and radial deviation. (From Putz-Anderson, V., 1994. *Cumulative Trauma Disorders: A Manual for Musculoskeletal Diseases of the Upper Limbs*, London: Taylor & Francis. With permission.)

the thumb extensor tendon, there may be the possibility of de Quervain's disease. Note, however, that there may be a possibility of a false positive error, because over the years physicians may have misdefined Finkelstein's test (Elliott, 1992).

In *Phalen's test* (Figure 6.5), the patient holds the wrist in hyperflexion for 1 min. Pain, tingling, or numbness radiating distally throughout the median distribution of the hand is a positive sign that carpal tunnel syndrome may be present (Phalen, 1966; Gellman et al., 1986). A reverse Phalen's test involves wrist and finger extension held for 1 min. The consequent wrist extension may cause larger increases in carpal canal pressure than for wrist flexion in the normal Phalen's test and the resulting pain and tingling symptoms are again a positive sign of carpal tunnel syndrome (Robert et al., 1994).

Similar positive signs may be found in *Tinel's test*, in which the median nerve at the wrist is tapped (Tine, 1915; Steward and Eisen, 1978; Buch-Jaeger and Foucher, 1994). In *Adson's test*, the patient is seated with the head extended and turned to the affected side. If on raising the affected arm and taking a deep breath, the pulse at the wrist becomes weaker, thoracic outlet syndrome may be present (Adson and Coffey, 1927).

Each of the above diagnostic tests for evaluating carpal tunnel syndrome evokes a subjective response from the patient with varying sensitivity and specificity (see Chapter 8). Their sensitivity varies widely from 32 to 89% and the specificity from 72 to 84% (Ghavanini and Haghighat, 1998). As such, they should not be interpreted as an unequivocal diagnosis, but as part of a set of tools that lead to the final diagnosis.

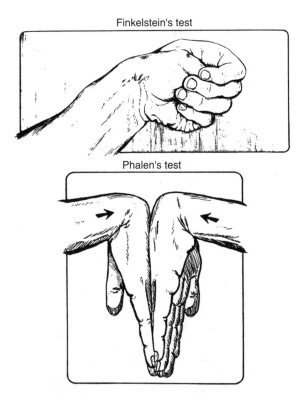

FIGURE 6.5
Finkelstein's and Phalen's tests for diagnosing wrist MSDs. (From Putz-Anderson, V., 1994. *Cumulative Trauma Disorders: A Manual for Musculoskeletal Diseases of the Upper Limbs*, London: Taylor & Francis. With permission.)

More complete or accurate diagnosis of the specific nerve disorder may fall to specialized laboratory tests. For example, if some of the above signs indicate carpal tunnel syndrome, further diagnostic tests can be done to identify whether the impaired nerve is truly the median nerve. The three main nerves innervating the hand, the radius, median and ulnar nerves, have separate and distinct innervation areas (Figure 6.6). The affected area may have tingling or numbness or decreased sensation, which may be evaluated by a *two-point discrimination test*. Impaired individuals may be able to distinguish two points from a single point only when they are at least 5 mm apart (Dellon and Kallman, 1983; Shurr et al., 1986). Similarly, reduced sensitivity to vibration at various frequencies and intensities (Dellon, 1983; Lundborg et al., 1986), to standardized pressures (Bell, 1990), and to temperatures (Arezzo et al., 1986) are further indications of innervation problems. Other potential diagnostic tests include grip and pinch strength compared to normative data (Mathiowetz et al., 1985) and efficiency of muscular contraction (Chaffin et al., 1980). Of course, all these procedures require honest cooperation by the patient.

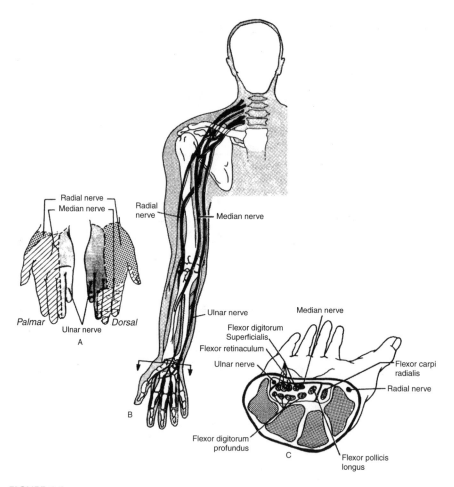

FIGURE 6.6
Median, radial, and ulnar nerve innervation patterns. (From Armstrong, T.J., 1983. *An Ergonomics Guide to Carpal Tunnel Syndrome*, Akron, OH: American Industrial Hygiene Association. With permission.)

A direct measurement of nerve conduction velocities and resultant slowing (discussed in detail in Section 7.4) is considered by many the "gold standard" in clearly diagnosing the appropriate nerve disorder. By measuring the velocity of median nerve and comparing it to the velocity of the ulnar nerve, a more rigorous diagnosis can be made. Note, however, that all of the median nerve entrapment syndromes (carpal tunnel, anterior interosseous, pronator teres, cubital tunnel) show quite similar nerve response, and palpation may be required to further isolate the specific disorder.

Electromyographic (EMG) techniques can also be used to assess muscle activity while radiographs and dye-induced arthrograms can be used examine bones and joints. Similarly, magnetic resonance imaging (MRI) can be used to provide images, based on the realignment hydrogen atoms to the energy supplied by specific radio frequency waves of soft tissues such as tendons and ligaments. Even though expensive, the idea is to provide as much diagnostic information in localizing the specific disorder as possible, so as to avoid unneeded surgery. Further details on medical diagnosis and various testing procedures can be found in Parker and Imbus (1992) or Putz-Anderson (1994).

The basic medical treatment philosophy should be to assist the patient with the most effective treatment plan at minimal cost, side effects, and disruption of life, and allow the patient to return to work and normal life as quickly as possible and with minimal pain. Therefore, the treatment strategy should follow a plan using the simplest approaches first, termed conservative treatments, and progressing toward more elaborate treatments with surgery as the last resort. Conservative treatments include the restriction of motion and splinting, applying heat and/or cold, medications and injections, and special exercises.

The purpose of restriction of motions is to avoid the activities that cause pain or stress the injured body part. This can be achieved by work restrictions, avoiding specific tasks on a job or, perhaps, changing the job altogether, or in placing the worker on an alternative or a light-duty job. Splints may be used to restrict extreme motions or support specific body parts in a neutral posture of lower stress. This will reduce pain for the worker and, in effect, decrease inflammation and swelling for the critical area. For example, in carpal tunnel syndrome, wrist splints may be used to maintain the wrist in a neutral posture but allow the fingers and thumbs to move. Splints are perhaps best used a night, to avoid falling asleep with a deviated posture. During the working day, if the job has not been specifically redesigned for the injured worker, there could be a chance for more stress and greater injury if the worker tries to fight the splint in performing the typically large ROM required on assembly or other types of jobs. Furthermore, extended splinting with limited muscle or joint inactivity could result in loss of muscle tone or joint ROM.

Heat and cold are used to relieve and facilitate the healing process. Ice, if applied immediately after an acute injury or overuse strain, reduces pain and swelling. Heat should be only used after 24 or 48 h, to increase the blood flow to the muscles and tendons in the injured area. It can be superficial, such as heat packs or hot baths, or deep heating from ultrasound. If heat is applied earlier, it will tend to increase bleeding and swelling and aggravate the healing process.

Medication is given to reduce pain and fight inflammation. Although inflammation is a natural response of the body to injury, it can slow the healing process. Aspirin is the cheapest and most commonly used drug that serves this purpose. Unfortunately, some individuals do not tolerate high doses of aspirin and suffer side effects of heartburn and gastrointestinal problems. Several relatively new nonsteroidal anti-inflammatory drugs have been developed as alternatives to aspirin. Unfortunately, most require a prescription, are quite costly, and may not eliminate the side effects completely.

Two are now available over the counter, ibuprofen (e.g., Motrin®) and naproxen sodium (i.e., Aleve). Injections of even stronger corticosteroids into the inflamed site offer the most effective relief, but are limited in the number of times they can be used. Injections of lidocaine or botulism may be useful in blocking selected pathways for various focal dystonias (Kaji, 2000).

Although somewhat counterintuitive, special exercise programs with stretching tend to promote increased circulation, increased ROM, and decreased muscle tension. These programs are most effective in recovering from shoulder injuries and will also tend to prevent further muscle strains. For hand and wrist disorders, care should be taken, since exercise may aggravate the existing condition. Note that these conservative approaches are most beneficial when pursued in parallel with an effective job redesign program.

6.4   Epidemiologic Approach to MSDs

6.4.1   Introduction to Epidemiology

Epidemiology, in the traditional sense, is the branch of medicine that studies epidemic diseases. Normally, this would not be of concern to the industrial ergonomist; however, to identify, understand, and control occupational risk factors leading to the development of workplace MSDs (which can be considered a form of disease and is sometimes termed *morbidity*), it is important to understand and utilize epidemiological techniques. Epidemiological studies can be of many forms with many different variables: directionality of exposure to the risk factors, types of data collection methods, timing of data collection, types and availability of subjects, number of observations made, etc. Two basic facets, manipulation and randomization, determine the design of the research approach. Manipulation of the study factor means that the experimenter can control exposure. In a traditional study, rats may be exposed to specific levels and durations of a carcinogen. In a workplace study, this may be more difficult to control. Randomization of the study subjects is a process in which chance (e.g., random number tables) is used to assign subjects to exposure conditions. Again, this is easy to do for rats being exposed to a toxin, but is much more difficult to do in an industrial environment, given worker choice, seniority, and union requirements.

The various permutations of the two factors produce three different general study types: experimental, quasi-experimental, and observational studies (Table 6.2). Experimental studies have the greatest control over both the factor of interest and the subjects involved. Because this factor can be directly manipulated, these are also called *intervention studies,* and because they commonly involve testing new drugs or therapies in a medical environment, they are also referred to as *clinical trials.* As shown in Figure 6.7, the procedures for

TABLE 6.2

Types of Epidemiological Studies

General Type	M	R	Experimental Unit/Design	Rigor (Precision)	Time Duration	Cost	Specific Type (Analysis)	Best For:	Worst For:
Experimental (Intervention)	Yes	Yes	Selected individuals	Tight	Relatively short (days, weeks)	High	Clinical trials (many)	Statistical rigor Intervention control	Cost and effort Ethical concerns
Quasi-experimental (Intervention)	Yes	No	Population subsets	Less tight	Long (months)	Med	Community studies (see cohort)	Large database Public education	Time and effort Loss of subjects
Observational	No	No	Individuals in two groups (with and without exposure)	Less tight	Long (several observations, longitudinal)	Med	Cohort studies = Prospective (RR, IR)	Clear cause and effect Accurate risk and exposure data	Time and effort Loss of subjects
			Individuals in two groups (with and without outcome)	Loose (unless well matched)	One observation (surveys and records)	Low	Case-control (OR)	Rare disorders Small groups	Selection bias Risk and exposure estimates
			Individuals sorted into four groups	Very loose	One observation (survey)	Very low	Cross-sectional (p, OR?)	Quick, simple study Identifying risk factors	Temporality, validity survivor bias

Note: M = manipulation, R = randomization, RR = risk ratio, IR = incidence rate, OR = odds ratio, p = prevalence.

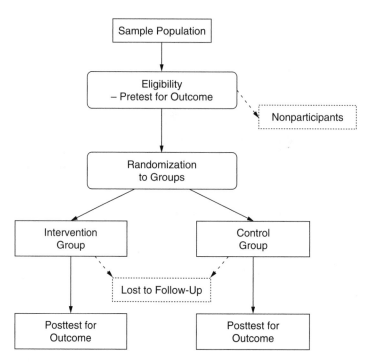

FIGURE 6.7
Schematic diagram of a clinical trial intervention study.

clinical trials include screening a sample population for eligibility with a pretest to eliminate those individuals already having the outcome of interest, e.g., disease or MSD. Then individuals are randomly assigned to one of two study groups: an intervention group and a control group. Finally, the outcome of interest is measured in both groups to see the efficacy of the intervention. However, as mentioned previously, because of cost and ethical issues (e.g., people cannot be forced to be exposed to a risk factor), these types of studies may not be possible for the industrial ergonomist.

Quasi-experimental studies involve the manipulation of the study factor but not randomization of study subjects (Figure 6.8). These typically are community interventions oriented toward education and behavioral changes at the population level, and, at best, the communities may be randomly assigned or not assigned to the intervention. Thus, study factors may involve control of alcohol use, cessation of smoking, driver safety, or control of dietary behavior. The interventions may be focused on targeted populations, i.e., individuals at risk for heart attacks or young teens at risk for drug use, or may be mandated by state law, i.e., seat belt use, driver blood alcohol levels, etc. However, the populations may not be well controlled, i.e., not all individuals follow the suggested procedures or all states do not follow the same levels of exposure, etc., and, thus, the quasi-experimental nature.

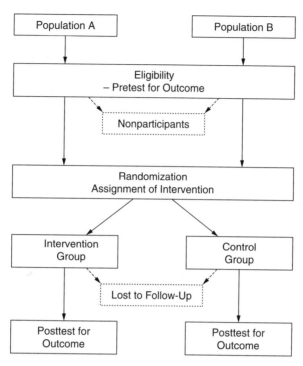

FIGURE 6.8
Schematic diagram of a community trial intervention study.

As a first observation, the above experimental types of studies may not seem an option for the industrial ergonomist. However, in practice, ergonomists do perform intervention studies, either in the mode of a clinical trial or a community trial. If a true randomization of subjects to either study group is restricted or completely lacking, the study then assumes the form of a community trial. For example, it is not uncommon that one plant is willing to undergo an intervention, e.g., an ergonomics program or an exercise program, while another plant is not. However, the plants or communities may not truly be randomly assigned treatments and the validity of the results may be confounded with other factors. In terms of analysis purposes, the study then assumes the shape of a prospective/cohort study discussed shortly.

Observational studies make careful measurements of patterns of exposure of musculoskeletal injuries in given populations to draw inferences about *etiology* or the development of the injury. There are three main types of observational studies, all based on the 2×2 contingency table shown in Table 6.3. This table cross-classifies exposure states and outcome status and allows one to tabulate individuals in various categories. Note that the outcome status is either having an MSD or not having the disorder. Of a total number of n subjects, a have been exposed to a particular risk factor and have shown

TABLE 6.3

The 2×2 Contingency Table (r_i = row, c_j = column)

Outcome Status	Exposure to Risk Factor		
	Yes	No	Total
Yes	a	b	$r_1 = a + b$
No	c	d	$r_2 = c + d$
Total	$c_1 = a + c$	$c_2 = b + d$	$n = a + b + c + d$

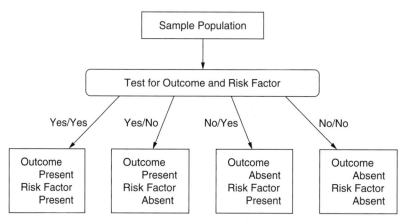

FIGURE 6.9

Schematic diagram of a cross-sectional study.

signs of the disorder, c have been exposed but are still healthy, b have not been exposed but have the disorder, and d have not been exposed and are healthy. A total of $a + b$ have the disorder while $c + d$ can be considered healthy, or at least are not yet showing signs of the disorder. A total of $a + c$ have been exposed while $b + d$ have not been exposed. These four values are known as *marginal totals* and will permit calculation of various probabilities and risk values. This table also serves as a point of reference in classifying the various types of observational studies.

In a *cross-sectional study*, or *prevalence study*, the ergonomist starts by selecting a sample of subjects (n) and then determining their distribution in terms of exposures and outcomes (Figure 6.9 and Table 6.4). This is most typically done as a survey of individuals in a single observation, i.e., a snapshot of time. Because exposure and outcome histories are collected simultaneously, one depends on the recall of the subjects to establish which of the risk factor exposures or outcomes came first. This is frequently unreliable due to a long time lag and lack of specialized knowledge of the part of the subject. Consequently, cross-sectional studies are most useful in identifying risk factors or in establishing prevalence of a relatively frequent disorder with a long duration or of one that is not often reported, such as is the case for work-related MSDs

TABLE 6.4

The 2×2 Contingency Table Leading to a Cross-Sectional Study (subject selection →→)

Outcome Status	Exposure to Risk Factor		Total
	Yes	No	
Yes (cases)	a	b	$r_1 = a + b$
No (noncases)	c	d	$r_2 = c + d$
Total	$c_1 = a + c$	$c_2 = b + d$	$n = a + b + c + d$

(WRMSDs). It can thus be considered as a "fishing expedition" on which to base more rigorous studies. Another problem is that only a small subset of the total population is examined, which is typically based on convenience of the ergonomist or the willingness to participate. Therefore, the results may not be valid for the full population. A better approach would be use a *stratified sampling* approach, in which the population is divided into mutually exclusive strata with random sampling performed within each stratum. However, practically, this might be quite difficult to accomplish in an industrial setting, with individuals refusing to participate.

In a *case-control study*, the ergonomist uses the basic premise that a disorder does not occur randomly but, rather, in a logical pattern that reflects the underlying etiology. Therefore, two groups are selected: *cases*, in which everyone has the disorder $(a + b)$ and *controls*, a comparable group in which everyone is free of the disorder $(c + d)$ (Figure 6.10 and Table 6.5). The ergonomist then seeks to identify possible causes of the disorder by finding out how the two groups differ. Because the disorder most likely does not occur randomly, the case group must have been exposed to some occupational risk factor that the control group was not exposed to. Therefore, one is progressing from effect to a possible cause. However, causality cannot be definitely established because of the lack of a time sequence. Among some of the other potential problems is the determination of cases. If the criteria are too broad, some individuals of the case group may not truly have the disorder. If the criteria are too restrictive, there may be too few cases to statistically analyze.

The selection of controls, termed *matching*, is similarly, if not more, critical. The closer the control group is to the case group in terms of age, gender, education, fitness, working skills, job titles, etc., the more likely one is to ascribe differences in disorder status to the exposure of interest. The closeness of this matching can easily be checked through the use of t-tests. If the two groups are not statistically different in various characteristics, then they should be reasonably well matched. Case-control studies are most useful for evaluating rarely occurring disorders or ones with a small number of cases. Similar to cross-sectional studies, the unit of observation and analyses is the individual, and data collection can be survey or more in-depth information sources such as employee, health insurance, or medical records.

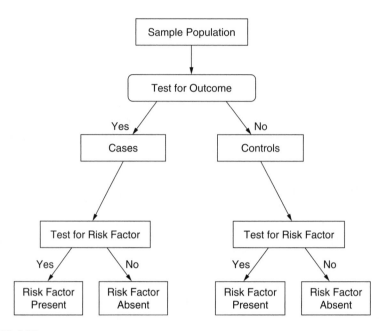

FIGURE 6.10
Schematic diagram of a retrospective case-control study.

TABLE 6.5

The 2×2 Contingency Table Leading to a Case-Control Study
(outcome-based selection →→)

Outcome Status	Exposure to Risk Factor		Total
	Yes	**No**	
Yes (cases)	a	b	$r_1 = a + b$
No (controls)	c	d	$r_2 = c + d$
Total	$c_1 = a + c$	$c_2 = b + d$	$n = a + b + c + d$

To eliminate the problems of recall and examine the effect of causality directly, a *cohort study* is used. It starts with a group of subjects who lack a history of the outcome but still are at risk for it (Figure 6.11). The exposure of interest is determined for each individual of the group, i.e., the cohort, and the group is followed for an extended period of time into the future to

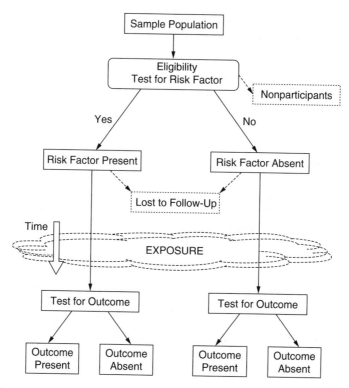

FIGURE 6.11
Schematic diagram of a prospective cohort study.

TABLE 6.6

The 2×2 Contingency Table Leading to a Cohort Study
(sample selection → ①, finding effect from cause ···→ ②)

Outcome Status	Exposure to Risk Factor		Total
	Yes	**No**	
Yes (cases)	a	b	$r_1 = a + b$
No (noncases)	c ②	② d	$r_2 = c + d$
Total	$c_1 = a + c$	$c_2 = b + d$	$(n) = a + b + c + d$
		①	

document the incidence of the outcome in the exposed and non-exposed individuals ($a + c$ and $b + d$ in Table 6.6). Because of this, it can be thought of as going from cause to effect and is good for demonstrating causation, the direct opposite of progression in the case-control study. Because of the progression in time, this type of study is also referred to as a *prospective* or *longitudinal study*. Another distinguishing feature of a cohort study is that at least two observations are made: an initial observation to determine exposure status and eligibility into the group and a second to determine the number of incident cases of the outcome that develop over the given time period (① and ② in Table 6.6). In this case, it is a one-sample cohort study, with the proportion being exposed determined on analysis of the first observation point. In a multisample cohort study, two or more select subgroups are chosen, an exposed cohort ($a + c$) and a non-exposed, comparison cohort ($b + d$). However, because of the selection procedure, the frequency of exposure in the population cannot be determined. Also, cohort studies are not suitable for rare disorders or ones with a long latency, because of the need for a large baseline sample or for a long study period. As in the case-control study, the cohort groups should be as matched as possible and the unit of observation and analyses is the individual. Data collection can involve both surveys and secondary data sources.

Sometimes cohort studies can be *retrospective* or historical. In a retrospective study, the investigation starts after both the exposure and outcome have occurred, as opposed to a prospective study, in which the outcome occurs after the exposure is measured. Typically, a retrospective study would examine the medical records of two similar working populations, one of which has the outcome and another that does not, over the course of several years to find differences in exposure between the two groups. The advantage is that all the exposures have already occurred and the conclusions can be drawn more rapidly than in a prospective study.

Although classically intervention studies are experimental, in practice, intervention studies also refer to prospective cohort studies that investigate the course of a control action on the development, or more likely, the reduction, of an MSD. Workers are assigned to the intervention group at random and then followed to determine the proportion of those exposed who the develop the outcome as compared to the proportion of those unexposed, the non-intervention group. Further details on epidemiological studies can be found in Sorock and Courtney (1996), Friis and Sellers (1996), Greenberg et al. (1996), and Woodward (1999). The ergonomist may also find the summary of the different features for each type of observational study in Table 6.7 useful for selecting the appropriate approach.

6.4.2 Statistical analyses

The statistical analyses and inferences based on the contingency table in Table 6.2 are basically the same for cross-sectional and case-control studies except for the interpretation of the results in view of the higher potential for bias for cross-sectional studies. For added interest and a practical application of the following statistical analyses, consider the injury data from a plant

TABLE 6.7

Detailed Comparison of the Three Types of Observational Studies
(+ = strength, – = weakness)

Feature	Cohort	Case-Control	Cross-Sectional
Survivor bias	+	–	–
Selection bias	+	+	–
Recall bias	+	–	–
Loss to follow-up	–	+	+
Temporality	+	–	–
Time and effort	–	+	+
Cost	–	+	+

TABLE 6.8

Association of Musculoskeletal Injuries and
Exposure to Vibration from Power Tools

Musculoskeletal Injuries	Exposure to Vibration		
	Yes	No	Total
Yes (cases)	9	39	48
No (noncases)	14	134	148
Total	23	173	196

using power tools shown in Table 6.8. The hypothesis or association of
interest is whether vibration is a risk factor for developing WRMSDs.

Considering the data as from a cross-sectional study, the simplest statistics
to calculate are various measures of *prevalence*, where p_a and p_b are the
proportions of existing number of MSD cases in the exposed and unexposed
groups, respectively. The sample estimates of p_a and p_b are obtained from

$$p_a = a/c_1 \quad \text{and} \quad p_b = b/c_2 \tag{6.1}$$

The prevalence difference (PD) for exposed vs. unexposed groups is

$$PD = p_a - p_b \tag{6.2}$$

The above, as they are only point estimates, do not allow for testing of
significance. For that, some form of interval estimation, such as a confidence
interval, is needed. The simplest calculation of the confidence interval is
based on the standard error approach, in which a $100(1 - \alpha)\%$ confidence
interval for PD is defined by

$$p_a - p_b \pm z_{\alpha/2} \left[p_a \left(1 - p_a\right)/c_1 + p_b \left(1 - p_b\right)/c_2 \right]^{1/2} \tag{6.3}$$

Other commonly used approaches for developing a confidence interval are described in Sahai and Khurshid (1966).

For the above vibration example in Table 6.8, the prevalence values are

$$p_a = 9/23 = 0.39 \quad \text{and} \quad p_b = 39/173 = 0.23 \tag{6.4}$$

while the prevalence difference is

$$PD = 0.39 - 0.23 = 0.16 \tag{6.5}$$

The 95% confidence interval (given that $z_{0.025}$ is 1.96) is

$$0.16 \pm 1.96\left[0.39 \times 0.61/23 + 0.23 \times 0.77/173\right]^{1/2} = 0.16 \pm 0.21 = \left(-0.05, \, 0.37\right) \tag{6.6}$$

Because the confidence interval overlaps 0, the difference in prevalence of MSDs between exposed and unexposed is not significant (at least not at an α of 5%) and vibration does not appear to be a risk factor.

One can also calculate the prevalence *odds ratio* (OR), which is the ratio of the prevalence odds for exposed vs. unexposed groups, defined as

$$OR = \frac{p_a/\left(1 - p_a\right)}{p_b/\left(1 - p_b\right)} = \frac{0.39/0.61}{0.23/0.77} = 2.2 \tag{6.7}$$

Another traditional analysis approach for contingency tables is the *chi square* (χ^2) in which the summation of difference between observed and expected values is calculated:

$$\chi^2 = \sum \frac{\left(o_i - e_i\right)^2}{e_i} \tag{6.8}$$

where
o_i = observed value
e_i = expected value

If the calculated value is larger than the test statistic $\chi^2_{\alpha/2}$ with

$$v = \left(r - 1\right)\left(c - 1\right) \tag{6.9}$$

degrees of freedom, then there is a significant difference between observed and expected values and significant association between outcome and exposure. Note that is the Pearson or ordinary chi square. Many epidemiologists use the Mantel–Haenszel (1959) chi square, especially for large sample approximation.

The expected values are calculated from the product of the intersecting column and row marginal probabilities times the total number of subjects:

$$e_a = \frac{c_1}{n} \times \frac{r_1}{n} \times n = \frac{c_1 r_1}{n} \tag{6.10}$$

Similarly,

$$e_b = \frac{c_2 r_1}{n} \tag{6.11}$$

$$e_c = \frac{c_1 r_2}{n} \tag{6.12}$$

$$e_d = \frac{c_2 r_2}{n} \tag{6.13}$$

Substituting these expressions into Equation 6.8 and simplifying yield

$$\chi^2 = \frac{n(ad - bc)^2}{c_1 c_2 r_1 r_2} \tag{6.14}$$

For this example, the value of chi square is

$$\chi^2 = \frac{200(9 \times 134 - 39 \times 14)^2}{23 \times 173 \times 48 \times 148} = 3.08 \tag{6.15}$$

and there are

$$v = (2-1)(2-1) = 1 \tag{6.16}$$

degree of freedom. The test statistic for an α of 5% is

$$\chi^2_{0.025} = 3.84 \tag{6.17}$$

Because the calculated value is less than the test statistic, then the association is not significant. Note, however, that if the number of subjects were doubled (e.g., more subjects were studied), then from Equation 6.14, the calculated chi square is 6.16 and becomes significant. This implies that chi square is an excellent measure of the significance of the association, but not at all useful as a measure of the degree of association.

One measure of the degree of association is the *phi coefficient*:

$$\phi = \left(\chi^2/n\right)^{1/2} \tag{6.18}$$

In this example, the value of the phi coefficient is

$$\phi = \left(3.08/1.96\right)^{1/2} = 0.125 \tag{6.19}$$

It can be interpreted as a correlation coefficient with values ranging between 0 and 1. Values below 0.4 or so, as a rule of thumb, are considered as having poor association.

For the more controlled cohort studies, there are several measures of quantifying risk for incurring the disorder. Because in this type of study there are two groups of individuals, one of which will incur the disorder in the future and the other of which will not incur the disorder, the calculation of risk is of interest. The first measure is the *risk ratio* or *relative risk* (RR), which relates the risks for MSDs for exposed and unexposed groups in a cohort study (i.e., since that is the design and direction of a cohort study as shown in Table 6.6). Among exposed individuals, the risk of an MSD is defined as

$$R_{exposed} = \frac{\text{exposed individuals incurring disorder}}{\text{all exposed individuals}} = \frac{a}{a+c} \tag{6.20}$$

Among unexposed individuals, the risk of an MSD is defined as

$$R_{unexposed} = \frac{\text{unexposed individuals incurring disorder}}{\text{all unexposed individuals}} = \frac{b}{b+d} \tag{6.21}$$

The risk ratio then becomes

$$RR = \frac{R_{exposed}}{R_{unexposed}} = \frac{a\left(b+d\right)}{b\left(a+c\right)} \tag{6.22}$$

The ratio assumes a value between 0 and ∞. A value greater than 1 indicates that the risk (or odds) is greater with exposure, a value of 1 indicates that the risk is the same for both groups, while a value less than 1 indicates that

TABLE 6.9

Guidelines for the Interpretation
of Risk Ratios and Odds Ratios

Value	Effect of Exposure
0.00–0.39	Strong benefit
0.40–0.59	Moderate benefit
0.60–0.89	Weak benefit
0.90–1.19	No benefit or effect
1.20–1.69	Weak hazard
1.70–2.59	Moderate hazard
≥2.60	Strong hazard

Source: Adapted from Greenberg (1986).

risk is less with exposure. Table 6.9 provides some general guidelines on interpreting the strength of association between exposure and the resulting disorder, but the true evaluation comes from a statistical analysis with the corresponding confidence interval.

Sometimes the risk ratio is converted to *attributable risk* (AR, also termed *etiologic fraction*):

$$AR = (RR - 1)/RR \tag{6.23}$$

which estimates the proportion by which the rate of the outcome among the exposed would be reduced if the exposure were eliminated. Note that in many cases a variety of factors may have contributed to the total outcome, so that the removal of one exposure does not reduce the outcome rate to zero. Rather, it provides a guide to the relative importance of the various study factors in reducing the outcomes.

The $100(1 - \alpha)\%$ confidence interval around the above point estimate of risk ratio can be calculated from the standard error (SE) of the risk ratio based on a Taylor series approximation (Sahai and Khurshid, 1996):

$$RR \; \exp\left(\pm z_{\alpha/2} \, SE\right) \tag{6.24}$$

where SE is defined by

$$SE = \left\{ \frac{c}{a(a+c)} + \frac{d}{b(b+d)} \right\}^{1/2} \tag{6.25}$$

Other commonly used test-based and exact approaches for developing a confidence interval are described in Sahai and Khurshid (1996).

For the vibration example, the risk ratio is

$$RR = \frac{9 \times 173}{39 \times 23} = 1.74 \tag{6.26}$$

and the standard error is

$$SE = \left\{ \frac{14}{9 \times 23} + \frac{134}{39 \times 173} \right\}^{1/2} = 0.296 \tag{6.27}$$

The 95% confidence interval then becomes

$$1.74 \exp\left(\pm 196 \times 0.296\right) = \left(0.97,\ 3.11\right) \tag{6.28}$$

Although the risk ratio value of 1.74, at first glance, seems to indicate a moderate hazard, the confidence interval encompasses the value of 1.0. Therefore, the risk ratio is not statistically significant and the risks to the exposed and unexposed groups are not significantly different.

Because the cohort study collects data prospectively, exposure time is available, from which an *incidence rate* (IR) can be calculated. An incidence rate reflects the number of new cases with respect to exposure time (*t*) in person hours or person days:

$$IR = a/t \tag{6.29}$$

It is somewhat similar to prevalence, which measures existing cases within a population. Given that the incidence rate is constant over time, the incidence rate is related to prevalence by the following relationship:

$$IR = \frac{p}{\left(1 - p\right)d} \tag{6.30}$$

where d = duration of the disorder.

In a case-control or in a retrospective study, the RR calculation would theoretically measure the risk of exposure to an antecedent risk, given the presence or absence of a disorder. However, this does not make logical sense, since the disease did not cause the risk. Therefore, the RR is usually not of interest for case-control studies and the odds ratio (OR) is a more useful measure of risk. The probability that the outcome of interest or a case was exposed to the risk factor can be expressed as the case exposure probability:

$$p_a = \frac{\text{exposed cases}}{\text{total cases}} = \frac{a}{a+b} \tag{6.31}$$

The probability for a case with no exposure is

$$p_b = \frac{\text{unexposed cases}}{\text{total cases}} = \frac{b}{a+b} \tag{6.32}$$

The overall odds of obtaining the outcome when the risk factor is present is then estimated by

$$p_a/p_b = a/b \tag{6.33}$$

Similarly, the odds of exposure among controls or those not having the outcome is

$$p_c/p_d = c/d \tag{6.34}$$

The odds ratio is then the odds of exposure for cases divided by odds of exposure for controls:

$$OR = \frac{a/b}{c/d} = \frac{ad}{bc} \tag{6.35}$$

The $100(1 - \alpha)\%$ confidence interval around the above point estimate can be calculated from the standard error of the odds ratio based on a Taylor series approximation (Sahai and Khurshid, 1996):

$$OR \exp\left(\pm z_{\alpha/2} SE\right) \tag{6.36}$$

where SE is defined by

$$SE = \left(1/a + 1/b + 1/c + 1/d\right)^{1/2} \tag{6.37}$$

Other commonly used test-based and exact approaches for developing a confidence interval are described in Sahai and Khurshid (1996).

Using the vibration exposure data of Table 6.8, the odds ratio is

$$OR = \frac{ad}{bc} = \frac{9 \times 134}{39 \times 14} = 2.21 \tag{6.38}$$

This value measures the association between the two characteristics of the study, MSDs and vibration, and can be interpreted to mean that the odds for a group of workers using power tools with vibration exposure to incur some type of MSD is over twice as great as a group of workers not similarly exposed. Note that it is identical in terms and value (except for round-off errors) to the prevalence odds ratio previously presented for a cross-sectional study (Eq. 6.7).

An argument has also been made that the odds ratio can be used as estimate of the incidence rate ratio, since both case and control groups only include only newly diagnosed or "incident" cases. Subjects can queried to exclude those who already had the disorder before the study period (Greenberg et al., 1996).

The standard error and 95% confidence interval around the point estimate of OR are

$$SE = \left(1/a + 1/b + 1/c + 1/d\right)^{1/2} = \left(1/9 + 1/39 + 1/14 + 1/134\right)^{1/2} = 0.464 \qquad (6.39)$$

$$OR\exp\left(\pm z_{\alpha/2}\, SE\right) = 2.21\exp\left(\pm 1.96 \times 0.464\right) = \left(0.89, 5.49\right) \qquad (6.40)$$

Because the confidence interval overlaps 1.0, the association could have possibly occurred by chance alone and the association is not statistically significant.

Note that, since cohort groups eventually either incur the outcome or remain outcome free, the same line of reasoning and odds ratio analysis as described above for case-control studies can also be utilized in cohort studies. The question then arises about the relationship between the odds ratio and risk ratio for cohort studies, as both measure the association between the two characteristics of interest. Comparing the definitions of the odds ratio and risk ratio:

$$OR = \frac{ad}{bc} \approx \frac{a\left(b+d\right)}{b\left(a+c\right)} = RR \qquad (6.41)$$

the two expressions will be mathematically very similar if the values of a and b are very small as compared to c and d, respectively, i.e., the prevalence of the outcome is very low or it is a very rare disorder. For the vibration example of Table 6.8, the odds ratio was 2.1 and the risk ratio was 1.74. These values are similar but not that close, because the corresponding prevalences ($p_a = 0.39$ and $p_b = 0.23$) were not that close to zero. This will typically be the case with WRMSDs, which in certain industries are actually quite prevalent.

There also has been some criticism of odds ratios, in that by taking the ratio as a measure of association, the base level of cases is lost. Thus, a large odds ratio for a small number of cases (e.g., an OR of 10 for 1000 cases) vs. a small odds ratio for a large number of cases (e.g., an OR of 2 for 1,000,000 cases) would obscure the real problem that there more than a million individuals suffering from some undesirable outcome. Several measures to correct this disparity are discussed in Fleiss (1981).

In summary, there are several common measures used in epidemiological studies: risk, prevalence, and incidence. However, there are variations in the units, interpretation, and applications of these measures. Incidence rates have units per time, whereas prevalence and risk have no units. Incidence rates and risk describe new occurrences of a disorder, whereas prevalence reflects existing cases of an already occurring disorder. Risk is most useful in predicting the proportion of a population that will incur the disorder over a specified period of time and thus can be used as an estimate of incidence rates. Incidence rates are preferred in predicting the rapidity of arising new cases while prevalence is preferred for quantifying the proportion of existing cases within a given population. Further information on various statistical techniques for epidemiological studies can be found in Fleiss (1981), Sahai and Khurshid (1996), and Woodward (1999). Again, Table 6.2 and Table 6.7 might be useful in sorting out these differences.

6.4.3 Multivariate Modeling

In epidemiological studies, the ergonomist is most concerned with finding which risk factors are related to the MSD and how they are related. Because there are likely several risk factors contributing to the disorder with potentially confounding effects, multivariate models permit the simultaneous evaluation of these risk factors with greatest computational and statistical efficiency. Implicitly, the risk factors are the independent x variables, which are potentially causing the negative outcome or the disorder, which is then the dependent y variable. The classical modeling approach would be to use a linear model of the form

$$y = \beta_0 + \beta_1 x_1 + \beta_2 x_2 + \ldots + \beta_n x_n + \varepsilon \qquad (6.42)$$

where
β = linear regression coefficients
ε = random error term

Although, mathematically, it is possible to use the above linear regression model for epidemiological analysis, there are several major problems with this approach. All are related to the basic fact that the independent outcome variable is typically either a binary variable with a value of 0 if no outcome occurs or a value of 1 if the outcome is present, or a proportion, representing a risk with a value in the range of 0 to 1. Therefore, the y–x relationship will most likely not be linear and the error distribution will not be the standard normal distribution. Proportions will typically arise from a binomial distribution. One remedial measure to linearize the regression and stabilize the

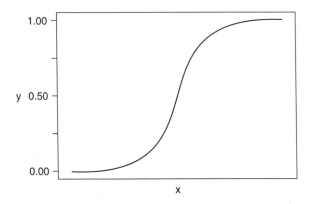

FIGURE 6.12
The logistic function.

error term variance is to transform the data. The arcsine square root is one suggestion (Woodward, 1999). However, this approach is only an approximation.

The best approach for binary variables is to use a *logistic* or *logit function* of the form:

$$y = \frac{1}{1+e^{-(\beta_0+\beta_1 x_1)}} \tag{6.43}$$

Its S-shape matches well both the binary or proportional form of the data (Figure 6.12). Equation 6.43 can be manipulated to the alternate form:

$$\ln\left[p/(1-p)\right] = \beta_0 + \beta_1 x_1 \tag{6.44}$$

Note that the left-hand side is the natural logarithm of the odds for a disorder, with probability p substituted for y. Thus, the logistic function forms a direct relationship between the logarithm of the odds of a disorder and the corresponding risk factors (Christensen, 1997).

As in linear regression analysis, the regression coefficients can be tested for statistical significance, under the hypothesis that $\beta_i = 0$, using the *Wald statistic* (W):

$$W = \beta_i / \text{SE}(\beta_i) \tag{6.45}$$

The Wald statistic follows the standard normal distribution and the null hypothesis can be rejected for either large positive or negative values of the test statistic (Jennings, 1986; Hosmer and Lemeshow, 1989).

The traditional approach to statistical model building is to seek the most parsimonious model that still explains the variability of the data. The inclusion of too many variables may cause confounding of variables and overfitting the model (i.e., too many variables as compared to the size of the data), resulting in unrealistically large coefficient estimates and correspondingly large standard errors. Furthermore, logistic regression with a large number of variables requires a considerable amount of computational time due to the iterations of the maximum likelihood function.

Therefore, a typical approach is to first conduct a multiple logistic regression concentrating on a single factor of interest. Termed "pseudo" univariate logistic regression, this allows one to find a smaller set of competent candidate variables for the final model. These variables are entered into full multiple logistic regression model through a forward stepwise algorithm, using a specified inclusion level for the Wald statistic. Once included, all variables are examined again to check if the one with largest probability (i.e., smallest z or W) should be removed at a specified exclusion level. Hosmer and Lemeshow (1989) recommend values in the range of 0.15 and 0.20 for inclusion to prevent excluding important variables from the model.

Once the model is complete (i.e., no more variables can be entered into the model) a goodness-of-fit test should be performed using one of several different measures. The Hosmer-Lemeshow (1989) statistic, H_c, based on a $2 \times m$ contingency table, and the Pearson chi square statistic in Equation 6.8 are perhaps easiest. An arbitrary number of groups, m, are chosen. Typically, m equals 10, corresponding to deciles of risk. The groups are defined by probabilities corresponding to values of $k/10$, with $k = 1, 2,\ldots10$ and the groups contain all subjects with estimated probabilities between adjacent cut points. Thus, the first group contains all subjects whose probability is ≤ 0.1, while the tenth group contains all those subjects whose probability is >0.9. Each group has two rows, corresponding to the outcome or to the lack of outcome. The observed values are the actual subject counts in the appropriate groupings. Estimates of the expected values are obtained by summing the estimated probabilities over all subjects in the outcome row in a group. For the lack of outcome row, the estimated expected value is obtained by summing, over all subjects in that group, one minus the estimated probability. The average expected value for each case is found by dividing the sums by the number of responses. The final calculation of the chi-square statistic in Equation 6.8 would have 20 entries for $m = 10$ and would be compared to the χ^2 with $m - 2$ or 8 degrees of freedom.

Now the model terms can be interpreted to make inferences about the study populations and occupational risk factors. For example, consider the simple model in Equation 6.44. Assume that the two populations are defined by the influence of one risk factor x_1. The control population was not exposed and x_1 is zero. Substituting into Equation 6.44 yields

$$\ln\left[p/\left(1-p\right)\right] = \beta_0 \tag{6.46}$$

By taking the antilog of both sides, the odds for the control population to incur the disorder becomes

$$p/(1-p) = e^{\beta_0} \qquad (6.47)$$

The case population is exposed to the risk factor and x_1 is one. Substituting into Equation 6.44 yields

$$\ln[p/(1-p)] = \beta_0 + \beta_1 \qquad (6.48)$$

Again, taking the antilog of both sides yields the odds for the case population to incur the disorder:

$$p/(1-p) = e^{\beta_0 + \beta_1} = e^{\beta_0} \times e^{\beta_1} \qquad (6.49)$$

The odds ratio for the case population as compared to the control population with regard to the risk factor becomes the ratio of Equations 6.47 and 6.49 and is simply

$$OR = e^{\beta_1} \qquad (6.50)$$

Thus, the odds ratio for any given risk factor can be found by taking the antilog of the corresponding coefficient. The $100(1 - \alpha)\%$ confidence interval for the odds ratio can be calculated using the standard error of the corresponding risk factor coefficient (Woodward, 1999):

$$e^{\beta_1 \pm z_{\alpha/2} SE(\beta_1)} \qquad (6.51)$$

As an example, consider You's (1999) case-control study of carpal tunnel syndrome. The most significant risk factors were age, wrist ratio, MSD history, and exposure of the hands to cold temperatures. The model coefficients β_i (all significant at $p < 0.05$) were 0.08, 0.32, 2.76, and 2.86, respectively, with corresponding standard errors of 0.042, 0.106, 0.933, and 1.193. The odds ratios for the cold temperature risk factor can be calculated simply from

$$e^{2.86} = 17.5 \qquad (6.52)$$

The 95% confidence interval is

$$e^{2.86 \pm 1.96 \times 1.193} = (1.68, \, 181.0) \qquad (6.53)$$

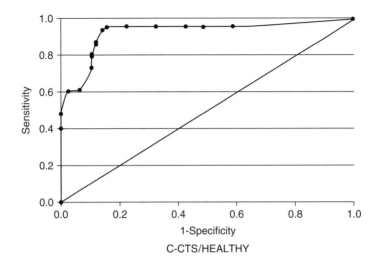

FIGURE 6.13

ROC curve for a carpal tunnel syndrome risk assessment model. (From You, H., 1999. The Development of a Risk Assessment Model for Carpal Tunnel Syndrome, Ph.D. thesis, University Park, PA: Pennsylvania State University. With permission.)

Because the confidence interval does not include the value of 1.0, the odds ratio is significant and one can conclude that workers exposed to cold temperatures will be considerably more likely (17.5 times, to be exact) to incur carpal tunnel syndrome as compared to unexposed workers. The odds ratios for the first three risk factors compute to values of 1.08, 1.37, and 15.76.

However, there are several other variables in the model and there could be possible interactions between the different risk factors as confounding effects. Also, the specific odds (rather than odds ratios) and confidence intervals for the odds can be calculated. However, this is a much more difficult procedure involving the variance-covariance matrix. Details for the above techniques can be found in Woodward (1999).

Other statistical techniques can be used to further ascertain the sensitivity, specificity, and validity of the model. These concepts are discussed in greater detail in Section 8.2 as the appropriateness, meaningfulness, or usefulness of a model or test to predict or quantify the actual risk that is incurred for a given individual while performing a given task in a given work environment. The plotting of *sensitivity* as a function of (1 − *specificity*) in a *receiver operating characteristic* (ROC) plot (Figure 6.13) can demonstrate that the models have a high power of discriminating cases from controls. The farther the ROC curve deviates from the diagonal line, the more discriminating the test. A test having a curve on the diagonal has equal chances of making a correct or incorrect decision. A perfect test would have an ROC curve going up the *y*-axis to a sensitivity of 1 and then going straight across parallel to the *x*-axis. The model plotted in Figure 6.13 shows a high level of discriminability, although not perfect. The actual value of discriminability, identified

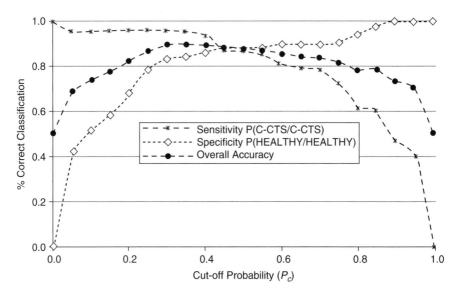

FIGURE 6.14

Classification performance of carpal tunnel syndrome risk assessment model. (From You, H., 1999. The Development of a Risk Assessment Model for Carpal Tunnel Syndrome, Ph.D. thesis, University Park, PA: Pennsylvania State University. With permission.)

as d', of the ROC curve can be computed by adding the two z-scores corresponding to the sensitivity and specificity at a specific cut-off criterion probability p_c. In this particular example, d' equals 2.51. It can vary from 0 to ∞, with larger values best (You, 1999; You et al., 2004).

A p_c is established to classify an individual into one of the two groups — if the probability of an individual belonging to the case group is greater than p_c, then the individual is classified into the case group; if less than p_c, then the individual is classified into the control group. For this particular study the determination of p_c was determined by the intersection of the specificity and sensitivity curves at roughly 0.50 (Figure 6.14). Note that for the overall model, the sensitivity is 87%, specificity is 88%, and accuracy is 88%.

The final step in model assessment is cross validation to determine the classification accuracy of the model. In lieu of selecting a new subject pool, the jack-knife method by Afifi and Clark (1996) creates a half-sized data set by choosing subject data elements randomly from both cases and controls in proportion to their original set size. Then, each of the above selected subjects is removed one at a time from the original data set, upon which a new multiple logistic regression model is created. A probability is estimated for each excluded participant using the corresponding logistic regression model and a classification is made for that excluded participant based on the new p_c. This new classification, as well as new sensitivity and specificity values, is compared to the original model. Obviously, this procedure requires considerable effort and computing resources. Figure 6.15 summarizes the

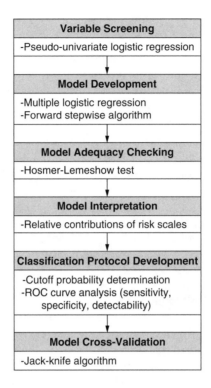

FIGURE 6.15
The development and validation procedure for a multivariate carpal tunnel syndrome risk assessment model. (From You, H., 1999. The Development of a Risk Assessment Model for Carpal Tunnel Syndrome, Ph.D. thesis, University Park, PA: Pennsylvania State University. With permission.)

various procedures and techniques used in the development of a multivariate model.

6.4.4 Quality of Epidemiological Research

For any study to adequately determine the work-relatedness of MSDs, several key criteria must be fulfilled. First, the study must show that there is an exposure, e.g., workers are being exposed to vibration while using power tools. Second, the study must show that the outcome of interest occurred, e.g., carpal tunnel syndrome has been diagnosed. Third and most importantly, *causality* or a direct association between exposure and the outcome must be shown. This association depends on several factors (Campbell and Stanley, 1966):

1. *Temporality.* The exposure precedes the outcome in time.
2. *Temporal contiguity,* or the timeliness of the precedence. The more temporally remote an exposure, the more likely other factors may affect the outcome.

3. *Covariance* of exposure and outcome. A reduction in the exposure should result in a reduction of the outcome.

4. *Congruity* of exposure and outcome. The direct association between levels of exposure and the levels of outcome is typically expressed as a *dose–response relationship*. In a linear relationship, a doubling of the dose would result in a doubling of the response. However, not all relationships are linear.

5. *Plausibility.* The likelihood that an association is compatible with a physiological mechanism, or that there is not some other plausible explanation 'or a confounding variable that is associated with both the exposure and the outcome.

The strength of this association can be evaluated by various measures discussed earlier: the odds ratio or relative risk ratio, consistency of the association across various subgroups, specificity of the association, and quantitative dose–response values.

More specifically, the general criteria mentioned above reflect in the following details to define a quality study:

1. In cohort studies, the inclusion or exclusion criteria for both exposed and non-exposed groups should be clearly defined. In case-control studies, the criteria for defining a case vs. a control must also be clearly defined. Similar criteria need to be identified for subdividing cases into work-related and non-work-related cases. This will increase statistical power and population validity.

2. Participation rates for groups or subgroups must exceed 70% or more. This will limit selection bias in the study.

3. Health outcome must be defined both by symptoms and a physical examination. The use of objective measures will limit the unreliability found in self-reports.

4. The investigators were blinded to health status when assessing exposure status, or vice versa. This will again limit selection bias.

5. The exposure measures were well defined and assessed independently. Again, self-reports tend to be less reliable than direct observations or actual measurements.

Unfortunately, not all the studies reviewed here fulfill all of the criteria. In fact, generally, few do. Typically, most studies were cross sectional, the simplest to implement, but having the least validity. However, these also tended to have large subject pools, which is good from a representative sample of the population standpoint. On the other hand, they tended to use less costly but more subjective approaches, job titles or self-reports, to evaluate exposures. In general, these studies were not rejected, because that would have eliminated a large proportion of studies. Also, many studies were not that rigorous in having high participation rates or using objective measures to evaluate outcomes. Therefore, as long as a study provided quantitative results (i.e., an OR, RR, or AR value) and fulfilled either the participation rate or outcome evaluation criteria, they were retained for further analyses.

These studies are summarized in Table 6.10 through Table 6.16 for neck MSD, shoulder MSD, elbow MSD, hand/wrist carpal tunnel syndrome, hand/wrist tendinitis, and hand/wrist vibration syndrome cases, with as much quantitative information as could be gleaned from the published information. Note that the attributable risk fraction was calculated with the OR as an estimate for the relative risk. As mentioned in Section 6.4.2, this approximation will be fairly accurate when the prevalence is low, roughly below 20 to 30%. A complete listing of all relevant MSD research studies with specialized categorizations can be found in the very detailed compendiums by NIOSH (1995, 1997), Kourinka and Forcier (1995), and the National Research Council (2001).

6.5 The Scientific Research and Evidence for Occupational Risk Factors

6.5.1 Neck Disorders

With regard to neck MSDs, studies from the United States have generally separated neck from shoulder disorders, whereas Scandinavian and Japanese studies have tended to lump the two together. This was based on the anatomical reasoning that many muscles act simultaneously on both the shoulder girdle and the upper spine. For the present discussions, both categories were combined. Overall prevalence ranges from 1.4% when diagnosed by physical findings to 4.9% when defined simply by symptoms alone (Hagberg and Wegman, 1987). Of the 30 studies examined and shown in Table 6.10, 23 found statistically significant effects for one or more contributory risk factors. With regard to repetition, defined as repetitive neck movements or repeated arm or shoulder motions, all four studies that could identify repetition as a separate factor found a significant positive association, with ORs ranging from 1.2 to 28.9 that accounted for an average of 72% of attributable risk. An additional 12 studies examined repetition but in conjunction with other variables. Of these, seven found statistically significant positive associations. Unfortunately, many studies primarily utilize hand/arm exposure assessments without specifically identifying neck or shoulder assessments. This gives rise to the possibility of misclassification errors. Also, because in most cases the studies were cross-sectional, temporality cannot be determined. However, several studies (Kiken et al., 1990; Baron et al., 1991; Hales et al., 1994)

TABLE 6.10

Summary of Epidemiological Studies Examining Neck MSDs

Reference	Type of Study	No. of Subjects	Study Population	Participation Rate > 70%	Physical Exam	Risk Factor	Risk Estimate (OR, RR)	Attributable Risk (%)	Exposure Assessment
Andersen and Gaardboe (1993a)	CS	1,482	Sewing machine operators	Yes	No	F, R	4.6*	78	Job titles
Andersen and Gaardboe(1993b)	CS	107	Sewing machine operators	Yes	Yes	F, R	6.8*	85	Job titles
Baron et al. (1991)	CS	281	Grocery scanners	No	Yes	F, R	2.00	—	Job titles
Bergqvist et al. (1995a)	CS	260	Office workers	Yes	No	P	4.4*	77	Observed
Bergqvist et al. (1995b)	CS	322	Office workers	Yes	Yes	R, C	6.9*	86	Self-reports
Bernard et al. (1994)	CS	973	Office workers	Yes	No	P, R	1.4*	29	Self-reports
Ekberg et al. (1994)	CC	746	Physician patients	Yes	No	P	4.8*	79	Self-reports
						R	15.6*	94	Self-reports
Ekberg et al. (1995)	CS	687	General population	Yes	No	R	1.2*	17	Self-reports
Hales and Fine (1989)	CS	112	Poultry processors	Yes	Yes	F, R	1.60	—	Job titles
Hales et al. (1994)	CS	518	Office workers	Yes	Yes	C	3.8*	74	Self-reports
Holmström et al. (1992)	CS	1,773	Construction workers	Yes	No	P	1.4–2.0*	29–50	Self-reports
Hünting et al. (1981)	CS	295	Office workers	NR	Yes	P, R	9.9*	90	Observed
Kamwendo et al. (1991)	CS	420	Office workers	Yes	No	C	1.6*	39	Self-reports
Kiken et al. (1990)	CS	294	Poultry processors	Yes	Yes	F, R	1.30	—	Job titles
Kukkonen et al. (1983)	CS	161	Office workers	NR	Yes	P, C	2.3*	57	Self-reports
Kuorinka and Koskinen (1979)	CS	206	Manufacturing	Yes	Yes	C	4.1*	76	Job titles
Linton and Kamwedo (1990)	CS	22,180	Industrial workers	Yes	No	C	3.5*	71	Self-reports

Study	Type of Study	Number of Subjects	Study population			Risk Factor	Risk Estimate	Participation Rate	
Luopajärvi et al. (1979)	CS	285	Assembly workers	Yes	Yes	F, R	1.60	—	Observed
Milerad and Ekenvall (1990)	CS	199	Dentists	Yes	No	P, R	2.1*	52	Self-reports
Ohlsson et al. (1995)	CS	214	Manufacturing	Yes	Yes	P, R	3.6*	72	Observed
Punnett et al. (1991)	CS	254	Meat packers	Yes	No	F, R	1.8 (males)	—	Observed
Rossignol et al. (1987)	CS	191	Office workers	Yes	No	R	4.6*	78	Self-reports
Schibya et al. (1995)	C	303	Sewing machine operators	Yes	No	C	3.3*	70	Self-reports
Tola et al. (1988)	CS	2,143	Machine operators	Yes	No	P	1.8*	44	Self-reports
Veiersted and Westgaard (1994)	C	30	Manufacturing	No	Yes	F	6.7*	85	Measured
Viikari–Juntura et al. (1991b)	C	154	General population	Yes	Yes	P	7.2*	86	Self-reports
						P	1.50	—	
Viikari–Juntura et al. (1994)	C	1,832	Machine operators	Yes	No	C	4.2*	76	Job titles
			Carpenters	Yes	No	C	3.0*	67	
Welch et al. (1995)	CS	47	Sheet metal workers	Yes	No	P	7.50	—	Self-reports
Wells et al. (1983)	CS	399	Mail carriers	Yes	No	F, P	2.6*	61	Self-reports
Yu and Wong (1996)	CS	151	Office workers	Yes	No	R	28.9*	97	Self-reports

Note: Some studies did not separate neck and shoulder disorders.

Type of Study: C = cohort, CC = case-control, CS = cross-sectional

Number of Subjects: Total of study population and referents or controls

Risk Factor: C= combination or many, F = force, P = posture, R = repetition, V = vibration

Participation Rate: NR = not reported

Risk Estimate: OR = odds ratio, RR = relative risk, * = $p \leq 0.05$.

defined outcome definition by excluding persons reporting symptoms prior to the job, ensuring that exposure preceded MSD occurrence. There were no studies that showed a clear dose–response relationship between repetition and neck MSDs. Plausibility that repetition is a risk factor for injury is found in sports injuries whereby low-load forces with high repetition result in a gradual deterioration of tissue strength from stress/strain deformation fatigue (Nicholas, 1990).

Posture, as a risk factor, has been generally defined either as an external load or as an internal force. Five of seven studies that isolated force separately from other risk factors found a significant positive association, with ORs ranging from 1.4 to 7.2, which accounted for 56% of the attributable risk (Table 6.11). If the two studies with nonsignificant effects are added in, then the attributable risk would drop to 42%. Four more studies examined posture but in conjunction with other variables, and all four found statistically significant positive associations. Temporality is most apparent in the prospective study of Veiersted and Westgaard (1994), in which workers developed MSDs within 6 to 51 weeks of starting work. Several studies (Rossignol et al., 1987; Andersen and Gaardboe, 1993a,b) found a dose–response relationship with prevalence or symptoms increasing with increased number of hours spent on task or the number of years at work, controlling for age. Plausibility for posture as a risk factor, indirectly through force, since the two are related, has been established by studies showing decreased blood flow, increased metabolite concentrations, and potential injury in near maximally contracted muscles (Larsson et al., 1990).

Most studies examined force in conjunction with other variables; in fact, only one study found a significant positive association with force as a single factor. Eight more studies examined force in combination, but only three of these found statistically significant positive associations. However, the combination of posture and force, especially in the form of static posture or static loading in extreme postures, causes an especially positive association with MSDs, accounting for up to 80% of attributable risk (Veiersted and Westgaard, 1994). Similar to repetition, there was no clear demonstration of temporality or a dose–response relationship. There was also no evidence that vibration had positive association with neck MSDs.

Overall, one can conclude, from Table 6.10 or the summary in Table 6.11, that there is evidence for positive association between repetition, posture, and force, individually, and neck-related MSDs. Interestingly, of the seven studies with nonsignificant associations, five relied on job titles or self-reports to assess exposure, while four of six studies that used direct observations or quantitative measurements to evaluate exposure had statistically significant positive associations between risk factors and MSDs. Therefore, one can conclude that the more objective the exposure assessment, the more likely a significant positive association can be found. Such associations are more easily visible for the neck as opposed to the other joints because of the large number of available studies performed.

TABLE 6.11

Summary of Tables 6.10 through 6.16 Showing Strength of Evidence for Contributory Risk Factors to MSDs

Upper Limb Area		Contributory Risk Factors									Conclusions Regarding Association of Risk Factors and MSDs
		Repetition		Posture		Force		Vibration		Combination	
		#Sig	OR	#Sig	OR	#Sig	OR	#Sig	OR	#Sig	OR	
Neck		4/4	1.2–29	5/7	1.4–7.2	1/1	6.7	0/0	—	15/20 1.4–9.9		Repetition, posture, force, and combinations thereof show positive associations
Shoulder		1/1	1.6	4/4	2.4–18	3/3	1.8–18	0/0	—	7/7 1.7–7.3		Combinations of repetition, posture, and force show strong positive associations
Elbow		1/1	2.8	2/2	4–37	1/2	6.7	1/1	4.9	5/9 1.7–6.7		Most individual and combinations of factors show positive associations
Hand/Wrist	Carpal tunnel syndrome	4/9	1.9–5.5	2/2	5.4–8.7	3/5	1.5–2.0	6/6	1.9–21	4/5 2.3–8.3		Vibration shows a very strong association, the combination of factors is also strong
	Tendinitis	0/1	—	1/1	3.7–6.2	0/0	—	0/0	—	5/5 2.5–17		The combination of risk factors shows strong positive associations
	Vibration syndrome	—	—	—	—	—	—	9/9	3.4–85	—	—	Vibration shows a very strong positive association

Note: #Sig = The number of studies showing significant results out of the total number studies in the given category.

OR = Odds ratios for the statistically significant studies.

6.5.2 Shoulder Disorders

For shoulder-related MSDs, repetition was defined by the number of pre-defined shoulder movements, the number of pieces handled per unit time, or some generalized characterization of repetitive work with the arm. The number of studies that examined repetition, or other risk factors individually, was rather limited (Table 6.12). However, repetition in combination with other risk factors showed an especially strong positive association with MSDs, with all five such studies showing statistically significant ORs ranging from 1.6 to 5.0 that accounted for an average attributable risk of 58%. Several studies of a cross-sectional design limited the number of cases in which the MSD was already present during exposure in order to suggest some temporality (Chiang et al., 1993; Ohlsson et al., 1994, 1995). For a dose–response relationship, Chiang et al. (1993) found significant increasing prevalences with increased repetition and Ohlsson et al. (1995) found increased MSDs with increased number of arm elevations and abductions. Plausibility is evidenced by Herberts et al.'s (1984) findings of fatigue in the supra- and infraspinatus muscles. This leads to the hypothesis that the rotator cuff muscles may develop high intramuscular pressures leading to impaired circulation in the muscles and tendons. The latter effect may also lead to inflammation and consequent tendinitis.

Four studies isolated posture separately from other risk factors and all found a significant positive association with ORs ranging from 2.4 to 18.3 and accounting for 81% of the attributable risk (Table 6.11). Three other studies found posture in combination with repetition to have statistically significant positive associations. In spite of the cross-sectional design of studies, elimination of workers with preexisting symptoms will improve the ability to detect temporality (Baron et al., 1991). Four studies found some evidence of a dose–response relationship, typically a higher OR for shoulder MSDs for individuals working longer hours (Bjelle et al., 1979; Baron et al., 1991; Ohlsson et al., 1994, 1995). Plausibility follows the same line of reasoning as for repetition (and force): more abducted arms place more pressure on the tendon and other tissues causing inflammation, microtrauma, and further problems.

Three studies isolated force separately from other risk factors and all found a significant positive association with ORs ranging from 1.8 to 18.3 and accounting for 72% of the attributable risk. Two other studies found force in combination with other variables to have statistically significant positive associations. Wells et al. (1983) found some evidence of temporality of carrying increased loads with incidence of shoulder disorders in mail carriers. For those carriers who experienced a weight increase as compared to the control group, the OR was 5.7 ($p < 0.05$) demonstrating a dose–response effect. Similarly Stenlund et al. (1992) found that, for the left shoulder, ORs increased with level of lifetime load lifted. This latter study was also the only one that examined the effects of vibration (in combination with force) on MSDs, finding a significant positive association. Overall, one can conclude, from Table 6.12 or

TABLE 6.12

Summary of Epidemiological Studies Examining Shoulder MSDs

Reference	Type of Study	No. of Subjects	Study Population	Participation Rate > 70%	Physical Exam	Risk Factor	Risk Estimate (OR, RR)	Attributable Risk (%)	Exposure Assessment
Andersen and Gaardboe (1993a)	CS	1,294	Sewing machine operators	Yes	No	C	7.3*	86	Job titles
Baron et al. (1991)	CS	281	Grocery scanners	No	Yes	F, R	3.9*	74	Job titles
Bjelle et al. (1979)	CC	51	Industrial workers	NR	Yes	P	10.6*	91	Measured
Chiang et al. (1993)	CS	207	Fish processors	Yes	Yes	F	1.8*	44	Measured
						R	1.6*	38	
English et al. (1995)	CC	1,576	General population	Yes	Yes	R, P	2.3*	57	Self-reports
Herberts et al. (1981)	CS	188	Shipyard welders, clerks	NR	Yes	P	18.3*	95	Job titles
Herberts et al. (1984)	CS	188	Shipyard welders, clerks	NR	Yes	F	18.3*	95	Job titles
		188	Plate workers	NR	Yes	F	16.2*	94	Job titles
Hoekstra et al. (1994)	CS	108	Office workers	Yes	No	P	5.1*	80	Self-reports
Milerad and Ekenvall (1990)	CS	199	Dentists	Yes	No	P	2.4*	58	Self-reports
Ohlsson et al. (1994)	CS	736	Fish processors	Yes	Yes	C	2.9–3.5*	66–71	Observed
Ohlsson et al. (1995)	CS	214	Manufacturing	Yes	Yes	P, R	5.0*	80	Observed
Sakakibara et al. (1995)	CS	52	Fruit pickers	Yes	Yes	P, R	1.7*	41	Observed
Stenlund et al. (1992)	CS	110	Rock blasters	Yes	Yes	F, V	2.2*	55	Self-reports
		109	Bricklayers	Yes	Yes	F, V	4.0*	75	Self-reports
Wells et al. (1983)	CS	399	Mail carriers	Yes	No	F	3.3–5.7*	70–82	Self-reports

Type of Study: C = cohort, CC = case-control, CS = cross-sectional

Number of Subjects: Total of study population and referents or controls

Risk Factor: C = combination or many, F = force, P = posture, R = repetition, V = vibration

Participation Rate: NR = not reported

Risk Estimate: OR = odds ratio, RR = relative risk, * = $p \leq 0.05$

the summary in Table 6.11, that there is evidence for a positive association between repetition, posture, and force and shoulder-related MSDs.

6.5.3 Elbow Disorders

There are relatively few studies examining risk factors and elbow MSDs (primarily epicondylitis). Repetition was typically defined by the number of cyclical elbow flexions/extensions, elbow pronations/supinations, or wrist motions that led to changes in the elbow region. Only one study for each of the risk factors (repetition, force, vibration) showed a significant positive association with MSDs (Table 6.13). There were two such studies for posture. However, nine studies showed combinations of risk factors to have positive associations with MSDs, five of which yielded statistically significant results with ORs ranging from 1.7 to 6.4 that accounted for 40% of the attributable risk (Table 6.11). As almost all of the studies were cross sectional, temporality cannot be easily determined. However, some dose–response relationship was shown by Baron et al. (1991) for number of hours worked per week, by Moore and Garg (1994) with respect to increasing strain on jobs, and Ritz (1995) with duration of exposure to stressful tasks. Plausibility is consistent with earlier clinical case studies and parallel sports research studies. Repetitive contractions of forearm extensors produce a force that is transmitted to the origin of the tendon on the lateral epicondyle. A chronic overload on the bone–tendon junction leads to microtrauma and inflammation. The lack of significance in many, especially cross-sectional, studies may result from a *survivor bias*. Only workers who are resistant to injury stay on the high exposure jobs, while those with MSDs shift to less stressful jobs. Overall, the majority of epidemiological studies support the hypothesis of repetitive, forceful work or repetitive flexions, extensions, pronations, or supinations leading to an increased risk of epicondylitis.

6.5.4 Hand/Wrist — Carpal Tunnel Syndrome

Vibration, as an individual risk factor, shows the strongest association with carpal tunnel syndrome cases, with all six studies showing statistically significant ORs ranging from 1.9 to 21.3 that accounted for an average of 80% of the attributable risk (Table 6.14; see Table 6.11). Because all studies used a dichotomous classification any dose–response relationship is difficult to determine. Also, there were no longitudinal studies to show temporality. The exact physiological mechanism for the development of carpal tunnel syndrome from vibration is not known because of the confounding factors of repetitive, forceful exertions typically found while using vibrating power tools. However, Taylor (1982) speculates that vibration injures peripheral nerves either directly by reducing tactile sensitivity or indirectly through the arterial vasoconstriction and the resulting ischemia of nerve tissue. The other

TABLE 6.13

Summary of Epidemiological Studies Examining Elbow MSDs

Reference	Type of Study	No. of Subjects	Study Population	Participation Rate > 70%	Physical Exam	Risk Factor	Risk Estimate (OR, RR)	Attributable Risk (%)	Exposure Assessment
Andersen and Gaardboe (1993a)	CS	1,205	Sewing machine operators	Yes	No	F, R	1.7	—	Job titles
Baron et al. (1991)	CS	270	Grocery scanners	No	Yes	F, R	2.3	—	Job titles
Bovenzi et al. (1991)	CS	96	Chain saw operators	NR	Yes	V	4.9*	80	Measured
Burt et al. (1990)	CS	836	Newspaper employees	Yes	No	R	2.8*	64	Observed
Byström et al. (1995)	CS	385	Auto assembly workers	Yes	Yes	C	0.7	—	Self-reports
Chiang et al. (1993)	CS	207	Fish processors	Yes	Yes	F, R	6.7* (males) 1.4 (females)	85	Measured
Hoekstra et al. (1994)	CS	108	Office workers	Yes	No	P	4.0*	75	Self-reports
Hughes et al. (1997)	CS	211	Smelter workers	No	Yes	P	37.0*	97	Observed
Kurppa et al. (1981)	C	862	Meat processors	Yes	Yes	F	6.7*	85	Observed
Luopajärvi et al. (1979)	CS	285	Food packers	Yes	Yes	C	2.7	—	Observed
Moore and Garg (1994)	CS	230	Pork processors	Yes	Yes	F, R	5.5*	82	Observed
Punnett et al. (1985)	CS	238	Garment workers	No	No	C	2.4*	58	Self-reports
Ritz (1995)	CS	290	Gas and water workers	NR	Yes	C	1.7–2.2*	41–55	Observed
Roto and Kivi (1984)	CS	162	Meatpackers	Yes	Yes	C	6.4*	84	Job titles
Viikari–Juntura et al. (1991a)	CS	709	Meatpackers	Yes	Yes	F	0.9	—	Observed

Type of Study: C = cohort, CC = case-control, CS = cross-sectional

No. of Subjects: Total of study population and referents or controls

Risk Factor: C = combination or many, F = force, P = posture, R = repetition, V = vibration

Participation Rate: NR = not reported

Risk Estimate: OR = odds ratio, RR = relative risk, * = $p \leq 0.05$

TABLE 6.14

Summary of Epidemiological Studies Examining Hand/Wrist Carpal Tunnel Syndrome Cases

Reference	Type of Study	No. of Subjects	Study Population	Participation Rate > 70%	Physical Exam	Risk Factor	Risk Estimate (OR, RR)	Attributable Risk (%)	Exposure Assessment
Barnhart et al. (1991)	CS	173	Ski fabricators	No	Yes	R	1.9–3.9*	47–75	Observed
Baron et al. (1991)	CS	175	Grocery scanners	No	Yes	F	3.7	—	Job titles
Bovenzi et al. (1991)	CS	96	Chain saw operators	NR	Yes	V	21.3*	95	Measured
Bovenzi (1994)	CS	1,148	Rock drillers and cutters	Yes	Yes	V	3.4*	71	Measured
Cannon et al. (1981)	CC	120	Aircraft engine workers	NR	Yes	V	7.0*	86	Measured
Chatterjee (1992)	CC	31	Rock drillers	Yes	Yes	V	10.9*	91	Measured
Chiang et al. (1990)	CS	207	Frozen food workers	Yes	Yes	Cold	1.9*	46	Observed
						R	1.9*	47	
Chiang et al. (1993)	CS	207	Fish processors	Yes	Yes	F	1.8*	44	Measured
						R	1.1	—	
deKrom et al. (1990)	CC	629	Hospital patients	Yes	Yes	P	5.4–8.7*	81–89	Self-reports
English et al. (1995)	CC	1,167	Hospital patients	Yes	Yes	P	1.8*	44	Self-reports
						R	0.4	—	
Feldman et al. (1987)	CS	586	Electronics workers	Yes	No	P, R	2.3*	56	Observed
Moore and Garg (1994)	CS	230	Pork processors	Yes	Yes	C	2.8	—	Observed
Morgenstern et al. (1991)	CS	1,058	Grocery workers	Yes	No	R	1.9	—	Self-reports

Reference	Type of Study	No. of Subjects	Study population	Participation Rate	Physical Exam	Risk Factor	Risk Estimate		Method
Nathan et al. (1988)	CS	471	Industrial workers	NR	Yes	F	1.7–2.0*	41–50	Self-reports
						R	1.0	—	
Nathan et al. (1992)	C	315	Industrial workers	No	Yes	F	1.5*	33	Self-reports
						R	1.1	—	
Osorio et al. (1994)	CS	56	Supermarket workers	Yes	Yes	F, R	8.3*	88	Observed
Punnett et al. (1985)	CS	238	Garment workers	No	No	C	2.7*	63	Self-reports
Schottland et al. (1991)	CS	178	Poultry processors	NR	Yes	C	1.7 LH	—	Job titles
							2.9* RH	65	
Silverstein et al. (1987)	CS	652	Industrial workers	Yes	Yes	F	2.9	—	Measured
						R	5.5*	82	
Tanaka et al. (1997)	CS	44,233	General population	Yes	No	P	5.5*	82	Self-reports
						V	1.9*	47	
Wieslander et al. (1989)	CC	177	Hospital patients	Yes	Yes	F	1.8*	44	Self-reports
						R	2.7*	63	
						V	6.1*	84	

Type of Study: C = cohort, CC = case-control, CS = cross-sectional

No. of Subjects: Total of study population and referents or controls

Risk Factor: C = combination or many, F = force, P = posture, R = repetition, V = vibration

Participation Rate, Physical Exam: NR = not reported

Risk Estimate: OR = odds ratio, RR = relative risk, * = $p \leq 0.05$, LH = left hand, RH = right hand three factors, repetition, posture, and force, individually show some evidence for a positive association with carpal tunnel syndrome. Four of nine studies found repetition individually to have a significant positive association with carpal tunnel syndrome. The lack of more significant results is again probably due to a survivor bias. In fact, Nathan et al. (1992) found that the highest risk group had a decrease in carpal tunnel syndrome prevalence over time. This could only occur as workers dropped out (and did not return) from the high-risk group as they incurred injuries. The expected temporality was reported by Feldman et al. (1987) who found increased median nerve motor latencies over time. For posture, individually, only two studies found significant positive associations with ORs ranging from 5.4 to 8.7. However, one study (English et al., 1995) confounded other upper limb joints with the wrist, while the second (Tanaka et al., 1997) was based purely on self-reports, which may limit the strength of the association. A dose–response effect was shown by deKrom et al. (1990) when workers suffered increased carpal tunnel syndrome with reportedly increased working hours.

In terms of force as risk factor, three of five studies found a significant positive association with ORs ranging from 1.5 to 2.0 and accounting for 42% of the attributable risk. However, in these and other studies force was typically combined with other exposure variables (repetition or awkward postures). Temporality is again difficult to ascertain from the cross-sectional nature of the studies. A dose–response relationship was shown individually only in Chiang et al. (1993) but more definitely when combined with repetition in Silverstein et al. (1987), Wieslander et al. (1989), and Osorio et al. (1994). The first study found an OR of 15.5 (or 94% attributable risk) for the combined effect. Plausibility is established by Rempel (1995) who found increased pressure in the carpal tunnel due to tendon forces from repetitive forceful exertions. This pressure in turn may reduce compress venules (which have weaker walls than arterioles), which causes an increasing capillary pressure and greater edema. If the edema becomes chronic, it may trigger fibrosis of nerve tissue. This hypothesis is supported by observations during carpal tunnel syndrome surgery of greater edema and vascular sclerosis and fibrosis (Rempel, 1995). Deviated or flexed wrist postures only further exacerbate the problem by potentially reducing the cross-sectional area of the tunnel and further increasing carpal pressure (Skie et al., 1990).

6.5.5   Hand/Wrist — Tendinitis

There were only seven epidemiological studies that examined physical risk factors associated with hand/wrist tendinitis. While force, repetition, and posture, individually, showed little evidence for a positive association with the incidence of hand/wrist tendinitis cases, the combination of these risk factors showed a very positive association. All five studies in the combination category (Table 6.15; see also Table 6.11) showed statistically significant ORs ranging from 2.5 to 17.0, with an average of 79% attributable risk. The only

TABLE 6.15

Summary of Epidemiological Studies Examining Hand/Wrist Tendinitis Cases

Reference	Type of Study	No. of Subjects	Study Population	Participation Rate > 70%	Physical Exam	Risk Factor	Risk Estimate (OR, RR)	Attributable Risk (%)	Exposure Assessment
Amano et al. (1988)	CS	204	Assembly line workers	NR	Yes	P	3.7–6.2*	73–84	Observed
Armstrong et al. (1987)	CS	652	Industrial workers	Yes	Yes	F, R	17.0*	94	Measured
Byström et al. (1995)	CS	385	Auto assembly workers	Yes	Yes	C	2.5*	60	Self-reports
Kuorinka and Koskinen (1979)	CS	236	Scissor makers	Yes	Yes	R	1.4	—	Observed
Kurppa et al. (1981)	C	765	Meat processors	Yes	Yes	C	14–38.5*	93–97	Observed
Luopajärvi et al. (1979)	CS	285	Food packers	Yes	Yes	C	4.1*	76	Observed
Roto and Kivi (1984)	CS	162	Meatpackers	Yes	Yes	C	3.1*	68	Job titles

Type of Study: C = cohort, CC = case-control, CS = cross-sectional

No. of Subjects: Total of study population and referents or controls

Risk Factor: C = combination or many, F = force, P = posture, R = repetition, V = vibration

Participation Rate: NR = not reported

Risk Estimate: OR = odds ratio, RR = relative risk, * = $p \leq 0.05$

prospective study by Kurppa et al. (1991) showed a significant increase in risk for injury with increasing time on the job indicating direct temporality. Armstrong et al. (1987) demonstrated strong evidence for a dose–response relationship in that the high-force, high-repetition group had a 17 times greater risk than the low-force, low-repetition group. However, somewhat contrary to the proportional role of stressors in carpal tunnel syndrome, the response of muscles and tendons to repetitive activity may be more like a U-shaped curve. Too little or too much activity may be harmful, but intermediate levels may be beneficial. These tissues have the ability to repair themselves, within reason. The difficulty is finding the threshold at which point overuse exceeds the ability of the tissue to repair the damage (Hart et al., 1995).

6.5.6   Hand/Arm — Vibration Syndrome

There is strong evidence of vibration showing a positive association with HAVS. All nine studies (see Table 6.11 and Table 6.16) showed statistically significant ORs from 3.4 to 85 with an average attributable risk of 87%. Although most of the studies are cross-sectional with a high possibility of recall bias and weakening temporality, many studies have indicated information about the latency period between initial exposure and the development of symptoms. This latency ranged from 0.7 to 17 years with a mean of 6.3 years. The one prospective study (Kivekäs et al., 1994) clearly showed an increased incidence rate of 14.7% in Finnish lumberjacks as compared to an incidence rate of only 2.3% in the referent group. In terms of a dose–response relationship, NIOSH (1989) examined the data of 23 cross-sectional studies and found a statistically significant linear relationship between vibration acceleration levels and prevalence of symptoms ($r = 0.67$, $p < 0.01$). As mentioned previously, plausibility has been established by many experts in that vibration injures peripheral nerves either directly, reducing tactile sensitivity, or indirectly, through the arterial vasoconstriction and the resulting ischemia of nerve tissue. Furthermore, if the blood vessels are damaged, they may become less sensitive to the reverse process, vasodilation, further exacerbating recovery from cold working conditions. In fact, there is some evidence that the walls of digital blood vessels may become permanently thickened in patients with HAVS (Takeuchi et al., 1986).

6.6   The Scientific Research and Evidence for Psychosocial Risk Factors

Psychosocial risk factors for upper limb MSDs have been studied less frequently than occupational risk factors, partly because there are fewer good objective measures of exposure and/or risk and partly because psychosocial

TABLE 6.16

Summary of Epidemiological Studies Examining Hand/Wrist Vibration Syndrome Cases

Reference	Type of Study	No. of Subjects	Study Population	Participation Rate > 70%	Physical Exam	Risk Factor	Risk Estimate (OR, RR)	Attributable Risk (%)	Exposure Assessment
Bovenzi et al. (1988)	CS	136	Rock drillers and cutters	NR	Yes	V	6.1*	83	Measured
Bovenzi (1994)	CS	855	Rock drillers and cutters	Yes	Yes	V	9.3*	89	Measured
Bovenzi et al. (1995)	CS	427	Forestry workers	Yes	Yes	V	6.2–32.3*	84–97	Measured
Kivekäs et al. (1994)	C	353	Lumberjacks	Yes	Yes	V	3.4–6.5*	71–85	Self-reports
Letz et al. (1992)	CS	271	Shipyard workers	Yes	No	V	5.0–40.6*	80–98	Self-reports
McKenna et al. (1993)	CS	92	Riveters		Yes	V	24.0*	96	Self-reports
Mirbod et al. (1994)	CS	2,979	Dental, industrial workers	NR	No	V	3.8*	73	Measured
Nagata et al. (1993)	CS	384	Chain-saw operators	NR	Yes	V	7.1*	86	Self-reports
Nilsson et al. (1989)	CS	150	Platers	Yes	Yes	V	14–85*	93–99	Measured

Type of Study: C = cohort, CC = case-control, CS = cross-sectional

No. of Subjects: Total of study population and referents or controls

Risk Factor: C = combination or many, F = force, P = posture, R = repetition, V = vibration

Participation Rate, Physical Exam: NR = not reported

Risk Estimate: OR = odds ratio, RR = relative risk, * = $p \leq 0.05$, LH = left hand, RH = right hand factors are measured at an individual level rather than a group level as for occupational factors, which limits the accuracy or precision of the measurements. Typically, psychosocial factors are separated into three subcategories. The first includes job and work environment factors that are not strictly physical and includes factors related to (1) job content, e.g., workload, control over the job, rest breaks, and other cyclical aspects, (2) work organization, e.g., supervision, interpersonal relationships, prestige, status, office hierarchy, etc., and (3) financial aspects, e.g., pay, benefits, vacation, equity issues, etc. The second category includes activities outside the work environment, e.g., exercise, a second job, family, child-care issues, etc. The third category includes individual characteristics such as genetic, e.g., gender, race, intelligence, and anatomical characteristics; social, e.g., social class, cultural background, educational level, and individual personality, i.e., attitudes toward work, attitudes toward life, susceptibility to stress and pain, etc. (Hurrell and Murphy, 1992).

Of the 19 studies that roughly fit previously discussed quality issues and include quantitative information (OR values and statistical calculations), most focused primarily on work environment factors rather than individual factors (Table 6.17). High workload, in a variety of forms including job pressures and lack of rest breaks, was the one factor that was most consistently associated with upper limb MSDs. Of the 19 studies, 12 found statistically significant positive associations. Somewhat counterintuitively, low workload in the form of monotonous work was also found to be a significant factor for MSDs in 5 of the 19 studies. Lack of control over the job was another factor that had significant positive associations with MSDs in 10 of the 19 studies.

Gender and age were the most common individual characteristics showing positive associations with MSDs, with females and older workers being typically more at risk. Outside-of-work factors showed few significant associations, perhaps because of the overlapping, confounding effects of many of these factors or because outside work situations may be exacerbated by work conditions (Sauter and Swanson, 1996). Positive associations were found for all types of MSDs, depending on which questions were asked about which type of symptoms. However, twice as many studies found significant positive associations with neck and shoulder disorders rather than with elbow, wrist, or hand disorders.

There is not a clear link between psychosocial factors and the etiology of MSDs. Some of the hypothesized explanations are as follows. An increased awareness of the problem leads to an increased perception and increased reporting. Increased muscle tension may lead to increased muscle strain or may exacerbate existing muscle strain, which may then develop into pain spasm cycles and a chronic problem (Bergkvist, 1984; Bongers et al., 1993; Sauter, and Swanson, 1996). The key would then be to break the cycle so that the initial pain and discomfort can be relieved. Finally, in a perverse way, the present system of workers' compensation may be a form of "incentive" that encourages workers to overreport symptoms (Frank et al., 1995).

Primarily because of the ease of administration of a survey as a snapshot in time, all but one study (Kvarnström, 1983) was cross-sectional. This, to some degree, limits the usefulness of the data and conclusions. Ideally, there should be more cohort (prospective) studies to truly identify the critical risk factors. Most studies used surveys or past medical records to establish the assessment of MSD outcome. Again, a worker's recall or subjective evaluation of pain or discomfort is not equivalent to a medically verified MSD. Finally, a wide variety of questionnaires or evaluations were used to classify psychosocial exposures. Ideally, only a few consistent measures should be used such that comparisons can be made between studies or data combined across studies to establish more significant conclusions. Nevertheless, there is still a clear positive association between psychosocial risk factors and MSDs in the upper limbs. This indicates the importance of not only modifying work-related physical sources of job stress but also the non-work-related sources of stress.

6.7 Iatrogenesis — A Contrarian View

Iatrogenesis refers to the argument, advocated by a small but vocal group of medical and public health researchers, that WRMSDs are merely an iatrogenic labeling of everyday pains. Iatrogenic is medically defined as resulting from the course of the professional activities of a physician, implying auto-suggestion from discussions, examinations, or treatments. In practice, iatrogenesis refers to the discounting of physical occupational risk factors in the development of MSDs, in favor of extraneous, sociological, or individual factors. Iatrogenesis was first proposed by Ferguson (1971a,b, 1973) as a form of "craft neuroses" or occupational disorders with a considerable amount of anxiety and other behavioral issues specific to a craft. The term first appeared in articles by Ferguson (1987) and Cleland (1987) to explain the rapid, almost epidemic-like, increase in RSIs (repetition strain injuries, the Australian term for WRMSDs) in the telecommunications industry in Australia in the early 1980s, which consequently earned the derogatory term "kangaroo paw" (Awerbuch, 1985). The same concept was soon appropriated and advanced in the United States by Hadler (1986, 1990, 1993).

Their basic arguments are multifold and fault a wide range of parties, including the medical establishment. In the current medical system, patients expect to be healthy; if not, there must be a specific reason for the illness or disorder. For lack of finding a specific cause or subjecting patients to endless and costly tests, rather than attempting to explain that the patient may have to endure nonspecific pain or discomfort for some time, the physician will assign a syndrome label. Next, the workers' compensation system is indicted for requiring structured responses (when they might not be easily available), encouraging overreporting, and extending disability periods (which may

TABLE 6.17

Summary of Epidemiological Studies Examining Psychosocial Factors and MSDs in the Upper Limbs

| Reference | Type of Study | No. of Subjects | Study Population (workers) | MSD Outcome Assessment | Associations with Upper Limb Outcomes (OR, * = p ≤ 0.05, + = positive but not significant) | | | | | | | |
| | | | | | Job and Work Environment | | | | | Individual | | |
					Job Dissatisfaction	High Workload	Monotonous Work	Low Job Control	Low Social Support	Sex	Age	Other
Bergqvist et al. (1995a,b)	CS	260	VDT	Survey, exam		U2.7* N7.4*		S3.2*	H4.5*	S7.1*	N2.1* H2.4	N4.0* glasses N6.4* children
Bernard et al. (1994)	CS	973	Newspaper	Survey		S1.5* Z1.4*		S1.6*Z1.4*				
Ekberg et al. (1994)	CC	746	General	MD exam		U3.8*		U16.5*		U16*		U3.7* smoker
Hales et al. (1994)	CS	553	Telecommunications	MD exam		Z2.3* N3.0* E2.4*	N4.2* E2.8*	S2.7* N3.5* E2.9*				E2.4* race
Houtman et al. (1994)	CS	5,865	General	Survey		M1.3*	M1.3*	M1.0		M1.6*	M4.0*	
Kamwendo et al. (1991)	CS	420	Clerical	Survey	U1.9*							
Karasek et al. (1987)	CS	8,700	White collar	Survey		M1.2*		M1.1*			M1.3*	
Kvarnström (1983)	CC	224	Fabrication	Medical records		S5.2*	S4.0*					S5* married
Lagerström et al. (1995)	CS	688	Female nurses	Survey		S1.7*	H1.6*	S1.7*				

Study	Type	No. of Subjects	Subjects	Exposure					
Leclerc et al. (1998)	CS	1,006	Industrial	MD exam	W1.4*			W2.2*	W2.3* well-being
Lemasters et al. (1998)	CS	552	Carpenters	Interview		S1.5 E1.4 Z1.5 Z1.5*	S1.9* E1.6 Z1.6*		
Magnavita et al. (1999)	CS	2,041	Sonographers	Survey			W1.6*		
Marcus and Gerr (1996)	CS	449	Female clerical	Survey		U2.5* EZ2*	U2.2*		
Pocekay et al. (1995)	CS	3,175	Semiconductor		O1.5*				O1.8* stress
Roquelaure et al. (1997)	CC	130	Blue-collar	Survey		O6.3*			
Silverstein et al. (1987)	CS	136	Casting	Interview				O4.8*	
Tola et al. (1988)	CS	3,221	Machinists, carpenters, clerical	Survey	U1.2*			U1.6*	
Toomingas et al. (1997)	CS	358	Male MMH Female clerical	Survey		S2.2* Z1.5		S3.2* Z1.8*	

Type of Study: C = cohort, CC = case-control, CS = cross-sectional

No. of Subjects: Total of study population and referents or controls

E = elbow, H = hand, M = overall muscle pains, O = overall MSDs, N = neck, S = shoulder, U = neck/shoulder combined, W = wrist, Z = hand/wrist combined (vast majority used self-reporting for exposure assessment)

also be the case for back pain; Hadler, 1986; Frank et al., 1995). It is also an adversarial system, in which if the condition is not improving rapidly, claimants cannot back out easily without casting doubt on their original claims and symptoms. The worker is indicted partially for being gullible and succumbing to general rumors or media alarms and partially for being greedy and seeking easy compensation. Ergonomists and other researchers are faulted for methodological problems in cross-sectional studies (which are the vast majority in the epidemiological studies cited in Section 6.5) in which prevalence or morbidity depends on reporting recall, volunteer biases, and difficulty in distinguishing between etiological and forecasting factors (Sackett, 1979). There are also sociological aspects such as sustained media interest and sensationalism, strong union support for "empowering the dispossessed," and, sometimes, an almost Luddite reaction to high-technology advancements (Arksey, 1998).

Similar to the "nature vs. nurture" concept in child development, there is probably some truth to the iatrogenic concept. Many of the above arguments can be found to occur, especially in extreme cases. Also, anecdotally (and from personal experience) there seems to be an increase in the reporting of MSDs upon completion of a symptom survey or participation in an ergonomics awareness program. This is only natural. Worker awareness has been increased and the person realizes there is a cause for the discomfort or pain that the person is already experiencing, making it easier to go to the plant nurse and report the problem. However, this increase in incidence rates is typically only a spike, which then should decrease below previous levels, once an ergonomics program has been implemented or, in the worst case, return to preexisting levels, once work returns to the status quo.

There are undoubtedly overlapping and confounding psychosocial and individual factors that exacerbate the development of MSDs by amplifying already existing strains and pains that normally result with many jobs. Unhappiness with the job, the supervision, pay, etc. were all shown to be contributory factors to MSDs. The key, however, is existing strains and pains. It would be unreasonable to expect that job unhappiness in itself would lead to MSDs. There has to be some underlying physical cause first. To completely eliminate the physical occupational stressors seems foolhardy at the least and potentially very costly, both to the company and to the individual workers. On the other hand, equal attention should also be given to the mental well-being of the worker. The company may be pleasantly surprised by increased productivity through increased worker motivation and the *Hawthorne effect* (Niebel and Freivalds, 2003).

Questions

1. Describe the etiology of tendon-related disorders.
2. What are some of the common tendon-related disorders?

3. Name several muscle disorders.

4. What is the etiology of muscle disorders? How are they different from tendon disorders?

5. What is a trigger point?

6. What are some of the possible causes of nerve disorders?

7. What is the carpal tunnel? What is the purpose of the flexor retinaculum?

8. What are some of the common nerve disorders?

9. What is the white finger syndrome? How is it related to Raynaud's syndrome?

10. What is bursitis? What occupation is typically associated with bursitis in the knee?

11. Compare and contrast rheumatoid arthritis and osteoarthritis.

12. Describe some of the medical tests used to diagnose WRMSDs in the upper limbs. What is the "gold standard" for such diagnostic tests?

13. What are some of the medical remedies used for treating WRMSDs?

14. What are the two key issues that influence the effectiveness of an epidemiological study?

15. What are the three main types of epidemiological studies? What are the trade-offs between these studies?

16. What is an intervention study? Why or why not may a cohort study be considered an intervention study?

17. What are the positive aspects and also the limitations of a cohort study?

18. What factor in a cohort study changes it from a retrospective to a prospective study? Give an example that could be used for WRMSDs in an industrial situation.

19. Compare and contrast case-control and cross-sectional studies. What is the key difference?

20. Which of the observational studies is best for showing causality? Why?

21. What is prevalence? How is statistical significance established for prevalence?

22. What is the basis for a chi square analysis?

23. What is a risk ratio and for what type of studies is it an appropriate analysis tool?

24. What is an odds ratio and for what type of studies is it an appropriate analysis tool?

25. How is statistical significance established for an odds ratio?

26. Compare and contrast a risk ratio to an odds ratio. How may they be similar?

27. What is attributable risk?

28. What is an incidence rate? How is it related to prevalence?

29. What is a logit function? What purpose does it serve in epidemiological studies?

30. What are some of the problems of multivariate modeling in epidemiological studies?

31. What are some of the ways of establishing the adequacy and validity of multivariate models?

32. What factors can be used to define causality in epidemiological research?

33. What are the occupational WRMSD risk factors that appear consistently across most epidemiological studies? Explain plausibility for each.

34. Which psychosocial and individual factors may contribute to upper limb WRMSDs? Explain plausibility for each of these.

35. What is iatrogenesis? Why may this be a factor in the reporting of WRMSDs?

36. How may the Hawthorne effect enter into the control of WRMSDs?

Problems

6.1. Show that Equations 6.8 and 6.14 are equivalent expressions.

6.2. A matched case-control study of power tool usage in an automotive assembly plant indicated that 190 of 320 workers using power tools experienced some sort of WRMSD symptoms, while only 10 of 70 unexposed workers showed similar symptoms.

   a. What is the odds ratio for power tool usage for WRMSD symptoms?

   b. Is this a statistically significant result?

6.3. A case-control study indicated that 15 of 100 workers exposed to high forces on the job exhibited WRMSD symptoms, while only 10 of 200 controls showed similar symptoms.

   a. What is the odds ratio for exposure?

   b. Is this a statistically significant result?

6.4. The Cool T-shirt Co. decided to evaluate the effects of an ergonomics program, which also included job rotation, rest breaks, and the elimination of its incentive program. After 2 years, in Plant A, with the ergonomics program, only 43 of 345 of sewing machine operators showed WRMSD symptoms, while, in Plant B, without an ergonomics program, 42 of 122 sewing machine operators showed WRMSD symptoms.

a. What type of epidemiological study was utilized?

b. What is the risk ratio for exposure?

c. Is this a statistically significant result?

6.5. A survey of 50 workers in a meatpacking plant regarding their working conditions (i.e., exposure to cold) and symptoms for white fingers yielded the following information:

11 were exposed to cold and had symptoms for white fingers

13 were exposed to cold but had no symptoms for white fingers

3 were not exposed to cold but had symptoms for white fingers

23 were not exposed to cold and had no symptoms for white fingers

a. What type of epidemiological study was used in the plant?

b. What are the implications (i.e., limitations) for this type of study?

c. What is the prevalence of white fingers in workers exposed to cold?

d. What is the prevalence of white fingers in workers not exposed to cold?

e. What is the odds ratio for incurring white fingers due to exposure to cold?

f. Is this a statistically significant result? Use $\alpha = 0.05$.

g. What does a chi square analysis indicate?

h. What is your overall conclusion regarding this plant?

6.6. Many workers in an electronics assembly plant have been reporting tingling sensations in the hand, which in many cases has been diagnosed as carpal tunnel syndrome. Initial observations indicate the use of high levels of pinch forces to insert wires into connectors. An ergonomist has suggested measuring the grip force ratio (force used divided by minimum force required) on a tracking task as a screening tool for carpal tunnel syndrome (the median nerve innervates the index finger) in addition to diagnostic testing of the carpal tunnel syndrome by a physician. Seven workers with strong symptoms of carpal tunnel syndrome are evaluated on the tracking task. Seven relatively similar symptom-free workers are also evaluated on the tracking task. The jobs of both sets of workers are studied for evidence of high pinch forces. The following data are obtained:

Carpal Tunnel Syndrome	Gender	Age	Wrist Circumference (mm)	Max Pinch Force (N)	Grip Force Ratio	Exposure to High Forces
Yes	M	35	184	101	7.4	Yes
Yes	F	35	168	69	7.7	Yes
Yes	F	57	156	43	10.0	Yes
Yes	F	45	187	80	6.0	Yes
Yes	F	56	193	54	4.0	No
Yes	F	29	145	48	5.6	No
Yes	M	43	189	69	7.2	Yes
No	M	31	168	68	5.0	No
No	F	40	159	80	4.6	No
No	F	62	161	40	5.0	Yes
No	F	45	153	48	4.6	No
No	F	47	151	50	5.4	Yes
No	F	33	166	51	3.8	No
No	M	45	174	83	3.2	No

a. What type of epidemiological study was used in the plant?

b. What are implications (i.e., limitations) for this type of study?

c. Are the groups well matched? (*Hint:* Perform a *t*-test on various characteristics.)

d. What is the prevalence of carpal tunnel syndrome in workers exposed to high pinch forces?

e. What is the prevalence of carpal tunnel syndrome in workers not exposed to high pinch forces?

f. What is the odds ratio for incurring carpal tunnel syndrome due to exposure of high pinch forces?

g. Is this a statistically significant result? Use $\alpha = 0.05$.

h. What does a chi square analysis indicate?

i. Is the grip force ratio a good screening tool for carpal tunnel syndrome? Consider a ratio over 6 to be excessive.

j. Does it appear that any of the individual characteristics (age, gender, wrist circumference, max pinch force) may predispose one to carpal tunnel syndrome? (*Hint:* Perform an odds ratio on a binary breakdown for each characteristic, e.g., consider 45 years a dividing line between young and old workers.)

k. What are your overall conclusions regarding this plant and study?

6.7. Develop a multiple logistic regression model for the data presented in Problem 6.6. Calculate the odds ratios and the respective confidence intervals for the significant factors.

References

Adson, A.W. and Coffey, J.R., 1927. Cervical rib: a method of anterior approach for relief of symptom by division of the scalenus anticus, *Annals of Surgery*, 85:839–857.

Afifi, A.A. and Clark, V., 1996. *Computer-Aided Multivariate Analysis*, 3rd ed., New York: Chapman & Hall.

Amano, M., Gensyo, U., Nakajima, H., and Yatsuki, K., 1988. Characteristics of work actions of shoe manufacturing assembly line workers and a cross-sectional factor-control study on occupational cervico-brachial disorders, *Japanese Journal of Industrial Health*, 30:3–12.

Andersen, J.H. and Gaardboe, O., 1993a. MSDs of the neck and upper limb among sewing machine operators: a clinical investigation, *American Journal of Industrial Medicine*, 24:689–700.

Andersen, J.H. and Gaardboe, O., 1993b. Prevalence of persistent neck and upper limb pain in a historical cohort of sewing machine operators, *American Journal of Industrial Medicine*, 24:677–687.

Arezzo, J.C., Shumburg, H.H., and Laudadio, C., 1986. Thermal sensitivity tester/device for quantitative assessment of thermal sense in diabetic neuropathy, *Diabetes*, 35:590–592.

Arksey, H., 1998. *RSI and the Experts, The Construction of Medical Knowledge*, London: UCL Press/Taylor & Francis.

Armstrong, T.J., 1983. *An Ergonomics Guide to Carpal Tunnel Syndrome*, Akron, OH: American Industrial Hygiene Association.

Armstrong, T.J. and Chaffin, D.B., 1978. An investigation of the relationship between displacements of the finger and wrist joints and the extrinsic finger flexor tendons, *Journal of Biomechanics*, 11:119–128.

Armstrong, T.J., Fine, L.J., Goldstein, S.A., Lifshitz, Y.R., and Silverstein, B.A., 1987. Ergonomic considerations in hand and wrist tendinitis, *Journal of Hand Surgery*, 12A:830–837.

Atroshi, I., Gummesson, C., Johnsson, R., Ornstein, E., Ranstam, J., and Rosen, I., 1999. Prevalence of carpal tunnel syndrome in a general population, *Journal of the American Medical Association*, 282:153–158.

Awerbuch, M., 1985. RSI or "kangaroo paw," *Medical Journal of Australia*, 142:237–238.

Backman, C., Boquist, L., Friden, J., Lorentzon, R., and Toolanen, G., 1990. Chronic Achilles paratenonitis with tendinosis: an experimental model in the rabbit, *Journal of Orthopaedic Research*, 8:541–547.

Barnhart, S., Demers, P.A., Miller, M., Longstreth, W.T., Jr., and Rosenstock, L., 1991. Carpal tunnel syndrome among ski manufacturing workers, *Scandinavian Journal of Work, Environment & Health*, 17:46–52.

Baron, S., Milliron, M., Habes, D., and Fidler, A., 1991. Hazard evaluation and technical assistance report: Shoprite Supermarkets, NJ, NY, NIOSH Report HHE 88-344-2092, Cincinnati, OH: U.S. Department of Health and Human Services, National Institute for Occupational Health and Safety.

Bell, J.A., 1990. Light touch — deep pressure testing using Semmes-Weinstein monofilaments, in Hunter, J.M., Mackin, E.J., and Callahan, A.D., Eds., *Rehabilitation of the Hand*, St. Louis: C.V. Mosby, 585–593.

Bergkvist, U., 1984. Video display terminals and health, *Scandinavian Journal of Work, Environment & Health*, 10:68–77.

Bergqvist, U., Wolfgast, E., Nilsson, B., and Voss, M., 1995a. MSDs among visual display terminal workers: individual, ergonomic, and work organizational factors, *Ergonomics*, 38:763–776.

Bergqvist, U., Wolfgast, E., Nilsson, B., and Voss, M., 1995b. The influence of VDT work on musculoskeletal disorders, *Ergonomics*, 38:754–762.

Bernard, B., Sauter, S., Fine, L.J., Petersen, M., and Hales, T., 1994. Job task and psychosocial risk factors for work-related musculoskeletal disorders among newspaper employees, *Scandinavian Journal of Work, Environment & Health*, 20:417–426.

Bjelle, A., Hagberg, M., and Michaelsson, G., 1979. Clinical and ergonomic factors in prolonged shoulder pain among industrial workers, *Scandinavian Journal of Work, Environment & Health*, 5:205–210.

Bongers, P.M., de Winter, C.R., Kompier, M.A.J, and Hildebrandt, V.H., 1993. Psychosocial factors at work and musculoskeletal disease, *Scandinavian Journal of Work, Environment & Health*, 19:297–312.

Bovenzi, M., 1994. Hand-arm vibration syndrome and dose–response relation for vibration-induced white finger among quarry drillers and stonecarvers. Italian Study Group on Physical Hazards in the Stone Industry, *Occupational and Environmental Medicine*, 51:603–611.

Bovenzi, M., Franzinelli, A., and Strambi, F., 1988. Prevalence of vibration-induced white finger and assessment of vibration exposure among travertine workers in Italy, *International Archives of Occupational and Environmental Health*, 61:25–34.

Bovenzi, M., Franzinelli, A., Mancini, R., Cannava, M.G., Maiorano, M., and Ceccarelli, F., 1995. Dose-response relation for vascular disorders induced by vibration in the fingers of forestry workers, *Occupational and Environmental Medicine*, 52:722–730.

Buch-Jaeger, N. and Foucher, G., 1994. Correlation of clinical signs with nerve conduction tests in the diagnosis of carpal tunnel syndrome, *Journal of Hand Surgery (Br)*, 19:720–724.

Burt, S., Hornung, R., and Fine, L., 1990. Hazard evaluation and technical assistance report: Newsday, Inc., Melville, N.Y., NIOSH Report HHE 89-250-2046, Cincinnati, OH: U.S. Department of Health and Human Services, National Institute for Occupational Health and Safety.

Byström, S., Hall, C., Welander, T., and Kilbom, Å., 1995. Clinical disorders and pressure-pain threshold of the forearm and hand among automobile assembly line workers, *Journal of Hand Surgery*, 20:782–790.

Campbell, D.T. and Stanley, J.C., 1966. *Experimental and Quasi-Experimental Designs for Research*, Chicago: Rand McNally.

Cannon, L.J., Bernacki, E.J., and Walter, S.D., 1981. Personal and occupational factors associated with carpal tunnel syndrome, *Journal of Occupational Medicine*, 23:255–258.

Chaffin, D.B., Lee, M.W., and Freivalds, A., 1980. Muscle strength assessment from EMG analysis, *Medicine and Science in Sports and Exercise*, 12:205–211.

Chang, K.Y., Ho, S.T., and Yu, H.S., 1994. Vibration induced neurophysiological and electron microscopical changes in rat peripheral nerves, *Occupational and Environmental Medicine*, 51:130–135.

Chattarjee, D., 1992. Workplace upper limb disorders: a prospective study with intervention, *Journal of Occupational Medicine*, 42:129–136.

Chiang, H., Chen, S., Yu, H., and Ko, Y., 1990. The occurrence of carpal tunnel syndrome in frozen food factory employees, *Kao Hsiung Journal of Medical Sciences*, 6:73–80.

Chiang, H., Ko, Y., Chen, S., Yu, H., Wu, T., and Chang, P., 1993. Prevalence of shoulder and upper-limb disorders among workers in the fish-processing industry, *Scandinavian Journal of Work, Environment & Health*, 19:126–131.

Christensen, R., 1997. *Log-Linear Models and Logistic Regression*, New York: Springer.

Cleland, L.G., 1987. RSI, a model of social iatrogenesis, *Medical Journal of Australia*, 147:236–239.

Conway, H. and Svenson, J., 1998. Occupational injury and illness rates, 1992–1996: why they fell, *Monthly Labor Review*, November:36–58.

Cornefjord, M., Sato, K., Olmarker, K., Rydevik, B., and Nordborg, C., 1997. A model for chronic nerve root compression studies. Presentation of a porcine model for controlled, slow-onset compression with analyses of anatomic aspects, compression onset rate, and morphologic and neurophysiologic effect, *Spine*, 22:946–57.

deKrom, M.C.T., Kester, A.D.M., Knipschild, P.G., and Spaans, F., 1990. Risk factors for carpal tunnel syndrome, *American Journal of Epidemiology*, 132:1102–1110.

Dellon, A.L., 1983. The vibrometer, *Plastic and Reconstructive Surgery*, 71:427–431.

Dellon, A.L. and Kallman, C.H., 1983. Evaluation of functional sensation in the hand, *Journal of Hand Surgery (Am)*, 8:865–870.

Dunham, W., Haines, G., and Spring, J.M., 1972. Bowler's thumb: ulnovolar neuroma of the thumb, *Clinical Orthopaedics*, 83:99–101.

Dyck, P.J., Lais, A.C., Giannini, C., and Engelstad, J.K., 1990. Structural alterations of nerve during cuff compression, *Proceedings of the National Academy of Sciences*, 87:9828–9832.

Ekberg, K., Björkqvist, B., Malm, P., Bjerre-Kiely, B., Karlsson, M., and Axelson, O., 1994. Case-control study of risk factors for disease in the neck and shoulder area, *Occupational and Environmental Medicine*, 51:262–266.

Ekberg, K., Karlsson, M., and Axelson, O., 1995. Cross-sectional study of risk factors for symptoms in the neck and shoulder area, *Ergonomics*, 38:971–980.

Elliott, B.G., 1992. Finkelstein's test: a descriptive error that can produce a false positive, *Journal of Hand Surgery (Br)*, 17B:481–482.

English, C.J. Maclaren, W.M., Court-Brown, C., Hughes, S.P.F., Porter, R.W., and Wallace, W.A., 1995. Relations between upper limb soft tissue disorders and repetitive movements at work, *American Journal of Industrial Medicine*, 27:75–90.

Faulkner, J.A., and Brooks, S.V., 1995. Muscle fatigue in old animals. Unique aspects of fatigue in elderly humans, *Advances in Experimental Medicine and Biology*, 384:471–480.

Faulkner, J.A., Brooks, S.V., and Zerba, E., 1990. Skeletal muscle weakness and fatigue in old age: underlying mechanisms, *Annual Review of Gerontology and Geriatrics*, 10:147–166.

Feldman, R.G., Travers, P.H., Chirico-Post, J., and Keyserling, W.M., 1987. Risk assessment in electronic assembly workers: carpal tunnel syndrome, *Journal of Hand Surgery*, 12A:849–855.

Ferguson, D., 1971a. Repetition injuries in process workers, *Medical Journal of Australia*, 2:408–412.

Ferguson, D., 1971b. An Australian study of telegraphists' cramp, *British Journal of Industrial Medicine*, 28:280–285.

Ferguson, D., 1973. A study of neurosis and occupation, *British Journal of Industrial Medicine*, 30:187–198.

Ferguson, D.A., 1987. "RSI": putting the epidemic to rest, *Medical Journal of Australia*, 147:213–214.

Finkelstein, J., 1939. Stenosing tendovaginitis at the radial styloid process, *Journal of Bone and Joint Surgery*, 12:509–540.

Fleiss, J.L., 1981. *Statistical Methods for Rates and Proportions*, New York: John Wiley & Sons.

Frank, J.W., Pulcins, I.R., Mickey, S.K., Shannon, H.S., and Stansfeld, S.A., 1995. Occupational back pain — an unhelpful polemic, *Scandinavian Journal of Work, Environment & Health*, 21:3–14.

Friis, R.H. and Sellers, T.A., 1996. *Epidemiology for Public Health Practice*, Gaithersburg, MD: Aspen Publishers.

Gellman, H., Gelberman, R.H., Tan, A.M., and Botte, M.J., 1986. Carpal tunnel syndrome: an evaluation of the provocative diagnostic tests, *Journal of Bone and Joint Surgery*, 68A:735–737.

Ghavanini, M.R. and Haghighat, M., 1998. Carpal tunnel syndrome: reappraisal of five clinical tests, *Electromyography and Clinical Neurophysiology*, 38:437–441.

Greenberg, R.S., 1986. Prospective studies, in S. Kotz and N.L. Johnson, Eds.. *Encyclopedia of Statistical Sciences*, Vol. 7, New York: John Wiley & Sons, 315–319.

Greenberg, R.S., Daniels, S.R., and Flanders, D.W., 1996. *Medical Epidemiology*, 3rd ed., New York: McGraw-Hill.

Hadler, N., 1986. Industrial rheumatology — the Australian and New Zealand experiences with arm pain and backache in the workplace, *Medical Journal of Australia*, 144:191–195.

Hadler, N., 1990. Cumulative trauma disorders, an iatrogenic concept, *Journal of Occupational Medicine*, 32:38–41.

Hadler, N., 1993. *Occupational Musculoskeletal Disorders*, New York: Raven Press.

Hagberg, M. and Wegman, D.H., 1987. Prevalence rates and odds ratios of shoulder-neck diseases in different occupational groups, *British Journal of Industrial Medicine*, 44:602–610.

Hales, T.R. and Fine, L., 1989. Hazard evaluation and technical assistance report: Cargill Poultry Division, Buena Vista, CA, NIOSH Report HHE 89-251-1997, Cincinnati, OH: U.S. Department of Health and Human Services, National Institute for Occupational Health and Safety.

Hales, T.R., Sauter, S.L., Petersen, M.R., Fine, L.J., Putz-Anderson, V., Schleifer, L.R., Ochs, T.T., and Bernard, B.P., 1994. Musculoskeletal disorders among visual display terminal users in a telecommunications company, *Ergonomics*, 37:1603–1621.

Hart, D.A., Frank, C.B., and Bray, R.C., 1995. Inflammatory processes in repetitive motion and overuse syndromes: potential role of neurogenic mechanisms in tendons and ligaments, in Gordon, S.L., Blair, S.J. and Fine, L.J., Eds., *Repetitive Motion Disorders of the Upper Extremity*, Rosemont, IL: American Academy of Orthopaedic Surgeons, 247–262.

Hedlund, U., 1989. Raynaud's phenomenon of fingers and toes of miners exposed to local and whole-body vibration and cold, *International Archives of Occupational & Environmental Health*, 61:457–461.

Herberts, P., Kadefors, R., Andersson, G., and Petersen, I., 1981. Shoulder pain in industry: an epidemiological study on welders, *Acta Orthopaedica Scandinavica*, 52:299–306.

Herberts, P., Kadefors, R., Högfors, C., and Sigholm, G., 1984. Shoulder pain and heavy manual labor, *Clinical Orthopaedics*, 191:166–178.

Hoekstra, E.J., Hurrell, J.J., and Swanson, N.G., 1994. Hazard evaluation and technical assistance report: Social Security Administration Teleservice Centers, Boston, MA, Fort Lauderdale, FL. NIOSH Report HHE 92-382-2450, Cincinnati, OH: U.S. Department of Health and Human Services, National Institute for Occupational Health and Safety.

Holmström, E.B., Lindell, J., and Moritz, U., 1992. Low back and neck/shoulder pain in construction workers: occupational workload and psychosocial risk factors, *Spine*, 17:663–671.

Hosmer, D.W. and Lemeshow, S., 1989. *Applied Logistic Regression*, New York: John Wiley & Sons.

Houtman, I.L.D., Bongers, P.M., Smulders, P.G.W., and Kompier, M.A.J., 1994. Psychosocial stressors at work and musculoskeletal problems, *Scandinavian Journal of Work, Environment & Health*, 20:139–145.

Howell, E. and Leach, R.E., 1970. Bowler's thumb, *Journal of Bone and Joint Surgery*, 52A:379–381.

Hughes, R.E., Silverstein, B.A., and Evanoff, B.A., 1997. Risk factors for work-related musculoskeletal disorders in an aluminum smelter, *American Journal of Industrial Medicine*, 32:66–75.

Hünting, W., Läubli, T.H., and Grandjean, E., 1981. Postural and visual loads at VDT workplaces, I. Constrained postures, *Ergonomics*, 24:917–931.

Hurrell, J.J. and Murphy, L.R., 1992. Psychological job stress, in Rom, W.N., Ed., *Environmental and Occupational Medicine*, 2nd ed., New York: Little, Brown, 675–684.

Jennings, D.E., 1986. Judging inferences adequacy in logistic regression, *Journal of the American Statistical Association*, 81:471–476.

Kaji, R., 2000. Facts and fancies on writer's cramp, *Muscle Nerve*, 23:1313–1315.

Kamwendo, K., Linton, S.J., and Moritz, U., 1991. Neck and shoulder disorders in medical secretaries. Part I. Pain prevalence and risk factors, *Scandinavian Journal of Rehabilitation Medicine*, 23:127–133.

Karasek, R.A., Gardell, B., and Lindell, J., 1987. Work and non-work correlates of illness and behaviour in male and female Swedish white collar workers, *Journal of Occupational Behavior*, 8:187–207.

Kiken, S., Stringer, W., and Fine, L.J., 1990. Hazard evaluation and technical assistance report: Perdue Farms, Lewistown, N.C.; Robersonville, N.C., NIOSH Report HHE 89-307-2009, Cincinnati, OH: U.S. Department of Health and Human Services, National Institute for Occupational Health and Safety.

Kivekäs, J., Riihimäki, H., Husman, K., Hänninen, K., Härkönen, H., Kuusela, T., Pekkarinen, M., Tola, S., and Zitting, A.J., 1994. Seven-year follow-up of white-finger symptoms and radiographic wrist findings in lumberjacks and referents, *Scandinavian Journal of Work, Environment & Health*, 20:101–106.

Kukkonen, R., Luopajärvi, T., and Riihimäki, V., 1983. Prevention of fatigue among data entry operators, in Kvalseth, T.O., Ed., *Ergonomics of Workstation Design*, London: Butterworth, 28–34.

Kuorinka, I. and Forcier, L., 1995. *Work Related Musculoskeletal Disorders (WMSDs): A Reference Book for Prevention*, London: Taylor & Francis.

Kuorinka, I. and Koskinen, P., 1979. Occupational rheumatic diseases and upper limb strain in manual jobs in a light mechanical industry, *Scandinavian Journal of Rehabilitation Medicine*, 5(Suppl. 3):39–47.

Kurppa, K., Viikari-Juntura, E., Kuosma, E., Huuskonen, M., and Kivi, P., 1991. Incidence of tenosynovitis or peritendinitis and epicondylitis in a meat-processing factory, *Scandinavian Journal of Work, Environment & Health*, 17:32–37.

Kvarnström, S., 1983. Occurrence of musculoskeletal disorders in a manufacturing industry with special attention to occupational shoulder disorders, *Scandinavian Journal of Rehabilitation Medicine*, 15(Suppl. 8):1–114.

Lagerström, M., Wenemark, M., Hagberg, M., and Hjelm, E.W., 1995. Occupational and individual factors related to musculoskeletal symptoms in five body regions among Swedish nursing personnel, *International Archives of Occupational & Environmental Health*, 68:27–35.

Larsson, S.E., Bodegard, L., Henriksen, K.G., and Öberg, P.A., 1990. Chronic trapezius myalgia: morphology and blood flow studied in 17 patients, *Acta Orthopaedica Scandinavica*, 61:394–398.

Lawrence, R.C., Helmick, C.G., Arnett, F.C., Deyo, R.A., Felson, D.T., Giannini, E.H., Heyse, S.P., Hirsch, R., Hochberg, M.C., Hunder, G.G., Lian, M.H., Pillemer, S.R., Steen, V.D., and Wolfe, F., 1998. Estimates of the prevalence of arthritis and selected musculoskeletal disorders in the United States, *Arthritis and Rheumatism*, 41:778–799.

Leclerc, A., Franchi, P., Cristofari, M.F., Delemotte, B., Mereau, P., Teyssier-Cotte, C., and Touranchet, A., 1998. Carpal tunnel syndrome and work organisation in repetitive work: a cross sectional study in France. Study Group on Repetitive Work, *Occupational & Environmental Medicine*, 55:180–187.

Lemasters, G.K., Atterbury, M.R., Booth-Jones, A.D., Bhattacharya, A., Ollila-Glenn, N., Forrester, C., and Forst, L., 1998. Prevalence of work related musculoskeletal disorders in active union carpenters, *Occupational & Environmental Medicine*, 55:421–427.

Letz, R., Cherniack, M.G., Gerr, F., Hershman, D., and Pace, P., 1992. A cross-sectional epidemiological survey of shipyard workers exposed to hand-arm vibration, *British Journal of Industrial Medicine*, 49:53–62.

Linton, S.J. and Kamwendo, K., 1989. Risk factors in the psychosocial work environment for neck and shoulder pain in secretaries, *Journal of Occupational Medicine*, 31:609–613.

Lowe, B.D. and Freivalds, A., 1999. Effect of carpal tunnel syndrome on grip force coordination on hand tools, *Ergonomics*, 42:550–564.

Lundborg, G., 1988. *Nerve Injury and Repair*, Edinburgh: Churchill Livingstone.

Lundborg, G., Lie-Stenström, A.K., Sollerman, C., Strömberg, T., and Pyykko, I., 1986. Digital vibrogram: a new diagnostic tool for sensory testing in compression neuropathy, *Journal of Hand Surgery*, 11A:693–699.

Luopajärvi, T., Kuorinka, I., Virolainen, M., and Holmberg, M., 1979. Prevalence of tenosynovitis and other injuries of the upper extremities in repetitive work, *Scandinavian Journal of Rehabilitation Medicine*, 5(Suppl. 3):48–55.

Magnavita, N., Bevilacqua, L., Mirk, P., Fileni, A., and Castellino, N., 1999. Work-related musculoskeletal complaints in sonologists, *Journal of Occupational and Environmental Medicine*, 41:981–988.

Malaviya, P., Butler, D.L., Boivin, G.P., Smith, F.N., Barry, F.P., Murphy, J.M., and Vogel, K.G., 2000. An *in vivo* model for load-modulated remodeling in the rabbit flexor tendon, *Journal of Orthopaedic Research*, 18:116–125.

Mantel, N. and Haenszel, W, 1959. Statistical aspects of the analysis of data from retrospective studies of disease, *Journal of National Cancer Institute*, 22:719–748.

Marcus, M. and Gerr, F., 1996. Upper extremity musculoskeletal symptoms among female office workers: associations with video display terminal use and occupational psychosocial stressors, *American Journal of Industrial Medicine*, 29:161–170.

Mathiowetz, V., Kashman, N., Volland, G., Weber, K., Dowe, M., and Rogers, S., 1985. Grip and pinch strength: normative data for adults, *Archives for Physical Medicine and Rehabilitation*, 66:69–72.

McComas, A., 1996. *Skeletal Muscle Form and Function*, Champaign, IL: Human Kinetics.

McCully, K.K. and Faulkner, J.A., 1985. Injury to skeletal muscle fibres of mice following lengthening contractions, *Journal of Applied Physiology*, 59:119–126.

McKenna, K., McGrann, S., Blann, A., and Allen, J., 1993. An investigation into the acute vascular effects of riveting, *British Journal of Industrial Medicine*, 50:160–166.

Milerad, E. and Ekenvall, L., 1990. Symptoms of the neck and upper extremities in dentists, *Scandinavian Journal of Work, Environment & Health*, 16:129–134.

Mirbod, S.M., Yoshida, H., Komura, Y., Fujita, S., Nagata, C., Miyashita, K., Inaba, R., and Iwata, H., 1994. Prevalence of Raynaud's phenomenon in different groups of workers operating hand-held vibrating tools, *International Archives of Occupational and Environmental Health*, 66:13–22.

Morgenstern, H., Kelsh, M., Kraus, J., and Margolis, W., 1991. A cross-sectional study of hand/wrist symptoms in female grocery checkers, *American Journal of Industrial Medicine*, 20:209–218.

Moore, J.S. and Garg, A., 1994. Upper extremity disorders in a pork processing plant: relationship between job risk factors and morbidity, *American Industrial Hygiene Association Journal*, 55:703–715.

Mosconi, T. and Kruger, L., 1996. Fixed-diameter polyethylene cuffs applied to the rat sciatic nerve induce a painful neuropathy: ultrasound morphometric analysis of axonal alterations, *Pain*, 64:37–57.

Nagata, C., Yoshida, H., Mirbod, S., Komura, Y., Fujita, S., Inaba, R., Iwata, H., Maeda, M., Shikano, Y., and Ichiki, Y., 1993. Cutaneous signs (Raynaud's phenomenon, sclerodactylia, and edema of the hands) and hand-arm vibration exposure, *International Archives of Occupational and Environmental Health*, 64:587–591.

Nathan, P.A., Meadows, K.D., and Doyle, L.S., 1988. Occupation as a risk factor for impaired sensory conduction of the median nerve at the carpal tunnel, *Journal of Hand Surgery*, 13B:167–170.

Nathan, P.A., Keniston, R.C., Myers, L.D., and Meadows, K.D., 1992. Longitudinal study of median nerve sensory conduction in industry: relationship to age, gender, hand dominance, occupational hand use, and clinical diagnosis, *Journal of Hand Surgery*, 17A:850–857.

National Research Council, 2001. Musculoskeletal Disorders and the Workplace, Washington, D.C.: National Academy Press.

Necking, L.E., Lundstrom, R., Dahlin, L.B., Lundborg, G., Thornell, L.E., and Friden, J., 1966. Tissue displacement is a causative factor in vibration-induced muscle injury, *Journal of Hand Surgery (Br)*, 21:753–757.

Nicholas, J.A., 1990. Clinical observations on sports-induced soft-tissue injuries, in Leadbetter, W.B., Buckwalter, J.A., and Gordon, S.L., Eds., *Sports-Induced Inflammation: Clinical and Basic Science Concepts*, Rosemont, IL: American Academy of Orthopaedic Surgeons, 143.

Niebel, B. and Freivalds, A., 2003. *Methods, Standards & Work Design*, 11th ed., New York: McGraw-Hill, 351–352.

Nilsson, T., Burström, L., and Hagberg, M., 1989. Risk assessment of vibration exposure and white fingers among platers, *International Archives of Occupational and Environmental Health*, 61:473–481.

NIOSH, 1989. Carpal Tunnel Syndrome: Selected References, Cincinnati, OH: National Institute for Occupational Safety and Health.

NIOSH, 1995. Cumulative Trauma Disorders in the Workplace: Bibliography. Report 95-119, Cincinnati, OH: National Institute for Occupational Safety and Health.

NIOSH, 1997. Musculoskeletal Disorders and Workplace Factors. Report 97-141, Cincinnati, OH: National Institute for Occupational Safety and Health.

Noonan, T.J., Best, T.M., Seaber, A.V., and Garrett, W.E., 1994. Identification of a threshold for skeletal muscle injury, *American Journal of Sports Medicine*, 22:257–261.

Ohlsson, K., Hansson, G.A., Balogh, I., Strömberg, U., Pålsson, B., Nordander, C., Rylander, L., and Skerfving, S., 1994. Disorders of the neck and upper limbs in women in fish processing industry, *Occupational and Environmental Medicine*, 51:826–832.

Ohlsson, K., Attewell, R., Pålsson, B., Karlsson, B., Balogh, I., Johnsson, B., Ahlm, A., and Skerfving, S., 1995. Repetitive industrial work and neck and upper limb disorders in females, *American Journal of Industrial Medicine*, 27:731–747.

Okutsu, I., Ninomiya, S., Hamanaka, I., Kuroshima, N., and Inanami, H., 1989. Measurement of pressure in the carpal canal before and after endoscopic management of carpal tunnel syndrome, *Journal of Bone and Joint Surgery*, 71A:679–683.

Olsen, N. and Nielsen, S.L., 1988. Vasoconstrictor response to cold in forestry workers: a prospective study, *British Journal of Industrial Medicine*, 45:39–42.

Osorio, A.M., Ames, R.G., Jones, J., Castorina, J., Rempel, D., Estrin, W., and Thompson, D., 1994. Carpal tunnel syndrome among grocery store workers, *American Industrial Hygiene Association Journal*, 25:229–245.

Parker, K.G. and Imbus, H.R., 1992. *Cumulative Trauma Disorders*, Chelsea, MI: Lewis Publishers.

Phalen, G.S., 1966. The carpal-tunnel syndrome, *Journal of Bone and Joint Surgery*, 48A, 211–228.

Pocekay, D., McCurdy, S.A., Samuales, S.J., Hammond, K., and Schenker, M.B., 1995. A cross-sectional study of musculoskeletal symptoms and risk factors in semiconductor workers, *American Journal of Industrial Medicine*, 28:861–871.

Praemer, A., Furner, S., Rice, D.P., 1999. *Musculoskeletal Conditions in the United States*, Rosemont, IL: American Academy of Orthopaedic Surgeons.

Punnett, L., Robins, J.M., Wegman, D.H., and Keyserling, W.M., 1985. Soft-tissue disorders in the upper limbs of female garment workers, *Scandinavian Journal of Work, Environment & Health*, 11:417–425.

Punnett, L., Fine, L.J., Keyserling, W.M., Herrin, G.D., and Chaffin, D.B., 1991. Back disorders and nonneutral trunk postures of automobile assembly workers, *Scandinavian Journal of Work, Environment & Health*, 17:337–346.

Putz-Anderson, V., 1994. *Cumulative Trauma Disorders: A Manual for Musculoskeletal Diseases of the Upper Limbs*, London: Taylor & Francis.

Reinstein, L., 1983. De Quervain's stenosing tenosynovitis in a video game player, *Archives of Physical Medicine and Rehabilitation*, 64:434–435.

Rempel, D., 1995. Musculoskeletal loading and carpal tunnel pressure, in Gordon, S.L., Blair, S.J., and Fine, L.J., Eds., *Repetitive Motion Disorders of the Upper Extremity*, Rosemont, IL: American Academy of Orthopaedic Surgeons, 123–133.

Ritz, B.R., 1995. Humeral epicondylitis among gas and waterworks employees, *Scandinavian Journal of Work, Environment & Health*, 21:478–486.

Robert, A.W., Cynthia, B., and Thomas, J.A., 1994. Reverse Phalen's maneuver as an aid in diagnosing carpal tunnel syndrome, *Archives of Physical Medicine and Rehabilitation*, 75:783–786.

Roquelaure, Y., Mechali, S., Dano, C., Fanello, S., Benetti, F., Bureau, D., Mariel, J., Martin, Y.H., Derriennic, F., and Penneau-Fontbonne, D., 1997. Occupational and personal risk factors for carpal tunnel syndrome in industrial workers, *Scandinavian Journal of Work, Environment & Health*, 23:364–369.

Rossignol, A.M., Morse, E.P., Summers, V.M., and Pagnotto, L.D., 1987. Video display terminal use and reported health symptoms among Massachusetts clerical workers, *Journal of Occupational Medicine*, 29:112–118.

Roto, P. and Kivi, P., 1984. Prevalence of epicondylitis and tenosynovitis among meatcutters, *Scandinavian Journal of Work, Environment & Health*, 10:203–205.

Rydevik, B., Lundborg, G., and Nordborg, C., 1976. Intraneural tissue reactions induced by internal neurolysis, *Scandinavian Journal of Plastic and Reconstructive Surgery*, 10:3–8.

Sackett, D.L., 1979. Bias in analytic research, *Journal of Chronic Diseases*, 32:51–63.

Sahai, H. and Khurshid, K., 1996. *Statistics in Epidemiology*, Boca Raton, FL: CRC Press.

Sakakibara, H., Miyao, M., Kondo, T., and Yamada, S., 1995. Overhead work and shoulder-neck pain in orchard farmers harvesting pears and apples, *Ergonomics*, 38:700–706.

Sauter, S.L. and Swanson, N.G., 1996. Psychological aspects of musculoskeletal disorders in office work, in Moon, S. and Sauter, S., Eds., *Psychosocial Factors and Musculoskeletal Disorders*, London: Taylor & Francis.

Schibye, B., Skov, T., Ekner, D., Christiansen, J., and Sjögaard, G., 1995. Musculoskeletal symptoms among sewing machine operators, *Scandinavian Journal of Work, Environment & Health*, 21:427–434.

Schottland, J.R., Kirschberg, G.J., Fillingim, R., Davis, V.P., and Hogg, F., 1991. Median nerve latencies in poultry processing workers: an approach to resolving the role of industrial "cumulative trauma" in the development of carpal tunnel syndrome, *Journal of Occupational Medicine*, 33:627–631.

Sheehy, M.P. and Marsden, C.D., 1982. Writer's cramp — a focal dystonia, *Brain*, 105: 461–480.

Shurr, D.G., Blair, W.F., and Bassett, G., 1986. Electromyographic changes after carpal tunnel release, *Journal of Hand Surgery (Am)*, 11:876–880.

Silverstein, B.A., Fine, L.J., and Armstrong, T.J., 1987. Occupational factors and the carpal tunnel syndrome, *American Journal of Industrial Medicine*, 11:343–358.

Simonsen, E.B.. Klitgaard, H., and Bojsen-Moller, F., 1995. The influence of strength training, swim training and ageing on the Achilles tendon and m. soleus of the rat, *Journal of Sports Sciences*, 13:291–295.

Sjøgaard, G. and Jensen, B.R., 1997. Muscle pathology with overuse, in Ranney, D., Ed., *Chronic Musculoskeletal Injuries in the Workplace*, Philadelphia: W.B. Saunders, 17–40.

Sjøgaard, G. and Søgaard, K., 1998. Muscle injury in repetitive motion disorders, *Clinical Orthopaedics and Related Research*, 351:21–31.

Skie, M., Zeiss, J., Ebraheim, N.A., and Jackson, W.T., 1990. Carpal tunnel changes and median nerve compression during wrist flexion and extension seen by magnetic resonance imaging, *Journal of Hand Surgery*, 15A:934–939.

Sommer, C., Gailbraith, J.A., Heckman, H.M., and Myers, R.R., 1993. Pathology of experimental compression neuropathy producing hyperesthesia, *Journal of Neuropathology and Experimental Neurology*, 52:223–233.

Sorock, G.S. and Courtney, T.K., 1996. Epidemiologic concerns for ergonomists: illustrations from the musculoskeletal disorder literature, *Ergonomics*, 39:562–578.

Stenlund, B., Goldie, I., Hagberg, M., Hogstedt, C., and Marions, O., 1992. Radiographic osteoarthrosis in the acromioclavicular joint resulting from manual work or exposure to vibration, *British Journal of Industrial Medicine*, 49:588–593.

Steward, J.D. and Eisen, A., 1978. Tinel's sign and the carpal tunnel syndrome, *British Medical Journal*, 2(6145):1125–1126.

Strömberg, T., Dahlin, L.B., Brun, A., and Lundborg, G., 1997. Structural nerve damage at wrist level in workers exposed to vibration, *Occupational and Environmental Medicine*, 54:307–311.

Takeuchi, T., Futatsuka, M., Imanishi, H., and Yamada, S., 1986. Pathological changes observed in the finger biopsy of patients with vibration-induced white finger, *Scandinavian Journal of Work, Environment & Health*, 12:280–283.

Tanaka, S., Wild, D.K., Seligman, P.J., Haperin, W.E., Behrens, V.J., and Putz-Anderson, V., 1995. Prevalence and work-relatedness of self-reported carpal tunnel syndrome among U.S. workers: analysis of the Occupational Health Supplement data of the 1988 National Health Interview Survey, *American Journal of Industrial Medicine*, 27:451–470.

Tanaka, S., Wild, D.K., Cameron, L., and Freund, E., 1997. Association of occupational and non-occupational risk factors with the prevalence of self-reported carpal tunnel syndrome in a national survey of the working population, *American Journal of Industrial Medicine*, 32:550–556.

Taylor, W., 1982. Vibration white finger in the workplace, *Journal of the Society of Occupational Medicine*, 32:159–166.

Taylor, W., Wasserman, D., Behrens, V., Reynolds, D., and Samueloff, S., 1984. Effect of the air hammer on the hands of stonecutters. The limestone quarries of Bedford, Indiana, revisited, *British Journal of Industrial Medicine*, 41:289–295.

Thun, M., Tanaka, S., Smith, A.B., Halperin, W.E., Lee, S.T., Luggen, M.E., and Hess, E.V., 1987. Morbidity from repetitive knee trauma in carpet and floor layers, *British Journal of Industrial Medicine*, 44:611–620.

Tine, J., 1915. Le signe du "fourmillement" dans les lésions des nerfs périphériques [Pins and needles' signs of peripheral nerve lesions], *Presse Médicale*, 23:388–389.

Tola, S., Riihimäki, H., Videman, T., Viikari-Juntura, E., and Häanninen, K., 1988. Neck and shoulder symptoms among men in machine operating, dynamic physical work and sedentary work, *Scandinavian Journal of Work, Environment & Health*, 14:299–305.

Toomingas, A., Theorell, T., Michelsen, H., and Nordemar, R., 1997. Associations between self-rated psychosocial work conditions and musculoskeletal symptoms and signs. Stockholm MUSIC I Study Group, *Scandinavian Journal of Work, Environment & Health*, 23:130–139.

Travell, J.G. and Simons, D.G., 1983. *Myofascial Pain and Dysfunction — The Trigger Point Manual*, Baltimore: Williams & Wilkins.

Veiersted, K.B. and Westgaard, R.H., 1994. Subjectively assessed occupational and individual parameters as risk factors for trapezius myalgia, *International Journal of Industrial Ergonomics*, 13:235–245.

Viegas, S.F. and Torres, F.G., 1989. Cherry pitter's thumb. Case report and review of the literature, *Orthopaedic Review*, 18:336–338.

Viikari-Juntura, E.J., Kurppa, K., Kuosma, E., Huuskonen, M., Kuorinka, I., Ketola, R., and Kanni, U., 1991a. Prevalence of epicondylitis and elbow pain in the meat processing industry, *Scandinavian Journal of Work, Environment & Health*, 17:38–45.

Viikari-Juntura, E.J., Vuori, J., Silverstein, B., Kalimo, R., Kuosma, E., and Videman, T., 1991b. A life-long prospective study on the role of psychosocial factors in neck-shoulder and low back pain, *Spine*, 16:1056–1061.

Viikari-Juntura, E.J., Riihimäki, H., Tola, S., Videman, T., and Mutanen, P., 1994. Neck trouble in machine operating, dynamic physical work and sedentary work: a prospective study on occupational and individual risk factors, *Journal of Clinical Epidemiology*, 47:1411–1422.

Warren, G.L., Hayes, D.A., Lowe, D.A., Prior, B.M., and Armstrong, R.B., 1993. Material fatigue initiates eccentric contraction-induced injury in rat soleus muscle, *Journal of Applied Physiology*, 464:477–489.

Welch, L.S., Hunting, K.L, and Kellogg, J., 1995. Work-related musculoskeletal symptoms among sheet metal workers, *American Journal of Industrial Medicine*, 27:783–791.

Wells, J.A., Zipp, J.F., Shuette, P.T., and McEleney, J., 1983. Musculoskeletal disorders among letter carriers, *Journal of Occupational Medicine*, 25:814–820.

Wieslander, G., Norback, D., Gothe, C.J., and Juhlin, L., 1989. Carpal tunnel syndrome (CTS) and exposure to vibration, repetitive wrist movements, and heavy manual work: a case-referent study, *British Journal of Industrial Medicine*, 46:43–47.

Wilks, S., 1878. *Lectures on Diseases of the Nervous System*, London: Churchill, 452–460.

Woo, S.L., Ritter, M.A., Amiel, D., Sanders, T.M., Gomez, M.A., Kuei, S.C., Garfin, S.R., and Akeson, W.H., 1980. The biomechanical and biochemical properties of swine tendons — long term effects of exercise on digital extensors, *Connective Tissue Research*, 7:177–183.

Woodward, M., 1999. *Epidemiology, Study Design and Data Analysis*, New York: Chapman & Hall.

You, H., 1999. The Development of a Risk Assessment Model for Carpal Tunnel Syndrome, Ph.D. thesis, University Park, PA: Pennsylvania State University.

You, H., Simmons, Z., Freivalds, A., Kothari, M.J., Naidu, S.H., and Young, R., 2004. The development of risk assessment models for carpal tunnel syndrome: a case-reference study, *Ergonomics*, 47:668–709.

Yu, I.T.S. and Wong, T.W., 1996. Musculoskeletal problems among VDU workers in a Hong Kong bank, *Occupational Medicine*, 46:275–280.

Yu, Z.S., Chao, H., Qiao, L., Qian, D.S., and Ye, Y.H., 1986. Epidemiologic survey of vibration syndrome among riveters, chippers and grinder in the railroad system of the People's Republic of China, *Scandinavian Journal of Work, Environment & Health*, 12:289–292.

7

Instrumentation

7.1 Introduction

Any biomechanics instrumentation or measurement technique, whether for research or industrial or in-the-field evaluations, must meet certain criteria for usefulness (Brand and Crowninshield, 1981; Chaffin et al., 1999):

1. The measured parameter should correlate accurately with the human function of interest, i.e., the instrument should be valid.
2. The measurement should be both accurate and repeatable, i.e., the instrument should be reliable.
3. The measurement should distinguish between normal and abnormal results; i.e., the instrument should be specific and sensitive.
4. The measurement should not significantly alter the function of interest.
5. The instrument or technique should be safe to use.
6. The instrument should be simple to use, relatively portable, relatively inexpensive, and insensitive to external noise.

The quantitative aspects of validity, reliability, sensitivity, and specificity are discussed in greater detail in Chapter 8. This chapter describes the different equipment and tools needed to evaluate human capability and capacities of the upper limbs, especially as related to likelihood of developing musculoskeletal disorders (MSDs). The practicality of these measurements with respect to the above criteria is also discussed.

7.2 Wrist and Finger Motion Measurement

7.2.1 Types of Measurement Devices

Various technologies for measuring wrist motions have been developed, but none has received universal acceptance. One such approach is based on videotape analysis of wrist motion. Developed by Armstrong et al. (1982), it utilizes a frame-by-frame analysis of videotape that records wrist flexion/ extension in one of five categories and radial/ulnar deviation in one of three categories. This method requires considerable time and effort because each individual frame must be analyzed manually, and yields absolute resolutions of only 30° for flexion/extension and 20° for radial/ulnar deviation. In addition, dynamic variables of the wrist, such as angular velocity and acceleration, are not easily obtainable with this type of analysis.

Another such method of wrist motion measurement was developed by Logan and Groszewski (1989) and utilizes an electromagnetic three-space-digitizer sensor system to obtain real-time, six degrees-of-freedom position information. Sensors determine specific x, y, z coordinates and θ, ϕ, ψ orientation angles with respect to a coordinate system based on a low-frequency magnetic field. Further analysis of these data provides flexion/extension, radial/ulnar deviation, and pronation/supination angles. Although this system provided useful information for a number of work tasks in the food processing industry, the system appeared to require an excessive amount of time for data acquisition and reduction and had limitations due to its instrumentation and magnetic noise.

Another very common approach is the simple goniometer with its output assessed electrically or mechanically. Typically, goniometers are relatively small and lightweight, offering quick and objective measurements of wrist joint motions (Nicole, 1987; Ojima et al., 1991; Hansson et al., 1996; Buchholz and Wellman, 1997). Numerous studies have already been performed using electrogoniometers (goniometers with electrical output) in laboratory, factory, and clinical settings. For example, Smutz et al. (1994) employed an electrogoniometer for measuring wrist posture in their ergonomic assessment of keyboard design. Moore et al. (1991) used the electrogoniometer to quantify wrist motion for ergonomic risk factors, and Ojima et al. (1991) performed a dynamic analysis of wrist circumduction using the electrogoniometer in the clinical field. However, in all these studies extensive calibration techniques were required.

Schoenmarklin and Marras (1993) developed an electromechanical goniometer to collect online data of wrist movements of flexion/extension, radial/ulnar deviation, and pronation/supination planes simultaneously. Further analyses of the data yielded angular velocity and acceleration. This wrist monitor was composed of two thin metal strips, placed on two adjacent segments with a rotary potentiometer placed at the center of the joint. This system produced relatively accurate and repeatable results. However, it was uncomfortable and obtrusive for hand motion.

There are several commercial goniometers (Biometrics Ltd, Gwent, U.K., and BIOPAC Systems, Inc., Santa Barbara, CA, http://www.biopac.com/) currently available for measuring both wrist flexion/extension and radial/ ulnar deviation, as well as forearm rotation of pronation/supination. These devices consist of two plastic end blocks that are separated by a flexible spring protecting a strain wire (Figure 7.1). The goniometers incorporate

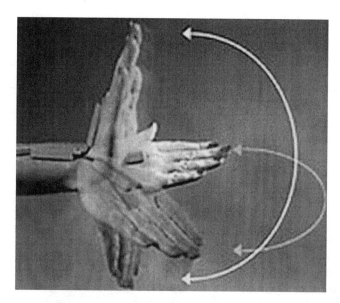

FIGURE 7.1
Flexible biaxial electrogoniometers. (Courtesy of BIOPAC Systems Inc., Santa Barbara, CA, http://www.biopac.com.)

gauge elements that measure bending strain along or around a particular axis. Biaxial goniometers measure orthogonal rotational axes simultaneously (e.g., wrist flexion/extension and radial/ulnar deviations), while torsiometers are used to measure angular twisting (e.g., forearm pronation/supination) as opposed to bending. Hansson et al. (1996), Rawes (1996), Bucholz and Wellman (1997), Spielholz (1998), and Marshall et al. (1999) have used biaxial goniometers and torsiometers to continuously measure wrist motions and forearm rotations.

One common problem of such biaxial devices is various types of measurement errors. When the forearm rotates, the distal and proximal end blocks do not rotate together, causing twist in the goniometer wire. The twist is primarily the result of the kinesiology of forearm rotation, in which the proximal end block of the goniometer is attached toward the middle of the forearm so that it rotates less than does the distal end block. The resulting twist leads to *crosstalk* and *zero drift* errors. Such common measurement errors occur as a result of the complexity of human joints and should be continually corrected. A summary of these measurement devices, with respective advantages and disadvantages, is given in Table 7.1.

7.2.2   Calibration Methods

Calibration typically occurs at several levels: the accuracy of the instrument in the measurement of a known fixed angle, the application errors, repeatability of measurements, and correction procedures for any errors. Buchholz

TABLE 7.1

Common Wrist Motion Measurement Devices

Measurement Device	Accuracy	Reliability	Cost	Advantages	Disadvantages
Videotape analysis	Low	Low	Low	Hard copy	Time intensive
3-D digitizer	High	High	High	Computer control	Problems with noise
Electromechanical goniometer	High	High	Low	Simple, direct measurement	Uncomfortable, intrusive
Flexible goniometers	High	High	Medium	Small, light, relatively unobtrusive Measure two planes simultaneously	Noise, crosstalk

and Wellman (1997) constructed a calibration fixture to allow accurate measurement of true angles in one wrist plane for various forearm rotations. The fixture consisted of a protractor element for measuring true wrist angles and a rotary element for controlling forearm rotation. They also developed correction procedures that included a slope transformation and zero drift transformation to adjust for errors due to crosstalk and zero drift. The equations of the slope-transformed values of flexion/extension (F/E_S) and radial/ulnar deviation (R/U_S) from goniometer measurements of flexion/extension (F/E_M) and radial/ulnar deviation (R/U_M) were

$$F/E_S = \left(F/E_M^2 + R/U_M^2\right)^{1/2}\left[\sin\left(\tan^{-1}\left\{\frac{F/E_M}{R/U_M}\right\}+\phi\right)\right] \tag{7.1}$$

$$R/U_S = \left(F/E_M^2 + R/U_M^2\right)^{1/2}\left[\cos\left(\tan^{-1}\left\{\frac{F/E_M}{R/U_M}\right\}+\phi\right)\right] \tag{7.2}$$

The angle ϕ is the twist in goniometer wire due to forearm rotation.

The second transformation of zero drift was made for corrected flexion/extension (F/E_C) and radial/ulnar deviation (R/U_C) angles from slope-transformed zero point averages of flexion/extension (F/E_0) and radial/ulnar deviation (R/U_0) angles as follows:

$$F/E_C = F/E_S + F/E_0 \tag{7.3}$$

$$R/U_C = R/U_S + R/U_0 \tag{7.4}$$

Based on the slope transformation and zero drift equations, they performed a nonlinear optimization minimizing the error and calculated true flexion/extension (F/E_T) and radial/ulnar deviation (R/U_T) angles:

$$\min \sum \left(\left| F/E_T - F/E_C \right| + \left| R/U_T - R/U_C \right| \right) \tag{7.5}$$

Hansson et al. (1996) introduced a test jig allowing independent setting of three planes of wrist angles, thus simulating the biomechanics of the wrist and forearm, and developed correction equations to induce actual wrist angles from recorded wrist angles as follows:

$$F/E' = S \times \cos \left(\phi - c\theta \right) \tag{7.6}$$

$$R/U' = S \times \sin \left(\phi - c\theta \right) \tag{7.7}$$

$$S = \left(F/E^2 + R/U^2 \right)^{1/2} \phi = \sin \left(R/U \right) \times \arctan \left(\frac{F/E}{R/U} \right) \tag{7.8}$$

where
F/E' = recorded flexion/extension angle
R/U' = recorded radial/ulnar deviation angle
F/E = actual flexion/extension angle
R/U = actual radial/ulnar deviation angle
θ = forearm rotation angle
c = a transducer-dependent constant

Ojima et al. (1991) measured the output of the electrogoniometer during wrist circumduction using a specially developed calibration apparatus. It consisted of a horizontal flat board and table, a universal joint at the end of the board, a metal straight bar joined to a universal joint, and a vertical board with a round hole and sliding side bar. The results showed that the measurement errors for flexion/extension and radial/ulnar deviation were within 4° and 1°, respectively, and that *hysteresis* was barely measurable, especially when subjects' forearms were fixed to eliminate forearm rotation.

Jang (2002) developed a calibration device (Figure 7.2) similar to Ojima et al. (1991) but used a simulated flexible ball joint rather than a human wrist. Static calibration of the Biometrics biaxial goniometer at nine different wrist flexion/extension angles and seven different radial/ulnar deviation angles produced an essentially linear ($r^2 = 0.999$, $p < 0.001$) relationship between true and measured angle. Nonrepeatabilities for flexion/extension and radial/ulnar deviation planes were 4.0 and 3.3%, respectively, while nonlinearities were 1.6 and 0.93%, respectively (Figure 7.3).

A dynamic calibration of the Biometrics biaxial goniometer was performed at two calibration fixture radii: 26.2 cm (maximum flexion or ulnar deviation angles = 37.5°) and 8.8 cm (maximum flexion or ulnar deviation angles = 14.4°). Although there was a very significant relationship ($r^2 = 0.998$, $p < 0.001$) between the true and measurement angles, there was a noticeable

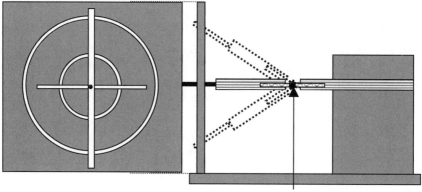

Three-dimensional universal joint

FIGURE 7.2
Calibration mockup for electrogoniometer testing. (From Jang, H., 2002. The Effects of Dynamic Wrist Workloads on Risks of Carpal Tunnel Syndrome, Ph.D. dissertation, University Park, PA: Pennsylvania State University. With permission.)

disparity with the goniometer overestimating the true flexion/extension angles by approximately 2° and true radial/ulnar deviation angles by 1.08° (i.e., wider circles; Figure 7.4).

7.2.3   Static Measurements — Range of Motion

The static components of the wrist joint typically include postural information such as position, and range of motion (ROM) measured in each plane of the wrist joint. The ROM of body joints is obviously an important factor in assessment of body mobility. Table 7.2 provides such static wrist ROM data.

These reported maximal wrist angles are very similar to each other. Generally, maximum wrist angles of flexion/extension are much larger than those of radial/ulnar deviation, and maximum ulnar deviation and supination angles are much larger than maximum radial deviation and pronation angles, respectively. Wrist angles under static conditions are much larger than those found under dynamic conditions, when measured from the beginning to the end of maximal dynamic movement. Schoenmarklin and Marras (1993) rationalized that the subjects might have focused more on the exertion and less on the maximal range of motion in dynamic movements.

Another consideration of static wrist joint measurements is forearm posture. Maximum wrist angles increase as the arm and shoulder muscles are used to rotate the forearm and hand. Therefore, when measuring the maximum range of motion in the wrist joint, the location and fixation of the arm and shoulder must be carefully constrained and documented.

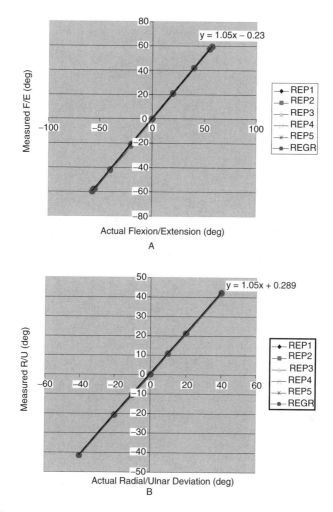

FIGURE 7.3

True and goniometer-measured angles during static calibration. (A) Flexion/extension plane, (B) radial/ulnar deviation plane. (From Jang, H., 2002. The Effects of Dynamic Wrist Workloads on Risks of Carpal Tunnel Syndrome, Ph.D. dissertation, University Park, PA: Pennsylvania State University. With permission.)

7.2.4 Dynamic Measurements — Angular Velocity and Acceleration

Dynamic components of the wrist typically include angular velocity and angular acceleration. Unfortunately, until fairly recently these have not been studied in detail. Schoenmarklin and Marras (1993) first established an important database on maximum dynamic capability in the three planes of wrist joint. Table 7.3 shows the maximum angular velocities and accelerations as a function of direction of movement.

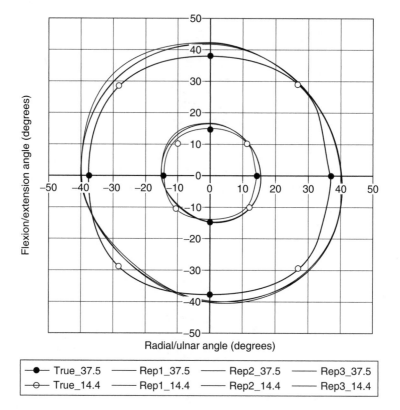

FIGURE 7.4

True and goniometer-measured angles during dynamic calibration. (From Jang, H., 2002. The Effects of Dynamic Wrist Workloads on Risks of Carpal Tunnel Syndrome, Ph.D. dissertation, University Park, PA: Pennsylvania State University. With permission.)

TABLE 7.2

Maximum Range of Motion Data of the Wrist Joint

| Previous Studies | Maximum Wrist Angle (°) | | | | | |
	Flexion	Extension	Radial Deviation	Ulnar Deviation	Pronation	Supination
Boone and Azen (1979)	76	75	19	33	—	—
Bonebrake et al. (1990)	86	62	34	68	105	120
Schoenmarklin and Marras (1993)	62	57	21	28	81	101
Marshall et al. (1999)	67	73	21	47	—	—

Table 7.3 reveals that maximum angular velocity and acceleration of pronation/supination plane are much higher than those for flexion/extension, and maximum angular velocity and acceleration of flexion/extension movements

TABLE 7.3

Maximum Angular Velocity and Acceleration as a Function of Movement Direction

Variables		Flexion/ Extension		Radial/Ulnar Deviation		Pronation/ Supination	
		F→E	E→F	R→U	U→R	P→S	S→P
Velocity	Dominant hand	−914	1,049	−436	356	−2,202	1,898
(°/s)	Nondominant hand	−926	1,069	−447	378	−2,072	1,784
Acceleration	Dominant hand	−12,007	16,092	−7,640	5,055	−45,034	36,336
(°/s²)	Nondominant hand	−12,051	16,020	−7,473	5,393	−39,367	33,217

Source: Schoenmarklin, R.W. and Marras, W.S., 1993. *International Journal of Industrial Ergonomics,* 11:207–224. With permission.

are much greater than those for radial/ulnar deviation movements. The magnitude of dynamic wrist capability depends on the movement direction in each plane as shown in Table 7.3. Flexion movement (from extreme extension angle to flexion, $E \rightarrow F$), ulnar movement ($R \rightarrow U$), and supination movement ($P \rightarrow S$) generate greater maximum angular velocities and accelerations than opposing movements. Schoenmarklin and Marras (1993) indicated that high dynamic capabilities of the flexion and supination movements were probably due to the greater biomechanical potentials of flexor and supinator muscles rather than of the extensor and pronator muscles, respectively. Also, the greater peak velocity and acceleration of ulnar movement were probably attributable to the effect of gravity.

Several studies have attempted to use the angular velocity and acceleration variable as potential risk factors in their epidemiological research (Marras and Schoenmarklin, 1993; Hansson et al., 1996; Marklin and Monroe, 1998; Serina et al., 1999). These values are summarized in Table 7.4.

Marras and Schoenmarklin (1993) performed a quantitative surveillance study on the factory floor. Based on a total of 40 subjects from eight industrial plants, wrist deviation, angular velocity, and acceleration variables were measured in three planes of wrist movements using dichotomous WRMSD risk levels (low and high risk). Table 7.4 indicates that the mean and maximum positions, angular velocity, and acceleration values of high-risk tasks are generally much higher than these of low-risk tasks in all three planes of wrist movements. Besides, angular velocity and acceleration appear to distinguish WRMSD risk levels more reliably than wrist deviation. The angular velocity and acceleration measures in high-risk tasks showed increases of 46.2 and 67.1%, respectively, over the same measures in low-risk tasks. These results show the importance of dynamic components on assessing WRMSD risk.

Hansson et al. (1996) investigated the position and angular velocity variables for tasks in the fish processing industry as means for characterizing static and dynamic properties of wrist movements. The results indicated that wrist deviations in fish processing tasks are much smaller than those in the low-risk tasks reported by Marras and Schoenmarklin (1993). However, the

TABLE 7.4

Mean and Peak Wrist Positions and Angular Velocity and Acceleration
in the Three Planes

Previous Studies	Variable	Task	F/E Mean	F/E Peak	R/U Mean	R/U Peak	P/S Mean	P/S Peak
Marras and Schoenmarklin (1993)	Position	High risk	−12.0[b]	6.6	−6.7	4.7	8.3	47.4
		Low risk	−10.1	4.4	−7.6	10.1	2.5	37.4
	Angular velocity	High risk	42	174	26	116	91	449
		Low risk	29	120	17	77	68	300
	Angular acceleration	High risk	824	4,471	494	3,077	1,824	11,291
		Low risk	494	2,588	301	1,759	1,222	7,169
Hansson et al. (1996)	Position	Fish processing	−1	n.a.	12	n.a.	n.a.	n.a.
	Angular velocity	Fish processing	61	142	36	84	n.a.	n.a.
Marklin and Monroe[a] (1998)	Angular velocity	Bone trimming	45	239	30	156	100	540
	Angular acceleration	Bone trimming	844	4,895	578	3,593	1872	12,522
Serina et al. (1999)	Position	Typing	−21.7	n.a.	−16.7	n.a.	86.8	n.a.
	Angular velocity	Typing	24	n.a.	12	n.a.	13	n.a.
	Angular acceleration	Typing	306	n.a.	134	n.a.	168	n.a.

[a] Data are maximum values among three intervals.
[b] "−" denotes extension and ulnar deviation.

angular velocities for F/E and R/U planes were 45 and 39%, respectively, higher than those for high-risk tasks. Serina et al. (1999) found that mean angular velocities and accelerations of typing tasks were similar to those of industrial tasks reported by Marras and Schoenmarklin (1993). In a clinical application, Ojima et al. (1991) found that angular-velocity/wrist-angle loci for healthy men were larger than for patients with carpal tunnel syndrome (CTS).

These studies demonstrate the need for measuring dynamic aspects (i.e., angular velocity and acceleration) of wrist motions as potential contributing risk factors for WRMSDs. Also, it is important to measure all three planes of wrist motions (flexion/extension, radial/ulnar deviation, and pronation/supination) simultaneously for best results.

7.3   Pressure and Force Distribution Measurements

7.3.1   Early Pressure Devices

In one of the earliest, simplest, nonquantitative approaches Swearingen et al. (1962) sat a subject on absorbent paper placed over an inked cloth. The density of ink transferred indicated a crude measure of pressure intensity. A similar approach was used by Fellows and Freivalds (1991) to identify critical areas on a tool handle for a more specific placement of pressure sensors. Subjects dipped their hands in fingerpaint and grasped the tool handle. Areas of highest pressure maintained the least amounts of paint, which spread to the areas of lowest pressure. Similarly, Dillon (1981) used strips of wax placed on top of the seat cushion. Lighter, ectomorphic individuals produced narrower and deeper indentations than heavy, endomorphic individuals. Lindan et al. (1965) used a bed of mechanical springs with more than 1000 sensors at 1.4 cm intervals to measure the whole-body pressure distribution. In a slightly different approach, thermography, with greater weight on a given area allowing less body heat to escape, was used to establish relatively nonquantitative pressure distributions (Trandel et al., 1975). However, reactive hyperemic thermal flare-ups distorted the results. Also, all of these approaches are relatively crude, with problems in repeatability, resolution, and accuracy.

For quantitative data, a large matrix of numerous sensors that can individually measure pressure is needed. The earliest such systems used mechanical valves with compressed air (Houle, 1969) or in a cruder approach without valves, plunger-activated liquid-filled manometers (Jürgens, 1969). Unfortunately, the major disadvantage with these systems is the need for a large apparatus with numerous relatively large pressure-gauge elements and a relatively large, mechanical control system. Later use of smaller sensors (Mooney et al., 1971), electronic controls and switches (Garber et al., 1978), and air as the pressure sensing medium (Bader et al., 1984) reduced some of the bulk in this approach. Based on the further work of Bader and Hawken (1986), the commercially available Talley Pressure Monitor (Talley Medical, Romsey, Hampshire, U.K.; http://www.talleymedical.co.uk/) was developed. Further testing (Ferguson-Pell and Cardi, 1991; Gyi et al., 1998) indicated high accuracy and repeatability as compared to force-sensing resistor systems but also several limitations: large (20 mm) sensor sizes, static measurements requiring at least 1 min of scanning, and relatively few sensors yielding poor resolution of the pressure distribution. The main advantage of pressure bladders is the ability to measure peak forces regardless of the orientation of the force.

Optical systems based on the prototype developed by Elftman (1934) have been used for both foot pressure (Betts et al., 1980; Franks et al., 1983) and seated pressure measurements (Mayo-Smith and Cochran, 1981; Kadaba et al., 1984; Treaster and Marras, 1987; Shields and Cook, 1988). This approach uses an acrylic sheet covered with a beaded silicone rubber baromat (Biomechanics, LeMesa, CA) incorporated into the seat pad or seat back. The working principle is based on differences in the optical properties of the acrylic–air and acrylic–rubber interfaces. A fluorescent light is attached along one edge of the acrylic sheet. The light enters the sheet but cannot be reflected out unless the baromat contacts the sheet. The greater the pressure on the rubber baromat, the more the beads deform and the more light is refracted from the acrylic sheet. The refracted light is photographed with a camera located either below the seat pan or reflected out with a mirror to a stationary camera. Processing of the refracted light is crucial for resolution, which has ranged from 9 levels using color (Shields and Cook, 1988) to 256 levels (Treaster and Marras, 1987) using direct digitization of the video signal and the available levels of gray scales on the video system. One problem with this system is the creep that occurs in all viscoelastic materials. If pressure is applied for a significant length of time (on the order of a half minute depending on the type of rubber used), then due to the continuous deformation of the rubber in contact with the acrylic, increased light output will occur for the same applied pressure (Betts et al., 1980). This will especially be a problem for dynamic measurements, such as measuring restlessness during long-term sitting.

Hertzberg (1972) developed a "pressure-measuring blanket" that consisted of an array of closely spaced thin flexible capacitors, each 1 cm² in area. Increased pressure was measured by a change in capacitance. This approach was improved by Drummond et al. (1982) who incorporated microprocessor control with a matrix of 64 strain-gauge resistive transducers instead of capacitors. Although quantitative specifications were not provided, the resistive transducers appeared to provide better sensitivity than the capacitors. However, the resistive transducers were fabricated onto an aluminum plate and then attached to a second aluminum base plate. Such a device is only useful for pressure measurements on a hard, uncontoured surface.

7.3.2 Force Sensing Electronic Components

The development of a new, lighter, and more flexible type of sensor provided more opportunities for pressure measurement applications. This force-sensing resistor (FSR) (Interlink Electronics, Camarillo, CA, http://www.interlinkelectronics.com; or in Europe, Electrade GmbH, Gräfelfing, Germany, http://www.electrade.com/html/FSRtm.htm) consists of two sheets of polymer film, with conductive interdigitating fingers and the other with a conductive film overlying the fingers, separated by a spacer. Applying a force to the resulting sandwich causes the resistance between the two contact surfaces to decrease, which can be measured through a voltage divider (Fellows and Freivalds, 1989). The force–resistance relationship is quite nonlinear (Figure 7.5, note the log-log scale) and, therefore, the sensors need to be calibrated carefully (Park, 1999). Because FSRs are quite flexible, one of the first applications involved measuring grip pressure distributions for different types of tool handle surfaces (Fellows and Freivalds, 1991) as well as seat pressure distributions with a matrix of 32 FSRs placed between two thin sheets of plastic and placed on the seat pans of two different automobile seats (Figure 7.6; Yun et al., 1992). A similar but larger mat of 225 sensors was used to model seating comfort in a car seat (Gross et al., 1994) and also to measure seated postural shifts (Fenety et al., 1994, 2000).

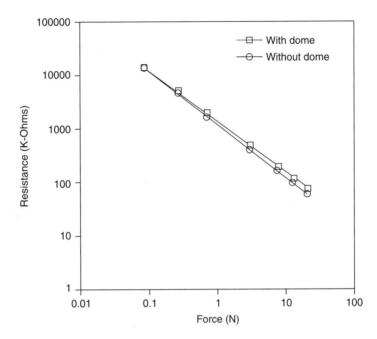

FIGURE 7.5

Force sensor calibration curves. (From Park, S.K., 1999. The Development of an Exposure Measurement System for Assessing Risk of Work-Related Musculoskeletal Disorders, Ph.D. thesis, University Park, PA: Pennsylvania State University. With permission.)

Although convenient and inexpensive, FSRs have several problems. Although termed "force sensing," they, in fact, measure pressure or force per unit area. Localized or directed applications of a force to a relatively large sensor will not yield a correct value. Also, directionality of the forces, including shear loading, as well as bending the sensor, can produce errors. To create a sensor that responds to force rather than pressure, Jensen et al. (1991) developed the method of forming an epoxy dome over the sensing area to better direct the applied forces to the sensor. This also helped stiffen the sensor area and keep it rigid during loading.

Park (1999) performed detailed calibration studies on UniForce FSRs (Figure 7.7, now available as Flexiforce sensors from Tekscan, Inc., South Boston, MA, http://www.tekscan.com/flexiforce.html), finding repeatability ranging from 87 to 94% for domed and 75 to 91% for undomed sensors, considerably worse than the 95% claimed by the manufacturer. Repeatability was worst for lowest forces. Also, there was a tendency for the sensor to flatten the logarithmic relationship by approximately 6% per day of usage (Figure 7.8). Once sensor performance drops below a given threshold (reference line in Figure 7.8) and fails to provide good calibration, the sensor can be considered to have failed. Park (1999) estimated failure to occur in 19 days for undomed sensors and 34 days for domed sensors.

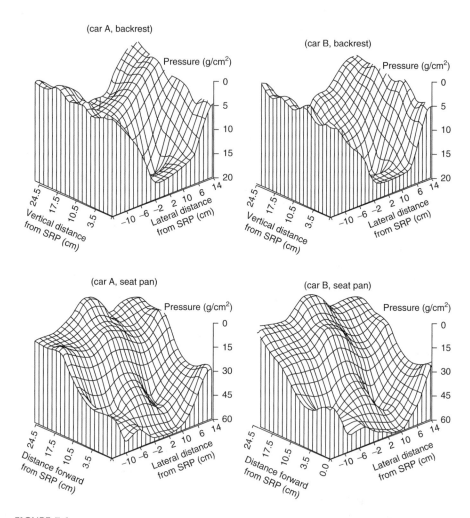

FIGURE 7.6
Pressure distribution curves for automobile seat pans and seat backs. (From Yun, M.H. et al., 1992. In Kumar, S., Ed., *Advances in Industrial Ergonomics and Safety IV*, London: Taylor & Francis, 403–410. With permission.)

The concept of the domed force sensor was further expanded by Carvalho and Radwin (1996). By sandwiching the traditional FSR between two layers of spring steel, placing the sandwich on an annular ring support, and covering it with a Torlon polymer dome, the usable force range was expanded by almost 100% and the resulting error was decreased by almost 50%. In another approach, Beebe et al. (1998) developed a completely new silicon-based force sensor with lower hysteresis and higher repeatability than the original sensor.

Another type of pressure sensor can be formed from piezoelectric film, which produces an electric current during displacement. Sorab et al. (1988)

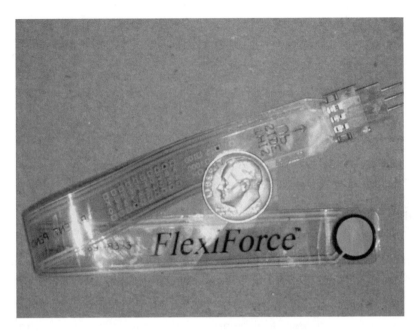

FIGURE 7.7
A FlexiForce force-sensing resistor. (Courtesy of Tekscan, Inc., http://www.tekscan.com/flex-iforce.html.)

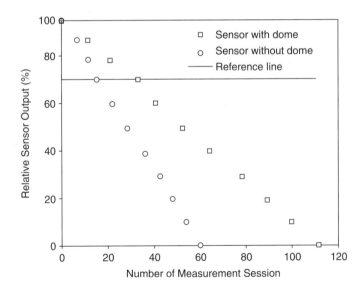

FIGURE 7.8
Force-sensing resistor decay. (From Park, S.K., 1999. The Development of an Exposure Measurement System for Assessing Risk of Work-Related Musculoskeletal Disorders, Ph.D. thesis, University Park, PA: Pennsylvania State University. With permission.)

used a piezoelectric sensor attached directly to a surgeon's hands to measure finger forces during delivery of newborns. However, the material is very fragile and, due to the transient nature of the electric signal, would serve poorly in static pressure measurements.

More recently, the force-sensing technology has been expanded to ready-made pressure sensing mats (Tekscan, Inc., South Boston, MA, http://www.tekscan.com/flexiforce.html). Two thin, flexible polyester sheets, with electrically conductive electrodes deposited in perpendicular directions (i.e., rows for one and columns for the other), sandwich an intermediate layer with semiconductive ink. A grid pattern is formed, creating a sensing location at each intersection. With an applied force, there is electrical resistance change at each of the intersecting points of the grid pattern, which can be mapped to create a pressure distribution pattern. Because the grid lines can be as close as 0.5 mm, there can be more than 170 sensors per square centimeter, establishing a very high-resolution matrix, albeit at a considerable cost. Primary applications have been for in-the-shoe pressure measuring systems (Woodburn and Helliwell, 1997), pressure measurements under burn garments (Mann et al., 1997), and also for seat pan pressure distributions for wheelchair users (Ferguson-Pell and Cardi, 1993). However, the system showed considerable hysteresis (±20%), creep (19%), and poor repeatability, but was liked by clinicians for its real-time display capabilities (Ferguson-Pell and Cardi, 1993).

A variation of the above resistive matrix approach is a conductive rubber sheet, which has the unique property in that it conducts electric current when compressed but acts as insulator when the pressure is released (Yokohama Image System Co. Ltd, Technical Development Center, Kanagawa, Japan, http://www.y-i-s.co.jp/CSAEnglish.html). Thus, in a gross sense it acts as a switching function, but when used carefully, its electrical resistance varies according to the applied pressure. The method has been used to measure pressure distributions within the wrist (Hara et al., 1992) and to evaluate comfort while lying on different types of bedding (http://www.hql.or.jp/gpd/eng/www/nwl/n14/ergo.html).

Another recent product that provides a highly detailed pressure distribution is the Fuji pressure film (Fuji Medical Systems, Stamford CT, http://www.prescale.com/E/E_index.htm). Pressure-sensitive film is constructed of a color-developing layer and a microcapsule layer sandwiched between a polyethylene terephthylate (PET) bases. The film comes in several pressure ranges. Once exposed to pressure, the film changes color and the resultant color pressure density is established with a specially designed densitometer, reading areas down to 1 mm. Typical applications so far have been for measuring occlusal forces in dental surgery (Harada et al., 2000), joint forces (Konrath et al., 1999), but not seating distributions. Although this approach appears to be quite sensitive for distribution, there has been some concern over error of 10 to 15% in the pressure readings, due to the contact pressure exceeding the film threshold or due to the rate of pressure loading (Hale and Brown, 1992). Using multiple ranges of film simultaneously showed considerable variations in readings due to the stacking order and interactions of the microcapsule layers and may not completely solve the first problem (Atkinson et al., 1998). Calibrating the film with the same rate of loading as anticipated experimentally may alleviate the second problem (Haut, 1989).

A comparison of various pressure and force distribution measurement systems, in terms of cost, accuracy, advantages, and disadvantages, is given in Table 7.5. Resolution has not been addressed, as the systems provide either continuous or discrete distributions. For the discrete systems, the resolution depends on how many sensors have been used. Only qualitative assessments have been made, because very few studies have provided quantitative data on reliability, validity, etc.

7.3.3 Integrated Touch Glove System

Yun et al. (1997) developed an integrated system, termed the "touch glove," to coordinate and facilitate real-time hand motion and grip force measurements in the field. The main component is the Cyberglove by Virtual Technologies of Palo Alto, CA (http://www.immersion.com/products/3d/interaction/overview.shtml). The Cyberglove uses a total of 22 strain-gauge sensors — three bend sensors and one abduction sensor per finger to measure finger flexion/extension and abduction/adduction angles — and two sensors at the wrist. In conjunction with a Polhemus magnetic sensor, the position of the hand with respect to a reference is also established. Analog signals for the strain gauges are digitized via an analog-to-digital (A/D) converter on the host computer. For a typical application, an 8-bit A/D converter (0 to 255 point) provides sufficient accuracy to map the appropriate ROM in degrees (<140°) for the fingers. For greater accuracy, 12-bit A/D converters will be more than sufficient. A device similar to that described in Section 7.2.2 but for the fingers would be needed to calibrate the glove.

The second component for the touch glove system is a force sensor matrix, consisting of 12 FSRs described in Section 7.3.2, overlaying the Cyberglove. Although the number of sensors and their locations are freely changeable, the current system utilizes sensors on the distal and metacarpal phalanges of each finger, except for the thumb, where only one sensor is attached to the distal phalanx. Three other sensors are placed on the thenar and hypothenar eminences, as shown in Figure 7.9. The location for the sensors was determined by the rough contact area a hand produces by gripping a cylindrical handle sprayed with paint following the procedures of Fellows and Freivalds (1991). The fully integrated touch glove holding a hand tool is shown in Figure 7.9.

The touch glove was then utilized in a set of laboratory calibration experiments to measure joint angles and finger forces as a function of handle diameter (Yun, 1994; Yun et al., 1997). The results indicated, as could be

TABLE 7.5

Comparison of Pressure and Force Distribution Measurement Systems

Type of Measurement	Distribution	Accuracy	Cost	Advantages	Disadvantages
Paint, wax, heat	Continuous	Low	Low	Simple and inexpensive	Not easily quantified
Baromat, optical scan	Continuous	Medium	Medium	Quantification of continuous data	Rubber creep, data conversion
Pneumatic, hydraulic	Discrete	High	Medium	Directionality unimportant	Cumbersome equipment
Force sensing resistors	Discrete	Medium	Low	Simple, inexpensive, easy to apply	Directionality, daily calibration
Pressure mats	Discrete	High	High	High resolution, many shapes	Cost, repeatability, hysteresis
Pressure film	Continuous	Medium	Medium	Nonintrusive	Sensitive to rate of loading

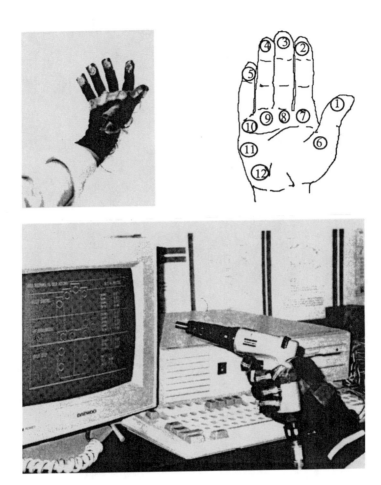

FIGURE 7.9
Sensor distribution on touch glove system. (From Yun, M.H., 1994. A Hand Posture Measurement Systems for the Analysis of Manual Tool Handling Tasks, Ph.D. dissertation, University Park, PA: Pennsylvania State University. With permission.)

hypothesized, that finger flexion angles decreased as grip diameter increased (Figure 7.10). Force distribution results (Figure 7.11) indicated that the fingertip forces were greater than metacarpal forces, thumb fingertip forces increased with increasing grip diameter, little fingertip forces decreased with increasing grip diameter, while the finger tip forces for middle fingers remained roughly constant. These results and the touch glove system were the bases for further research on optimal handle diameter (see Section 9.3.2) and handle shapes (see Section 9.3.3). The system has also been used successfully in the field measuring pinch forces during warehouse handling of glass windshields (Lowe and Freivalds, 1997).

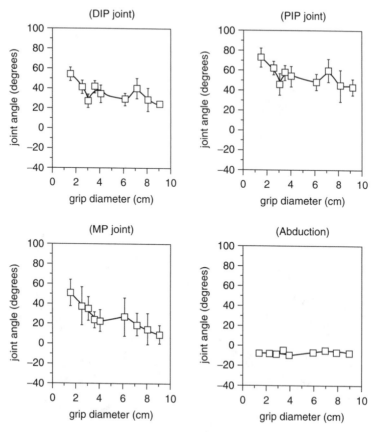

FIGURE 7.10
Index finger joint angles as a function of grip diameter. (From Yun, M.H. et al., 1997. *IEEE Transactions on Systems, Man, and Cybernetics, Part B: Cybernetics*, 27:835–846. With permission.)

7.4   Nerve Conduction Measurements

7.4.1   Basic Concepts

Currently, the most reliable technique for diagnosing and assessing the severity of CTS is nerve conduction assessment (Kembel, 1968; Melvin et al., 1973; Jackson and Clifford, 1987; Stevens, 1987; Kimura, 1989; Ghavanini and Haghighat, 1998). Electromyographic (EMG) instrumentation (see Section 7.5) is used to measure and quantify nerve conduction parameters, such as latency, amplitude, duration and conduction velocity, by measuring the time required for an electrical impulse to travel from a stimulus site to the measurement site, typically on the median nerve. The results are then compared against reference values, which have been established for both healthy and

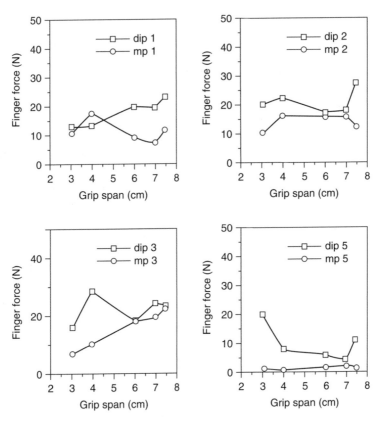

FIGURE 7.11

Finger forces as a function of grip diameter. (From Yun, M.H. et al., 1997. *IEEE Transactions on Systems, Man, and Cybernetics, Part B: Cybernetics*, 27:835–846. With permission.)

symptomatic populations. Patients with CTS show prolonged median motor nerve latency and/or decreased median motor nerve amplitude as compared with normal subjects (Simpson, 1956; Thomas, 1960; Kimura, 1979, 1989). Similarly, such patients also demonstrate a prolonged median sensory nerve latency and/or decreased amplitude (Kembel, 1968; Felsenthal and Spindler, 1979; Kimura and Ayyar, 1985; Stevens, 1987).

The conceptual pathophysiological explanation for such changes in median nerve conduction is based on various models (Moore et al., 1991; Tanaka and McGlothin, 1993; Hagberg et al., 1995; Werner and Armstrong, 1997) leading to the following scenario. Occupational risk factors such as forceful exertion, repetitive motions, and awkward postures may cause muscular fatigue and discomfort to the carpal tunnel at wrist during work. If sufficient recovery time is provided after such, the fatigue and discomfort are short-lived. However, if work is continued despite fatigue and discomfort, the tendons may become strained due to inadequate lubrication and signs of inflammation and swelling may appear within carpal tunnel

(Sissons, 1979). Tendon structures are especially susceptible, as tendon sheaths appear to require a much longer recovery time than muscles. This swelling causes a further increase in the carpal tunnel pressure.

With sufficient increase in pressure, local venous congestion occurs within the vascular structure of the nerve, as well as ischemia in the arterioles nourishing the nerve, leading to endoneurinal edema (Sunderland, 1976). The role of neural ischemia is supported by the relatively rapid recovery from acute CTS after carpal tunnel release surgery and or the development of CTS symptoms by artificially restricting blood flow to the nerve with the pneumatic tourniquet test (Moore, 1992). The neural edema further increases the effect of the original compression, thus creating a vicious circle. If this condition persists for a prolonged period of time, it leads to progressive long-term axonal deterioration resulting in the characteristic symptoms for CTS, numbness, tingling, and pain in the areas corresponding to distribution of the nerves (Tanaka and McGlothlin, 1993). Mechanical pressure to the nerve, on the other hand, causes direct histologic changes to the nerve, including thinning or shearing of the myelin under the area of compression (Armstrong, 1994).

7.4.2 Nerve Stimulation and Recording

Since Simpson (1956) first measured median nerve latency in patients with CTS, the technique has been continually improved in its sensitivity and specificity for CTS diagnosis. However, the technique basically still consists of two components: sensory nerve conduction with stimulating and recording electrodes on the median nerve (or other nerve of interest) and motor nerve conduction with stimulating electrodes on the nerve and recording electrodes in the muscles innervated by that nerve.

Either surface or needle electrodes may be used to stimulate the nerve. Stimulating electrodes consist of a *cathode* (negative pole) and an *anode* (positive pole). As the current flows between them, negative charges that accumulate under the cathode depolarize the nerve and form an action potential (see Section 3.3). Most commercially available stimulators provide a probe that mounts the cathode and the anode at a fixed distance, usually 2 to 3 cm apart. The anode must be placed proximal to the cathode while stimulating (Figure 7.12).

The pulses of moderate intensity are used to adjust the positions of the cathode until further relocation causes no change in the size of the muscle action potential. With the cathode at the best stimulating site, one then defines the maximal intensity that just elicits a maximal potential. Increasing the stimulus another 20 to 30% supramaximal, then, guarantees the activation of all the nerve axons innervating the recorded muscle (but does not further increase the muscle potential).

Surface stimulations of 0.1 ms duration, and 100 to 300 V or 5 to 40 mA intensity are usually sufficient to fully activate a healthy nerve but cause no

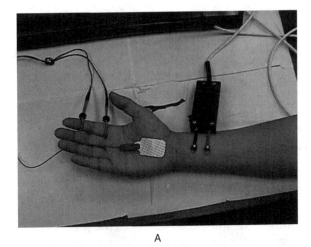

A

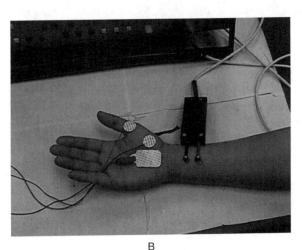

B

FIGURE 7.12
Setup for median nerve conduction studies: (A) sensory nerve (antidromic), (B) motor nerve (orthodromic). (From Jang, H., 2002. The Effects of Dynamic Wrist Workloads on Risks of Carpal Tunnel Syndrome, Ph.D. dissertation, University Park, PA: Pennsylvania State University. With permission.)

particular risk to an ordinary patient. Special care to safeguard the patient includes proper grounding and the placement of the stimulator with a sufficient distance from a pacemaker or other implanted electronic devices (AAEE, 1984). Stimulation by a needle electrode inserted subcutaneously close to the nerve requires much less current than surface stimulation to elicit the same response. The anode may be a surface electrode located on the skin or a second needle electrode inserted in the vicinity of the cathode.

Recording the response potentials again requires a pair of surface electrodes or needle electrodes, the cathode and the anode. With this arrangement, the propagating action potential, originating under the cathode, gives rise to a simple biphase waveform with initial negativity. Surface electrodes, in general, are better than needle electrodes for recording a compound motor nerve action potential in assessing contributions from all discharging units, because its onset latency indicates the conduction time of the fastest fibers, whereas its amplitude is approximately proportional to the number of available axons. The use of a needle electrode improves the recording from small atrophic muscles because the needle electrode registers only a small portion of the muscle action potential with less interference from neighboring discharges.

Routine recording of the sensory nerve action potential, in general, is performed with surface ring electrodes, which provide adequate and reproducible information non-invasively. (Tashjian et al., 1987; Jackson and Clifford, 1989; Kimura, 1989; Burnham and Steadward, 1994). Some, however, prefer needle electrodes placed perpendicular to the nerve to improve the resolution, and to improve the signal-to-noise ratio (Rosenfalck, 1978). Sensory studies are usually performed with filters set at 20 Hz to 2 kHz while motor studies are usually performed with filters set at 2 Hz to 10 kHz.

The nerve can be stimulated either in the normal conduction direction, termed *orthodromic*, or in the reverse direction, termed *antidromic*. For example, in a sensory nerve fiber, stimulation at a distal point and recording proximal to the point of stimulation is orthodromic nerve conduction. If the process is reversed by stimulating the sensory nerve fibers proximal to the recording points, then the technique is an antidromic nerve conduction (Figure 7.13A). This is also sometimes termed distal nerve conduction.

The major advantage of an orthodromic technique is that only sensory fibers are stimulated and recorded. It has also been suggested that orthodromic nerve conduction parameters are less affected by change of temperature (Chodoroff et al., 1985). The primary advantage of the antidromic technique is a larger response amplitude compared to the orthodromic technique because the digital nerves lie nearer the surface. The amplitude of the sensory nerve action potential is essential to establish the severity of CTS and its progress. MacDonell et al. (1990) reported the antidromic technique is a more sensitive method for assessing mild CTS.

The conventional site for stimulation of both sensory and motor nerves is the wrist (Figure 7.13B). At the wrist, the cathode may be placed 3 cm proximal to the crease of the wrist (Kimura, 1989). Alternative techniques use a fixed distance from the recording electrode, most commonly 12 to 14 cm (DiBenedetto et al., 1986; Jackson and Clifford, 1989; Carroll, 1987). Sensory potentials can be recorded from the first, second, or third digits with surface ring electrodes usually placed around the proximal (cathode) and distal interphalangeal joints (anode), at a fixed distance of 4 cm between cathode and anode (Dumitru and Walsh, 1988) (Figure 7.13A). Motor potentials are recorded at the abductor pollicis brevis muscle at the base of the thumb (Figure 7.13B). Table 7.6 describes the common sites of electrode placement for the median, ulnar, and radial nerves.

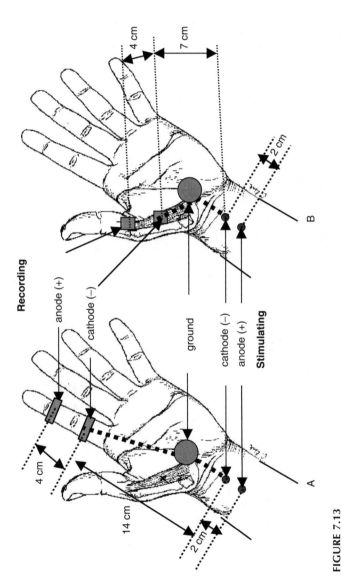

FIGURE 7.13

Electrode placements for median nerve conduction studies: (A) sensory nerve (antidromic), (B) motor nerve (orthodromic). (From Jang, H., 2002. The Effects of Dynamic Wrist Workloads on Risks of Carpal Tunnel Syndrome, Ph.D. dissertation, University Park, PA: Pennsylvania State University. With permission.)

TABLE 7.6

Common Electrode Placements for Nerve Conduction Studies

Nerve	Fibers	Stimulation Site			Recording Site		
		Cathode	Anode	Distance	Cathode	Anode	Ground Site
Median	Motor	Fixed distance from recording electrode mostly 7–8 cm, or 3 cm proximal to the distal crease at wrist	2–3 cm proximal to cathode	7–8 cm	The belly of the abductor pollicis brevis (APB) at thumb	The tendon of abductor pollicis brevis (APB) at thumb	Palm (metacarpal phalanges of third digit)
	Sensory	Fixed distance from recording electrode mostly 12–14 cm, or 3 cm proximal to the distal crease at wrist	2–3 cm proximal to cathode	12–14 cm	Proximal interphalangeal joints (PIP) of second or third digits	Distal interphalangeal (DIP) joints or 4 cm distal to cathode	Palm (metacarpal phalanges of third digit)
Ulnar	Motor	Fixed distance from recording electrode mostly 7–8 cm, or 3 cm proximal to the distal crease at wrist	2 cm proximal to cathode	7–8 cm	Belly of the abductor digiti minimi (ADM)	Tendon of the abductor digiti minimi (ADM), 3 cm distally	Palm (metacarpal phalanges of third digit)
					Belly of the first dorsal interosseous muscle	Tendon of the first dorsal interosseous muscle	Dorsum side of palm
	Sensory	Fixed distance from recording electrode mostly 12–14 cm, or 3 cm proximal to the distal crease at wrist	2–3 cm proximal to cathode	12–14 cm	Proximal interphalangeal (PIP) joints of the fifth or fourth digits	Distal interphalangeal (PIP) joints of the fifth or fourth digits	Palm (metacarpal phalanges of third digit)
Radial	Motor	Forearm at lateral edge of the extensor carpi ulnaris (ECU) muscle 8–10 cm proximal to the styloid process	2 cm proximal to cathode	—	Monopolar needle electrode in the extensor indicis	Dorsum of hand laterally	Posterior forearm, 4 to 5 cm proximal to distal crease at wrist
	Sensory	Lateral edge of the radius in the distal forearm	2–3 cm proximal to cathode	—	Metacarpal phalangeal (MP) joint of first digit	Intercarpal (IP) joints of first digit	Posterior forearm, 4 to 5 cm proximal to distal crease at wrist

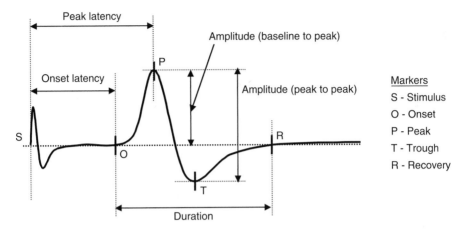

FIGURE 7.14

Typical median nerve conduction waveform. (From Jang, H., 2002. The Effects of Dynamic Wrist Workloads on Risks of Carpal Tunnel Syndrome, Ph.D. dissertation, University Park, PA: Pennsylvania State University. With permission.)

7.4.3 Response Measures

Typical nerve conduction measures are identified in the sample response waveform shown in Figure 7.14. *Onset latency* (SO, in ms) is the time between nerve stimulation and the initial response detected at the active recording electrode. *Peak latency* (SP, in ms) is time between nerve stimulation and peak response detected at the active recording electrode. The amplitude of the waveform (in mV for motor NCS, μV for sensory NCS) can be measured between the baseline and negative peak (OP) or between the negative peak and the positive peak (PT). The duration of the waveform (in ms) is the time between the initial deviation from the baseline and the ultimate return to the baseline (OR). The conduction velocity (in m/s) is calculated by dividing stimulated nerve length by the peak latency.

For motor nerve conduction studies, latency consists of two components: (1) nerve conduction time from the stimulus point to the nerve terminal and (2) neuromuscular transmission time from the axonal terminal to the motor end plate, including the time required for generation of muscle action potentials. Thus, onset latency is a measure of the fastest conducting motor fibers (Kimura, 1989). To calculate the pure motor nerve conduction velocity, one must eliminate the time for neuromuscular transmission and generation of muscle action potentials. The difference between the two latency responses elicited at two separate points excludes the two components common to both stimuli. Thus, it represents the time necessary for the nerve impulse to travel between the two stimulus points. The motor nerve conduction velocity is derived as the ratio between the distance from one point of stimulation (Site A) to the next (Site B) and the corresponding latency difference between them.

TABLE 7.7

Normal Values for Median Motor Nerve Conduction

Authors	Onset Latency (ms)		Amplitude (mV)		Conduction Velocity (m/s)	
	Normal	Abnormal (>2 SD)	Normal	Abnormal (<2 SD)	Normal	Abnormal (<2 SD)
Burnham and Steadward (1994)	3.63 ± 0.28	4.2	12.8 ± 4.0	4.6	59.6 ± 3.7	52.0
Jackson and Clifford (1989)	3.2 ± 0.27	3.8	12.6 ± 3.22	6.1	—	—
Kimura (1989)	3.49 ± 0.34	4.2	—	—	48.8 ± 5.3	38.0
Kimura (1979)	3.6 ± 0.36	4.3	—	—	49.0 ± 5.7	37.4
Melvin et al. (1973)	3.7 ± 0.3	4.5	13.2 ± 5.0	3.0	56.7 ± 3.8	48.9
Thomas et al. (1967)	3.4 ± 0.48	4.4	—	—	59.1 ± 5.2	48.5
Johnson and Olsen (1960)	—	—	—	—	53.0 ± 6.4	40.0
Average	3.5	4.2	12.9	4.6	54.7	44.7

Note: All data are antidromic.

The reliability of results depends on accuracy in determining the length of the nerve segment, estimated with the surface distance along the course of the nerve. Unlike motor latency, which includes neuromuscular transmission, sensory latency consists only of the nerve conduction time from the stimulus point to the recording electrode. Therefore, stimulation of the nerve at a single site is enough for calculation of sensory nerve conduction velocity, which is calculated by dividing stimulated nerve length by onset latency.

Patients with CTS, compared with normal individuals, have been shown to have prolonged median motor nerve latencies, decreased median motor nerve amplitudes (Simpson, 1956; Thomas, 1960; Kimura, 1979, 1989) and decreased median motor nerve conduction velocities in the presence of CTS (Thomas, 1960; Kimura, 1979; Kimura and Ayyar, 1985). However, even normal values (Table 7.7) show considerable variability, with distal onset latency usually ranging between 3.2 and 3.7 ms, motor nerve amplitude ranging between 12.6 and 13.2 mV, and conduction velocity ranging between 48.8 and 59.6 m/s. The upper limits for normal subjects and lower limits for CTS diagnosis are usually defined as mean plus two standard deviations, yielding values of 4.5 ms for latency, 3.0 mV for amplitude, and 32.4 m/s for conduction velocity. However, it is important to note that there was considerable variability in distal median motor nerve conduction parameters reported by these investigators, with various experimental settings, different room and skin temperatures, and a variety of conduction distances.

Similar to median motor nerve studies, the results of median sensory nerve conduction studies indicated that between 49 and 66% of patients with CTS demonstrate a prolonged median sensory peak latency, a reduced median sensory nerve amplitude, or even a complete absence of sensory nerve action potential between the wrist and a specific digit (Kemble, 1968; Felsenthal and Spindler, 1979; Kimura and Ayyar, 1985; Stevens, 1987). Most researchers used the index finger for stimulation or recording, but some used the middle finger. Normal values (Table 7.8) indicate that distal onset latency ranges between 2.5 and 2.8 ms, peak latency ranges between 3.0 and 3.2 ms, sensory nerve amplitude ranges between 32.9 and 44.9 mV, and conduction velocity ranges between 56.2 and 58.3 m/s. The upper limits for normal subjects and lower limits for CTS diagnosis are again defined as mean plus two standard deviations, yielding values of 3.5 ms for onset latency, 4.0 ms for peak latency, 0 mV for amplitude, and 44.4 m/s for conduction velocity.

7.4.4 Limitations

There are a variety of factors that influence nerve conduction parameters and that need to be carefully controlled or noted to avoid false-positive CTS diagnoses based on erroneous interpretation of nerve conduction measurement. These factors include skin temperature and age and, perhaps, gender and body mass index.

Skin temperature has a profound effect on nerve conduction parameters (Baysal et al., 1993; Letz and Gerr, 1994). As the skin temperature decreases, the nerve conduction action potential recorded from a nerve demonstrates an increased amplitude and prolonged latency. Tashjian et al. (1987) reported that the antidromic median sensory nerve latency was delayed by 0.06 ms/° with cooling, and median sensory nerve amplitude was found to increase with upper extremity cooling with the antidromic technique by 3.5 µV/°. Lee et al. (1993) claim that this temperature effect on latency may be as large as 0.1 ms/°. Conversely, nerve impulses conduct faster at higher body temperature. The conduction velocity increases almost linearly, by 2.4 m/s/° as the temperature measured near the nerve increases form 29 to 38°C (Johnson and Olsen, 1960).

Correction factors for skin temperature are typically employed only when wrist temperature exceeds normal ranges, defined as 29.6 to 33.4°C (Halar et al., 1983). However, to improve the sensitivity of nerve conduction studies, Jackson and Clifford (1989) suggested applying correction factors when the skin temperature measured at the wrist midline exceeded 31.0°C.

Slowing of median nerve function occurs naturally with increasing age although not necessarily leading to the development of CTS (Nathan et al., 1988, 1992). Specifically, median sensory nerve conduction velocity decreases by as much as 1.3 m/s per decade of age (Stetson et al., 1992; Letz and Gerr., 1994). Similarly, sensory nerve conduction velocity has been shown to decline by 1 m/s per decade (Chodoroff et al., 1985).

Effects of the body mass index on median nerve conduction are conflicting. Nathan et al. (1992) reported a strong positive correlation, while Letz and Gerr (1994) reported a small negative association between measures. If other variables are carefully accounted for, then gender differences in median nerve conduction parameters have been minimal (Nathan et al., 1988, 1992; Stetson et al., 1992; Robinson et al., 1993).

TABLE 7.8

Normal Values for Median Sensory Nerve Conduction

Authors	Onset Latency (ms)		Peak Latency (ms)		Amplitude (µV)		Conduction Velocity (m/s)	
	Normal	Abnormal (>2 SD)	Normal	Abnormal (>2 SD)	Normal	Abnormal (<2 SD)	Normal	Abnormal (<2 SD)
Burnham and Steadward (1994)	—	—	—	—	44.9 ± 14.8	15.1	58.3 ± 5.7	46.7
Jackson and Clifford (1989)	2.47 ± 1.2	2.7	3.16 ± 0.16	3.5	32.9 ± 10.4	11.9	—	—
Kimura (1989)	2.84 ± 3.4	3.5	—	—	38.5 ± 15.6	7.1	56.2 ± 5.8	44.4
Kimura (1979)	2.82 ± 2.8	3.4	—	—	41.3 ± 19.3	2.5	57.3 ± 6.9	45.1
Melvin et al. (1973)	—	—	3.2 ± 0.2	3.8	41.6 ± 25.0	0.0	56.9 ± 4.0	48.7
Johnson and Melvin (1967)	—	—	3.0 ± 0.4	4.0	—	—	—	—
Average	2.7	3.2	3.1	3.8	39.8	7.3	57.2	46.2

Note: All data are antidromic.

To improve the sensitivity of nerve conduction tests and to clarify the confounding effects of a generalized peripheral neuropathy, clinicians have suggested comparing median nerve conduction to ulnar or radial nerve conduction. Felsenthal and Spindler (1979) performed a 14-cm antidromic sensory nerve action potential technique to index finger and little finger for comparison of median and ulnar nerve. They concluded that a difference greater than 0.46 ms between median and ulnar sensory nerve peak latencies in the same hand was suggestive of CTS. Similarly, Johnson et al. (1981) and Jackson and Clifford (1989) recommended differences of median and ulnar peak latency of 0.3 and 0.35 ms, respectively, suggestive of CTS.

Johnson et al. (1987) established a comparison study of median to radial sensory nerve in thumb with a 10-cm antidromic sensory nerve action potential technique. They concluded that a peak latency disparity of greater than 0.4 ms between median and radial is suggestive of CTS because 93% of normal subjects demonstrated a difference of 0.4 ms or less. Carroll (1987) and Jackson and Clifford (1989) also reported differences of 0.3 to 0.4 ms as suggestive of CTS. Normal ulnar and radial sensory conduction values to be used in comparison with median nerve values are summarized in Table 7.9. Note that the amplitude and conduction velocity of the little finger are slightly larger and faster than for the ring finger.

7.5   Electromyography

As discussed in Chapter 3, the neuromuscular system consists of many muscles, each containing many motor units, each of which consists of a nerve innervating a collection of muscle fibers. For the muscle to produce force, these motor units need to be recruited according to the size principle, from the smallest to the largest, and from lower to higher thresholds. To recruit a given motor unit, nerve action potentials proceed from the cell body (which has received similar action potentials, either from higher centers in the central nervous system or from other neurons in the peripheral nervous system), along the axon, across the synapse to each of the corresponding muscle fibers. There, through depolarization of the cell membrane, a similar muscle action potential is generated, which passes along the muscle fiber, depolarizing the membranes of sarcoplasmic reticulum, releasing calcium ions to promote the cross-bridging of thick and thin filaments, and, ultimately, causing force production in the muscle. For a muscle twitch, a few small motor units may be involved at relatively low firing frequencies with a small amount of muscle action potential. For maximum muscle contraction, all the motor units need to be recruited at tetanic frequencies, resulting in a high level of muscle action potentials or electrical activity in the muscle. This muscle

TABLE 7.9

Normal and Abnormal Values for Ulnar and Radial Sensory Nerve

Nerve	Authors	Latency (ms)		Amplitude (µV)		Conduction Velocity (m/s)	
		Normal	Abnormal (>2 SD)	Normal	Abnormal (<2 SD)	Normal	Abnormal (<2 SD)
Ulnar nerve	Burnham and Steadward (1994)	—	—	26.7 ± 9.8 (Digit 4)	7.1	55.7 ± 4.7 (Digit 4)	46.3
				42.7 ± 18.0 (Digit 5)	6.7	58.1 ± 5.7 (Digit 5)	46.7
	Kimura (1989)	2.54 ± 0.29 (Digit 5)	3.12	35.0 ± 14.7 (Digit 5)	5.6	54.8 ± 5.3 (Digit 5)	44.2
Radial nerve	Burnham and Steadward (1994)	—	—	—	—	59.4 ± 5.6 (Digit 1)	48.2
	Kimura (1989)	2.37 ± 0.22 (Digit 1)	2.81	13.0 ± 7.5 (Digit 1)	0.0	58.0 ± 6.0 (Digit 1)	46.0

electrical activity, termed *electromyography* or EMG for short, can be measured by placing electrodes either on the surface of the skin or within the muscle and suitably amplifying and processing the signal. Because the electrical activity varies with the amount of motor unit recruited and thus the force produced by the muscle, EMG is a good measure of muscle force production, especially in occupational activities, where the force cannot be measured directly without interfering with the task at hand. However, over time as the muscle fatigues, force production drops, but motor unit recruitment and corresponding electrical activity increases. Therefore, EMG is also very useful in quantifying localized muscle fatigue.

7.5.1 EMG Instrumentation

The most crucial step in measuring a noise-free electrical signal is the proper attachment of electrodes to the individual. This can be either *invasive*, within the muscle, by using needle electrodes, or *noninvasive*, on the surface of the skin over the belly of the muscle of interest, by using surface electrodes. Needle electrodes yield a more sensitive signal, to the point of even isolating individual motor units. However, because they are invasive, they typically require the supervision of a medically trained expert and, thus, are better suited for a clinical setting rather than an industrial setting. Surface electrodes, as noninvasive, do not require such medical supervision and, as they are slightly less sensitive to electrical noise, are better suited to an industrial environment. They should be high-quality silver/silver-chloride electrodes used in conjunction with specialized electrode paste to improve the electrical conductance. However, to achieve as low an *electrical impedance* as possible (and reduce the effect of electrical noise), it is also important to prepare the subject by shaving the individual's hair, abrading the skin to remove the dry, scaling surface layer, rubbing electrode paste into the skin to further reduce skin resistance, and letting the electrode paste "soak" into the skin for 10 to 20 min before the start of experimentation. By such means it is often possible to decrease skin resistance from values as high as 200,000 Ω to as low as 5,000 Ω.

The electrodes can be attached either in a *unipolar* or *bipolar* mode. In the unipolar mode, one active electrode is attached over the belly of the muscle to obtain the largest signal possible from the greatest number of motor units. The reference and ground electrodes are placed on nearby bony parts with minimal electrical activity. In the bipolar mode, the two active electrodes are placed over different areas of the muscle to obtain a differential reading, with the ground again placed on a bony part. The unipolar mode is best suited for industrial applications, in which overall muscle force is being estimated, while the bipolar mode is used for muscular dysfunction in clinical applications.

Next, the electrodes should be inserted into a small portable preamplifier worn on the subject as close as possible to the measuring site. By reducing the length of the electrode leads it is possible to minimize noise received from the *antenna effect* and to minimize motion artifacts. Amplification of the desired signal close to the origin also reduces the effects of any electrical noise added later in the circuitry. The preamplifier should have a high input impedance, up to 100 M or at least 100 times the electrode impedance. The preamplifier should also contain a fuse or some other circuitry to limit faulty circuits.

The preamplified signal is next sent to an amplifier for further amplification (preferably variably controlled) and preprocessing. The amplifier should have a high *common-mode signal-to-noise rejection ratio* of at least 80 to 90 dB. This serves to reduce input lead capacitance differences and electrical noise from 60 Hz line current or other electrical instruments or machines in the vicinity. The amplifier should have wide, preferably adjustable, *bandwidth*, on the order of 10 to 1000 Hz and an adjustable notch filter (or two) to reduce noise at critical frequencies, such as 60 Hz. The amplifier output levels should be in the range of the ±5 V expected for A/D converters on computers.

Foulke et al. (1981) developed one such EMG measuring system for industrial use that meets the above criteria. It uses a commercially available but slightly modified AC voltmeter to provide both instantaneous raw outputs compatible with computer input as well as an RMS (root-mean-square) signal processor (discussed in Section 7.5.2). The system has been successfully used in several industrial studies of hand-intensive work potentially leading to WRMSDs (Armstrong et al., 1982; Freivalds, 1990; Park et al., 1991). Further details on surface EMG and EMG instrumentation can be found in Basmajian and De Luca (1985), Cram et al. (1988), NIOSH (1990), DeLuca (1997), and Chaffin et al. (1999).

7.5.2   EMG Analysis

The raw EMG signal can be analyzed in one of four different approaches based on the variables analyzed and the complexity of the analysis: EMG amplitude, EMG frequency, EMG-force relationships, and amplitude probability distributions. The simplest and most straightforward analysis is to process the raw signal through an EMG system, similar to that described in Section 7.5.1, and obtain an *RMS signal* defined as extracting the square root of the mean of the function squared:

$$\text{EMG}_{\text{RMS}} = \left\{ \frac{1}{T} \int_0^T v^2(t)\,dt \right\}^{1/2} \tag{7.9}$$

where $v(t)$ = raw voltage signal and T = time period for the periodic signal.

In practice, many amplifiers or processors may not produce an exact RMS value, but will produce a *smoothed-rectified signal* close in value. Note that rectification, or creating positive values from negative values, is comparable to squaring the function and then taking the square root. Smoothing through a resistor-capacitor (RC) circuit with a time constant of

$$\tau = \frac{1}{RC} \tag{7.10}$$

is comparable to integration. Note also that the term *integrated EMG* applies to EMG values obtained by charging a capacitor (Bigland and Lippold, 1954). It does not correspond to the smooth-rectified or RMS EMG, which rises or falls, depending on the raw signal, as opposed to the integrated EMG, which would continually rise until the capacitor is discharged.

As would be expected from the general description of EMG at the beginning of Section 7.5, the relationship of EMG_{RMS} to muscle force is monotonically increasing and provides the basis for estimating muscle tension during an activity. This relationship was first observed by Lippold (1952) and characterized as a direct linear relationship (Bigland and Lippold, 1954). Later, more detailed analyses led to observations of a nonlinear upward trend (Nightingale, 1960; Zuniga and Simmons, 1969), while others claimed a nonlinear downward trend (Milner-Brown et al., 1973; Kosarov and Gydikov, 1976).

Figure 7.15 may explain the controversy. There are two simultaneous events occurring during force production. Initially as a motor unit is recruited, successive twitches increase the force rapidly as the firing rate also increases rapidly. With more action potentials the contribution to the amplitude of the EMG signal increases, yielding an upward slope (slope 1 in Figure 7.15). Near tetanic frequency, the force levels off at the maximum tension level for the motor unit, and the firing frequency, although still increasing, becomes cyclical, at which point the RMS value changes little and the contribution to the EMG amplitude decreases with a shallower slope (slope 2 in Figure 7.15). This process is termed *rate coding* (Milner-Brown et al., 1973). Simultaneously, additional motor units are also recruited. However, based on the size principle, each additional motor unit is larger, producing more force, but is also recruited at a higher threshold, with higher frequency and larger muscle action potentials and contributing more to EMG amplitude (slopes 3 and 4 in Figure 7.15).

Complicating matters further is that electrode position on the muscle can also affect EMG (Zuniga et al., 1970) while, from Chapter 3, muscle size, length, and velocity affect force development. Therefore, most force prediction models (Cholewicki and McGill, 1994; Granata and Marras, 1995) take the general form of

$$F = g \times f_1 \times f_v \times EMG_{RMS} \tag{7.11}$$

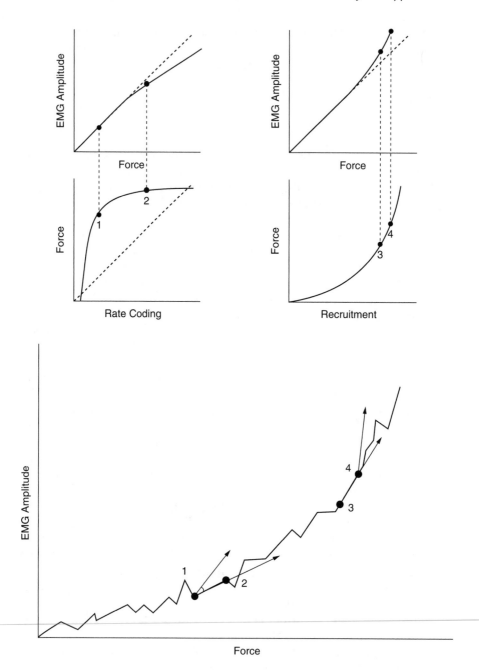

FIGURE 7.15
Theoretical basis for EMG amplitude-force relationship (see text for explanation).

where
F = predicted muscle force
g = gain factor for a given muscle, individual, etc.

f_l = scaling factor for muscle length
f_v = scaling factor for velocity of muscle contraction

The gain factor g is very critical and methods for determining it, especially for multiple-muscle systems, have been formulated (Cholewicki and McGill, 1994). Thus, in most cases, it is important to standardize the shape of the EMG amplitude–force relationship for a given individual, a given muscle, or a specific activity. Then this curve can be used to reasonably estimate the forces required to perform other more complex activities by that same person.

To compare across individuals or tasks, a frequently used practice is to normalize the EMG signal for each muscle or subject as follows:

$$\text{EMG}_{\text{Norm}} = \frac{\text{EMG}_i - \text{EMG}_{\text{Min}}}{\text{EMG}_{\text{Max}} - \text{EMG}_{\text{Min}}} \qquad (7.12)$$

where
EMG_i = EMG signal at time i
EMG_{Min} = minimum EMG signal, typically taken at rest
EMG_{Max} = maximum EMG signal obtained from that muscle

Normalization allows EMG values to be compared across a variety of conditions. For example, electrode placement could vary from muscle to muscle, day to day, or individual to individual. Normalization then allows data to be compared as relative values across muscles, days, individuals, or other factors of interest. However, one needs to be careful in using this technique on dynamic exertions, which could lead to large errors, if the normalization is performed at an arbitrary muscle or joint position. Instead, any normalization of an EMG signal taken at a given joint angle must be normalized with minimum and maximum EMG signals taken at the same joint angle (Mirka, 1991).

Note that, as a muscle fatigues, individual motor units may reduce the level of force production or even completely drop out, even though the motoneuron is still firing and muscle action potentials are still being created. As the result, for a given level of force production, EMG amplitude increases (Lippold et al., 1961) and the EMG amplitude–force relationship shown in Figure 7.15 shifts upward. If EMG amplitude is found to increase over the course of a working shift for the same activity, then one could surmise that muscle fatigue is occurring. From Chapter 3, it would be expected that muscle fatigue would occur once static muscle forces exceeded 15% of maximum voluntary contraction (MVC), i.e., the point at which the blood flow to the muscle starts being occluded, reducing the amount of oxygen supplied to the working muscle.

In addition, during fatigue, as motor units drop out, the frequency characteristics of the EMG signal will also change, leading to the second type of EMG analysis. As discussed in Chapter 3, the larger motor units are higher frequency, faster twitch, and more fatigable, while the smaller motor units are lower frequency, slower twitch, and more fatigue resistant. Thus, there

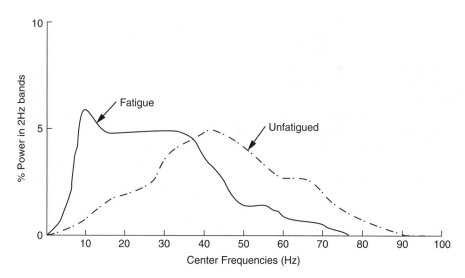

FIGURE 7.16
Average EMG power spectrum with reference to fatigue. (Adapted from Chaffin, 1973.)

is a tendency for the fast fatigable motor units to drop out first, leaving behind the slower, more fatigue-resistant motor units in the active pool. Consequently, there is a drop in the frequency characteristics of the EMG signal or a downward shift in the mean power of the signal that serves as a clear measure of the occurrence of muscle fatigue (Figure 7.16) (Chaffin, 1969, 1973). Again, the frequency characteristics vary with many of the same factors that affect EMG amplitude but, with careful control, *frequency analysis* can be a useful tool for biomechanical studies (Herberts et al., 1980; Hagberg, 1981; Hansson et al., 1992). Typically, the raw EMG is filtered appropriately, digitally sampled (twice as fast as the highest frequency of interest), and processed with a fast Fourier transform to produce a *power spectrum* (IEEE, 1967; Bergland, 1969). As an alternative to software analysis, there are also a variety of commercially available spectrum analyzers.

The shape of the EMG amplitude–force curve is the basis for the third type of EMG analysis. deVries (1968) postulated that the functional state of muscle may be better assessed by examining the slope of the EMG amplitude–force curve, termed the *efficiency of electrical activity*, rather than assessing muscle strength alone, which may be influenced by psychological factors such as motivation. deVries (1968) found that the slope decreased with improved muscle function for athletes and increased with disuse atrophy. Whereas deVries (1968) only considered linear slopes, Chaffin et al. (1980) expanded the concept to the more common nonlinear formulation and used a two-part piecewise linear regression to model the Type I and Type II motor units (Figure 7.17). This type of EMG analysis was then found to be successful in correctly identifying 21 of 22 individuals who were either "faking" or providing sincere muscular exertions and in significantly ($r^2 = 0.6$, $p < 0.001$) predicting their true MVC.

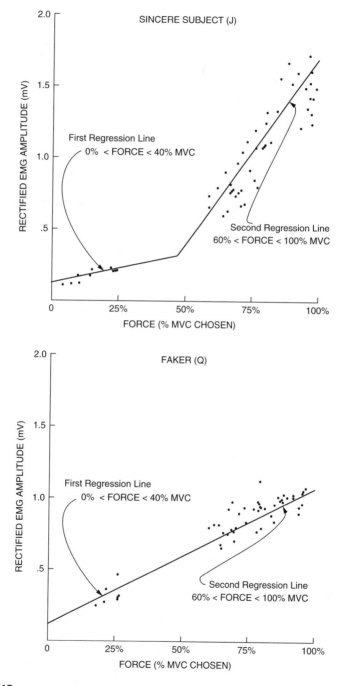

FIGURE 7.17
Piecewise regression analysis of EMG amplitude-force relationship. (From Chaffin, D.B. et al., 1980. *Medicine and Science in Sports and Exercise*, 12:205–211. With permission.)

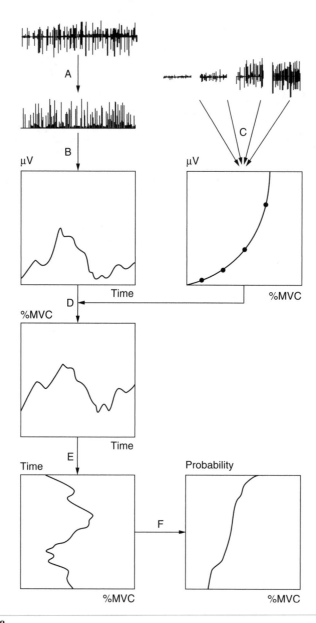

FIGURE 7.18
Formation of the amplitude distribution function (see text for details). (From Jonsson, B., 1978. *Scandinavian Journal of Rehabilitation Medicine*, 10(Suppl. 6):69–74. With permission.)

The fourth type of EMG analysis, developed by Jonsson (1978), is the most involved in that it combines several of the above techniques into one measure. The smooth-rectified EMG signal from a manual task over a given time period (Figure 7.18, steps A, B, D) is compared to a previously developed individual-specific EMG amplitude–force curve (step C) to produce a force

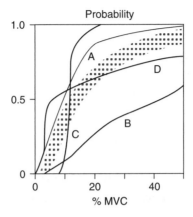

FIGURE 7.19

Application of the amplitude distribution function to manual tasks (see text for details). (From Jonsson, B., 1978. *Scandinavian Journal of Rehabilitation Medicine*, 10(Suppl. 6):69–74. With permission.)

over time curve (step E). The resulting force data are then sorted by amplitude in ascending order to produce a cumulative probability distribution termed the amplitude distribution function (step F). Figure 7.19 depicts the resulting amplitude distribution function when applied to a variety of manual tasks in comparison to recommended exertion levels (shaded arc). Task A depicts an acceptably low muscular load on the trapezius muscle when using a light tool. Tasks B, C, and D all place excessively high muscular loading, Task C at the static loading level (roughly 8 to 10% MVC), Task D at the peak levels, while Task B, throughout the full range of exertion.

This technique has since been used by a several other researchers (Hagberg, 1979; Linderhed, 1993) but, perhaps, has been less popular because of its complexity and extreme limits. The static loading recommended by Jonsson (1978) of 2 to 5% MVC is much lower than the Rohmert (1960) 15% MVC level discussed in Chapter 3 and could be difficult to achieve in many industries. Further details on EMG analyses can be obtained from Desmedt (1973), NIOSH (1990), and Kumar and Mital (1996).

Questions

1. What are the characteristics needed for a "good" measurement system?
2. Compare and contrast common motion measurement systems.
3. What are crosstalk, zero drift, and hysteresis?
4. Compare and contrast force distribution measurement systems.
5. Discuss the problem of force vs. pressure measurements found in many force distribution measurement systems. How may a force-sensitive sensor be improved in this regard?

6. What is the conceptual explanation for changes in nerve conduction found in many WRMSDs?

7. Describe the equipment and procedures used in nerve conduction velocity measurement.

8. What is the difference between orthodromic and antidromic stimulation? When would each be used?

9. What is the difference between onset and peak latency? Which would be preferred and why?

10. What are some of the factors that may limit the validity and reliability of nerve conduction velocity measurements?

11. Describe the equipment and procedures used to record EMG.

12. How do common-mode rejection ratios, bandwidth, and filtering affect the EMG signal?

13. How may EMGs be used to estimate muscle force?

14. Compare and contrast RMS, smooth-rectified, and integrated EMG signals.

15. Why are EMG signals sometimes normalized?

16. What information does frequency analysis of an EMG signal provide?

17. What is efficiency of electrical activity? Why is the curve non-linear?

18. Explain the usefulness of distribution analysis for EMG signals.

Problems

1. Calculate the RMS value for a sinusoid with a peak-to-peak amplitude of 1 mV.

2. Calculate the normalized value for a 0.1 mV response in the signal of Problem 7.1.

References

AAEE, 1984. *Guidelines in Electrodiagnostic Medicine*, Rochester, MN: Professional Standard Committee, American Association of Electromyography and Electrodiagnosis.

Armstrong, T.J., 1994. *Cumulative Trauma Disorders of the Hand and Wrist: Ergonomic Guides*, Akron, OH: American Industrial Hygiene Association.

Armstrong, T.J., Foulke, J.A., Joseph, B.S., and Goldstein, S.A., 1982. Investigation of cumulative trauma disorders in a poultry processing plant, *American Industrial Hygiene Association Journal*, 43:103–116.

Atkinson, P.J., Newberry, W.N., Atkinson, T.S., and Haut, R.C., 1998. A method to increase the sensitive range of pressure sensitive film, *Journal of Biomechanics*, 31:855–859.

Bader, D.L. and Hawken, M.B., 1986. Pressure distribution under the ischium of normal subjects, *Journal of Biomedical Engineering*, 8:353–357.

Bader, D.L., Gwilliam, J., Newson, T., and Harris, J.D., 1984. Pressure mapping at the interface, *Care: Science and Practice*, 8:67–69.

Basmajian, J.V. and De Luca, C.J., 1985. *Muscles Alive: Their Functions Revealed by Electromyography*, 5th ed., Baltimore: Williams & Wilkins.

Baysal, A.I., Chang, C.W., and OH, S.J., 1993. Temperature effects on nerve conduction studies in patients with carpal tunnel syndrome, *Acta Neurologica Scandinavica*, 88:213–216.

Beebe, D.J., Denton, D.D., Radwin, R.G., and Webster, J.G., 1998. Silicon-based tactile sensor for finger-mounted applications, *IEEE Transactions on Biomedical Engineering*, 45:151–159.

Bergland, G.D., 1969. A guided tour of the fast Fourier transform, *IEEE Spectrum*, July:41–52.

Betts, R.P., Duckworth, T., Austin, I.G., Crocker, S.P., and Moore, S., 1980. Critical light reflection at a plastic/glass interface and its application to foot pressure measurements, *Journal of Medical Engineering and Technology*, 4:136–142.

Bigland, B. and Lippold, O.C.J., 1954. The relation between force, velocity, and integrated electrical activity in human muscles, *Journal of Physiology*, 123:214–224.

Bonebrake, A.R., Fernandez, J.E., Marley, R.J, Dahalan, J.B., and Kilmer, K.J., 1990. A treatment for carpal tunnel syndrome: evaluation of objective and subjective measures, *Journal of Manipulative and Physiological Therapeutics*, 13, 507–520.

Boone, D.C. and Azen, S.P., 1979. Normal range of motion in joints of male subjects, *Journal of Bone and Joint Surgery*, 61, 756–759.

Brand, R.A. and Crowninshield, R.D., 1981. Comment on criteria for patient evaluation tools, *Journal of Biomechanics*, 14:655.

Buchholz, B. and Wellman, H., 1997. Practical operation of a biaxial goniometer at the wrist joint, *Human Factors*, 39:119–129.

Burnham, R.S. and Steadward, R.D., 1994. Upper extremity peripheral nerve entrapments among wheelchair athletes, *Archives of Physical Medicine and Rehabilitation*, 75:519–524.

Carroll, G., 1987. Comparison of median and radial nerve sensory latencies in the electrophysiological diagnosis of carpal tunnel syndrome, *Electroencephalography and Clinical Neurophysiology*, 68:101–106.

Carvalho, A.A. and Radwin, R.G., 1996, New method for extending the range of conductive polymer sensors for contact force, *International Journal of Industrial Ergonomics*, 17:285–290.

Chaffin, D.B., 1969. Surface EMG frequency analysis as a diagnostic tool, *Journal of Occupational Medicine*, 11(3):109–115.

Chaffin, D.B., 1973. Localized muscle fatigue — definition and measurement, *Journal of Occupational Medicine*, 15(4):346–354.

Chaffin, D.B., Lee, M., and Freivalds, A., 1980. Muscle strength assessment from EMG analysis, *Medicine and Science in Sports and Exercise*, 12:205–211.

Chaffin, D.B., Andersson, G.B.J., and Martin, B.J., 1999. *Occupational Biomechanics*, 3rd ed., New York: John Wiley & Sons.

Chodoroff, G., Tashjian, E., and Ellenberg, M., 1985. Orthodromic vs antidromic sensory nerve latencies in healthy persons, *Archives of Physical Medicine and Rehabilitation*, 66:589–591.

Cholewicki, J. and McGill, S.M., 1994. EMG assisted optimization: a hybrid approach for estimating muscle forces in an indeterminate biomechanical model, *Journal of Biomechanics*, 27:1287–1289.

Cram, J.R., Kasman, G.S., and Holtz, J., 1988. *Introduction to Surface Electromyography*, Gaithersburg, MD: Aspen Publishers.

DeLuca, C.J., 1997. The use of surface electromyography in biomechanics, *Journal of Applied Biomechanics*, 13:135–163.

Desmedt, J.E., Ed., 1973. *New Development in Electromyography and Clinical Neurophysiology*, Basel, Switzerland: Karger.

deVries, H.A., 1968. Efficiency of electrical activity as a physiological measure of the functional state of muscle tissue, *American Journal of Physical Medicine*, 47:10–22.

DiBenedetto, M., Mitz, M., Klingbeil, G., and Davidoff, D.D., 1986. New criteria for sensory nerve conduction especially useful in diagnosing carpal tunnel syndrome, *Archives of Physical Medicine and Rehabilitation*, 67:586–589.

Dillon, J., 1981. The role of ergonomics in the development of performance tests for furniture, *Applied Ergonomics*, 12:169–175.

Drummond, D.S., Narechania, R.G., Rosenthal, A.N., Breed, A.L., Lange, T.A., and Drummond, D.K., 1982. A study of pressure distributions measured during balanced and unbalanced sitting, *Journal of Bone and Joint Surgery*, 64A:1034–1039.

Dumitru, D. and Walsh, N., 1988. Practical instrumentation and common sources of error, *American Journal of Physical Medicine and Rehabilitation*, 67:55–65.

Elftman, H., 1934. A cinematic study of the distribution of pressure in the human foot, *Anatomical Record*, 59:481–487.

Fellows, G.L. and Freivalds, A., 1989. The use of force sensing resistors in ergonomic tool design, *Proceedings of the Human Factors Society*, 33:713–717.

Fellows, G.L. and Freivalds, A., 1991. Ergonomic evaluation of a foam rubber grip for tool handles, *Applied Ergonomics*, 22:225–230.

Felsenthal, G. and Spindler, H., 1979. Palmer conduction time of median and ulnar nerves of normal subjects and patients with carpal tunnel syndrome, *American Journal of Physical Medicine and Rehabilitation*, 58:131–138.

Fenety, P.A., MacLeod, D., and Crouse, J., 1994. Use of a pressure mat to continuously measure seated postural shifts, *Proceedings of the 12th Triennial Congress of the International Ergonomics Association*, Vol. 2, Mississauga, Ontario, Canada: Human Factors Association of Canada, 92–94.

Fenety, P.A., Putnam, C., and Walker, J.M., 2000. In-chair movement: validity, reliability and implications for measuring sitting discomfort, *Applied Ergonomics*, 31:383–393.

Ferguson-Pell, M. and Cardi, M.D., 1991. Evaluation of three advanced pressure mapping systems for clinical applications in seating and positioning, *Annals of Biomedical Engineering*, 19:643.

Ferguson-Pell, M. and Cardi, M.D., 1993. Prototype development and comparative evaluation of wheelchair mapping system, *Assistive Technology*, 5:788–791.

Foulke, J.A., Goldstein, S.A., and Armstrong, T.J., 1981. An EMG preamplifier system for biomechanical studies, *Journal of Biomechanics*, 14:437–438.

Franks, C.I., Betts, R.P., and Duckworth, T., 1983. Microprocessor-based image processing system for dynamic foot pressure studies, *Medical & Biological Engineering & Computing*, 21:566–572.

Freivalds, A., 1990. Pinching forces sustained during lens polishing operations, *International Journal of Industrial Ergonomics*, 6:261–266.

Garber, S.L., Krouskop, T.A., and Carter, R.E., 1978. A system for clinically evaluating wheelchair pressure-relief cushions, *American Journal of Occupational Therapy*, 32:565–570.

Ghavanini, M.R. and Haghighat, M., 1998. Carpal tunnel syndrome: reappraisal of five clinical tests, *Electromyography and Clinical Neurophysiology*, 38:437–441.

Granata, K.P. and Marras, W.S., 1995. An EMG-assisted model of trunk loading during free-dynamic lifting, *Journal of Biomechanics*, 28:1309–1317.

Gross, C.M., Goonetilleke, R.S., Menon, K.K., Banaag, J.C.N., and Nair, C.N., 1994. The biomechanical assessment and prediction of seat comfort, in Lueder, R. and Noro, K., Eds., *Hard Facts about Soft Machines: The Ergonomics of Seating*, London: Taylor & Francis, 231–253.

Gyi, D.E., Porter, M., and Robertson, N.K.B., 1998. Seat pressure measurement technologies: considerations for their evaluation, *Applied Ergonomics*, 27:85–91.

Hagberg, M., 1979. The amplitude distribution of surface EMG in static and intermittent static muscular performance, *European Journal of Applied Physiology*, 40:265–272.

Hagberg, M, 1981. Work load and fatigue in repetitive arm elevation, *Ergonomics*, 24:543–555.

Hagberg, M., Silverstein, B., Wells, R., Smith, M.J., Hendrick, H.W., Carayon, P., and Perusse, M., 1995. *Work-Related Musculoskeletal Disorders, WMSDs: A Reference Book for Prevention*, London: Taylor & Francis.

Halar, E.M., DeLisa, J.A., and Soine, T.L., 1983. Nerve conduction studies in upper extremities: skin temperature corrections, *Archives of Physical Medicine and Rehabilitation*, 64:412–416.

Hale, J.E. and Brown, T.D., 1992. Contact stress gradient detection limits of pressensor film, *Journal of Biomechanical Engineering, Transactions of the ASME*, 114:352–357.

Hansson, G.A., Strömberg, U., Larsson, B., Ohlsson, K., Balogh, I., and Moritz, U., 1992. Electromyographic fatigue in neck/shoulder muscles and endurance in women with repetitive work, *Ergonomics*, 35:1341–1352.

Hansson, G.A., Balogh, I., Ohlsson, K., Rylander, L., and Skerfving, S., 1996. Goniometer measurement and computer analysis of wrist angles and movements applied to occupational repetitive work, *Journal of Electromyography and Kinesiology*, 6:23–35.

Hara, T., Horii, E., An, K.N., Cooney, W.P., Linscheid, R.L., and Chao, E.Y., 1992. Force distribution across wrist joint: application of pressure sensitive conductive rubber, *Journal of Hand Surgery*, 17:339–347.

Harada, K., Watanabe, M., Ohkura, K., and Enomoto, S., 2000. Measure of bite force and occlusal contact area before and after bilateral split ramus osteotomy of the mandible using a new pressure-sensitive device: a preliminary report, *Journal of Oral Maxillofacial Surgery*, 58:370–373.

Haut, R., 1989. Contact pressures in the patello-femoral joint during impact loading on the human flexed knee, *Journal of Orthopaedic Research*, 7:272–280.

Herberts, P., Kadefors, R., and Broman, H., 1980. Arm positioning in manual tasks: a electromyographic study of localized muscle fatigue, *Ergonomics*, 23:655–665.

Hertzberg, H.T.E., 1972. *The Human Buttocks in Sitting: Pressures, Patterns, and Palliatives,* SAE Technical Paper 720005, Warrendale, PA: Society of Automotive Engineers.

Houle, R.J., 1969. Evaluation of seat devices designed to prevent ischemic ulcers in paraplegic patients, *Archives of Physical Medicine and Rehabilitation,* 50:587–594.

IEEE, 1967. Special issue on fast Fourier transform and its application to digital filtering and spectral analysis, *IEEE Transactions on Audio and Electroacoustics,* AU-15:1–117.

Jackson, D.A. and Clifford, J.C., 1989. Electrodiagnosis of mild carpal tunnel syndrome, *Archives of Physical Medicine and Rehabilitation,* 70:199–204.

Jang, H., 2002. The Effects of Dynamic Wrist Workloads on Risks of Carpal Tunnel Syndrome, Ph.D. dissertation, University Park, PA: Pennsylvania State University.

Jensen, T.R., Radwin, R.G., and Webster, J.G., 1991. A conductive polymer sensor for measuring external finger forces, *Journal of Biomechanics,* 24:851–858.

Johnson, E.W. and Melvin, J.L., 1967. Sensory conduction studies of median and ulnar nerves, *Archives of Physical Medicine and Rehabilitation,* 48:25–30.

Johnson, E.W. and Olsen. K.J., 1960. Clinical value of motor nerve conduction velocity determination, *Journal of the American Medical Association,* 172:2030–2035.

Johnson, E.W. and Terebuh, B.M., 1997. Sensory and mixed nerve conduction studies in carpal tunnel syndrome, *Physical Medicine and Rehabilitation Clinics of North America,* 8:477–501.

Johnson, E.W., Wells, R.M., and Duran, R.J., 1962. Diagnosis of carpal tunnel syndrome, *Archives of Physical Medicine and Rehabilitation,* 43:414–419.

Johnson, E.W., Kukla, R., and Wongsam P., 1981. Sensory latencies to the ring finger: normal values and relation to carpal tunnel syndrome, *Archives of Physical Medicine and Rehabilitation,* 62:206–208.

Johnson, E.W., Sipski, M., and Lammertse, T., 1987. Median and radial sensory latencies to digit I: normal values and usefulness in carpal tunnel syndrome, *Archives of Physical Medicine and Rehabilitation,* 68:140–141.

Jonsson, B., 1978. Quantitative electromyographic evaluation of muscular load during work, *Scandinavian Journal of Rehabilitation Medicine,* 10(Suppl. 6):69–74.

Jürgens, H.W., 1969. Die Verteilung des Körperdrucks auf Sitzfläche und Rückenlehne als Problem der Industrieanthropologie, [Distribution of body weight on the seat pan and seat back as an ergonomics problem], *Ergonomics,* 12:198–205.

Kadaba, M.P., Ferguson-Pell, M.W., Palmieri, V.R., and Cochran, G.V.B., 1984. Ultrasound mapping of the buttock-cushion interface contour, *Archives of Physical Medicine and Rehabilitation,* 65:467–469.

Kembel, F., 1968. Electrodiagnosis of the carpal tunnel syndrome, *Journal of Neurology, Neurosurgery and Psychiatry,* 31:23–27.

Kimura, J., 1979. The carpal tunnel syndrome — localization of conduction abnormalities within the distal segment of the median nerve, *Brain,* 102:619–635.

Kimura, J., 1989. *Electrodiagnosis in Diseases of Nerve and Muscle: Principles and Practice,* 2nd ed., Philadelphia: Davis.

Kimura, J. and Ayyar, D.R., 1985. The carpal tunnel syndrome: electrophysiological aspects of 639 symptomatic extremities, *Electroencephalography and Clinical Neurophysiology,* 25:151–164.

Konrath, G.A., Hamel, A.J., Guerin, J., Olson, S.A., Bay, B., and Sharkey, N.A., 1999. Biomechanical evaluation of impaction fractures of the femoral head, *Journal of Orthopaedic Trauma,* 13:407–413.

Kosarov, D. and Gydikov, A., 1976. Dependence of the discharge frequency of motor units in different human muscles upon the level of the isometric muscle tension, *EMG Clinical Neurophysiology*, 16:293–306.

Krouskop, T.A., Williams, R., Krebs, M., Herszkowicz, I., and Garber, S., 1985. Effectiveness of mattress overlays in reducing interface pressures during recumbency, *Journal of Rehabilitation Research and Development*, 22:7–10.

Kumar, S. and Mital, A., 1996. *Electromyography in Ergonomics*, London: Taylor & Francis.

Lee, H.J., DeLisa, J.A., and Bach, J.R., 1993. The effect of temperature on antidromic median sensory conduction, *Electromyography and Clinical Neurophysiology*, 33:125–128.

Letz, R. and Gerr, F., 1994. Covariates of human peripheral nerve function: nerve conduction velocity and amplitude, *Neurotoxicology and Teratology*, 16:95–104.

Lindan, O., Greenway, R.M., and Piazza, J.M., 1965. Pressure distribution on the surface of the human body: I. Evaluation in lying and sitting positions using a "bed of springs and nails," *Archives of Physical Medicine*, 46:378–385.

Linderhed, H., 1993. A new dimension to amplitude analysis of EMG, *International Journal of Ergonomics*, 11:243–247.

Lippold, O.C.J., 1952. The relation between integrated action potentials in a human muscle and its isometric contraction, *Journal of Physiology*, 117:492–499.

Lippold, O.C.J., Redfearn, J.W.T., and Vuo, J., 1961. The electromyography of fatigue, *Ergonomics*, 4:121–131.

Logan, S.E. and Groszewski, P., 1989. Dynamic wrist motion analysis using six degree of freedom sensors, *Biomedical Sciences Instrumentation*, 25:213–220.

Lowe, B.D and Freivalds, A., 1997. Analyses of glove types and pinch forces in windshield glass handling, in B. Das, Ed., *Advances in Occupational Ergonomics and Safety*, Amsterdam: IOS Press, 477–480.

MacDonell, R.A., Schwartz, M.S., and Swash, M., 1990. Carpal tunnel syndrome — which finger should be tested? An analysis of sensory conduction in digital branches of the median nerve, *Muscle and Nerve*, 13:601–606.

Mann, R., Yeong, E.K., Moore, M.L., and Engrav, LH., 1997. A new tool to measure pressure under burn garments, *Journal of Burn Care & Rehabilitation*, 18:160–163.

Marklin, R. W. and Monroe, J.F., 1998. Quantitative biomechanical analysis of wrist motion in bone trimming jobs in the meat packing industry, *Ergonomics*, 41:227–237.

Marras, W.S. and Schoenmarklin, R.W., 1993. Wrist motions in industry, *Ergonomics*, 36:341–351.

Marshall, M.M., Mozrall, J.R., and Shealy, J.E., 1999. The effects of complex wrist and forearm posture on wrist range of motion, *Human Factors*, 41:205–213.

Mayo-Smith, W. and Cochran, G.V.B., 1981. Wheelchair cushion modification: device for locating high-pressure regions, *Archives of Physical Medicine and Rehabilitation*, 62:135–136.

Melvin, J.L., Schuchmann, J.A., and Lanese, R.R., 1973. Diagnostic specificity of motor and sensory nerve conduction variables in the carpal tunnel syndrome, *Archives of Physical Medicine and Rehabilitation*, 54:69–74.

Milner-Brown, H.S., Stein, R.B., and Yemm, R., 1973. Changes in firing rate of human motor units during linearly changing voluntary contractions, *Journal of Physiology*, 230:371–390.

Mirka, G.A., 1991. The quantification of EMG normalization error, *Ergonomics*, 34:343–352.

Mooney, V., Einbund, M.J., Rogers, J.E., and Stauffer, E.S., 1971. Comparison of pressure distribution qualities in seat cushions, *Bulletin of Prosthetic Research*, 10–15:129–143.

Moore, A., Wells, R., and Ranney, D., 1991. Quantifying exposure in occupational manual tasks with cumulative trauma disorder potential, *Ergonomics*, 34:1433–1453.

Moore, J.S., 1992. Carpal tunnel syndrome, *Occupational Medicine: State of the Art Reviews*, 7:741–763.

Nathan, P.A., Meadows, K.D., and Doyle, L.S., 1988. Relationship of age and sex to sensory conduction of the median nerve at the carpal tunnel and association of slowed conduction with symptoms, *Muscle and Nerve*, 11:1149–1153.

Nathan, P.A., Keniston, R.C., Myers, L.D., and Meadows, K.D., 1992. Longitudinal study of median nerve sensory conduction in industry — relationship to age, gender, hand dominance, occupational hand use and clinical diagnosis, *Journal of Hand Surgery*, 17A:850–857.

Nicole, A.C., 1987. A flexible electrogoniometer with wide spread applications, in Jonsson, B., Ed., *International Series on Biomechanics: Biomechanics X*, Champaign, IL: Human Kinematics, 1029–1033.

Nightingale, A., 1960. Relationship between muscle force and EMG in stand-at-ease position, *Annals of Physical Medicine*, 5:187–191.

NIOSH, 1990. Surface Electromyography Procedures Manual for Use in the Industrial Setting, Morgantown, WV: National Institute for Occupational Safety and Health.

Ojima, H., Miyake, S., Kumashiro, M, Togami, H., and Suzeki, K., 1991. Dynamic analysis of wrist circumduction: a new application of the biaxial flexible electrogoniometer, *Clinical Biomechanics*, 6:221–229.

Park, D., Yun, M.H., and Freivalds, A., 1991. Knife replacement studies at an automobile carpet manufacturing plant, in *Proceedings of the Human Factors Society, 35th Annual Meeting*, Santa Monica, CA: The Human Factors and Ergonomics Society, 848–852.

Park, S.K., 1999. The Development of an Exposure Measurement System for Assessing Risk of Work-Related Musculoskeletal Disorders, Ph.D. thesis, University Park, PA: Pennsylvania State University.

Rawes, M.L., Richardson, J.B., and Dias, J.J., 1996. A new technique for the assessment of wrist movement using a biaxial flexible electrogoniometer, *Journal of Hand Surgery*, 21:600–603.

Robinson, L.R., Rubner, D.E., Wahl, P.W., Fujimoto, W.Y., and Stolov, W.C., 1993. Influences of height and gender on normal nerve conduction studies, *Archives of Physical Medicine and Rehabilitation*, 74:1134–1138.

Rohmert, W., 1960. Ermittlung von Erholungspausen für Statische Arbeit des Menschen [Determination of recovery times for human static work], *Internationale Zeitschrift für angewandte Physiologie einschliesslich Arbeitsphysiologie*, 18:123–164.

Rosenfalck, A., 1978. Early recognition of nerve disorders by near-nerve recording of sensory action potentials, *Muscle and Nerve*, 1:360–367.

Schoenmarklin, R.W. and Marras, W.S., 1993. Dynamic capabilities of the wrist joint in industrial workers, *International Journal of Industrial Ergonomics*, 11:207–224.

Serina, E.R., Tal, R., and Rempel, D., 1999. Wrist and forearm postures and motions during typing, *Ergonomics*, 42:938–951.

Shields, R.K. and Cook, T.M., 1988. Effect of seat angle and lumbar support on seat buttock pressure, *Physical Therapy*, 68:1682–1686.

Simpson, J.A., 1956. Electrical signs in the diagnosis of carpal tunnel and related syndromes, *Journal of Neurology, Neurosurgery and Psychiatry,* 19:275–280.

Sissons, H.A., 1979. Diseases of joints, tendon sheaths, bursae and other soft tissues, in Symmers, W.S., Ed., *Systemic Pathology,* 2nd ed., Vol. 5, New York: Churchill Livingston, 2492–2493.

Smutz, P., Serina, E., and Rempel, D., 1994. A system for evaluating the effects of keyboard design on force, posture, comfort and productivity, *Ergonomics,* 37:1649–1660.

Sorab, J., Allen, R.H., and Gonik, B., 1988. Tactile sensory monitoring of clinician-applied forces during delivery of newborns, *IEEE Transactions of Biomedical Engineering,* 35:1090–1093.

Spielholz, P., 1998. Development of an electrogoniometer calibration procedure for measurement of wrist angle and forearm rotation, in Kumar, S., Ed., *Advances in Occupational Ergonomics and Safety,* 499–502.

Stetson, D.S., Albers, J.W., Silverstein, B.A., and Wolfe, R.A., 1992. Effects of age sex and anthropometric factors on nerve conduction measures, *Muscle and Nerve,* 15:1095–1104.

Stevens, J.C., 1987. The electrodiagnosis of carpal tunnel syndrome, *Muscle and Nerve,* 10:99–113.

Sunderland, S., 1976. The nerve lesion in the carpal tunnel syndrome, *Journal of Neural Neurosurgery and Psychiatry,* 39:615–626.

Swearingen, J.J., Wheelwright, C.D., and Garner, J.D., 1962. An Analysis of Sitting Areas and Pressures of Man, Rep. 62-1, Oklahoma City, OK: U.S. Civil Aero-Medical Research Institute.

Tanaka, S. and McGlothlin, J.D., 1993. A conceptual quantitative model for prevention of work-related CTS, *International Journal of Industrial Ergonomics,* 11:181–193.

Tashjian, E.A., Ellenberg, M.R., Gross, N., Chodoroff, G., and Honet, J.C., 1987. Temperature effect on antidromic and orthodromic sensory nerve action potential latency and amplitude, *Archives of Physical Medicine and Rehabilitation,* 68:549–552.

Thomas, P.K., 1960. Motor nerve conduction in the carpal tunnel syndrome, *Neurology,* 10:1045–1050.

Trandel, R.S., Lewis, D.W., and Verhonick, P.J., 1975. Thermographical investigation of decubitus ulcers, *Bulletin of Prosthetic Research,* 10–24:137–155.

Treaster, D.E. and Marras, W.S., 1987. Measurement of seat pressure distributions, *Human Factors,* 29:563–575.

Webb Associates, 1978. Anthropometric Source Book: Vol. I; Anthropometry for Designers, NASA Reference Publication 1024.

Werner, R.A. and Armstrong, T.J., 1997. Carpal tunnel syndrome: ergonomic risk factors and intracarpal canal pressures, in Johnson, E.W., Ed., *Carpal Tunnel Syndrome,* Philadelphia: W.B. Saunders.

Woodburn, J. and Helliwell, P., 1997. Observations on the F-scan in-shoe pressure measuring system, *Clinical Biomechanics,* 12:S16.

Yun, M.H., 1994. A Hand Posture Measurement Systems for the Analysis of Manual Tool Handling Tasks, Ph.D. dissertation, University Park, PA: Pennsylvania State University.

Yun, M.H., Donges, L., and Freivalds, A., 1992. Using force sensitive resistors to evaluate driver seating comfort, in Kumar, S., Ed., *Advances in Industrial Ergonomics and Safety IV,* London: Taylor & Francis, 403–410.

Yun, M.H., Cannon, D., Freivalds, A., and Thomas, G., 1997. An instrumented glove for grasp specification in virtual-reality based point-and-direct telerobotics, *IEEE Transactions on Systems, Man, and Cybernetics, Part B: Cybernetics*, 27:835–846.

Zuniga, E.N. and Simmons, D.G., 1969. Nonlinear relationship between averaged EMG potential and muscle tension in normal subjects, *Archives of Physical Medicine and Rehabilitation*, 50:613–620.

Zuniga, E.N., Truong, X.T., and Simons, D.G., 1970. Effects of skin electrode position of averaged electromyographic potentials, *Archives of Physical Medicine and Rehabilitation*, 51:264–272.

8

Job and Worksite Analysis

8.1 The Need for Job Analysis

Chapter 6 has presented data from epidemiological studies that identified WRMSD risk factors such as force, posture, repetition, etc. These risk factors were primarily identified through statistical analysis of musculoskeletal injury records, tracking of injuries back to specific jobs, and detailed surveys of workers. Such approaches collectively form a system of *passive surveillance* but may not provide necessary information in sufficient detail.

A more *active surveillance* approach utilizes job and worksite analysis by trained ergonomists and provides more detailed information on worker postures, forces produced during work, the number of repetitions performed during a shift, etc. that will assist the analyst in identifying specific occupational risk factors. Such an active approach may identify potential problems or stressful conditions before workers develop symptoms severe enough to require medical treatment, potentially saving the company medical costs and lost time and wages.

Such a job or worksite analysis involves a systematic evaluation of the tasks, the duties, the workplace, the tools, and the working conditions necessary to perform the job in a satisfactory manner and may include many of the measurements, techniques, and instruments described in Chapter 7. The results of such a structured approach should be a quantitative or semi-quantitative evaluation of the risks involved with the particular job, with perhaps even a final risk score. This approach then lends itself to job redesign by providing a seminumerical guide for the reduction of the overall risk score. A consequent reduction of WRMSD risk and potential decrease in injuries and medical costs are the anticipated final goals for such job and worksite analysis.

8.2   Reliability and Validity of Assessment Tools

8.2.1   Basic Concepts

Before any of the posture or task analyses and WRMSD risk assessment tools are to be used in either screening jobs or assigning workers to appropriate jobs, there arise concerns regarding the accuracy and precision of the observations, measurements, or analyses associated with these techniques and tools. An ergonomist would hope that these tools have characteristics of both *validity* and *reliability*.

Validity refers to the appropriateness, meaningfulness, and usefulness of a tool or survey to measure what it is supposed to measure. For example, a given WRMSD risk assessment tool is supposed to measure and quantify the actual risk that is incurred for a given individual while performing a given task in a given work environment. A valid assessment tool will allow the ergonomist to make useful inferences about an individual working on a given job. There can be different types of validity; the simplest is *face* or *content validity*. This refers to the content or format of the tool, which, on its face level, should measure what it is intended to measure. Thus, the content of any risk assessment survey or checklist should include basic questions on the amount of time worked, the number and types of motions involved, the force levels exerted, the types of tools or equipment handled, etc. Such content validity is typically determined by opinion or judgment such as by a panel of experts.

A second type of validity is *criterion* or *predictive validity* and refers to the relationship of scores obtained using the tool and actual WRMSD injuries incurred, which is the true criterion for considering a particular job risky. However, the whole purpose of these tools is to be able to predict or identify the risky jobs ahead of time before the actual injuries are incurred. Predictive validity can be determined by correlating model risk predictions with actual job injury rates. The third type of validity is *construct validity* and refers to physiological or psychological construct or characteristic being measured by the tool. It is most important in a basic theoretical research sense and perhaps less so to a practicing ergonomist in an industrial setting. Whereas the researcher might be interested in identifying all of the factors — force, frequency, posture, etc. — that lead to potential injuries, the industrial ergonomist may be interested only in identifying the risky jobs. Construct validity is more difficult to quantify, and researchers may spend many years adjusting and fine-tuning a prediction model.

Reliability refers to the consistency or stability of a measure, i.e., how consistent are the scores or values obtained by two different analysts on the same job, or how the scores vary over time, i.e., is learning occurring? The importance of a reliable tool is obvious; an ergonomist could not use a tool or questionnaire that gives an unreliable measure of job risk, because, then, any job redesigns or worker reassignments would be meaningless as they would not be based on the variables expected.

8.2.2 Reliability of Assessments

One can consider that any assessment consists of a true value superimposed with a random variable due to measurement errors. Because measurement errors are always present to some degree in research, it is important to be able to quantify the amount of variation or errors to be expected. The simplest measure of such variability is the *coefficient of variability* (CV) for a series of repeated measurements:

$$CV = s/\bar{x} \tag{8.1}$$

where s = standard deviation of the measurements and $\bar{x}$ = mean of the measurements. Typically, the CV should be less than 10%, with 5% even better.

More formal estimates of measurement errors are expressed as a *correlation* or *reliability coefficient*. For example, one common error component to be quantified is consistency over time, referred to as *test-retest reliability*. To assess this type of reliability, the same analysis is performed on the same jobs with a certain amount of intervening time. The two sets of scores are correlated using the standard *Pearson product moment correlation coefficient* (Currier, 1984):

$$r = \frac{\Sigma x_i y_i - \Sigma x_i \Sigma y_i/n}{\left[\Sigma x_i^2 - \left(\Sigma x_i\right)^2/n\right]^{1/2}\left[\Sigma y_i^2 - \left(\Sigma y_i\right)^2/n\right]^{1/2}} \tag{8.2}$$

where
x_i = scores from the first analysis
y_i = scores from the second analysis
n = number of jobs analyzed

The resulting correlation coefficient will range from 0 to ±1. A correlation coefficient of zero indicates no relationship between the two applications of the analysis and a very poor tool to be used for job analysis. A correlation coefficient of +1 indicates a perfect relationship and a very reliable analysis tool (very unlikely in real life). A score of –1 indicates a perfect inverse relationship. This would be very unlikely in these testing or analysis scenarios but could happen in a theoretical statistical sense between two unknown variables. Typically, for a tool to be reliable, the correlation coefficient should be roughly 0.9.

Typically, the longer the time interval between measurements, the lower the correlation coefficient and the lower the reliability. This would indicate that something has changed over time; perhaps the analyst has forgotten key aspects of using the tool, or perhaps more training is required, or perhaps the job or person being analyzed has changed. On the other hand, reliability is typically increased, if there are several similar questions examining a particular variable of interest, especially for those with psychosocial aspects and more subjective evaluations. Although no universally acceptable levels of reliability have been established, one appropriate scheme was suggested by Currier (1984). Values greater than 0.9 can be considered high reliability, values between 0.8 and 0.9 good reliability, values between 0.7 and 0.8 fair reliability, and values below 0.7 poor reliability.

For situations where it is impractical to administer the same test to the same individuals (e.g., when workers may become sensitized to questions regarding pain or psychosocial aspects), an alternative approach to test-retest reliability is the *split-half procedure*. Two halves of a survey are scored separately for each person and a correlation coefficient is calculated for the two sets of scores. The level of the correlation indicates the degree to which the two halves provide the same results and, thus, describes the internal consistency of the survey. The reliability coefficient for the full survey is computed using the *Spearman–Brown prophecy formula* (Fraenkel and Wallen, 1996), which for an exact split formulation is

$$r_{tot} = \frac{2r_{1/2}}{1 + r_{1/2}} \tag{8.3}$$

where r_{tot} = reliability for the full survey and $r_{1/2}$ = correlation coefficient for one half the survey. A relatively low correlation coefficient of 0.8 for one half the survey would result in an overall reliability coefficient of 0.889 for the full survey. This demonstrates an important principle of reliability. The reliability of a survey can be increased by increasing its length with additional items similar to the original items.

Three other statistical approaches can be used for internal consistency checks. Two are not, strictly speaking, statistical tests, but computational formulas for a test's reliability from Kuder–Richardson (1937), specifically their formulas 20 and 21:

$$r = \frac{n}{n-1} \times \left\{ 1 - \frac{\Sigma p (1-p)}{s^2} \right\} \tag{8.4}$$

$$r = \frac{n}{n-1} \times \left\{ 1 - \frac{\bar{x}(1-\bar{x}/n)}{s^2} \right\} \tag{8.5}$$

where
n = number of items on test
r = estimate of test's reliability
p = proportion passing a given item
s^2 = variance of test
$\bar{x}$ = mean score of test

Equation 8.4 (Kuder–Richardson formula 20) is the most robust estimate of a test's reliability but requires more complex summations of test takers' proportion of passing items. Equation 8.5 (Kuder–Richardson formula 21) is considerably simpler to calculate but uses a more conservative assumption that all test items have the same difficulty. Note that for surveys or WRMSD risk assessments, "passing" would constitute exceeding a certain critical threshold value for risk for a given item. For example, if the mean score on a WRMSD screening survey with 40 items is 30, with a variance of 10, the reliability would be

$$r = \frac{40}{39} \times \left\{ 1 - \frac{30\left(1 - 30/40\right)}{10} \right\} = 0.256 \tag{8.6}$$

This reliability score of 0.256 is quite low considering that a value of 0 indicates no relationship and a value of 1 indicates perfect correlation. Many commercially available achievement tests in education (not for predicting WRMSD) have reliability coefficients exceeding 0.9 on the Kuder–Richardson formulas. Even classroom tests may have reliability coefficients exceeding 0.7 (Fraenkel and Wallen, 1996). The overall conclusion for this sample WRMSD screening test is that it would be quite unreliable and provide little use in identifying critical jobs or individuals who might be susceptible to WRMSD.

A variation of Kuder–Richardson formula 20 (Equation 8.4) was developed by Cronbach (1951) and is termed *Cronbach's alpha*. Its primary application is for tests or screening surveys where scoring is not simply right or wrong and more than one answer may be possible. It is formulated as

$$\alpha = \frac{n}{n-1} \times \left\{ 1 - \frac{\Sigma s_i^2}{s_t^2} \right\} \tag{8.7}$$

where
s_i^2 = variance of item scores
s_t = variance of test scores
α = estimate of test's reliability

8.2.3 Reliability of Analysts

Another measure of the reliability and validity of an assessment is the amount of agreement between analysts. If the agreement between analysts is high, then there is a possibility, but not a guarantee, that the scoring reflects the measure or factor that it is meant to score. If their agreement is low, the usefulness of that assessment is very limited, because even the experts cannot agree what is being measured or scored. The simplest index of agreement is the overall proportion of agreement:

$$p_o = a + d \tag{8.8}$$

where
p_o = proportion of observations agreeing
a = proportion of observations in desired category agreeing
d = proportion of observations in opposite category agreeing

There may be several complicating factors in using proportions of observers agreeing. For one, one of the categories may be quite rare, so that either a or d will be very likely quite large and thus inflate the value of p_o. Also, some degree of agreement is to be expected by chance alone. With pure random guessing, with $a = b = c = d = 0.25$ (Table 8.1), Equation 8.8 yields a p_o of 0.5. Therefore, there needs to be a way of correcting for chance. This was accomplished by Cohen (1960) with the *kappa statistic* (κ) defined as

$$\kappa = \frac{p_o - p_e}{1 - p_e} \tag{8.9}$$

where
p_o = proportion of agreement observed
p_e = proportion of agreement expected by chance

For most purposes, values of kappa greater than 0.8 may be considered excellent agreement beyond chance, values between 0.6 and 0.8 substantial agreement, values between 0.4 and 0.6 moderate agreement, and values below 0.4 (even including possible negative values) poor agreement (Landis and Koch, 1977). Note that, although kappa is an improvement over simple proportionality of agreement, it works best with dichotomous data. Grouping of continuous data into categories for the convenience of the analyst is not valid. The principal weakness of kappa is that it measures the frequency of exact agreement rather than the degree of approximate agreement.

A weighted kappa (Cohen, 1968) was developed to address this problem. However, the weighted kappa has its own set of problems, in that it allows the weights to be of arbitrary magnitude, distorting the resulting statistic (Maclure and Willett, 1987). Standardizing the weights alleviates this problem and results in the weighted kappa becoming equivalent to Cronbach's alpha (Equation 8.7). Further information on interrater agreement can be found in Fleiss (1981). Note that the above discussion applies only to ordinal data or ranking. For continuous data measurements, as might be expected in a thorough exposure assessment tool, standard statistical approaches, such

TABLE 8.1

Wrist Posture Counts

	Analyst B	
Analyst A	Ulnar Deviation	Neutral Position
Ulnar deviation	34 ($a = 34/50$)	5 ($b = 5/50$)
Neutral position	1 ($c = 1/50$)	10 ($d = 10/50$)

as analysis of variance, are more appropriate. Even when continuous data are grouped into ordinal categories, serious errors can arise with the kappa statistic. Only time sample data should be used with the kappa statistic (Maclure and Willett, 1987).

Example 8.1: Measurement of the Amount of Agreement between Analysts

Consider a simple example of two analysts counting body postures, specifically whether the right wrist is in ulnar deviation (Table 8.1). The analysts examine videos of 50 workers on an electronic assembly job. Their evaluation of the 50 workers yields the following data, with a, b, c, and d being proportions of the various combinations of interrater agreement.

The overall proportion of agreement is

$$p_o = 34/50 + 10/50 = 0.88 \tag{8.10}$$

The proportion agreement by chance is calculated from the revised contingency table where the expected values are the products of the intersection of the respective column and row totals divided by the grand total, similar to Equation 6.10. The resultant expected values for agreement, by row, are 27.3, 11.7, 7.7, and 3.3, respectively. The overall proportion agreement by chance is then

$$p_o = 27.3/50 + 3.3/50 = 0.612 \tag{8.11}$$

Correcting for chance agreement, the kappa statistic yields

$$\kappa = \frac{p_o - p_e}{1 - p_e} = \frac{0.88 - 0.612}{1 - 0.612} = 0.691 \tag{8.12}$$

In either case, there is substantial agreement between analysts.

For continuous data, in which analysts give specific values of angle, force, or frequency, as opposed to categorical data, other methodologies need to be used. For two analysts, the two sets of scores can be simply correlated using the Pearson product moment correlation of Equation 8.2. For more than two analysts, *intraclass correlations* based on analysis of variance (ANOVA) of the data are utilized (Shrout and Fleiss, 1979). In a typical scenario *a* analysts evaluate *b* jobs. In Case 1 each job is evaluated by a different set of *a* analysts, randomly selected from a larger population of analysts. In Case 2, a random sample of *a* analysts is randomly selected from a larger population of analysts. Each analyst then evaluates the same jobs. A very specific Case 3 could also be considered, in which the *a* analysts are the only analysts of interest. However, typically, the results of any job analysis instrument would need to be generalized over a larger population of analysts and, therefore, Case 3 will not be considered.

Case 1 is analyzed as a one-way ANOVA yielding the intraclass correlation coefficient:

$$ICC_1 = \frac{MS_{job} - MSE}{MS_{job} + (a-1)MSE} \tag{8.13}$$

where
ICC_1 = intraclass correlation coefficient for Case 1
MS_{job} = between-jobs mean square
MSE = within-jobs mean square or mean square error
a = number of analysts

Case 2 is analyzed as a two-way ANOVA, yielding the intraclass correlation coefficient:

$$ICC_2 = \frac{MS_{job} - MSE}{MS_{job} + (a-1)MSE + a(MS_{analyst} - MSE)/b} \tag{8.14}$$

where
ICC_2 = intraclass correlation coefficient for Case 2
$MS_{analyst}$ = between-analyst mean square
b = number of jobs

ICC_2 will typically be smaller than ICC_3 because of the added random effects of analysts and generalizability to a larger population of analysts. Similarly, ICC_1 will typically be smaller than ICC_2 because of the added variability due to a larger pool of analysts. Example 8.2 may help clarify the ICCs between Case 1 and 2. More details on intraclass correlation coefficients and Case 3 can be obtained from Shrout and Fleiss (1979).

TABLE 8.2

Frequency of Wrist Deviations

Job No.	Analyst	Analyst	Analyst
1	2	5	8
2	1	3	2
3	4	6	8
4	1	2	6
5	5	6	9
6	2	4	7
7	6	8	12
8	3	5	8

Example 8.2: Calculation of Intraclass Correlation Coefficients

Consider the frequency of wrist deviations for eight different jobs shown in Table 8.2. For Case 1, consider each job scored by a different set of three analysts. A one-factor (jobs) ANOVA on wrist deviation frequencies yields

Source	Degrees of Freedom	Sum of Squares	Mean Squares	F-value	p-value
Job	7	91.96	13.14	2.22	0.088
Error	16	94.67	5.92		
Total	23	186.63			

The intraclass correlation coefficient for Case 1 from Equation 8.13 is

$$\text{ICC}_1 = \frac{\text{MS}_{job} - \text{MSE}}{\text{MS}_{job} + (a-1)\text{MSE}} = \frac{13.14 - 5.92}{13.14 + (2)5.92} = \frac{7.22}{24.98} = 0.29 \quad (8.15)$$

For Case 2, consider the same three analysts scoring all eight jobs. A two-factor (jobs and analysts) ANOVA on wrist deviation yields

Source	Degrees of Freedom	Sum of Squares	Mean Squares	F-value	p-value
Job	7	91.96	13.14	14.24	0.001
Analyst	2	81.75	40.88	44.30	0.001
Error	14	12.92	0.92		
Total	23	186.63			

The intraclass correlation coefficient for Case 2 from Equation 8.14 is

$$\text{ICC}_2 = \frac{\text{MS}_{job} - \text{MSE}}{\text{MS}_{job} + (a-1)\text{MSE} + a(\text{MS}_{analyst} - \text{MSE})/b} \quad (8.16)$$

$$= \frac{13.14 - 0.92}{13.14 + (2)0.923 + 3(40.88 - 0.92)/8} = \frac{12.22}{29.97} = 0.41$$

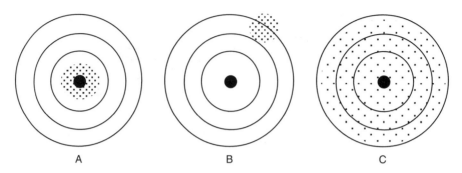

FIGURE 8.1
Comparison of accuracy and precision using the bull's-eye analogy. (A) Good accuracy and good precision. (B) Good precision but not accurate. (C) Poor precision, maybe accurate (hard to judge).

8.2.4 Accuracy and Precision

Another way of examining validity and reliability is in the engineering context of *accuracy* and *precision* or *resolution*. An instrument is considered accurate if measurements are made with small errors or small deviations from the "true value." This can be considered in the context of target shooting. A rifle is considered accurate if it hits the bull's-eye or has a very small deviation from the center (Figure 8.1A). Similarly, an instrument may be considered as precise or having a high resolution if it can detect very small quantities. In terms of target shooting, if the rifle produces a very small scatter, it is considered precise. However, it might not be scattered around the bull's-eye, in which case, it is not very accurate and needs to be resighted (Figure 8.1B). The opposite case, although it may be hard to interpret, is in which the rifle may be accurate, hitting the target, but with a large scatter. It may be accurate, but the lack of precision makes it difficult to judge the accuracy (Figure 8.1C). Obviously, the best scenario is for the rifle to be both accurate and precise, i.e., hitting the bull's-eye with a small scatter (Figure 8.1A). Thus, accuracy is similar to validity and precision is similar to reliability. Note that it is possible to have reliability without validity, but not validity without reliability. Further information on developing valid and reliable tests can be found in a variety of research methodology texts in both psychology and education (Thorndike and Hagen, 1977; Fraenkel and Wallen, 1996; Kerlinger and Lee, 2000). Table 8.3 may also be useful in identifying appropriate procedures for determining the reliability of a screening tool.

There are several other measures that indicate the usefulness of an assessment tool. *Sensitivity* refers to the assessment tool's ability to identify injurious jobs, i.e., jobs that will result in injuries in the future. It can be expressed as the fraction of injurious jobs that are correctly identified as injurious from Table 8.4 or from the *signal-detection theory* analogy shown in Figure 8.2:

$$\text{Sensitivity} = \frac{\text{True positives}}{\text{True positives} + \text{False negatives}} \times 100\% = \frac{a}{a+c} \times 100\% \quad (8.17)$$

TABLE 8.3

Sources of Variation and Procedures for Estimating the Reliability
of an Assessment Instrument

Sources of Variation		Procedure	Specific Test
Instrument itself	Test-retest reliability (confounded with variation within testees)	Basic — give identical instrument twice within short time span	Pearson correlation coefficient r (Equation 8.2).
	Internal consistency (still confounded with variation between testees)	Better — divide instrument into equal halves and give both to testees	Split-half procedure, Pearson r (Equation 8.2) and Spearman-Brown prophecy r (Equation 8.3)
	Internal consistency (still confounded with variation between testees)	Better — give full instrument to testees	Kuder-Richardson r (Equation 8.4 and 8.5) or Cronbach α (Equation 8.7), ICC_1 (Equation 8.12).
Variation over time (effect of learning or sensitization of testees)		Give identical instrument two or more times over time period of interest	Pearson correlation coefficient r (Equation 8.2)
Variation in analysts, interrater agreement		Compare scores obtained by two or more analysts	Kappa (Equation 8.9), ICC_2, (Equation 8.13)

TABLE 8.4

Classification Table for Test Results and the "True" Status of a Disorder

Test Result	The "Truth"		Total	
	Disorder	**No Disorder**	**Total**	
Positive	a = true positives	b = false positives	$a + b$	$\dfrac{a}{a+b} = \dfrac{\text{positive}}{\text{predictive value}}$
Negative	c = false negatives	d = true negatives	$c + d$	$\dfrac{d}{c+d} = \dfrac{\text{negative}}{\text{predictive value}}$
Total	$a + c$	$b + d$	$n = a + b + c + d$	
	$\dfrac{a}{a+c}$ = sensitivity	$\dfrac{d}{b+d}$ = specificity		$\dfrac{a+d}{a+b+c+d}$ = accuracy

In this analogy, safe jobs would score low on an assessment tool's risk rating and injurious jobs would have a high rating. Obviously, there would be a distribution of scores within safe jobs as well as for injurious jobs, with considerable overlap between the two distributions. The central vertical line represents the criterion level, at which point, based on the risk score, a job is classified as either safe or injurious. Thus, some jobs, even though they may score low on a risk assessment tool's rating, could still cause injuries. Being scored low, they would not be classified as injurious and would result

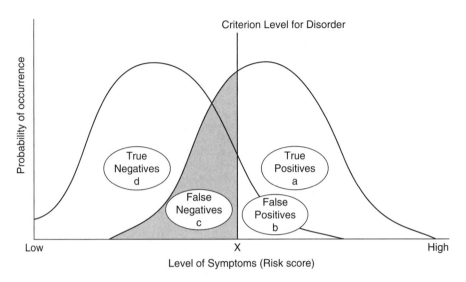

FIGURE 8.2
Signal-detection analogy for an assessment tool risk score.

in false negatives. Similarly, some safe jobs having no injuries may still be scored with a high value and would result in false positives. Correctly identified injurious jobs would be true positives and correctly identified safe jobs would be true negatives.

Specificity refers to the assessment tool's ability to correctly identify safe jobs and would be expressed as

$$\text{Sensitivity} = \frac{\text{True negatives}}{\text{True negatives} + \text{False positives}} \times 100\% = \frac{d}{d+b} \times 100\% \quad (8.18)$$

Note that changing the criterion level to increase the sensitivity of the test will result in a trade-off with an increase of false positives.

The *positive predictive value* of an assessment tool is its ability to predict which jobs will result in future musculoskeletal injuries, or

$$\text{Predictive value} = \frac{\text{True positives}}{\text{True positives} + \text{False negatives}} \times 100\%$$

$$\qquad\qquad (8.19)$$

$$= \frac{a}{a+b} \times 100\%$$

Another, less commonly used measure, is accuracy. It measures the degree of agreement between an assessment tool and the *gold standard* (the best tool):

$$\text{Accuracy} = \frac{\text{True positives} + \text{True negatives}}{\text{Grand total}} = \frac{a+d}{a+b+c+d} \times 100\% \quad (8.20)$$

Unfortunately, there are few data on the sensitivity, specificity, or predictive value for many of the assessment tools. These tools are simply not accurate enough to categorize all of the contributing risk factors. Or from another perspective, there is simply too much variability in the jobs and the individuals working on these jobs, which, at this point in time, are not understood well enough with the existing models to be accurately assessed.

8.2.5 Applications

The above issues of validity and reliability are very important in developing an exposure assessment instrument. Reliability will depend very much on the type of information sought and how it is collected. Self-reported information on work history, job titles, and job duration can typically be considered reliable and valid with kappa values between 60 and 70% (Rona and Mosbech, 1989; Östlin et al., 1990). Questions on general physical activity, perhaps even gross postures, have reliability coefficients of 0.70 to 0.87 and can be considered sufficiently reproducible (Wiktorin et al., 1996). For more detailed information regarding level of activities and more detailed postures, reliability becomes worse, with intraclass correlation coefficients ranging between 0.24 and 0.69 (Spielholz et al., 1999). Correlation coefficients between such questionnaire data and validation criteria (typically analysis of job videotapes or direct instrumented measurements) become much worse, between 0.1 and 0.3 (Lamb and Brodie, 1990; Ainsworth et al., 1993; Wiktorin et al., 1996; Spielholz et al., 2001). Even basic working postures or their durations as reported on questionnaires can vary by as much as 34% from direct observation data (Baty et al., 1986) and have kappa values as low as 45% (Rossignol and Baetz, 1987).

In terms of WRMSD symptom severity, self-administered questionnaires have shown high test-retest reliabilities (Pearson correlation coefficient of $r = 0.91$) and internal consistencies (Cronbach alpha of $\alpha = 0.89$) (Levine et al., 1993). However, when such self-reported information is correlated to direct clinical evaluations, the correlations drop considerably. For two-point discrimination tests and monofilament tests the Spearman-Brown correlation coefficient ranged from $r = 0.12$ to $r = 0.42$ (Levine et al., 1993), while for direction nerve conduction latencies the Pearson correlation coefficient ranged from $r = 0.46$ to $r = 0.53$ (You et al., 1999). The highest correlations were obtained with primary symptoms of numbness, tingling, and nocturnal sensations as opposed to secondary symptoms of pain, weakness, and clumsiness.

In general, there is a tendency for the self-reported data to overestimate exposure (i.e., duration, force, postural angles) as compared to direct measurements, which Spielholz et al. (2001) attributes to a lack of adjustment of the psychophysical rating scale on the part of the workers. Also, the rank ordering of self-reported data was similar to the rank ordering of direct measurements. Although both of these observation may allow the potential

readjustment of self-reported data to yield more reliable and valid occupational risk assessments, the easiest approach may still be to use the simplest
and most basic questions that will be understood by the general working
population.

One would suspect that trained observers or analysts would provide more
reliable data. Keyserling and Witting (1988) were the first to examine the
agreement of expert ratings. Five experts rated ten jobs at three levels. Perfect
agreement was found in only 30% of the cases which, assuming perfect
agreement by chance to be less than 1%, yields a kappa of 0.29. This is only
fair agreement according to the Landis and Koch (1977) scale. If consensus
agreement (i.e., three of five scores are identical) is considered, then 87.5%
of the cases were in "agreement."

Genaidy et al. (1993) and Baluyutt et al. (1995) examined the reliability of
visually estimating postural angles from videotapes. In general, the absolute
error was almost 10°, with flexion/extension angles and lower back and neck
postures easiest to estimate and wrist and elbow postures most difficult to
estimate. Also, interestingly, estimates of angles exhibited a range effect;
smaller angles were overestimated while larger angles were underestimated.

Burt and Punnett (1999) had two analysts evaluate postures for 70 jobs.
Exact agreement between analysts ranged from a low of 26% for shoulder
elevation to a high of 99% for wrist flexion. However, once chance agreement
was introduced through a kappa statistic, the proportion of agreement was
much lower, from 0.0 (with even a couple of slightly negative values) to a
high of 0.55. Of the 18 posture assessments only 2 exceeded the 0.4 threshold
for moderate agreement, with the rest fair or poor agreement. The reason
for the relatively high percentage of basic agreement but low kappa was
explained by the fact that some of the postures were observed rarely, therefore artificially increasing the probability that the two analysts would indicate the some posture. On the other hand, Burt and Punnett (1999) reasoned
that a low value of kappa may be useful in deterring analysts from using
an exposure assessment tool that has not been properly evaluated over a
wide range of conditions.

In terms of force estimation, van der Beek et al. (1992) had two observers
rate truck driver postures and force exertions at three levels. Interobserver
reliability of force was 0.95 with a kappa of 0.81. Similarly, deLooze et al.
(1994) examined two analysts rating loads in nine different manual material
handling tasks. Interobserver reliability after 1 week of practice was 0.76
with a kappa of 0.68. However, reliability with directly recorded values for
load was lower at 0.63 with a kappa of 0.50. Their conclusion was that
observations of the task may not be valid.

A better approach may be for the subject to estimate the task force through
a simulated contraction on a measurement instrument (Kotani, 1995). In the
study, 20 subjects exerted various levels of a required task force on an
instrumented tool. After each exertion, the subjects attempted to replicate

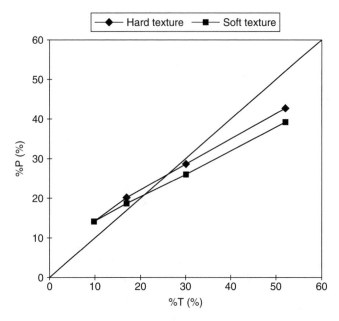

FIGURE 8.3

Relationship between task force on tool (%T) and perceived force on a grip dynamometer (%P) for different textures. (From Kotani, K., 1995. Modeling Perception and Production of Force as a Means of Estimating Force Requirements in Industrial Tasks, Ph.D. dissertation, University Park, PA: Pennsylvania State University. With permission.)

the exact force level on a grip dynamometer. The relationships between the task force on the tool and the perceived force for the grip dynamometer were significantly linear (mean $r^2 = 0.84$, $p < 0.001$) with a slight overestimation for low forces and a larger underestimation for high forces (Figure 8.3). Interestingly, tool grip texture and wrist deviation significantly affected perceived force.

In general, interobserver reliability can be influenced by a variety of factors. The sequence of postures and activities can be memorized from one analysis session to another resulting in a learning effect. This problem can be minimized if sufficient time is given between sessions or if a variety of jobs are analyzed in a random order. Obviously, the reverse effect must also be taken into account. The analysts should be trained sufficiently well that any learning effects with regard to the assessment tool have leveled off. Interobserver reliability will also tend to decrease as the complexity of the assessment tool increases. The larger number of simultaneously observed categories, the greater the variance in the responses that can be expected. A good review of the types of information that can be obtained and the various problems that can be expected to occur in observational analysis and exposure assessment is found in Kilbom (1994).

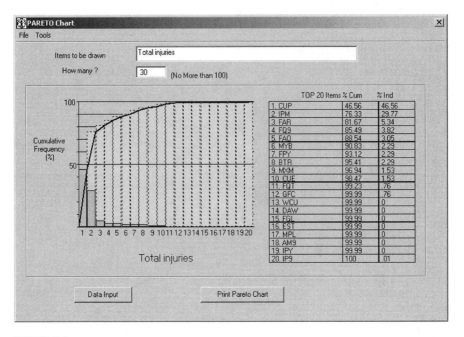

FIGURE 8.4

Pareto distribution of injuries; 20% of jobs account for 80% of the injuries.

8.3 Initial Identification of Musculoskeletal Injury Problems

8.3.1 Initial Steps

The first step in evaluating the scope of WRMSDs in the workplace is a thorough review of existing medical, safety, and insurance records. In the United States, regulations issued by Occupational Safety and Health Administration (OSHA) require that most employers maintain records of work-related injuries and disorders. These are maintained on the standard OSHA 300 log, which is subject to review by OSHA inspectors as well as open to employees and union representatives. In addition, the company will most likely keep more detailed records for each injury or disorder, both for medical and workers' compensation purposes. Therefore, there will be a variety of data sources available for an initial attempt at identifying the problem.

One tool that may be useful in identifying problem areas is the *Pareto analysis* (named after the Italian economist Vilfredo Pareto, 1848–1923). Items of interest (e.g., injuries in Figure 8.4) are identified and measured on a common scale and are then arranged in ascending order, creating a cumulative probability distribution. Typically, 80% or more of the total activity is accounted for by 20% of the ranked items; consequently, the technique is sometimes called the 80–20 rule. For example, in Figure 8.4, 81% of total injuries occur on three job titles, or less than 20% of all job titles. (In Vilfredo Pareto's original application, more than 80% of wealth was concentrated in less than 20% of individuals.) Theoretically, the ergonomist concentrates the greatest effort on those few jobs that produce most of the problems and return the greatest benefit for the amount of effort or money invested. In many cases, the Pareto distribution can be transformed to a straight line using a lognormal transformation, from which further quantitative analyses can be performed (Herron, 1976).

8.3.2 Surveys and Subjective Ratings

In many cases, medical records are incomplete or may not reflect the true nature of the problem. Many workers may be hesitant to report relatively minor arm pain at the workplace, thinking that it is not work related, and have it treated by their family physician. However, these may be the first signs of an oncoming epidemic that should be caught early on; therefore, the next step should be to survey the workers. Questionnaires and surveys have been developed for this purpose. Note, however, that these surveys rely on the worker's recognition of the problem and willingness to respond. Therefore, unless special steps are taken, such as anonymity of responses and lack of retribution on the part of management, the response may be biased.

8.3.2.1 Symptom Surveys

A typical questionnaire, developed by OSHA (1990), is shown in Figure 8.5. The questions are designed to disclose the nature, location, and severity of the symptoms. Questions are also needed to determine whether the workers have received treatment for any previous musculoskeletal injuries and whether they have other conditions that may exhibit similar symptoms, such as arthritis, diabetes, thyroid disorders, gout, kidney disease, menstrual problems, pregnancy, and use of oral contraceptives. Thus, such a questionnaire is typically termed a *symptom survey.*

8.3.2.2 Body Discomfort Maps

Another common tool for surveying workers is the *body discomfort map* developed by Corlett and Bishop (1976) (Figure 8.6). The worker marks each body part where pain or discomfort is experienced and then rates the level of that pain on a *visual analogue scale* (VAS). The VAS is typically a 10-cm line drawn on a piece of paper with end points of 0 (nothing at all) to 10 (almost maximum), on which the subject is asked to indicate the degree of perceived pain by putting a mark on the line (Neely et al., 1992). The use of such a subjective rating for pain has been found to be both valid and reliable (Reading, 1980; Price et al., 1983).

Symptoms Survey

Date_____

Department_____ Job title _____

Number of years on this job _____ Previous job _____

1) Have you had any pain and discomfort during the last year?   Yes   No

If yes, check area: Neck ____ Shoulder ____ Elbow/forearm ____ Hand/wrist ____ Fingers ____
Upper back ____ Low back ____ Thigh/knee ____ Lower leg ____ Ankle/feet ____

2) Please put a check by the word(s) that best describe your problem:
　　　____ Aching　　　____ Numbness　　　____ Tingling
　　　____ Burning　　　____ Pain　　　____ Weakness
　　　____ Cramping　　____ Swelling　　　____ Loss of color
　　　____ Stiffness　　　____ Other

3) When did you first notice the problem? _____

4) How long does each episode last? (Mark an X along the line)

1 hour　　1 day　　　1 week　　　1 month　　　　　　　　　6 months

5) What do you think caused the problem? _____

6) Have you had this problem in the last 7 days?   Yes   No

7) How would you rate this problem now? (Mark an X along the line)

None　　　　　　　　　　　　　　　　　　　　　　　Unbearable

8) How would you rate this problem at its worst? (Mark an X along the line)

None　　　　　　　　　　　　　　　　　　　　　　　Unbearable

9) Have you had medical treatment for this problem?   Yes   No

If no, why not? _____
If yes, where and when did you receive treatment? _____
If yes, did the treatment help?   Yes   No

10) How much time have you lost in the last year because of this problem? _____

11) How many days in the last year were you on restricted or light duty because of this problem? _____

Please comment on what you think would improve your symptoms.

_____
_____
_____

FIGURE 8.5
Typical symptoms survey questionnaire. (From OSHA, 1990.)

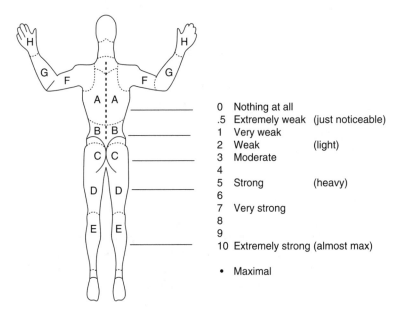

FIGURE 8.6
Body discomfort map with ratings of perceived pain. (Adapted from Corlett and Bishop, 1976; Borg, 1982.)

8.3.2.3   *Subjective Ratings*

An alternative but comparable rating scale is the Borg (1982) *category ratio scale* (CR-10) with several verbal anchors, originally designed for muscular exertion (Figure 8.6), which may provide a higher level of precision than the VAS (Cameron, 1996). However, the VAS may be preferred by workers who do not have the time to read and to consider the anchor points individually (Ulin et al., 1990). Also, the VAS may not impose the need to exceed a threshold of sensation intensity at each level before proceeding to the next level, as do the category ratio scales such as the CR-10 (Wilson and Jones, 1989). This type of approach has been used successfully by a number of researchers to assess postural discomfort (Boussenna et al., 1982; Kuorinka, 1983; Bhatnagar et al., 1985; Harms-Ringdahl, 1986; Saldana et al., 1994) or the identification of WRMSDs in the workforce (Buckle et al., 1984).

Overall, such a visual map with rating scales is an especially useful tool for situations in which the working population may not be native born or does not have sufficient English skills to read lengthy instructions or questions. This approach can also provide crude quantitative measures. By counting the number of times each body part was marked and dividing by the number of total responses, a rough measure of the incidence of the problem is obtained. Furthermore, the mean level of the perceived pain ratings provides a rough measure of the severity of the problem.

8.3.2.4   Nordic Questionnaire

One comprehensive questionnaire that utilizes both body discomfort maps and detailed questions to elicit further information is the Nordic Questionnaire (Kuorinka et al., 1987). It consists of a general survey with specific sections for various body parts (Figure 8.7). Test-retest reliabilities for samples of 20 workers showed identical responses on 77 to 100% of the questions and validity tests between a physiotherapist and 82 workers showed identical responses on 87 to 100% of the questions. The Nordic Questionnaire has been used quite successfully in identifying potentially injurious situations in many studies (Dickinson et al., 1992; Deakin et al., 1994; Bru et al., 1994; Hagen et al., 1998).

8.3.3   Limitations of Surveys

Note that the results of any such questionnaires or surveys must be interpreted with caution. Workers may be hesitant to provide true and accurate responses. Pain tolerance varies considerably between individuals. Also, there are many technical factors that enter into the proper design, validation, and analyses of surveys. Some are discussed in Section 8.2, but others include the reading level of the respondents, the length and wording of the surveys, written or oral response, etc. Further details on survey design can be obtained from Warwick and Lininger (1975) and Berdie et al. (1986). Note also that this is only the starting point in identifying the problem. More in-depth worksite analyses will be necessary to identify the source of these WRMSDs.

8.4   Gross Posture and Task Analyses

8.4.1   Early Recording of Postures

Poor postures, as mentioned in Chapter 6, can be major factors in the cause of musculoskeletal injuries. However, the accurate recording of postures is not an easy matter. Systems for recording postures were developed as early as the 17th century for choreography. Current variations of such systems, the Labanotation and Benesh notation, require several months of diligent training to achieve suitable skill and speed. These, obviously, would not be suitable for widespread use in industry or even more-detailed laboratory use.

A simpler system for defining a posture numerically was developed by Priel (1974). It noted the position and angle of each joint with respect to a reference level and independent of other joint positions. The angles were estimated in orthogonal planes in roughly 15° increments. The system is simple and can be learned quickly but requires a considerable number of data entries on the forms to obtain the final *posturegram*.

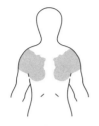

SHOULDER

How to answer the questionnaire: By shoulder trouble is meant ache, pain or discomfort in the shaded area. Please concentrate on this area, ignoring any trouble you may have in adjacent parts of the body. There is a separate questionnaire for other areas of discomfort.

Please answer by putting a cross in the appropriate box—one cross for each question. You may be in doubt as to how to answer, but please do your best anyway.

9. Have you ever had shoulder trouble (ache, pain or discomfort)?

   1 No   2 Yes   ☐

If you answered No to Question 9, do not answer Questions 10–17.

10. Have you ever hurt your shoulder in an accident?

   1 No   2 Yes, my right shoulder
            3 Yes, my left shoulder
            4 Yes, both shoulders   ☐

11. Have you ever had to change jobs or duties because of shoulder trouble?

   1 No   2 Yes   ☐

12. Have you had shoulder trouble during the last 12 months?

   1 No   2 Yes, in my right shoulder
            3 Yes, in my left shoulder
            4 Yes, in both shoulders   ☐

If you answered No to Question 12, do not answer Questions 13–17.

13. What is the total length of time that you have had shoulder trouble during the last 12 months?

   1 1–7 days
   2 8–30 days
   3 More than 30 days, but not every day
   4 Every day   ☐

14. Has shoulder trouble caused you to reduce your activity during the last 12 months?

   a. Work activity (at home or away from home)?

      1 No   2 Yes   ☐

   b. Leisure activity?

      1 No   2 Yes   ☐

15. What is the total length of time that shoulder trouble has prevented you from doing your normal work (at home or away from home) during the last 12 months?

   1 0 days
   2 1–7 days
   3 8–30 days
   4 More than 30 days   ☐

16. Have you been seen by a doctor, physiotherapist, chiropractor or other such person because of shoulder trouble during the last 12 months?

   1 No   2 Yes   ☐

17. Have you had shoulder trouble at any time during the last 7 days?

   1 No   2 Yes, in my right shoulder
            3 Yes, in my left shoulder
            4 Yes, in both shoulders   ☐

FIGURE 8.7
The shoulder section of the Nordic Questionnaire for analysis of musculoskeletal symptoms. (From Kuorinka, I. et al., 1987. *Applied Ergonomics*, 18:233–237. With permission.)

8.4.2 OWAS

Another readily learned procedure is the Ovaco Working Posture Analysis System (OWAS) developed at the Finnish Institute of Occupational Health for use in the steel industry (Karhu et al., 1977, 1981). The system uses a two-step procedure, the first of which collects data at regular intervals using

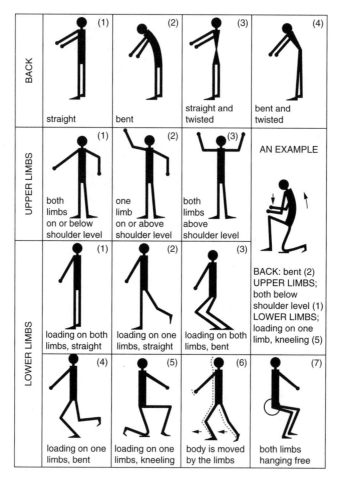

FIGURE 8.8
The OWAS posture assessment tool. (From Karhu, O. et al., 1977. *Applied Ergonomics*, 8, 199–201. With permission.)

a three-digit code based on the posture categories given in Figure 8.8. For example, the code 215 would represent a worker with a bent back, with both arms below shoulder level, and kneeling. A later version incorporates three levels of loading (<10 kg, <20 kg, and >20 kg).

The second step analyzes the data to provide frequency distributions of the postures, and rates the work phases into four levels of "action" categories, with category 4 the worst. Although somewhat simplistic, OWAS does provide a means of recording and categorizing working postures rather quickly. Also, test-retest correlations are very high, $r = 0.97$ to $r = 1.0$ (Mattila et al., 1993). Unfortunately, little detail is given to the upper limbs. An interesting extension of OWAS to the construction industry was formulated by Buchholz et al. (1996).

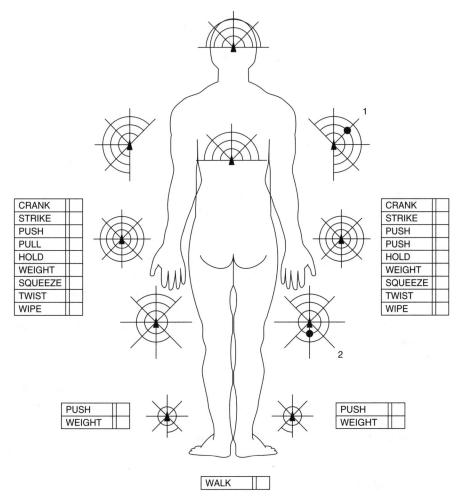

FIGURE 8.9

The posture targeting tool. (From Corlett, E.N. et al., 1979. *Ergonomics*, 22:357–366. With permission.)

8.4.3 Posture Targeting

A slightly more detailed approach for recording postures at random times during the workday was developed by Corlett et al. (1979). Termed *posture targeting*, the analyst records the body part angle on the body diagram shown in Figure 8.9 by blackening in the appropriate area on a target-like concentric circle arrangement. The first concentric circle represents 45° angular displacement from the standard anatomical position, while each succeeding circle is another 45° increment in displacement. The "target" itself represents azimuth angles in the coronal plane. For example, point 1 in Figure 8.9 indicates the arm is at 90° flexion (pointing horizontally) at 45° from the midsagittal plane. Point 2 indicates the wrist is in 45° extension. Note that repeated observations over time could create a series of points or even a blackened area, indicating a range of movement or static postures. The procedure can be learned in less than an hour and provides test-retest correlations as high as $r = 0.67$ to $r = 0.88$. The approach allows the analyst to identify the most frequent and potentially most stressful postures for more detailed biomechanical analysis and can be combined with worker reports of musculoskeletal pain to provide a comprehensive workplace evaluation (Corlett and Manenica, 1980).

8.4.4   RULA

The above posture targeting system of Corlett et al. (1979) was later refined by McAtamney and Corlett (1993) and Corlett (1995) into the rapid upper limb assessment or *RULA*. Upper limb postures (Group A) from Figure 8.10 for the left or right side are combined per Table 8.5A to yield an upper limb score. This score is adjusted upward by one point if the posture is mainly static, and by one, two, or three points if a 2 to 10 kg intermittent load, 2 to 10 kg static load, or >10 kg load is handled, respectively. The same procedure is repeated for trunk and leg postures (Group B) from Figure 8.10 and combined per Table 8.5B to yield a trunk score. This score is similarly corrected and then added to the upper limb score to yield a final grand score as a rudimentary musculoskeletal injury risk level with values above 5 requiring changes (Table 8.6). RULA has shown good correlation with self-reported musculoskeletal discomfort (Hedge et al., 1995; Kilroy and Dockrell, 2000) and has since been expanded to the whole body, the Rapid Entire Body Assessment (REBA) (Hignett and McAtamney, 2000).

8.4.5   Video Posture Analyses

These early systems were primarily relatively simple pencil-and-paper posture recording systems relying on visual observations. For more detailed analyses both a permanent record and finer breakdown or categorization are required. Armstrong et al. (1979, 1982) developed one such system for the upper extremities. First, the job was recorded either on film (as done by the authors) or on videotape (current approach). Next, the analyst selected frames at frequent, regular intervals and recorded shoulder, elbow, and wrist angles and hand posture according to one of six grasp specifications as shown in Figure 8.11. Also, measures of hand forces were obtained indirectly from observation of forearm muscle EMG. The method was quite successful in identifying stressful tasks in poultry processing and later in the garment industry (Punnett and Keyserling, 1987), but at a relatively high cost of effort, several minutes per frame or several hours per minute of videotape.

Other similar videotape approaches include (1) the VIRA (Persson and Kilbom, 1983; Kilbom et al., 1986), which utilized two perpendicular cameras,

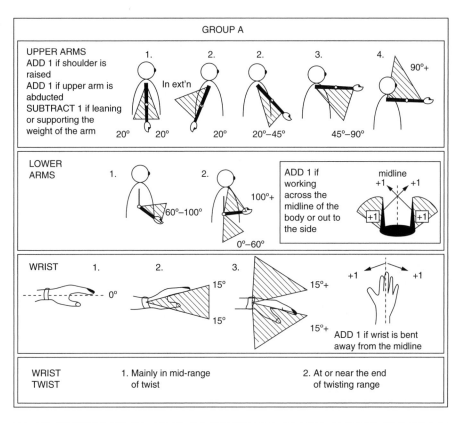

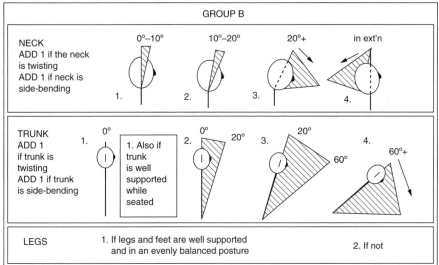

FIGURE 8.10

The RULA posture assessment tool. (From McAtamney, L. and Corlett, E.N., 1993. *Applied Ergonomics*, 24, 91–99. With permission.)

TABLE 8.5A

Upper Limb Posture Score (Group A) from the RULA Posture Assessment Tool

Upper Arm	Lower Arm	Wrist Posture Score							
		1		**2**		**3**		**4**	
		W. 1	Twist 2	W. 1	Twist 2	W. 1	Twist 2	W. 1	Twist 2
1	1	1	2	2	2	2	3	3	3
	2	2	2	2	2	3	3	3	3
	3	2	3	3	3	3	3	4	4
2	1	2	3	3	3	3	4	4	4
	2	3	3	3	3	3	4	4	4
	3	3	4	4	4	4	4	5	5
3	1	3	3	4	4	4	4	5	5
	2	3	4	4	4	4	4	5	5
	3	4	4	4	4	4	5	5	5
4	1	4	4	4	4	4	5	5	5
	2	4	4	4	4	4	5	5	5
	3	4	4	4	5	5	5	6	6
5	1	5	5	5	5	5	6	6	7
	2	5	6	6	6	6	7	7	7
	3	6	6	6	7	7	7	7	8
6	1	7	7	7	7	7	8	8	9
	2	8	8	8	8	8	9	9	9
	3	9	9	9	9	9	9	9	9

Source: McAtamney, L. and Corlett, E.N., 1993. *Applied Ergonomics*, 24:91–99. With permission.

TABLE 8.5B

Trunk/Neck/Leg Posture Score (Group B) from the RULA Posture Assessment Tool

Neck Posture Score	Trunk Posture Score											
	1		**2**		**3**		**4**		**5**		**6**	
	Legs 1	Legs 2	Legs 1	Legs 2	Legs 1	Legs 2	Legs 1	Legs 2	Legs 1	Legs 2	Legs 1	Legs 2
1	1	3	2	3	3	4	5	5	6	6	7	7
2	2	3	2	3	4	5	5	5	6	7	7	7
3	3	3	3	4	4	5	5	6	6	7	7	7
4	5	5	5	6	6	7	7	7	7	7	8	8
5	7	7	7	7	7	8	8	8	8	8	8	8
6	8	8	8	8	8	8	8	9	9	9	9	9

Source: McAtamney, L. and Corlett, E.N., 1993. *Applied Ergonomics*, 24:91–99. With permission.

a four-part categorization scheme for the shoulder and neck, and computer assistance to record time spent in the posture, and (2) the Keyserling (1986) one-camera approach for trunk and shoulder angles with computer tabulation. The advantage of the latter approach is that the film can be run in real

TABLE 8.6

Grand Score Table

Upper Limb	Trunk/Neck/Leg Score (B)						
Score (A)	1	2	3	4	5	6	7+
1	1	2	3	3	4	5	5
2	2	2	3	4	4	5	5
3	3	3	3	4	4	5	6
4	3	3	3	4	5	6	6
5	4	4	4	5	6	7	7
6	4	4	5	6	6	7	7
7	5	5	6	6	7	7	7
8	5	5	6	7	7	7	7

Source: McAtamney, L. and Corlett, E.N., 1993. *Applied Ergonomics*, 24:91–99. With permission.

time, saving considerable time over frame-by-frame analysis. Also, inexperienced analysts could be trained in 2 h and show very good consistency between observations.

Further automation of upper limb posture analysis was implemented by Yen and Radwin (2002) using the Armstrong et al. (1982) classification scheme and a computer-controlled VCR. (Further information on the multimedia video task analysis, or MVTA, computer system is available at http://mvta.engr.wisc.edu/mvta.htm.) The average difference among analysts for average joint angle was 11.4°. An alternative approach using spectral analysis of goniometric data (previously presented in Radwin and Lin, 1993, and Yen and Radwin, 1999) was much more consistent (average joint deviation angle was only 0.9°) and took only 16% of the time to perform than did manual ratings by analysts. Even considering the additional time needed for setting up the instrumentation, total spectral analysis time was 77% of manual analysis time. However, no overall risk assessment was provided.

8.4.6 Task Analyses

Several other posture classification systems were developed as part of a general job or task analysis system. The first of these is the AET job analysis method of Rohmert and Landau (1983) and a later variation in the form of PLIBEL (Kemmlert, 1995). Later approaches to continuously record and classify postural changes have utilized the capabilities of personal computers (PCs). The first was a relatively crude classification of gross postures without specifying exact angles by Foreman et al. (1988). Later approaches became more detailed by either specifying more accurately joint angles, the Portable Ergonomic Observation (PEO) method by Fransson-Hall et al. (1995), or by categorizing the loads involved, the Task Recording and Analysis on Computer (TRAC) method by van der Beek et al. (1992). Although quite detailed, some such as ARBAN (Holzman 1982; Wangenheim et al., 1986) are essentially computerized versions of the previously mentioned body discomfort

ANALYST: _____
DATE: _____

JOB: _____
HAND: *RIGHT/LEFT*

UPPER EXTREMITY POSTURES AND WORK ELEMENT RECORDING SHEET

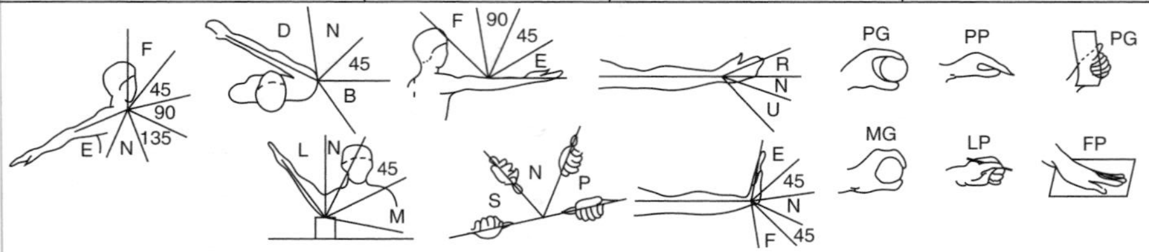

FIGURE 8.11

Upper extremity postures and work element recording sheet. (From Armstrong, T.J. et al., 1982. *American Industrial Hygiene Association Journal*, 43:103–116. With permission.)

map with a rating for perceived effort using the CR-10 scale at each of the body locations used to identify ergonomic hazards on a job. However, by providing a mean value of the summated ratings, ARBAN is also a coarse overall WRMSD risk assessment instrument.

Note that all the above systems focus primarily on gross posture and/or general task analysis and typically neglect the upper limbs and the key factors leading to WRMSDs in the upper limbs. One exception to this is Sperling et al.'s (1993) cube model for classifying hand tool work. It categorizes three factors, force, precision, and time, at three levels, during hand tool usage and then defines acceptable limits. Although it does not strictly define a risk level for developing WRMSDs in the upper limbs, the cube model is a step in the right direction. More detailed reviews of different postural assessment techniques are provided by Genaidy et al. (1994), Juul-Kristensen et al. (1997), and Kilbom (1994). For convenience, the main posture assessment instruments are summarized and categorized by characteristics in Table 8.7.

8.5 Quantitative Upper Limb WRMSD Risk Assessment Tools

8.5.1 Checklists

One of the first risk assessment tools developed specifically for identifying upper limb WRMSD was an Upper Extremity Checklist (Figure 8.12) with questions grouped into five sections relating to repetitiveness, mechanical contact stresses, forceful exertions, awkward postures, and hand tool usage (Stetson et al., 1991; Keyserling et al., 1993). Some questions required a simple binary response, corresponding to no/zero and yes, while others required categorization into a three-level scale, corresponding to zero/insignificant, moderate, and substantial ergonomic exposures. Once the checklist was completed, the total number of nonzero responses was summed to produce an overall stress score. The authors, however, emphasized that because of the qualitative nature of the responses and user interpretation of stressors the checklist was designed primarily as a screening tool to identify critical jobs for later analyses and to view the overall risk score with caution.

The checklist was utilized by plant personnel on four worksites to evaluate 335 jobs and was considered a quick but effective screening tool (Keyserling et al., 1993). However, when the checklist was compared to results of expert (defined as "university personnel with extensive experience") analyses, the percent of analysts agreeing on the various categories ranged from a low of 39% to a high of 90%, or in terms of the kappa statistic (Equation 8.9), from a low of –22% to a high of 80%. Only two of seven categories score a kappa in the range of substantial agreement. The poor agreement was attributed to exposure variability because the checklist and expert analyses were often spaced months apart with different workers observed, perhaps using different methods.

TABLE 8.7

Categorization of Posture Assessment and Gross Task Analysis Instruments (in order of complexity)

Type of Instrument (Key Ref.)	Equipment Used	Posture Levels of Categorization	Force	Frequency	Learning Time	Analysis Time	Test-Retest Reliability	Validity (With Standard)
Posture Recording via Sampling	*Paper/pencil*	*Gross postures*						
Posturegram (Priel, 1974)	Paper/pencil	Sh 6-Ro, Sh 8-A/A, Sh 8-F/E, El 4-Ro, El 6-F/E, Wr 3-F/E	—	—	Long	Medium	—	—
OWAS (Karhu et al., 1977)	Paper/pencil	Sh 3-F/E and trunk angles	3 levels	% time	5 days	Short	$0.74 < r < 0.99$*	—
Posture targeting (Corlett et al., 1979)	Paper/pencil	Nominally 4 × 8 categories, but, in practice, infinite combinations	—	—	1 h	Medium	$0.67 < r < 0.88$*	Upper arm $r = 0.32$*, lower arm $r = 0.08$ NS
RULA (McAtamney and Corlett, 1993)	Paper/pencil	Sh 5-F/E, Sh A/A, El 3-F/E, Wr 3-F/E, Wr 3-R/U	4 levels	2 levels	Medium	Short	—	—
Continuous Posture Recording	*Video*	*Micro postures*						
Armstrong (1979, 1982)	1 camera, PC	Sh 5-F/E, Sh 4-A/A, Sh 4-Ro, El 4-F/E, El 2-Ro, Wr 5-F/E, Wr 3-R/U, 6 grasps	From EMG	Cycle time # grasps	Medium	Very long	—	—

VIRA (Persson et al., 1983)	2 cameras, PC	Sh 5-F/E, Sh 4-A/A	—		Cycle time ½ h	Medium	6% error *	—
Keyserling (1986)	1 camera, PC	Sh 3-F/E and trunk angles	—		Cycle time 20 h	Medium	Time, $r = 0.98$*; Posture $r = 0.95$*	Time, $r = 0.99$*
Wrigley et al. (1991)	1 camera, PC	Infinite, true motion analysis	—		Medium	Medium	$r = 0.99$*	Difference = 1.4°
MVTA (Yen and Radwin, 2002)	1 camera, PC	Either Armstrong (1982) or infinite	—		Cycle time Medium	Long or short	—	Diff = 11.4° or 0.9°
Task (Risk) Analysis								
Gross postures								
AET (Rohmert and Landau, 1983)	Paper/pencil	Arm, hand/finger, trunk	5 levels	5 levels		Long	Good if trained	—
ARBAN (Holzmann, 1982)	Video, PC	El 3-Ro × 4-F/E, similar for other joints	Borg-CR10		Cycle time Long	Long	Good if trained	—
TRAC (van der Beek et al., 1992)	Pocket PC	4 for arms and trunk, legs	3 levels		Short	Medium	$0.24 < r < 0.89$	$r = 0.98$*, posture
PEO (Fransson-Hall et al., 1995)	Pocket PC video helps	Sh 2-F/E, wrist, neck, trunk,	Loads lifted	Cycle time # events	Cycle time 10 h	Medium	Time, r *; Frequency, r NS	$r = 0.5$*, for posture

Abbreviations: Sh = shoulder, El = elbow, Wr = wrist, A/A = abduction/adduction, F/E = flexion/extension, R/U = radian/ulnar deviation, Ro = rotation, — = unknown or not applicable,* = significant at $p < 0.05$, NS = not significant at $p > 0.05$.

UPPER EXTREMITY CHECK LIST

Worker Information

Which hand is the operator's dominant hand? (circle one)

Left Hand   Right Hand   Both Hands

Circle a *, √ or o to answer each question below.

Repetitiveness	**No**	**Yes**
1. Does the job involve repetitive use of the hands and wrists? Answer "yes" if either of the following is true:	o	*

   a. The work cycle is less than 30 s long, or

   b. The hands repeat the same motions/exertions for more
       than ½ of the work cycle

Mechanical Stress   **Left Hand   Right Hand**

2. Do hard or sharp objects, tools, or parts of the workstation put localized pressure on the:	no	yes	no	yes	element(s)
a. back or side of the fingers?	o	√	o	√	_____
b. palm or base of the hand?	o	√	o	√	_____
c. forearm or elbow?	o	√	o	√	_____
d. armpit?	o	√	o	√	_____
3. Is the pain or base of the hand used as a striking tool (like a hammer)?	o	√	o	√	_____

Force

4. Does the worker lift, carry, push or pull objects weighing more than 4.5 kg (10 lb)?	o	√	o	√	_____
5. Does operator grip an object or a tool that has a smooth, slippery (no texture or hand holds to reduce slipping)?	o	√	o	√	_____
6. Is the tip of a finger or thumb used as a pressing or pushing tool?	o	√	o	√	_____

7. Check box if no gloves are worn   ☐
   and skip this question.

If the operator wears gloves, do the gloves hinder gripping?	o	√	o	√	_____

FIGURE 8.12
Upper extremity checklist. (From Keyserling, W.M. et al., 1993. *Ergonomics*, 36:807–831. With permission.)

UPPER EXTREMITY CHECK LIST (continued)

	Left Hand			Right Hand			
	no	some	more than ⅓ cycle	no	some	more than ⅓ cycle	element(s)
8. Does operator grip or hold a part or a tool that weighs more than 2.7 kg (6 lb) per hand?	o	√	*	o	√	*	_____

Posture

9. Is a pinch grip used?	o	√	*	o	√	*	_____
10. Is there wrist deviation?	o	√	*	o	√	*	_____
11. Is there twisting, rotating or screwing motion of the forearm?	o	√	*	o	√	*	_____
12. Is there reaching down and behind the torso?	o	√	*	o	√	*	_____
13. Is an elbow used at or above mid-torso level?	o	√	*	o	√	*	_____

Tools, Hand-Held Objects and Equipment

14. Is vibration from the tool or object transmitted to the operator's hand?	o	√	*	o	√	*	_____
15. Does cold exhaust air blow on the hand or wrist?	o	√	*	o	√	*	_____
16. Is a finger used in a rapid triggering motion?	o	√	*	o	√	*	_____

	no	yes	no	yes	
17. Is the tool or object unbalanced?	o	√	o	√	_____
18. Does the tool or object jerk the hand?	o	√	o	√	_____

List all tools, objects and equipment used to answer Questions 14–18

Total Score = _____ − _____
　　　　　　　(No. of *'s)　　　(No. of √'s)

Comments:

FIGURE 8.12 (continued)

8.5.2   Strain Index

Moore and Garg (1995) proposed a more quantitative job analysis method-ology based on physiological considerations and job risk factors, which yielded a final risk score. Termed the Strain Index (SI), six task variables — intensity of exertion, duration of exertion, efforts per minute, wrist posture, speed of exertion, and duration of task — were rated on an ordinal five-point exposure scale (Table 8.8). The ratings were converted to six multipliers from Table 8.9, which when multiplied together yield the final SI score. For example, a task with 20% maximum voluntary contraction (MVC) exertions over 60% of one cycle, with 12 efforts per minute, with 18° ulnar deviations, at 95% of normal pace for a full 8-hour shift would yield ratings of 2, 4, 3, 3, 3, and 4 from Table 8.8, respectively. These ratings convert to multipliers of 3.0, 2.0, 1.5, 1.5, 1.0, and 1.0 from Table 8.9, respectively, and, when multiplied together, yield a final SI score of 13.5. SI scores above 5.0 were considered to be potentially hazardous.

The authors tested the SI methodology on data from an earlier study in a pork processing plant (Moore and Garg, 1994). The SI correctly identified 11 of 12 jobs associated with WRMSD morbidity and all 13 jobs not associated with WRMSDs. The relative risk was 11.7 greater for the hazardous jobs (as defined by the SI) as opposed to the jobs deemed safe. A later study on 28 turkey processing jobs (Knox and Moore, 2001) established sensitivity, specificity, and positive predictive values for the SI of 0.86, 0.79, and 0.92, respectively.

8.5.3   OCRA

A more detailed exposure assessment tool for upper limbs, termed the OCRA exposure index, was proposed by Occhipinti (1998). The final exposure index is a ratio of the number of motions (termed technical actions) performed in repetitive tasks during a shift to the number of recommended or allowed motions for that shift. The categorization of motions follows a procedure developed by Colombini (1998), shown in Figure 8.13. The calculation of the number of allowed motions is a fairly complex procedure involving multi-pliers for various risk factors (see tables in Figure 8.14) that is somewhat analogous to those in the SI of Moore and Garg (1995):

$$A_r = F_r \sum_1^n CF \times F_f \times F_p \times F_a \times D \tag{8.21}$$

where

A_r = total number of motions recommended during shift
F_r = multiplier for the lack of recovery period during the shift
CF = reference number of motions per minute (typically 30)
F_f = multiplier for the force risk factor
F_p = multiplier for the posture risk factor
F_a = multiplier for additional elements of risk
D = duration of each repetitive task in minutes

TABLE 8.8

Strain Index Rating Criteria

Rating	Intensity of Exertion (%MVC)	Duration of Exertion (% of cycle)	Efforts per min	Wrist Posture (worst case)			Speed of Work (% speed rating)	Duration per day (hours)
				Extension	Flexion	Ulnar Dev.		
1	<15	<10	<4	0–10	0–5°	0–10°	<80	<1
2	16–30	10–29	4–8	11–25°	6–15°	11–15°	81–90	1–2
3	31–50	30–49	9–14	26–40°	16–30°	16–20°	91–100	2–4
4	51–75	50–79	15–19	41–55°	31–50°	21–25°	101–115	4–8
5	>75	≥80	≥20	>55°	>50°	>25°	>115	>8

Source: Adapted from Moore and Garg (1995).

TABLE 8.9

Strain Index Multiplier Table (for Table 8.8)

Rating	Intensity of Exertion	Duration of Exertion	Efforts per min	Wrist Posture	Speed of Work	Duration per day
1	1	0.5	0.5	1.0	1.0	0.25
2	3	1.0	1.0	1.0	1.0	0.50
3	6	1.5	1.5	1.5	1.0	0.75
4	9	2.0	2.0	2.0	1.5	1.00
5	13	3.0	3.0	3.0	2.0	1.50

Source: Adapted from Moore and Garg (1995).

Biomechanics of the Upper Limbs

UPPER LIMB: ☑ RIGHT ☐ LEFT

TASK INVOLVEMENT: *OPERATING A LEVER*

		POSTURAL SCORE IN CYCLE/TASK (A+B=MAX 16)

SHOULDER POSITIONS AND MOVEMENT

|_0_|_0_|_0_|A2 CYCLE

0° 60° 20°

0° 60° 20°

0° 0°

- MOVEMENTS IN EXTREME ARTICULAR RANGE: THEY LAST: ☐ 1/3, ☐ 2/3, ☐ 3/3 of cycle/task time
- STEREOTYPE MOVEMENTS (score 4):
  ☑ Performs work gestures of the same type involving the shoulder for more than 50% of the cycle/task time. |_4_|B1
- STATIC POSTURES (score 4):
  ☐ Keeps the arm raised (unsupported) at an angle more than 60° or in extension, for at least 10 sec consecutively once every cycle (short cycle: inf. 30 sec). For longer cycle time increase proportionally the time of the static contraction.
  ☐ Keeps the arm raised (unsupported) at an angle of:
  ☐ 60° for more than 1 min
  ☐ 40° for more than 2 min
  ☐ 20° for more than 3 min

|_0_|_4_| SHOULDER

ELBOW MOVEMENTS

|_0_|_0_|_0_|A2 CYCLE

RANGE
2 Score
0°

0°

SUPINATION PRONATION

- MOVEMENTS IN EXTREME ARTICULAR RANGE: THEY STAND: ☐ 1/3, ☐ 2/3, ☐ 3/3 of cycle/task time
- LACK OF VARIATION (score 4): ☑ Performs work gestures of the same type involving the elbow for at least 50% of the cycle. |_4_|B2

|_0_|_4_| ELBOW

WRIST POSITION AND MOVEMENTS

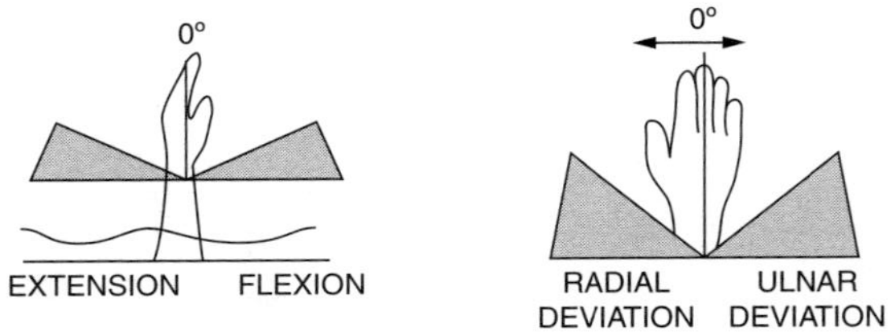

EXTENSION   FLEXION   RADIAL DEVIATION   ULNAR DEVIATION

0°   0°

– MOVEMENTS IN EXTREME ARTICULAR RANGE: THEY LAST: ☐ 1/3, ☐ 2/3, ☐ 3/3 of cycle/task time
– LACK OF VARIATION (score 4):
☑ Performs work gestures of the same type involving the wrist for at least 50% of the cycle.
☐ Keeps the wrist flexed or extended (at an angle of over 45°) or deviated laterally (ulna or radius) for at least 50% of cycle/task time.

|_0_|_0_|_0_|A3 CYCLE

|_0_|_4_| WRIST/HAND

TYPE OF GRIP AND FINGER MOVEMENTS

TIME OF THE GRIP AND FINGER POSITION   SCORE

						SCORE
[ ] TIGHT GRIP (1.5 cm)	☐ 1/3,	☐ 2/3,	☐ 3/3	2
[ ] PINCH	☐ 1/3,	☐ 2/3,	☐ 3/3	3
[ ] PALMAR GRIP	☐ 1/3,	☐ 2/3,	☐ 3/3	4
[ ] HOOK GRIP	☐ 1/3,	☐ 2/3,	☐ 3/3	4
[ ] KEYING	☐ 1/3,	☐ 2/3,	☐ 3/3	1
[ ] WIDE GRIP (4–5 cm)	☐ 1/3,	☐ 2/3,	☑ 3/3	….
[ ]	☐ 1/3,	☐ 2/3,	☐ 3/3	….
[ ]	☐ 1/3,	☐ 2/3,	☐ 3/3	

|_4_|B3

|_1_|_1_|_1_|_1_|A4 SCORE

LACK OF VARIATION (score 4):
[1] Performs work gestures of the same type involving the same finger(s) for at least 50% of the cycle.
[2] Holds an object in a pinch or palmar (or hook) grip for at least 50% of the cycle.

|_0_|B4

|_0_|_4_| GRIP/HAND

FIGURE 8.13
Upper limb postures for the OCRA index of exposure. (From Colombini, D., 1998. *Ergonomics*, 41:1261–1289. With permission.)

Part A. *Summary of data for calculating index of exposure to repetitive movements of the upper limbs.*

| Department or line .... | Station or task .... | Shift .... |

Characterization of repetitive tasks performed during shift

	A	B	C	D
• duration of task in shift (min)				
• mean cycle duration (s)				
• action frequency (no. of actions/min)				
• total actions in task				

• total actions in shift
(sum of A, B, C, D) [ ] A_e

Characterization of non-repetitive tasks performed during shift

	X	Y	X
• duration (min)			
• comparable to recovery			
• not comparable to recovery			

Total no. of minutes of non-repetitive
task comparable to recovery

min [ ]

Characterization of breaks during shift

• duration of meal break (min)
• other breaks
• total duration of other breaks (min)

Time-wise distribution of tasks and breaks in shift
(describe exact sequence of tasks and breaks, and their relative duration in minutes)

1 h

No. of hours in shift featuring lack of recovery times, N = _____

	A	B	C	D	
• minutes spent with previous adequate recovery periods					D_{re}
• minutes spent without previous adequate recovery periods					D_{so}

FIGURE 8.14
Worksheet for the calculation of the OCRA index of exposure. (From Occhipinti, E., 1998. *Ergonomics*, 41:1290–1311. With permission.)

Part B. *Calculation of the index of exposure (IE) for the left upper limb.*

	A	B	C	D	tasks
• **Action frequency constant** (no. of actions/min)	30	30	30	30	C.F.

• **Force factor** (perceived effort)   ×

BORG	0.5	1	1.5	2	2.5	3	3.5	4	4.5	%
FACTOR		1	0.85	0.75	0.65	0.55	0.45	0.35	0.2	0.1	0.01

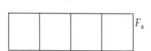 F_s

×

• **Posture factor**

SCORE	0–3	4–7	8–11	12–15	16
FACTOR	1	0.70	0.60	0.50	0.33

SH [ ]	SH [ ]	SH [ ]	SH [ ]	(*)select
EL [ ]	EL [ ]	EL [ ]	EL [ ]	lowest factor
WR [ ]	WR [ ]	WR [ ]	WR [ ]	among elbow,
HA [ ]	HA [ ]	HA [ ]	HA [ ]	wrist
				and hand
(*)	(*)	(*)	(*)	F_p
[——]	[——]	[——]	[——]	

• **Additional items factor**   ×

0	4	8	12
1	0.95	0.90	0.80

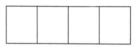 F_a

×

• **Duration of repetitive task** (min)

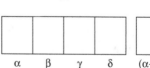

=

π

• **No. of recommended actions per**
repetitive task and totals
(partial result without recovery factor)   α   β   γ   δ   (α+β+γ+δ)

• **Factor for lack of recovery time**
    (No. of hours without adequate recovery)

NO. HOURS	0	1	2	3	4	5	6	7	8
FACTOR	1	0.90	0.80	0.70	0.60	0.45	0.25	0.10	0

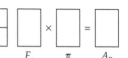

F_c π A_R

$$IE = \frac{\text{Total no. of actions observed in the repetitive tasks}}{\text{Total no. of recommended actions}} = \frac{A_e}{A_r} = \boxed{}$$

FIGURE 8.14 (continued)

The final index of exposure (IE) is then

$$IE = A_e/A_r \qquad (8.22)$$

where A_e = total number of motions observed during the repetitive tasks.

Theoretically, when IE scores are below one, the exposures can be considered acceptable. As the index increases above one, the exposure becomes increasingly hazardous. However, Occhipinti (1998) adopted a three-level classification scheme analogous to the green/amber/red colors of a traffic light. For IE scores below 0.75 (green region), the exposure is acceptable. IE scores ranging between 0.75 and 4.00 (amber region) are borderline significant and need to be monitored more closely. IE scores above 4.00 (red area) are considered significant with corrections to the workplace required.

OCRA was validated over the course of eight studies involving 462 exposed and 749 non-exposed workers (Grieco, 1998). Linear regression by job category of the OCRA IE score with a normalized damage index, total number of WRMSDs divided by the total number of limbs at risk (because some workers had multiple disorders or even multiple disorders for a given limb), yielded a significant correlation ($r^2 = 0.72$, $p = 0.004$). A log transformation yielded an even better relationship ($r^2 = 0.88$, $p = 0.0002$). Although fairly complicated, the OCRA model seems to show promise.

8.5.4 Recent Developments

There has also been ongoing activity by a committee of the American National Standards Institute (ANSI Z-365) to standardize methodology for assessing upper limb WRMSD risks through the use of checklists. Although several working drafts have been released, no definitive methods or tools have been recommended so far. On the other hand, the American Conference on Government Industrial Hygienists has just released a new threshold level value (TLV) to be used in the reduction of WRMSDs (Figure 8.15; ACGIH, 2002). Peak force is estimated by the Borg (1982) CR-10 scale or as a fraction of %MVC, while hand activity level is estimated from a 10-point linear scale with verbal anchors ranging from 0, hands idle most of the time, to 10, rapid steady motion. The top line is the TLV, while the bottom line is an action limit for implementing corrective measures. As this is a new measure, no data are currently available on its reliability or validity.

8.6 Data-Driven Upper Limb WRMSD Risk Index

Another upper limb WRMSD risk assessment index, similar to OCRA, was developed by Seth et al. (1999). However, two main differences distinguish

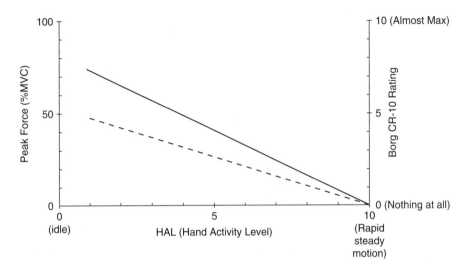

FIGURE 8.15
The TLV for reduction of WRMSDs based on hand activity level. The top line is the TLV, the bottom line is an action level. (Adapted from ACGIH, 2002.)

this tool, termed the CTD Risk Index (available at http://www.ie.psu.edu/courses/ie552/CTDriskindex.htm), from the others previously discussed. First, wrist posture data collected with the Yun et al. (1997) integrated touch glove system (see Section 7.3.3) were fed directly into the model. Second, WRMSD data from industry were used to develop the regression coefficients of the final model to yield a predicted incidence rate. The risk assessment model is presented here in a step-by-step approach.

Wrist deviation and arm rotation cause a significant grip strength decrement as compared to a neutral wrist posture. These effects, from the data of Terrell and Purswell (1976), Imrahn (1991), and Hallbeck et al. (1992), were expressed as equations for MVC for power grip and various pinches produced in five wrist positions (neutral, flexion, extension, radial and ulnar deviation) and in three arm rotations (pronation, midposition, and supination) (Table 8.10). Inputting the appropriate parameters yields the variable *Force Capacity Wrist*. Similarly, force decrements occur for both power and pinch grip depending on the grip span utilized. This effect again can be quantified from the data of Greenberg and Chaffin (1976) and Petrofsky et al. (1980) to yield average grip span strength decrements for spans ranging from 0 to 11 cm as shown in Table 8.11. Inputting the appropriate parameters yields the variable *Grip Span Force*.

Repeated exertions will result in muscle fatigue and reduced capacity for further exertions. This effect can be quantified from the data of Schutz (1972) as the maximum *%MVC Allowed* for a particular wrist motion based on the exertion time for the motion and the time between exertions or motions. If the *%MVC Required* to perform the motion is greater than that allowed as calculated below (*%MVC Allowed*), then a penalty is assessed to that motion.

TABLE 8.10

Force Capacity Wrist Equations

Grip Type	Wrist Position	%MVC as a Function of Wrist Angle A (degrees)
Power	Flexion/Extension/Pronation	$-.0113A^2 + .1826A + 88$
Power	Flexion/Extension/Midposition	$-.0114A^2 + .1308A + 99$
Power	Flexion/Extension/Supination	$-.0112A^2 + .0979A + 100$
Power	Radial/Ulnar Deviation/Pronation	$-.0337A^2 + .025A + 99$
Power	Radial/Ulnar Deviation/Midposition	$-.0538A^2 + .275A + 88$
Power	Radial/Ulnar Deviation/Supination	$-.0338A^2 + .075A + 100$
Lateral Pinch	Flexion/Extension/Supination	$-.0124A^2 + .1905A + 100$
Lateral Pinch	Radial/Ulnar Deviation/Pronation	$-.0409A^2 + .1525A + 100$
Chuck Pinch	Flexion/Extension/Supination	$-.0158A^2 + .2191A + 98$
Chuck Pinch	Radial/Ulnar Deviation/Pronation	$-.0626A^2 + .1275A + 98$
2-Point Pinch	Flexion/Extension/Supination	$-.0114A^2 + .1423A + 72.4$
2-Point Pinch	Radial/Ulnar Deviation/Pronation	$-.00535A^2 + 72.4$

TABLE 8.11

Grip Span Force Equations

Grip Type	%MVC as a Function of Grip Span Width (G in cm)
Power	$-.3624G^3 + 4.6865G^2 - 3.6186G + 14.4$
Lateral Pinch	$-.8308G^2 + 3.0288G + 97.59$
Chuck Pinch	$-.2363G^2 - .7093G + 100.22$
2-Point Pulp Pinch	$-.3931G^2 + 1.6383G + 99.22$

$$\%\text{MVC Allowed} = \left[.9503\,\text{TW}^{-0.394} \times \text{TR}^{0.2246} \times \text{MW}^{0.258} \times 0.475\right] \times 100 \quad (8.23)$$

where

TW = work time of grip or motion (min)
TR = rest time between grips or motions (min)
MW = time worked during one shift (min)

For each motion a *Force Capacity* is calculated as the product of *Force Capacity Wrist* and *Grip Span Force*:

$$\text{Force Capacity} = \text{Force Capacity Wrist} \times \text{Grip Span Force}/100 \quad (8.24)$$

%MVC Required$_{Adj}$ is calculated based on *%MVC Required* to perform the motion and the previously calculated *Force Capacity*. *%MVC Required* is typically found by dividing the subjective job force requirement to the operator's MVC.

$$\%\text{MVC Required}_{Adj} = \%\text{MVC Required}/\text{Force Capacity} \times 100 \quad (8.25)$$

The $\%MVC\ Required_{Adj}$ is then compared to the $\%MVC\ Allowed$ for Equation 8.23. If the $\%MVC\ Allowed$ is greater than the $\%MVC\ Required_{Adj}$, then no penalty is assessed to that hand motion and that motion will have a *Force Frequency Score (FFS)* of one. If the $\%MVC\ Allowed$ is less than the $\%MVC\ Required_{Adj}$, then the FFS_i for that individual motion is calculated as follows:

$$FFS_i = n \times \%\text{MVC Required}_{Adj}/\%\text{MVC Allowed} \quad (8.26)$$

where n = number of hand motions per job cycle.

The FFS_i values for each individual hand motion are then summed to obtain an overall force frequency score:

$$FFS = \sum FFS_i \times N/10{,}000 \quad (8.27)$$

where N = number of job cycles per shift.

The scaling factor of 10,000 is the NIOSH (Hales et al., 1989) maximum recommended number of damaging wrist motions that can be performed in an 8-h shift. The model then assesses which hand has a higher overall *FFS* and uses that value for further calculations.

Gross torso posture of a worker while performing a job is important because awkward postures can lead to fatigue. The resulting fatigue, defined as *%Endurance Capacity*, can be quantified in a manner similar to Equation 8.23:

$$\%\text{Endurance Capacity} = \left\{ 1 - \left[\begin{array}{c} 1.0996 \times F_{MVC}^{1.863} \times \text{TW}^{0.734} \\ \times \text{TR}^{-.413} \times \text{MW}^{0.481} \end{array} \right] \right\} \times 100 \quad (8.28)$$

where
TW   = work time posture held (min)
TR   = rest time between postures (min)
MW   = minutes worked during one shift (min)
F_{MVC} = relative weight, weight held divided by 51 lb (from the NIOSH Lifting Equation; Waters et al., 1993)

Five postures are considered: neck and back flexion, elbow and shoulder flexion, and shoulder abduction. For simplicity's sake (and difficulty interpreting angles from job videotapes), *Points* are assigned to various angles as follows: for back flexion 0 to 10° = 0, 10 to 20° = 1, 20 to 45° = 2, and >45° = 3 points; for neck flexion 0 to 30° = 0, 30 to 45° = 1, 45 to 60° = 2, and >60° = 3 points;

for elbow flexion/extension (with a 90° bent elbow being considered the neutral posture) 10° flexion to 30°extension = 0, everything else is 1 point; for shoulder flexion 0 to 20° = 0, 20 to 45° = 1, 45 to 90° = 2, and >90° = 3 points; and for shoulder abduction 0 to 30° = 0, 30 to 60° = 1, 60 to 90° = 2, >90° = 3 points.

The *Posture Score* for each body part is obtained by multiplying the point value by the *%Endurance Capacity* (Equation 8.28) and dividing the product into 50, which is considered the limit for acceptable fatigue or endurance:

$$\text{Posture Score} = 50 / (\%\text{Endurance Capacity} \times \text{Points}) \qquad (8.29)$$

The *Overall Posture Score* (OPS) is the maximum of individual *Posture Scores* for each joint.

The final risk score is a weighted average *FFS* (Equation 8.2.7) and *OPS* in the form of a predicted incidence rate (*IR*) normalized to 200,000 exposure hours:

$$IR = -3.41\,FFS + 1.87\,OPS \qquad (8.30)$$

Regression of predicted incidence rates against the actual incidence rates experienced on 24 industrial jobs in the garment and the printing industry (involving a total of 288 workers) yielded a significant ($p < 0.001$) linear regression with $r^2 = 0.52$. As a comparison, Moore and Garg's (1995) SI yielded a nonsignificant ($p = 0.2$) regression with $r^2 = 0.17$ as did also the proposed ANSI Z-365 checklist ($r^2 = 0.22$). The only limitations found were for very short cycle jobs (typically under 4-s cycle times), in which any error in miscounting motions could be amplified into a large error for the final predicted incidence rate.

Novice ergonomists (university graduate students) required at least several trials in becoming proficient with the risk assessment model. However, by the 5th trial, average time required for job analysis had decreased to 12 min and test-retest reliability was up to $r^2 = 0.72$. A simplified verison of this risk index has been developed into a paper-and-pencil checklist for use in industry (Figure 8.16), with values greater than 1.0 indicating risk for injury. However, it has not been validated or checked for reliability.

Note that the roughly 48% of the variance unaccounted for was thought to be due to individual differences such as gender, age, physical fitness, etc. and the psychosocial risk factors discussed in Section 6.6. This leads to the need for further modeling efforts utilizing the multivariate tools discussed in Section 6.4.3 (You, 1999).

For convenience, the main upper limb WRMSD risk assessment instruments are summarized in Table 8.12. Also, many of these risk assessment instruments are available as part of an Upper Extremity Assessment tools package from NexGen Ergonomics, Inc. (6600 Trans Canada Highway, Suite 750, Pointe Claire, Quebec, Canada, http://www.nexgenergo.com/).

CTD Risk Index

Job Title:	VCR Counter No.:		Date:	
Job Description:	Department:		Analyst:	
Cycle Time (in minutes; obtain from videotape)				①
$\#Cycle/Day = \dfrac{(480 - Lunch - Breaks)}{CycleTime} =$		②a	③ Larger of ②a or ②b:	
# Parts/Day (if known)		②b		
# Handmotions/Cycle			④	
# Handmotions/Day (③ × ④)			⑤	
Frequency Factor (Divide ⑤ by 10,000) =				

(Circle appropriate condition)	Points			
	0	1	2	3
Working Posture	Sit	Stand		
Hand Posture 1: Pulp Pinch	No	Yes		
Hand Posture 2: Lateral Pinch	No	Yes		
Hand Posture 3: Palm Pinch	No	Yes		
Hand Posture 4: Finger Press	No	Yes		
Hand Posture 5: Power Grip	Yes	No		
Type of Reach	Horizontal	Up/Down		
Hand Deviation 1: Flexion	No	Yes		
Hand Deviation 2: Extension	No	Yes		
Hand Deviation 3: Radial Dev.	No	Yes		
Hand Deviation 4: Ulnar Dev.	No	Yes		
Forearm Rotation	Neutral	In/Out		
Elbow Angle	=90°	≠90°		
Shoulder Abduction	0	<45°	<90°	>90°
Shoulder Flexion	0	<90°	<180°	>180°
Back/Neck Angle	0	<45°	<90°	>90°
Balance	Yes	No		
Total the Points for the Circled Conditions			⑥	
Posture Factor (Divide by ⑥ by 10) =				

Grip or Pinch Force Used on Task	⑦	lbs.	⑨ Divide ⑦ by ⑧:
Max Grip or Pinch Force	⑧	lbs.	
Force Factor (Divide ⑨ by .15) =			

(Circle appropriate condition)	Points			
	0	1	2	3
Sharp Edge	No	Yes		
Glove	No	Yes		
Vibration	No	Yes		
Type of Action	Dynamic	Intermittent	Static	
Temperature	Warm	Cold		
Total the Points for the Circle Conditions			⑩	
Miscellaneous Factor (Divide ⑩ by 3) =				

CTD Risk Index = .3 × (Frequency + Posture + Force Factors) + .1 × (Miscellaneous Factor)

CTD Risk Index = .3 × (+   +   ) + .1 × (   )   =

FIGURE 8.16

A simple CTD risk index. (From Niebel, B. and Freivalds, A., 2003. *Methods, Standards, and Work Design*, New York: McGraw-Hill. With permission.)

TABLE 8.12

Categorization of Upper Extremity WRMSD Risk Assessment Instruments (in order of complexity)

Type of Instrument (Key Ref.)	Equipment Used	Posture (No. of Levels)	Force (No. of Levels)	Frequency (No. of Levels)	Duration per Cycle	Overall Duration	Learning Time	Analysis Time	Test–Retest Reliability	Validity (with Standard)
TLV (ACGIH, 2002)	Paper, pencil	—	10 levels	10 levels	—	One	Very short	Very short	—	—
Upper Extremity Checklist (Keyserling et al., 1993)	Paper, pencil	3 levels	2 levels	2 or 4 levels (2 variations)	2 levels	None	Short	Short	—	$\kappa > 0.7$, 2 of 7; $\kappa < 0.4$, 5 of 7
Strain Index (Moore and Garg, 1995)	Paper, pencil	5 levels	5 levels	5 levels	5 levels	5 levels	Short	Medium	—	86% sensitivity 79% specificity
OCRA (Grieco, 1998; Occhipinti, 1998)	Paper, pencil	2 or 3 levels	10 levels	Count number of motions	5 levels	8 levels	Medium	Medium	—	$r^2 = 0.88$, $p = 0.0002$
CTD Risk Index (Seth et al., 1999)	Touch glove, videotape, PC	Torso, arms = 4 levels, wrist = continuous	Continuous	Count number of motions	Continuous	Continuous	Medium	Medium	$r = 0.72$	$r^2 = 0.52$, $p = 0.001$

Abbreviations: Sh = shoulder, El = elbow, Wr = wrist, A/A = abduction/adduction, F/E = flexion/extension, R/U = radian/ulnar deviation, Ro = rotation, — = unknown or not applicable, * = significant at $p < 0.05$, NS = not significant at $p > 0.05$.

Questions

1. What is the difference between passive and active surveillance? What implications does that have for a research study?
2. What is validity and how can it be further defined?
3. What is reliability and how can it be measured?
4. What does a correlation coefficient of –1 mean? Does it mean that assessment tool under evaluation is worthless?
5. What is a split-half procedure and why is it needed?
6. How can the reliability over time of an assessment tool be established?
7. How can the reliability of an assessment tool between analysts be established?
8. What is the purpose of the kappa statistic? That is, what are its benefits?
9. What procedures can be used to establish the agreement between items or analysts given continuous data?
10. Compare and contrast the two classes of interclass correlation coefficients.
11. Compare and contrast accuracy and precision.
12. How do accuracy and precision of a test relate to the validity and reliability of a test?
13. What is the difference between the sensitivity and specificity of a test?
14. How does signal detection theory relate to the effectiveness of an assessment tool?
15. Discuss the trade-offs of self-reports as compared to direct measurements of occupational risk factors.
16. How does the predictive value of a risk assessment tool vary according to the prevalence of the WRMSD?
17. How may one initially identify the scope of WRMSDs in a workplace?
18. What is the purpose of symptom surveys? Describe some typical approaches.
19. Describe some of the different posture analysis tools. What are the advantages and disadvantages of each?
20. What are the trade-offs in using a paper-and-pencil posture analysis tool such as RULA as opposed to a video-based tool such as VIRA or MVTA?
21. Discuss the trade-offs between using a simple risk assessment instruments such as the ACGIH (2002) TLV and the more complex OCRA?

Problems

8.1. On a 40-question test, the mean passing score is 35 and the variance is 5. What is the Kuder–Richardson measure of reliability for this test?

8.2. A new risk assessment tool is being developed to identify the risk for WRMSDs. In a study, 300 workers are screened by physicians for WRMSDs, yielding 100 confirmed cases. The risk assessment tool yields 200 positives, of which 50 are true positives. Calculate the sensitivity, specificity, and predictive value of this tool.

8.3. A new test is being compared with the gold standard measurement with the following results:

	Gold Standard	
New Test	+	−
+	22	2
−	8	73

What are the sensitivity and specificity?

8.4. Two analysts are comparing their results on a posture assessment tool.

	Analyst B	
Analyst A	+	−
+	82	9
−	8	2

a. What is the percentage agreement?

b. What is the kappa?

c. Is this a reliable tool? That is, is there reasonable agreement between analysts?

8.5. The prevalence of CTS in the general industry is approximately 1.5%. A large NIOSH study will screen approximately 10,000 workers. The sensitivity and specificity associated with this test is thought to be 22.9 and 99.8%, respectively.

a. What is the positive predictive value of this test?

b. What is the negative predictive value of this test?

8.6. An analyst counts the number of deviated wrist motions for eight jobs on April 2 and then repeats the analysis for the same eight jobs on April 19.

a. What is the test-retest reliability for this analysis?

b. What is a potential problem with this approach?

c. How could it be corrected?

Job No.	April 2	April 19
1	2	3
2	1	2
3	4	6
4	1	2
5	5	6
6	2	4
7	6	8
8	3	5

8.7. Two analysts separately estimated the forces required to perform ten different jobs.
   a. What is the Pearson product moment correlation coefficient?
   b. What is the interclass correlation coefficient (Case I)?
   c. Is there good agreement between the analysts?

Job No.	Analyst A	Analyst B
1	20	50
2	10	30
3	40	60
4	10	20
5	50	60
6	20	40
7	60	80
8	40	30
9	60	30
10	30	50

8.8. The ratings of perceived exertion for six different jobs are given below.
   a. Given that four analysts were picked randomly for each job, find a measure of agreement for their ratings.
   b. Given that the same four analysts rated each job, find a measure of agreement for their ratings.
   c. Which approach gives better reliability? Why? Discuss the implications of the results.

Jobs	Analysts			
	A	B	C	D
1	9	2	5	8
2	6	1	3	2
3	8	4	6	8
4	7	1	2	6
5	10	5	6	9
6	6	2	4	7

8.9. Evaluate the following eight jobs, focusing on the right hand and assuming a grip force as stated (videoclips available at http://www.ie.psu.edu/courses/ie327/design.htm): (1) stamping extrusions — 30% MVC; (2) stamping end coupling — 15% MVC; (3) flashlight assembly — 15% MVC; (4) union assembly M 15% MVC; (5) hospital bed rail assembly M 30% MVC; (6) stitching garments — 30% MVC; (7) labeling garments — 15% MVC; (8) cut and tack (garments) — 30% MVC.

    a. Use RULA to evaluate upper limb posture.

    b. Use the ACGIH (2002) TLV limits to evaluate WRMSD risk.

    c. Use the SI to evaluate WRMSD risk.

    d. Use the CTD Risk Index to evaluate WRMSD risk.

    e. Use the simplified CTD Risk Index (Figure 8.16) to evaluate WRMSD risk.

    f. How do the SI, CTD Risk Index, and simplified CTD Risk Index scores compare?

References

ACGIH, 2002. *2002 TLVs and BEIs*, Cincinnati, OH: American Conference of Governmental Industrial Hygienists.

Ainsworth, B.E., Jacobs, D.R., Leon, A.S., Richardson, M.T., and Montoye, H.J., 1993. Assessment of the accuracy of physical activity questionnaire occupational data, *Journal of Occupational Medicine*, 35:1017–1027.

Armstrong, T.J., Chaffin, D.B., and Foulke, J.A., 1979. A methodology for documenting hand positions and forces during manual work, *Journal of Biomechanics*, 12:131–133.

Armstrong, T.J., Foulke, J.A., Joseph, B.S., and Goldstein, S.A., 1982. Investigation of cumulative trauma disorders in a poultry processing plant, *American Industrial Hygiene Association Journal*, 43:103–116.

Baluyutt, R., Genaidy, A.M., Davis, L.S., Shell, R.L., and Simmons, R.J., 1995. Use of visual perception in estimating static postural stresses: magnitudes and sources of error, *Ergonomics*, 38:1841–1850.

Baty, D., Buckle, P.W., and Stubbs, D.A., 1986. Posture recording by direct observation, questionnaire assessment and instrumentation: a comparison based on a recent field study, in Corlett, E.N., Wilson, J., and Manenica, I., Eds., *The Ergonomics of Working Postures*, London: Taylor & Francis, 283–292.

Berdie, D.R., Anderson, J.F., and Niebuhr, M.A., 1986. *Questionnaires: Design and Use*, 2nd ed., Metuchen, N.J: Scarecrow Press.

Bhatnagar, V., Drury, C.G., and Schiro, S.G., 1985. Posture, postural discomfort, and performance, *Human Factors*, 27:189–199.

Borg, G.A.V., 1982. Psychophysical bases of perceived exertion, *Medicine and Science in Sports and Exercise*, 14:377–381.

Boussenna, M., Corlett, E.N., and Pheasant, S.T., 1982. The relation between discomfort and postural loading at the joints, *Ergonomics*, 25:315–322.

Bru, E., Mykletun, R. J., and Svebak, S., 1994. Assessment of musculoskeletal and other health complaints in female hospital staff, *Applied Ergonomics*, 25:101–105.

Buchholz, B., Paquet, V., Punnett, L., Lee, D., and Moir, S., 1996. PATH: a work sampling-based approach to ergonomic job analysis for construction and other non-repetitive work, *Applied Ergonomics*, 27:177–187.

Buckle, P.W., Stubbs, D.A., and Baty, D., 1984. Musculoskeletal disorders, and discomfort. and associated work factors, in Corlett, E.N., Wilson, J., and Manenica, I., Eds., *The Ergonomics of Working Postures*, London: Taylor & Francis, 19–30.

Burt, S. and Punnett, L., 1999. Evaluation of interrater reliability for posture observations in a field study, *Applied Ergonomics*, 30:121–135.

Cameron, J.A., 1996. Assessing work-related body-discomfort: current strategies and a behaviorally oriented assessment tool, *International Journal of Industrial Ergonomics*, 18:389–398.

Cohen, J., 1960. A coefficient of agreement for nominal scales, *Educational and Psychological Measurement*, 20:37–46.

Cohen, J., 1968. Weighted kappa: nominal scale agreement with provision for scaled disagreement or partial credit, *Psychological Bulletin*, 70:213–220.

Colombini, D., 1998. An observational method for classifying exposure to repetitive movements of the upper limbs, *Ergonomics*, 41:1261–1289.

Corlett, E.N, 1995. The evaluation of posture and its effects, in Wilson, J. and Corlett, E.N., Eds., *The Evaluation of Human Work*, 2nd ed., London: Taylor & Francis, 663–699.

Corlett, E.N. and Bishop, R.P., 1976. A technique for assessing postural discomfort, *Ergonomics*, 19:175–182.

Corlett, E.N. and Manenica, I., 1980. The effects and measurement of working postures, *Applied Ergonomics*, 11:7–16.

Corlett, E.N., Madeley, S.J., and Manenica, I., 1979. Posture targetting: a technique for recording working postures, *Ergonomics*, 22:357–366.

Cronbach, L.J., 1951. Coefficient alpha and the internal structure of tests, *Psychometrika*, 16:297–334.

Currier, D.P., 1984. *Elements of Research in Physical Therapy*, Baltimore, MD: Williams & Wilkins.

Deakin, J.M., Stevenson, J.M., Vail, G.R., and Nelson, J.M., 1994. Use of the Nordic Questionnaire in an industrial setting: a case study, *Applied Ergonomics*, 25:182–185.

deLooze, M.P., Toussaint, H.M., Ensink, J., and Mangnus, C., 1994. The validity of visual observations to assess posture in a laboratory-simulated, manual material-handling task, *Ergonomics*, 37:1335–1343.

Dickinson, C.E., Campion, K., Foster, A.F., Newman, S.J., O'Rourke, A.M.T., and Thomas, P.G., 1992. Questionnaire development: an examination of the Nordic Musculoskeletal Questionnaire, *Applied Ergonomics*, 23:197–201.

Fleiss, J.L., 1981. *Statistical Methods for Rates and Proportions*, 2nd ed., New York: John Wiley & Sons, 212–236.

Foreman, T.K., Davies, J.C., and Troup, J.D.G., 1988. A posture and activity classification system using a microcomputer, *International Journal of Industrial Ergonomics*, 2:285–289.

Fraenkel, J.R. and Wallen, N.E., 1996. *How to Design and Evaluate Research in Education*, 3rd ed., New York: McGraw-Hill, 153–169.

Fransson-Hall, C., Gloria, R., Kilbom, Å., and Winkel, J., 1995. A portable ergonomic observation method (PEO) for computerized on-line recording of postures and manual handling, *Applied Ergonomics*, 26:93–100.

Genaidy, A., Al-Shedi, A.A., and Karwowski, W., 1994. Postural stress analysis in industry, *Applied Ergonomics*, 25:77–87.

Genaidy, A.M., Simmons, R.J., Guo, L., and Hidalgo, J.A., 1993. Can visual perception be used to estimate body part angles? *Ergonomics*, 36:323–329.

Greenberg, L., and Chaffin, D.B., 1976. *Workers and Their Tools: A Guide to the Ergonomics of Hand Tools and Small Presses*, Midland, MI: Pendell.

Grieco, A., 1998. Application of the concise exposure index (OCRA) to tasks involving repetitive movements of the upper limbs in a variety of manufacturing industries: preliminary validations, *Ergonomics*, 41:1347–1356.

Hagen, K.B., Magnus, P., and Vetlesen, K., 1998. Neck/shoulder and low-back disorders in the forestry industry: relationship to work tasks and perceived psychosocial job stress, *Ergonomics*, 41:1510–1518.

Hales, T., Habes, D., Fine, L., Hornung, R., and Boiano, J., 1989. Health Hazard Evaluation Report, Bennett Industries, Peotone, IL, HETA 89-146-2049, Cincinnati, OH: National Institute of Occupational Safety and Health.

Hallbeck, M.S., Kamal, M.S., and Harmon, P.E., 1992. The effects of forearm posture, wrist posture and hand on three peak pinch force types, in *Proceedings of the Human Factors and Ergonomics Society 36th Annual Conference*, Santa Monica, CA: Human Factors and Ergonomics Society, 801–805.

Harms-Ringdahl, K., 1986. On assessment of shoulder exercise and load-elicited pain in the cervical spine. Biomechanical analysis of load — EMG — methodological studies of pain provoked by extreme position, *Scandinavian Journal of Rehabilitation Medicine*, Suppl. 14:1–40.

Hedge, A., McCrobie, D., Land, B., Morimoto, S., and Rodriguez, S., 1995. Healthy keyboarding: effects of wrist rests, keyboard trays, and a present tiltdown system on wrist posture, seated posture, and musculoskeletal discomfort, in *Proceedings of the Human Factors and Ergonomics Society 39th Annual Conference*, Santa Monica, CA: Human Factors and Ergonomics Society, 630–634.

Herron, D., 1976. Industrial engineering applications of ABC curves, *Transactions of the American Institute of Industrial Engineers*, 8:210–218.

Hignett, S. and McAtamney, L., 2000. Rapid Entire Body Assessment (REBA), *Applied Ergonomics*, 31:201–205.

Holzmann, P., 1982. ARBAN — a new method for analysis of ergonomic effort, *Applied Ergonomics*, 13:82–86.

Imrahn, S.N., 1991. The influence of wrist posture on different types of pinch strength, *Applied Ergonomics*, 22:379–384.

Juul-Kristensen, B., Fallentin, N., and Ekdahl, C., 1997. Criteria for classification of posture in repetitive work by observation methods: a review, *International Journal of Industrial Ergonomics*, 19:397–411.

Karhu, O., Kansi, P., and Kourinka, I., 1977. Correcting working postures in industry: a practical method for analysis, *Applied Ergonomics*, 8:199–201.

Karhu, O., Härkönen, R., Sorvali, R., and Vepsäläinen, P., 1981. Observing working postures in industry: examples of OWAS application, *Applied Ergonomics*, 12:13–17.

Kemmlert, K., 1995. A method assigned for the identification of ergonomic hazards — PLIBEL, *Applied Ergonomics*, 26:199–211.

Kerlinger, F.N. and Lee, H.B., 2000. *Foundations of Behavioral Research*, New York: Harcourt College Publishers.

Keyserling, W.M., 1986. Postural analysis of the trunk and shoulders in simulated real time, *Ergonomics*, 29:569–583.

Keyserling, W.M. and Witting, S.J., 1988. An analysis of experts ratings of ergonomic stress, *International Journal of Industrial Ergonomics*, 2:291–304.

Keyserling, W.M., Stetson, D.S., Silverstein, B.A., and Brouwer, M.L., 1993. A checklist for evaluating ergonomic risk factors associated with upper extremity cumulative trauma disorders, *Ergonomics*, 36:807–831.

Kilbom, Å., 1994. Assessment of physical exposure in relation to work-related musculoskeletal disorders — what information can be obtained from systematic observations? *Scandinavian Journal of Work, Environment & Health*, 20:30–45.

Kilbom, Å., Persson, J., and Jonsson, B., 1986. Risk factors for work-related disorders of the neck and shoulder — with special emphasis on working postures and movements, in Corlett, E.N., Wilson, J., and Manenica, I., Eds., *The Ergonomics of Working Postures*, London: Taylor & Francis, 44–53.

Kilroy, N. and Dockrell, S., 2000. Ergonomic intervention: its effect on working posture and musculoskeletal symptoms in female biomedical scientists, *British Journal of Biomedical Sciences*, 57:199–206.

Knox, K. and Moore, J.S., 2001. Predictive validity of the Strain Index in turkey processing, *Journal of Occupational and Environmental Medicine*, 43:451–462.

Kotani, K., 1995. Modeling Perception and Production of Force as a Means of Estimating Force Requirements in Industrial Tasks, Ph.D. dissertation, University Park, PA: Pennsylvania State University.

Kuder, G. F. and Richardson, M.W., 1937. The theory of the estimation of test reliability, *Psychometrika*, 2:151–160.

Kuorinka, I., 1983. Subjective discomfort in a simulated repetitive task, *Ergonomics*, 26:1089–1101.

Kuorinka, I., Jonsson, B., Kilbom, Å., Vinterberg, H., Biering-Sørensen, F., Andersson, G., and Jørgensen, K., 1987. Standardised Nordic questionnaires for the analysis of musculoskeletal symptoms, *Applied Ergonomics*, 18:233–237.

Lamb, K.L. and Brodie, D.A., 1990. The assessment of physical activity by leisure-time physical activity questionnaire, *Sports Medicine*, 10:159–180.

Landis, R. and Koch, G.G., 1977. The measurement of observer agreement for categorical data, *Biometrics*, 33:159–174.

Levine, D.W., Simmons, B.P., Koris, M.J., Daltroy, L.H., Hohl, G.G., Fossel, A.H., and Katz, J.N., 1993. A self-administered questionnaire for the assessment of severity of symptoms and functional status in carpal tunnel syndrome, *Journal of Bone and Joint Surgery*, 75A:1585–1592.

Maclure, M., and Willett, W.C., 1987. Misinterpretation and misuse of the kappa statistic, *American Journal of Epidemiology*, 126:161–169.

Mattila, M., Karwowski, W., and Vilkki, M., 1993. Analysis of working postures in hammering tasks on building construction sites using the computerized OWAS method, *Applied Ergonomics*, 24:405–412.

McAtamney, L. and Corlett, E.N., 1993. RULA: a survey method for the investigation of work-related upper limb disorders, *Applied Ergonomics*, 24:91–99.

Moore, J.S. and Garg, A., 1994. Upper extremity disorders in a pork processing plant: relationships between job risk factors and morbidity, *American Industrial Hygiene Association Journal*, 55:703–715.

Moore, J.S. and Garg, A., 1995. The strain index: A proposed method to analyze jobs for risk of distal upper extremity disorders, *American Industrial Hygiene Association Journal*, 56:443–458.

Neely, G., Ljundggren, G., Sylvén, C., and Borg, G., 1992. Comparison between the visual analogue scale (VAS) and category ratio scale (CR-10) for the evaluation of leg exertion, *International Journal of Sports Medicine*, 13:133–136.

Niebel, B. and Freivalds, A., 2003. *Methods, Standards, and Work Design*, New York: McGraw-Hill.

Occhipinti, E., 1998. OCRA: a concise index for the assessment of exposure to repetitive movements of the upper limbs, *Ergonomics*, 41:1290–1311.

OSHA, Occupational Safety and Health Administration, 1990. Ergonomics Program Management Guidelines for Meatpacking Plants, Washington, D.C.: Bureau of National Affairs.

Östlin, P., Wärneryd, B., and Thorslund, M., 1990. Should occupational codes be obtained from census data or from retrospective survey data in studies in occupational health? *Social Indicators Research*, 23:231–246.

Persson, J. and Kilbom, Å., 1983. *VIRA — en enkel videofilmteknik för registering och analys av arbetsställningar och rörelser — Undersökningsrapport*, [VIRA — a simple video technique for recording and analyzing working postures and motions — Research Report], Solna, Sweden: Arbetsmiljöinstitutet.

Petrofsky, J.S., Williams, C., Kamen, G., and Lind, A.R., 1980. The effect of handgrip span on isometric exercise performance, *Ergonomics*, 23:1129–1135.

Price, D.D., McGrath, P.A., Rafii, A., and Buckingham, B., 1983. The validation of visual analogue scales as ratio scale measures for chronic and experimental pain, *Pain*, 17:45–56.

Priel, V.Z., 1974. A numerical definition of posture, *Human Factors*, 16:576–584.

Punnett, L. and Keyserling, W.M., 1987. Exposure to ergonomic stressors in the garment industry: application and critique of job-site work analysis methods, *Ergonomics*, 30:1099–1166.

Radwin, R.G. and Lin, M.L., 1993. An analytical method for characterizing repetitive motion and postural stress using spectral analysis, *Ergonomics*, 36:379–389.

Reading, A.E., 1980. A comparison of pain rating scales, *Journal of Psychosomatic Research*, 24:119–124.

Rohmert, W. and Landau, K., 1983. *A New Technique of Job Analysis*, London: Taylor & Francis.

Rona, R.J. and Mosbech, J., 1989. Validity and repeatability of self-reported occupational and industrial history from patients in EEC countries, *International Journal of Epidemiology*, 18:674–679.

Rossignol, M. and Baetz, J., 1987. Task-related risk factors for spinal injury: validation of a self-administered questionnaire on hospital employees, *Ergonomics*, 30:1531–1540.

Saldana, N., Herrin, G.D., Armstrong, T.J., and Franzblau, A., 1994. A computerized method for assessment of musculoskeletal discomfort in the workforce: a tool for surveillance, *Ergonomics*, 37:1097–1112.

Schutz, R.K., 1972. Cyclic Work-rest Exercises Effect on Continuous Hold Endurance Capability, Ph.D. dissertation, Ann Arbor: University of Michigan.

Seth, V., Weston, R.L., and Freivalds, A., 1999. Development of a cumulative trauma disorder risk assessment model for the upper extremities, *International Journal of Industrial Ergonomics*, 23:281–291.

Shrout, P.E. and Fleiss, J.L., 1979. Intraclass correlations: uses in assessing rater reliability, *Psychological Bulletin*, 86:420–428.

Sperling, L., Dahlman, S., Wikström, L., Kilbom, Å., and Kadefors, R., 1993. A cube model for the classification of work with hand tools and the formulation of functional requirements, *Applied Ergonomics*, 24:212–220.

Spielholz, P., Silverstein, B., and Stuart, M., 1999. Reproducibility of a self-report questionnaire for upper extremity musculoskeletal disorder risk factors, *Applied Ergonomics*, 30:429–433.

Spielholz, P., Silverstein, B., Morgan, M., Checkoway, H., and Kaufman, J., 2001. Comparison of self-report, video observation and direct measurement methods for upper extremity musculoskeletal disorder physical risk factors, *Ergonomics*, 44:588–613.

Stetson, D.S., Keyserling, W.M., Silverstein, B.A., and Leonard, J.A., 1991. Observational analysis of the hand and wrist: a pilot study, *Applied Occupational and Environmental Hygiene*, 6:927–937.

Terrell, R. and Purswell, J.L, 1976. The influence of forearm and wrist orientation on static grip strength as a design criterion for hand tools, in *Proceedings of the Human Factors and Ergonomics Society 36th Annual Conference*, Santa Monica, CA: Human Factors and Ergonomics Society, 28–32.

Thorndike, R.L. and Hagen, E.P., 1977. *Measurement and Evaluation in Psychology and Education*, New York: John Wiley & Sons.

Ulin, S.S., Ways, C.M., Armstrong, T.J., and Snook, S.H., 1990. Perceived exertion and discomfort versus work height with a pistol-shaped screwdriver, *American Industrial Hygiene Association Journal*, 51:588–594.

van der Beek, A.J., van Gaalen, L.C. and Frings-Dresen, M.H.W., 1992. Working postures and activities of lorry drivers: a reliability study of on-site observation and recording on a pocket computer, *Applied Ergonomics*, 23:331–336.

Wangenheim, M., Samuelson, B., and Wos, H., 1986. ARBAN — a force ergonomic analysis method, in Corlett, E.N., Wilson, J., and Manenica, I., Eds., *The Ergonomics of Working Postures*, London: Taylor & Francis, 243–255.

Warwick, D.P. and Lininger, C.A., 1975. *The Sample Survey: Theory and Practice*, New York: McGraw-Hill.

Waters, T.R., Putz-Anderson, V., Garg, A., and Fine, L., 1993. Revised NIOSH equation for the design and evaluation of manual lifting tasks, *Ergonomics*, 36:749–776.

Wiktorin, C., Hjelm, E.W., Winkel, J., and Köster, M., 1996. Reproducibility of a questionnaire for assessment of physical load during work and leisure time, *Journal of Occupational and Environmental Medicine*, 38:190–201.

Wilson, R.C. and Jones, P.W., 1989. A comparison of the visual analogue scale and modified Borg scale for the measurement of dyspnea during exercise, *Clinical Science*, 76:277–282.

Wrigley, T.V., Green, R.A., and Briggs, C.A., 1991. Microcomputer video image processing technology in working posture analysis, *Applied Ergonomics*, 22:2–8.

Yen, T.Y. and Radwin, R.G., 1999. Automated job analysis using upper extremity biomechanical data and template matching, *International Journal of Industrial Ergonomics*, 25:19–28.

Yen, T.Y. and Radwin, R.G., 2002. A comparison between analysis time and inter-analyst reliability using spectral analysis of kinematic data and posture classification, *Applied Ergonomics*, 33:85–93.

You, H., 1999. The Development of a Risk Assessment Model for Carpal Tunnel Syndrome, Ph.D. thesis, University Park, PA: Pennsylvania State University.

You, H., Simmons, Z., Freivalds, A., Kothari, M.J., and Naidu, S.H., 1999. Relationships between clinical symptom severity scales and nerve conduction measures in carpal tunnel syndrome, *Muscle & Nerve*, 22:497–501.

Yun, M.H., Cannon, D., Freivalds, A., and Thomas, G., 1997. An instrumented glove for grasp specification in virtual-reality based point-and-direct telerobotics, *IEEE Transactions on Systems, Man, and Cybernetics, Part B: Cybernetics*, 27: 835–846.

9

Hand Tools

9.1 Introduction

9.1.1 Historical Development of Tools

Tools are as old as the human race itself. The hands and feet could be considered tools given to humans by nature. However, tools as we know them were developed as extensions of the hands and feet to reinforce the range, strength, and effectiveness of these limbs. Thus, early humans, by picking up a stone, could make the fist heavier and harder, to produce a more effective blow. Similarly, by using a stick, a longer and stronger arm was created.

The exact time when humans began to use and to make tools is not known. Leaky (1960), during his excavations in Africa, uncovered evidence that more than a million years ago the prehistoric human was already a toolmaker using stones for chipping and bones for leather work. Similarly, Napier (1962, 1963) indicated that with changing tasks, such as converting from the power to precision grip, there was a similar change in the anatomy of the hand as well as development of tools. An important milestone occurred when the stone tool was provided with a handle some 35,000 years ago. The addition of the handle increased the range and speed of action and increased the kinetic energy for striking tasks (Drillis, 1963). A still later change in tool development occurred with the change in tasks from food gathering to food production. New tools were required and developed accordingly. Surprisingly, many of these tools, with minor improvements and refinements, are still in use today. The reasons for such stagnation could be twofold: either the tool reached an optimal form very quickly with no room for improvement or there was no impetus for further improvement. The latter is the resigned view that, because a tool has been used by so many people for so many years, no further improvement is possible. The former view is obviously not true, as Lehmann (1953) noted the existence of more than 12,000 different styles of shovels in Germany in the 1930s, all essentially used for the same task. Indeed, the last great change in tool development occurred with the start of the Industrial Revolution with a change in task from food production to manufacturing of goods.

9.1.2 Tools and Musculoskeletal Injuries

The parallel development of tools with changing technology has given rise to another problem. The current technology explosion has proceeded too quickly to permit the gradual development of tools appropriate for the new industrial tasks. The instant demands for new and specialized tools to match the needs of technology has, in many cases, bypassed the testing needed to fit these tools to the human users. This has resulted in a variety of hand-tool-generated work stressors — high force, high repetition, poor posture — leading to cumulative trauma and chronic problems, reducing productivity, disabling individuals, and increasing medical costs in the plant (Rothfleisch and Sherman, 1978; Cannon et al., 1981; Silverstein et al., 1987).

Approximately 6% of all compensable work injuries and 10% of all industrial injuries in the United States are caused by the use of hand tools (Mital and Sanghevi, 1986; Aghazadeh and Mital, 1987). This means more than 73,000 injuries involving at least one work day lost, amounting to over $10 billion annually in costs (Bureau of Labor Statistics, 1995). The most injured body parts by both nonpowered and powered hand tools were the upper extremities (59.3 and 51.0%, respectively) followed by back, trunk, and lower extremities. Fingers accounted for 56% of upper extremity injuries or about 30% of all body parts (Aghazadeh and Mital, 1987).

9.1.3 General Tool Principles

An efficient tool has to fulfill basic requirements (Drillis, 1963):

1. It must perform effectively the function for which it is intended. Thus, an axe should convert a maximum amount of its kinetic energy into useful chopping work, separate cleanly wood fibers, and be easily withdrawn.

2. It must be properly proportioned to the body dimensions of the operator to maximize efficiency of human involvement.

3. It must be designed to the strength and work capacity of the operator. Thus, allowances must be made for the gender, training, and physical fitness of the operator.

4. It should not cause undue fatigue, i.e., it should not demand unusual postures or practices that will require more energy expenditure than necessary.

5. It must provide sensory feedback in the form of pressure, some shock, texture, temperature, etc. to the user.

6. The capital and maintenance cost should be reasonable.

9.2   General Biomechanical Considerations of Tools

9.2.1   Anatomy and Types of Grip

As discussed in Chapter 5, the human hand is a complex structure of bones, arteries, nerves, ligaments, and tendons. The fingers are controlled by the extensor carpi and flexor carpi muscles in the forearm. The muscles are connected to the fingers by tendons, which pass through a channel in the wrist formed by the bones of the back of the hand on one side and the transverse carpal ligament on the other. Through this channel, called the carpal tunnel, pass also various arteries and nerves. The bones of the wrist connect to two long bones in the forearm, the ulna and the radius. The radius connects to the thumb side of the wrist and the ulna connects to the little finger side of the wrist. The orientation of the wrist joint allows movement in only two planes, each at 90° to the other. The first movement plane gives rise to palmar flexion and dorsiflexion. The second movement plane gives rise to ulnar and radial deviation. The ulna and radius of the forearm connect to the humerus of the upper arm. The biceps brachii, brachialis, and bracho-radialis control elbow flexion and to some degree supination (outward rotation) of the wrist. The triceps acts as an elbow extensor.

A unique feature of the above upper extremity is the manual dexterity produced by the hand. Napier (1956) defined the prehensile movements of the human hand in terms of a power grip and a precision grip. In a *power grip* the tool, whose axis is more or less perpendicular to the forearm, is held in a clamp formed by the partly flexed fingers and the palm, with opposing pressure applied by the thumb (Figure 9.1). There are three subcategories of the power grip, differentiated by the line of action of force: (1) force parallel to the forearm, as in sawing; (2) force at an angle to the forearm, as in hammering; and (3) torque about the forearm, as when using a screwdriver. As the name implies, the power grip is used for power or for holding heavy objects (Bendz, 1974).

In a *precision grip*, the tool is pinched between the flexor aspects of the fingers and the opposing thumb. The relative position of the thumb and fingers determines how much force is to be applied and provides a sensory surface for receiving feedback necessary to give the precision needed. There are two types of precision grip (Figure 9.1): (1) internal, in which the shaft of the tool (e.g., knife) passes under the thumb and is thus internal to the hand; and (2) external, in which the shaft (e.g., pencil) passes over the thumb and is thus external to the hand (Konz and Johnson, 2000). The precision grip is used for control. There is also the hook grip, which is used to support weight by the fingers only, as in holding a box; a lateral pinch, as in holding a key; and a pulp or tip pinch, depending on whether the pulpy part or the nails of the fingers touch. A finer gradation of grips is also possible, as presented by Kroemer (1986). Note that all of these pinches have a significantly decreased strength capability as compared to the power grip (Table 9.1) and, therefore, large forces should never be applied using pinch grips.

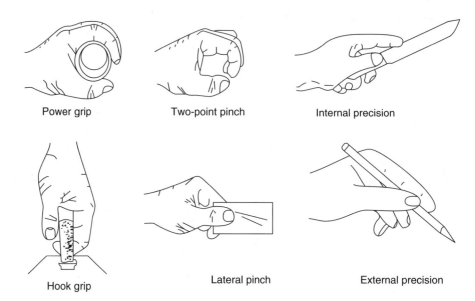

Power grip   Two-point pinch   Internal precision

Hook grip   Lateral pinch   External precision

FIGURE 9.1

Types of grip. (From Freivalds, A., 1999. In Karwowski, W. and Marras, W.S., Eds., *Occupational Ergonomics Handbook*, Boca Raton, FL: CRC Press, 461–478. With permission.)

TABLE 9.1

Relative Forces for Different Types of Grips

Grip	Male (N)	Female (N)	% of Power Grip
Power grip	400	228	100
Tip pinch	65	45	18
Pulp pinch	61	43	17
Lateral pinch	109	76	30

Source: Adapted from An et al. (1986).

9.2.2 The Biomechanics of a Power Grip

One theory of gripping forces has been described by Pheasant and O'Neill (1975) and by Grieve and Pheasant (1982). The hand gripping a cylindrical handle forms a closed system of forces in which portions of the digits and palm are used, in opposition to each other, to exert compressive forces on the handle (Figure 9.2). The strength of the grip (G) may be defined as the sum of all components of forces exerted normal to the surface of the handle:

$$G = \Sigma g \qquad\qquad (9.1)$$

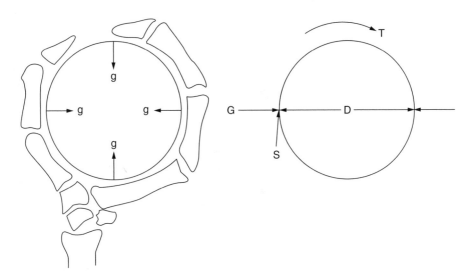

FIGURE 9.2
The mechanics of gripping. (From Freivalds, A., 1987. *International Reviews of Ergonomics*, 1:43–75. With permission.)

When exerting a turning action on the handle, the maximum torque, as given at the moment of hand slippage, is given by

$$T = S \cdot D \tag{9.2}$$

where T = torque, S = total frictional or shear force, and D = handle diameter, and where S can be defined by

$$S = \mu G \tag{9.3}$$

where μ = the coefficient of friction.

Thus, torque is directly dependent on handle diameter and indirectly on diameter squared, since the gripping force also depends on the circumference of the handle gripped. This was confirmed experimentally by Pheasant and O'Neill (1975). For thrusting motions in the direction of the long axis of the handle, the diameter is not involved and determination of maximum force is more complicated. For handles larger than the grip span diameter, the gripped area no longer increases in proportion of the diameter. An analysis of such conditions was performed by Replogle (1983) who concluded that for handles up to twice the grip span diameter the relative ungripped area of the handle increases, reducing the effective gripped area. Torque is then dependent on handle diameter as follows:

$$T = \frac{3d^2 (4 - d)}{(d + 2)^2} \tag{9.4}$$

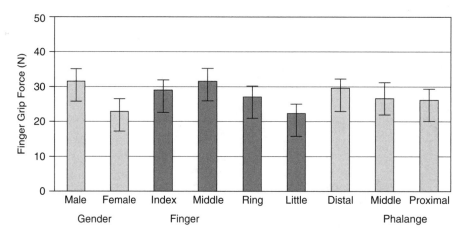

FIGURE 9.3
Finger forces by finger, phalange, and gender. (Adapted from Kong and Freivalds, 2003.)

where d = the ratio of handle diameter to grip span diameter. For larger handle diameters the expression for torque becomes much more complicated (Replogle, 1983).

The individual fingers do not contribute equally to force production in a power grip. The middle finger is the strongest at 28.7% of the grip force, followed by the index, ring, and little fingers, with percentage contributions of 26.5, 24.6, and 20.2%, respectively (Figure 9.3; Kong, 2001; Kong and Freivalds, 2003). Similar values have been found by An et al. (1978), Amis (1987), Ejeskar and Örtengren (1981), Chen (1991), and Radhakrishnan and Nagaravindra (1993).

These different finger force contributions may be explained by the mechanical characteristics of bone and muscle. From the bone point of view, the middle finger is at the center of the hand and longer than the others and, thus, may have mechanical advantage over the other fingers. The index and the ring fingers are located about the same distance from the center of the hand and, consequently, exert a similar amount of force. The little finger is the farthest from the center of the hand and, therefore, may have a mechanical disadvantage over the other fingers when gripping.

From the muscle point of view, each finger has different muscle characteristics such as mass, volume, and length of muscle fibers. Brand et al. (1981) reported that the mass or volume of muscle is proportional to the total work capacity and showed that the flexor digitorum superficialis (FDS) of the middle finger has the largest mass fraction of total weight, followed by the flexor digitorum profundus (FDP) of the middle finger. The FDS of the little finger has the lowest mass fraction. Ketchum et al. (1978) also reported that the FDS of the middle finger was strongest and the combined force of both the superficialis and the profundus tendons was also the strongest in the middle finger, followed by the index, ring, and little fingers.

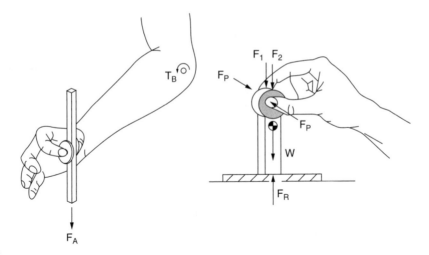

FIGURE 9.4
Forces of a precision grip. (From Lowe, B.D. and Freivalds, A., 1999. *Ergonomics*, 42:550–554. With permission.)

Phalange force distributions are also non-uniform. The force imposed by the distal phalange (35.9%) was significantly higher than that imposed by the middle (32.4%) and the proximal (31.7%) phalanges in the gripping task (Figure 9.3; Kong, 2001; Kong and Freivalds, 2003). These findings are confirmed by An et al. (1978), Amis (1987), Chao et al. (1989), and Lee and Rim (1990). Note that these results only apply to a gripping task. For a pulling task utilizing a power grip, a greater amount of the force is applied by the proximal (37.6%) and middle (33.6%) phalanges and a lesser amount by the distal phalange (28.8%) (Kong, 2001; Kong and Freivalds, 2003). Note also that female power grip force is roughly 70% of the male power grip force (Figure 9.3).

9.2.3 The Biomechanics of a Precision Grip

A precision or pinch grip can be modeled as follows (Figure 9.4). The application force (F_A) is transmitted to the work piece (in addition to the tool weight) through the axis of the tool. In static equilibrium, a reactive force (F_R) is directionally opposite and equal in magnitude to the application force plus the weight of the tool (W):

$$F_R = F_A + W \qquad (9.5)$$

When F_A is applied, the tendency for the reactive force, F_R, to push the tool upward through the grasp is resisted by the frictional forces (F_{f1} and F_{f2}) between the fingertip surfaces and tool grip surface material. The sum of these frictional forces must be greater than the force applied with the tool

(F_A) to resist the slip. In this paradigm, the frictional forces at each digit (F_f) are a result of the pinch forces normal to the tool surface (F_P) multiplied by the static coefficient of friction (μ) between the digital pulpar skin and the tool grip surface material. Further, the forces applied by the thumb and index finger are equal in magnitude and opposite in direction (due to net zero horizontal translation of the tool) so that the total frictional force downward is equal to $2\mu F_P$:

$$F_{f1} + F_{f2} \geq F_R - W \qquad (9.6)$$

$$2\mu F_p \geq F_R - W \qquad (9.7)$$

Provided that the tool does not slip within the grip, $2F_{p(\text{task})}$ must be greater than the minimum pinch force required to prevent slip, $2F_{p(\text{slip})}$. At the instant of slip, $2F_{p(\text{slip})}$ is directionally opposite and equal in magnitude to ($F_R - W$), so the coefficient of friction can be defined by

$$2F_{P(\text{slip})}\mu = F_R - W \qquad (9.8)$$

$$\mu = \frac{F_R - W}{2F_{P(\text{slip})}} \qquad (9.9)$$

Conversely, if μ is known, calculation of the minimum required pinch force (pinch force at slip) as a function of reactive force F_R is

$$F_{p(\text{slip})} = \frac{F_R - W}{2\mu} \qquad (9.10)$$

The pinch force *safety margin* (SM) is defined as the excessive pinch force (sum of thumb and index finger force) exceeding the minimum pinch force resisting slip ($2F_{p(\text{slip})}$):

$$SM = 2F_{p(\text{task})} - 2F_{p(\text{slip})} \qquad (9.11)$$

$$SM = 2F_{p(\text{task})} - \frac{F_R - W}{\mu} \qquad (9.12)$$

The safety margin can be an unreliable measure of excess grip force because it relies on the skin coefficient of friction, which can be difficult to measure and generally is estimated. One can also define a *force ratio* as the ratio of grip to application forces. The force ratio is not dependent on unreliable estimates of frictional coefficients, but, because it is a unitless ratio, it cannot provide any information on the absolute magnitude of excess grip force.

9.2.4   Measurement of Skin Coefficient of Friction

The *coefficient of friction* between the digital pulpar skin and the grip surface has been measured by determining peak shear force as a function of normal (pinch) force (Buchholz et al., 1988). The subjects pinched, between alcohol-cleansed (to remove oils) thumb and index fingertips, an instrumented "tool." Based on visual feedback of force displayed on an oscilloscope, the subjects attempted to maintain a constant normal (pinch) force while slowly pulling upward on the clamped tool, which also measured axial force. As the upward pull force increased, the fingertip shear forces were estimated from axial forces on the tool. Eventually, the fingertips slipped, with the ratio of the maximum axial force immediately preceding the slip to the sum of the two normal forces yielding the coefficient of friction. The coefficients ranged approximately from 0.25 to 0.55 for different materials, with large inter- and intrasubject variabilities. Cloth and suede material exhibited higher values as compared to aluminum. Also, the coefficient of friction was inversely related to the pinch force applied by the digits, decreasing approximately 0.1 per each 30 N of pinch force. The calculation of the coefficient of friction is further complicated by the difficulties subjects had in maintaining a constant pinch force and avoiding the reflexive pinch force increase or a *slip reflex*, which occurs approximately 75 ms after the onset of slip between the fingertips and the object (Cole and Abbs, 1987; Johansson and Westling, 1987).

Later research found very similar results, but with significantly lower values of friction for older adults (Cole, 1991; Lowe and Freivalds, 1999). This could be attributed to the reduced eccrine sweat gland output (Cole, 1991), but with regular cleansing of the fingertip surfaces, this should not be a major factor. An alternative explanation may be related to skin deformation characteristics and changes in the viscoelasticity of the pulpar skin that may occur with age. Young skin viscoelastic properties deviate considerably from Amonton's laws (Comaish and Bottoms, 1971), which aging would only exacerbate. The deviations from Amonton's laws were demonstrated quite dramatically by Bobjer et al. (1993) in measuring coefficients of friction for textured and nontextured surfaces contaminated with oil and lard. In many conditions, they found coefficients of friction well above the theoretical limit of 1.0.

The results also presented trade-off problems for designers of hand tools. Smooth, nontextured handles produced highest coefficients of friction for clean hands ($\mu = 1.4$), but lowest coefficients of friction ($\mu = 0.2$) when the hands were contaminated, as one would reasonably expect. By adding texture, the friction was increased for contaminated conditions, perhaps by channeling them away. However, with normal (cleansed with alcohol) hands, any texture decreased the coefficient of friction, perhaps because of the decreased area of contact with the skin. Perhaps the optimum situation with acceptable coefficients of friction for all conditions (approximately uniform at μ = 0.75) were achieved with a coarse texture of alternating 2-mm ridges and 2-mm grooves (Bobjer et al., 1993).

9.2.5 Grip Force Coordination

Coordination was defined by Athènes and Wings (1989) as "the way in which different motor acts are coupled with regard to their temporal and spatial characteristics to allow for a more efficient motor performance." Neurophysiological studies of grip force coordination in simple lift and hold maneuvers have revealed that individuals apply a higher grip force than demanded by mechanical conditions (mainly friction) of the external object (Johansson and Westling, 1984: Westling and Johansson, 1984). The higher grip force represents a safety margin (Johansson, 1991), or buffer, against unanticipated perturbing forces or slip of the tools from the grip. The minimum ratio of grip force to the load force (external force demand) is governed by mechanical conditions of the hand–object interface and the force, which is transmitted through the grasped object to its external environment. The actual ratio of these forces is scaled above this minimum slip force to achieve an adequate margin of safety. The scaling of the ratio of these forces determines the efficiency of an individual's grip force coordination and represents a clear trade-off between maintaining a margin of safety and minimizing excess grip force on the object.

Under conditions in which there is impairment of the sensory nerves, such as anesthesia of the digital pulpy areas, subjects have experienced difficulties in modulating grip force in parallel with the load force (Johansson et al., 1992). Microneurographic recordings from the afferent tactile mechanoreceptors have shown that cutaneous feedback from these receptors is critical in transmitting information regarding the conditions preceding slip at the grip interface (Westling and Johansson, 1987). When the mechanoreceptors are anesthetized, individuals lose this feedback. Similarly, Cole (1991) observed force coordination impairments in elderly individuals that were attributed to an age-related decrement in tactile sensibility.

Compression neuropathies of the median nerve, such as carpal tunnel syndrome (CTS), result in decreased tactile sensitivity of the thumb and first digits (Jackson and Clifford, 1989) and could be hypothesized to consequently also degrade the ability to coordinate pinch grip, resulting in higher grip force levels. Reviews of epidemiological studies have suggested that force exertions exceeding 15 to 20% of an individual's maximum voluntary contraction (MVC) may be linked with musculoskeletal disorders (MSDs) (Kroemer, 1989, 1992). This suggestion appears to be based on previous findings that force exertions below 15% MVC are associated with an essentially infinite endurance time while recovery periods are needed for larger exertions (Monod and Scherrer, 1965; Rohmert, 1973).

The effects of a deficit in grip force coordination efficiency relative to a 15% MVC threshold are illustrated conceptually in Figure 9.5 (Lowe and

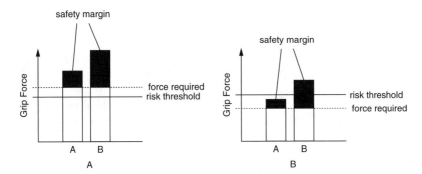

FIGURE 9.5
Conceptual model of the relationship between the required force, safety margin, and risk threshold. (A) Employee B exerts only 29% higher grip force on the tool, but the grip force exceeding the risk threshold is 83% higher than that of employee A. (B) Employee B's grip force, which exceeds the risk threshold, is attributable exclusively to a higher safety margin while employee A's grip force is below the risk threshold. (From Lowe, B.D. and Freivalds, A., 1999. *Ergonomics*, 42:550–554. With permission.)

Freivalds, 1999). Two individuals (A and B) of equivalent maximum strength may actually exert very different grip forces when performing identical tasks. The model illustrates that the employee who exerts a higher grip force as a result of reduced grip force coordination efficiency (higher safety margin) has an amplified risk. When the force requirement is below the risk threshold, an individual with reduced grip force coordination efficiency may apply a grip force above the threshold purely as a result of the safety margin. Those individuals who already are slightly impaired with a median nerve entrapment disorder would exhibit even higher grasp forces and would have even greater risk.

Grip coordination was tested further by Lowe and Freivalds (1999) with an instrumented hand tool (shown in Figure 9.4) on seven patients diagnosed with CTS and seven matched controls. The subjects were required to track a sinusoidal target force (varying both in amplitude and frequency between conditions) presented on an oscilloscope display by applying a tool application force (F_A). The application force and pinch force ($2F_P$) were recorded (Figure 9.6) and used to calculate two measures of grip coordination. The *modulation index* indicated the percentage of maximum pinch force as modulated between the minimum and maximum tool application force:

$$\text{Modulation index} = \frac{F_{P\max(t)} - F_{P\min(t)}}{F_{P\max(t)}} \tag{9.13}$$

The modulation index ranged from 0 (no grip force modulation) to 1 (most efficient grip force modulation). The force ratio represented the ratio of total grip force to the applied force, integrated over one period of the application force cycle:

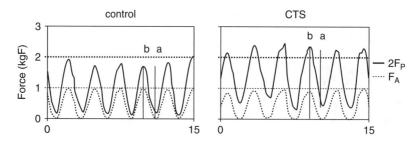

FIGURE 9.6
Grip force ($2F_P$) and application force (F_A) performance for a typical control group subject (left panel) and CTS group subject (right panel). The modulation index is the ratio of the lengths of line segments *a* (difference between maximum and minimum pinch forces) and *b* (peak pinch force). (From Lowe, B.D. and Freivalds, A., 1999. *Ergonomics*, 42:550–554. With permission.)

$$\text{Force ratio} = \int \frac{2F_{P(t)}dt}{F_{R(t)}} \tag{9.14}$$

On average, the CTS group exerted significantly higher pinch forces at equivalent levels of application force (Figure 9.7A) and modulated their grip force less (Figure 9.6), indicating a lower efficiency of grip force coordination. More specifically, the mean value for the modulation index was 12.4% lower for the CTS group, while the force ratio was 54% higher for the CTS group (Figure 9.7B). The link between median nerve compression and decreased grip coordination is hypothesized to be an adaptive, compensatory rescaling of the force ratio to a higher safety margin. The increased force ratio (and safety margin) serves as a larger buffer against localized slips, which may be "undetected" by a less sensitive afferent system. The higher grip forces indicate higher flexor tendon forces as they glide within the carpal tunnel, further aggravating the compression of the medium nerve through the tendon–pulley model (see Section 5.2). For example, Chao et al. (1976) estimated the flexor digitorum profundus tendon forces to be 4.32 times the external force measured at the fingertip. A 54% average increase in the force ratio for patients with CTS as compared to controls would now yield tendon forces as great as 6.5 times the external force, further accelerating the risk for further injury. However, by increasing the friction characteristics of the tool surface (in this case, suede material), the force ratio for the patients with CTS was reduced significantly, almost to the same level as found in controls (Lowe and Freivalds, 1999).

9.2.6 Static Muscle Loading

When tools are used in situations in which the arms must be elevated or tools must be held for extended periods, muscles of the shoulders, arms,

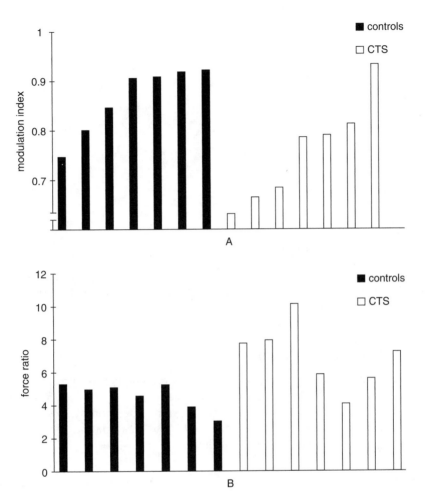

FIGURE 9.7
(A) Mean modulation indices. (B) Mean force ratios. Each bar is the subject's mean for 24 trials. (From Lowe, B.D. and Freivalds, A., 1999. *Ergonomics*, 42:550–554. With permission.)

and hands may be loaded statically, resulting in fatigue, reduced work capacity, and soreness. Abduction of the shoulder with corresponding elevation of the elbow will occur if work must be done with a straight tool on a horizontal workplace. An angled tool reduces the need to raise the arm (Eastman Kodak, 1983). A good example of such a tool is the redesigned soldering iron described by Tichauer and Gage (1977).

Prolonged work with arms extended can produce soreness in the forearm for assembly tasks done with force. By rearranging the workplace so as to keep the elbows at 90°, most of the problem can be eliminated (Figure 9.8). Similarly, continuous holding of an activation switch can result in fatigue of the fingers and reduced flexibility. Thus, tool activation forces should be kept low to reduce this loading, or a power grip bar instead of a single-finger

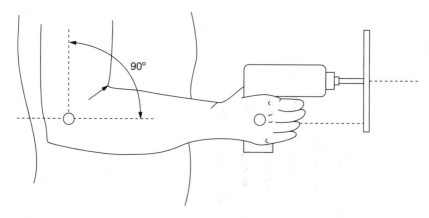

FIGURE 9.8
Optimum working posture with elbow bent at 90°.

trigger should be used. For a two-handled tool, a spring-loaded return saves the fingers from having to return the tool to its starting position (Eastman Kodak, 1983).

9.2.7   Awkward Wrist Position

As the wrist is moved from its neutral position there is loss of grip strength (Terrell and Purswell, 1970). Starting from a neutral wrist position, full pronation decreases grip strength by 12%, full flexion/extension by 25%, and full radial/ulnar deviation by 15% (Figure 9.9). This degradation of maximum grip strength available can be quantified by

$$\% \text{ Grip Strength} = 95.7 + 4.3\,PS + 3.8\,FE - 25.2\,FE^2 - 16.8\,RU^2 \quad (9.15)$$

where
PS = 1 if the wrist is fully pronated or supinated and 0 if in a neutral position
FE = 1 if the wrist is fully flexed or extended and 0 if in a neutral position
RU = 1 if the wrist is fully in radial or ulnar deviate and 0 if in a neutral position

Furthermore, awkward hand positions may result in soreness of the wrist, loss of grip, and, if sustained for extended periods of time, occurrence of WRMSDs. To reduce this problem, the workplace of the tools should be redesigned to allow for a straight wrist, i.e., lowering work surfaces and edges of containers, tilting jigs toward the hand, etc., using a pistol grip on knives (Armstrong et al., 1982), using a pistol handle on powered tools for vertical surfaces and in-line handles for horizontal surfaces (Armstrong, 1983), and putting a bend in the tool handle to reflect the axis of grasp such as the Tichauer and Gage (1977) pliers.

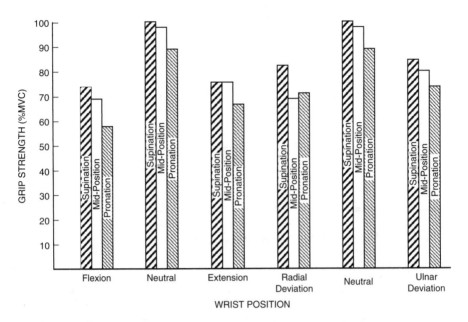

FIGURE 9.9
Grip strength as a function of wrist and forearm position. (Adapted from Terrell and Purswell, 1976.)

9.2.8 Tissue Compression

Often in the operation of a hand tool considerable force is applied by the hand. Such actions can concentrate considerable compressive force on the palm of the hand or the fingers, resulting in ischemia, obstruction of blood flow to the tissues, and eventual numbness and tingling of the fingers. Handles should be designed to have large contact surfaces to distribute the force over a larger area or to direct it to less sensitive areas such as the tissue between the thumb and index finger. Similarly, finger grooves or recesses in tool handles should be avoided. Because hands vary considerably in size, the grooves will accommodate a fraction of the population (McCormick and Sanders, 1982).

9.2.9 Repetitive Finger Action

If the index finger is used excessively for operating triggers, symptoms of trigger finger develop. Trigger forces should be kept low, preferably below 10 N (Eastman Kodak, 1983), to reduce the load on the index finger. Two- or three-finger-operated controls are preferable. Finger strip controls are even better, because they require the use of more and stronger fingers. Absolute finger flexion strengths are shown in Table 9.2.

TABLE 9.2

Maximal Static Finger Flexion Forces

Digit	Max Force (N)	% of Force of Thumb
Thumb	73	100
Index	59	81
Middle	64	88
Ring	50	69
Little	32	44

Source: Adapted from Hertzberg (1973).

9.3   Handles for Single-Handled Tools

9.3.1   Handle Length

A cutout handle should be large enough to provide space for all four fingers. Hand breadth across the metacarpals ranges from 71 mm for a 5% female to 97 mm for a 95% male (Garrett, 1971). Thus, 100 mm may be a reasonable minimum, but 125 mm may be more comfortable (Konz and Johnson, 2000). Eastman Kodak (1983) recommended 120 mm. If the grip is enclosed or gloves are used, even larger openings are recommended. For an external precision grip, the tool shaft must be long enough to be supported at the base of the first finger or thumb. A minimum value of 100 mm is suggested (Konz and Johnson, 2000). For an internal precision grip, the tool should extend past the palm, but not so far as to hit the wrist (Konz and Johnson, 2000). It is interesting to note that screwdriver torque was experimentally found to be proportional to the handle grip length (Magill and Konz, 1986).

9.3.2   Handle Diameter

For a power grip on screwdrivers Rubarth (1928) recommended a diameter of 40 mm. Basing their recommendation on empirical judgments of stair rails, Hall and Bernett (1956) suggested 32 mm. Based on minimum EMG activity, Ayoub and LoPresti (1971) found a 51-mm handle diameter to be best. However, based on the maximum number of work cycles completed before fatigue and on the ratio of grip force to EMG activity, they suggested a 38-mm diameter. Pheasant and O'Neill (1975) found that muscle strength deteriorates when using handles greater than 50 mm in diameter. Rigby (1973), for full encirclement of the hand and heavy loads, recommended 38 mm. For handles on boxes, Drury (1980) found diameters of 31 to 38 mm to be best in terms of least reduction in grip strength. Using various handles of noncircular cross section, Cochran and Riley (1982, 1986b) found largest thrust forces in handles of 130-mm circumference (or 41.4-mm equivalent circular diameter) for both males and females. For manipulation, however, the smallest handles of 22 mm were found to be best (Cochran and Riley, 1983). Replogle (1983), in validating his gripping model, found maximum torques at twice the grip span diameter. With average spans of about 25 mm, this yields a handle diameter of 50 mm. Eastman Kodak (1983), based on company experiences, recommended 30 to 40 mm with an optimum of 40 mm for power grips and 8 to 16 mm with an optimum of 12 mm for precision grips.

Based on the above data, one could summarize that handle diameters should be in the range of 31 to 50 mm with the upper end best for maximum torque and the lower end for dexterity and speed. However, it would also be best to size the handle to each individual's hand. This was first succinctly observed by Fox (1957) in that a handle that allows some overlap between the thumb and index finger may be better than a larger handle that matches the individual's grip diameter. Grant et al. (1992) later confirmed that handles 1 cm smaller than the inside grip diameter maximized grip strength as compared to handles 1 cm larger or those matching the inside grip diameter.

Kong (2001) and Kong et al. (in press) went further by defining normalized handle size (NHS) as the ratio of the handle circumference to hand length, as measured from the wrist crease to the tip of the middle finger. In the study, 30 subjects, ranging from 5th percentile females to 95th percentile males, with hand lengths ranging from 160 to 205 mm, gripped a variety of handle sizes in several different tasks. This resulted in NHS ranging from 45 to 90%. Maximum grip forces and minimum subjective ratings of perceived exertion were obtained roughly in the range of 50 to 55% NHS or absolute handle sizes in the range of 30.6 to 39.2 mm, depending on the individual's hand length. A more detailed analysis indicated that a better match yet is for the handle size to conform to individual finger lengths, with the ratio of the handle circumference to the length of finger ranging from 90 to 110%. This would result in a handle that is of an asymmetrical double frustum shape, described further in the next section.

9.3.3 Handle Shape

As early as 1928, Rubarth investigated handle shape and concluded that, for a power grip, one should design for maximum surface contact so as to minimize unit pressure of the hand. Thus, a tool with a circular cross section was found to give largest torque. Pheasant and O'Neill (1975) concluded that the precise shape of handles was irrelevant and recommended simple knurled cylinders. Evaluation of handle shape on grip fatigue in manual lifting (which is a different action from that for tool use) did not indicate any significant differences in shapes (Scheller, 1983). Maximum pull force, however, was obtained with a triangular cross section, apex down. For thrusting forces, the circular cross section was found to be worst and a triangular best (Cochran and Riley, 1982). However, for a rolling type of

TABLE 9.3

Recommended Sizes for a Set of Four Double Frustum Handles

Handle Feature	Small	Medium	Large	Extra Large
Large top end	22.7	25.5	28.5	31.3
Connecting middle part	30.6	33.4	36.4	39.2
Small bottom end	12.7	15.4	18.4	21.3

manipulation, the triangular shape was slowest (Cochran and Riley, 1983). A more comprehensive study indicated that no one shape may be perfect, and that shape may be more dependent on the type of task and motions involved than initially thought (Cochran and Riley, 1986b). A rectangular shape of width:height ratios, from 1:1.25 to 1:1.50 appeared to be a good compromise. A further advantage of a rectangular cross section is that the tool does not roll when placed on a table (Konz and Johnson, 2000). It should also be noted that handles should not have the shape of a true cylinder except for a hook grip. For screwdriver type tools, the handle end is rounded to prevent undue pressure at the palm and for hammer type tools the handle may have some flattening curving to indicate the end of the handle.

In a departure from the circular, cylindrically shaped handles, Bullinger and Solf (1979) proposed a more radical design using a hexagonal cross section, shaped as two truncated cones joined at the largest ends. Such a shape fits the contours of the palm and thumb best in both precision and power grips and yielded highest torques (9 Nm) in comparison with more conventional handles. A more detailed study by Kong (2001) and Kong et al. (in press) identified four asymmetric double frustum cone handle sizes that would fit most of the adult population:

Small, corresponding to a 5th percentile female hand (160 mm)

Medium, corresponding to a 50th percentile female/5th percentile male hand (175 mm)

Large, corresponding to a 50th percentile male/95th percentile female hand (190 mm)

Extra large, corresponding to a 95th percentile male hand (205 mm)

The double frustum shape, with thick ends joined, allows one handle to fit all four fingers naturally. The index and middle fingers are larger; thus the slant of the top cone is less (6.9°) than for the bottom cone (15.4°). The total length of the handle is 130 mm, i.e., 65 mm for each cone. Specific diameters (mm) for each of the four handles are given in Table 9.3.

A final note on shape is that T-handles yield much better performance than straight screwdriver handles; Pheasant and O'Neill (1975) reported as much as 50% increase in torque. Optimum handle diameter was found to be 25 mm and optimum angle was 60°, i.e., a slanted T (Saran, 1973). The slant allows the wrist to remain straight and thus generate larger forces.

9.3.4 Texture and Materials

For centuries wood was the material of choice for tool handles. Wood was readily available, and easily worked. It has good resistance to shock and to thermal and electrical conductivity and has good frictional qualities even when wet. Because wooden handles can break and stain with grease and oil, there has been a shift to plastic and even metal. Plastic handles are typically knurled or cross-hatched with grooves to improve the hand/tool frictional interface (Pheasant and O'Neill, 1975).

Such grooved fiberglass handles were evaluated with respect to traditional wooden handles by Chang et al. (1999). Although the focus was primarily on weight and efficiency of shoveling, with hollow handles requiring 12% less energy expenditure than solid handles, the subjects rated the grooved fiberglass handles more acceptable than wooden handles in terms of tactile feeling and slipperiness.

Metal should be covered with rubber or leather to reduce shock and electrical conductance and increase friction (Fraser, 1980). Such a resilient covering may also aid in the reduction of hand discomfort. Fellows and Freivalds (1991) found that a 4-mm foam covering on wooden-handled garden tools provided a significantly more uniform grip force distribution and lower ratings of perceived discomfort as compared to plain wooden handles. Unfortunately, in most cases, the total grip forces were higher for the foam-covered handles due to an excessive deformation of the foam and a feeling of "loss of control" in the subjects. The authors hypothesized that a thinner layer of foam would have provided more control, but still maintained a better grip force distribution.

9.3.5 Angulation of Handle

As discussed in Section 9.2.7, deviations of the wrist from the neutral position under repetitive load can lead to a variety of cumulative trauma disorders as well as decreased grip strength (Figure 9.9). Therefore, angulation of tool handles, e.g., power tools, may be necessary so as to maintain a straight wrist. The handle should reflect the axis of grasp, i.e., about 78° from the horizontal, and should be oriented so that the eventual tool axis is in line with the index finger (Fraser, 1980). This principle was first applied to pliers (Figure 9.10) by Tichauer and Gage (1977) and then later to soldering irons, knives, and other tools.

An interesting extension of this concept has been promoted as Bennett's handle (Emanuel et al., 1980). Bennett developed this concept based on the angle formed by the index finger and the life line under the thumb. This angle of 19°, used for his handles, is claimed to maintain a straight wrist, generate increased strength, and control and reduce stress, shock, and fatigue (Bennett Ergonomic Labs, 1983). Bennett's claims initially were supported by anecdotal evidence of improved performance by various individuals (Emanuel et al., 1980). Since then, Konz and colleagues (Granada and Konz,

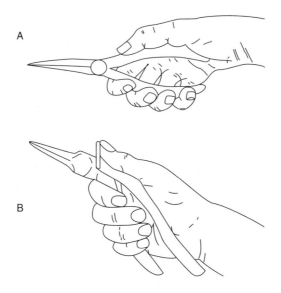

FIGURE 9.10

(A) Conventional pliers causing ulnar deviation. (B) Ergonomically redesigned pliers allowing the hand to work in line with the forearm. (From Freivalds, A., 1987. *International Reviews of Ergonomics*, 1:43–75. With permission.)

1981; Krohn and Konz, 1982; Konz and Streets, 1984; Konz, 1986) have conducted a variety of tests to evaluate the effectiveness of Bennett's handle on a hammer in comparison with a standard hammer. In the second study a variety of angled handles were evaluated and subjects rated a 10° bend as most preferred. In the third study, performance in driving nails was evaluated using various bent hammers. No performance difference was found. The 10° bend was again rated significantly higher. In the final study using a semantic-differential questionnaire, Konz (1986) concluded that although no significant performance effects were found, subjects preferred a slight (5 to 10°) bend rather than the 19° of Bennett's handle. An independent study by Knowlton and Gilbert (1983) used cinematography to evaluate a curved and conventional claw hammer. Bilateral grip strength was measured before and after a task, nail driving. The curved hammer produced a smaller strength decrement and caused less ulnar deviation than the hammer. Thus, a bent handle does give some benefits.

9.4 Handles for Two-Handled Tools

9.4.1 Grip Span

Grip strength and the resulting stress on finger flexor tendons vary with the size of the object being grasped. A maximum grip strength is achieved at

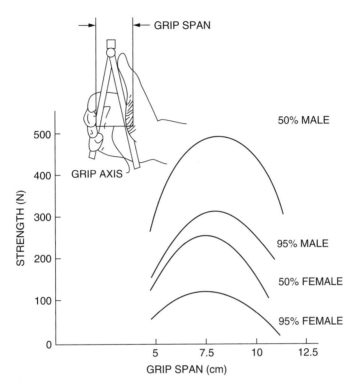

FIGURE 9.11
Grip strength capability for various grip spans. (From Greenberg, L. and Chaffin, D.B., 1976. *Workers and Their Tools*, Midland, MI: Pendell. With permission.)

about 45 to 80 mm (Pheasant and Scriven, 1983; Chaffin et al., 1999). The smaller values of 45 mm were obtained on a dynamometer with parallel sides (Pheasant and Scriven, 1983), whereas the larger values of 75 to 80 mm were obtained on a dynamometer with handles angled inward (Figure 9.9). This relationship can be modeled as

$$\% \text{ Grip Strength} = 100 - 0.11 * S - 10.2 * S^2 \qquad (9.16)$$

where S = given grip span minus optimum grip span in cm.

Also, as shown in Figure 9.11, there is quite a large variation in strength capacity over the population. To accommodate this population variability, maximal grip requirements should be limited to less than 90 N.

A similar effect is found for pinch strength (Figure 9.12). However, the overall four-point pulp pinch force is a much more reduced force level (approximately 17% of power grip; see Figure 9.10 for other types of pinches) and drops sharply beyond a 4- to 5-cm pinch span (Heffernan and Freivalds, 2000).

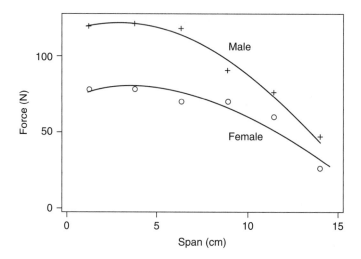

FIGURE 9.12
Pulp pinch strength capability for various grip spans. (Adapted from Heffernan and Freivalds, 2000.)

9.4.2 Gender

Female grip strength typically ranges from 50 to 67% of male grip strength (Konz and Johnson, 2000; Pheasant and Scriven, 1983; Chaffin et al., 1999); i.e., the average male can be expected to exert approximately 500 N while the average female can be expected to exert approximately 250 N. An interesting survey by Ducharme (1975) examined how tools and equipment that were physically inadequate for female workers hampered their performance. The worst offenders were crimpers, wire strippers, and soldering irons. Females have a twofold disadvantage — an average lower strength and an average smaller grip span. Ducharme concluded that women could be integrated more quickly and safely into the work if tools were designed to accommodate smaller dimensions.

On the other hand, Pheasant and Scriven (1983) challenged Ducharme's assertions based on their findings that optimal performance for both males and females occurred at similar conditions. Males had sufficient strength to overcome the deficiencies in tool design, which posed much greater problems for females.

9.4.3 Handedness

Alternating hands permits reduction of local muscle fatigue. However, in many situations this is not possible as the tool use is one-handed. Furthermore, if the tool is designated for the user's preferred hand, which for 90%

of the population is the right hand, then 10% are left out (Konz, 1974). Laveson and Meyer (1976) gave several good examples of right-handed tools that cannot be used by a left-handed person, i.e., a power drill with side handle on the left side only, a circular saw, and a serrated knife leveled on one side only.

A few studies have compared task performance using dominant and non-dominant hands. Shock (1962) indicated the nonpreferred hand grip strength to be 80% of the preferred hand grip strength. Miller and Freivalds (1987) found right-handed males to show a 12% strength decrement in the left hand while right-handed females showed a 7% strength decrement. Surprisingly, both left-handed males and females had nearly equal strengths in both hands. They concluded that left-handed subjects were forced to adapt to a right-handed world. Using time study ratings, Konz and Warraich (1985) found decrements, ranging from 9% for an electric drill to 48% for manual scissors, for ratings using the nonpreferred hand as opposed to the preferred hand.

9.5   Other Tool Considerations

9.5.1   Posture

A series of studies were performed by Mital and colleagues to examine various tool and operator factors on torque capability (Mital, 1985, 1986; Mital et al., 1985; Mital and Sanghavi, 1986). In general, unless the posture is extreme, i.e., standing vs. lying, torque exertion capability was not affected substantially. The height at which torque was applied had no influence on peak torque exertion capability. On the other hand, torque exertion capability decreased linearly with increasing reach distance. Another interesting requirement for proper tool usage is the volume or space envelope generated during operation of the tool. Comprehensive data on a variety of tools have been collected by Baker et al. (1960).

9.5.2   Weight

The weight of a hand tool will determine how long it can be held or used and how precisely it can be manipulated. For tools held in one hand with the elbow at 90° for extended periods of time, Greenberg and Chaffin (1976) recommend a load of no more than 2.3 kg. A similar value is suggested by Eastman Kodak (1983). For precision operations, tool weights greater than 0.4 kg are not recommended unless a counterbalanced system is used. Heavy tools, used to absorb impact or vibration, should be mounted on a truck to reduce effort for the operator (Eastman Kodak, 1983).

9.5.3   Gloves

Gloves are often used with hand tools for safety and comfort. Safety gloves are seldom bulky, but gloves worn in subfreezing climates can be very heavy and interfere with grasping ability. Wearing woolen or leather gloves may add 5 mm to the hand thickness and 8 mm to the handbreadth at the thumb, while heavy mittens add 25 and 40 mm, respectively (Damon et al., 1966). A study on the effects of wearing different gloves on manual performance was performed by Weidman (1970). Neoprene gloves slowed performance times by 12.5% over barehanded performance, terry cloth by 36%, leather by 45%, and PVC by 64%. In some cases, by protecting the hand, gloves could improve operational speed (Bradley, 1969a,b). On the other hand, gloves consistently reduced torque production (Swain et al., 1970). Thus, there is a trade-off to be considered between increased injury and reduced performance without gloves and reduced performance with gloves. Perhaps the tool should be redesigned even more.

9.5.4   Vibration

Vibration is a separate and very complex problem with powered hand tools. Vibration can induce white finger syndrome, the primary symptom of which is a reduction in blood flow to the fingers and hand due to vasoconstriction of the blood vessels. As a result there is loss of sensory feedback and decreased performance. The effect is dependent on the root-mean square (RMS) level of the vibration, characteristic frequencies, and individual susceptibility to the condition. It is a very complex and separate problem that is discussed in other sources (McCormick and Sanders, 1982).

9.5.5   Rhythm

The operation of hand tools involves repetition of a particular pattern of motion. A skilled operator acquires a basic motor pattern that will be most economical in terms of energy expenditure and is thus one attribute of skill. Once this pattern is established, it is continued with very consistent velocity and acceleration through kinesthetic and aural feedback. Optimum rhythms have been observed by Drillis (1963) as follows: filing, 78 strokes/min; chiseling, 60 strokes/min; shoveling, 14 to 17 strokes/min; and cranking, 35 revolutions/min.

9.5.6   Miscellaneous

Tools should not have protruding sharp edges or corners. Two-handed tools should have stop limits to limit closure of the tools and prevent pinching of the fingers. Locking tools should not engage until the tool closes to the point where the fingers cannot be inserted. Tool surfaces should have matted surfaces to reduce glare (Fraser, 1980). Further details on efficient tool design can be found in Freivalds (1999).

9.6 Agricultural and Forestry Tools

9.6.1 Shovels and Spades

Spades are used to cut turf and lift and turn soil, while shovels are used to lift, move, and toss loose soil or grain. The blade is fastened to the shaft through a socket, which, if stamped from a flat sheet, is generally rolled over to form a crimp known as a frog. This produces a compensating hollow in the back, yielding a hollow-back socket. The shaft may either taper to an end or have a handle. The handle traditionally has been of a T form, but more lately of a D form. Long spade shafts are generally 1.2 to 1.27 m long, while the short D handle is about 0.7 m long. The angle of the shaft with respect to the blade horizontal is called the lift and provides the tool with added leverage.

The task of shoveling was first examined scientifically at the Bethlehem Steel Works in 1898 (Taylor, 1913; Copley, 1923) by Taylor, who found that maximum performance was attained using a load of 9.7 kg. Since then, many studies have examined various aspects of shoveling. The results of these studies are summarized by the particular feature investigated.

9.6.1.1 Shoveling Rate

Most studies (Lehmann, 1953; Dressel et al., 1954; Müller and Karrasch, 1956; Wyndham et al., 1966) consistently agreed on a high rate of shoveling in the range of 18 to 21 scoops/min. Adjusted data from the two most complete studies (Lehmann, 1953; Müller and Karrasch, 1956) are plotted in Figure 9.13. Although quite different in other aspects, both data sets clearly show increasing efficiency with increasing shoveling rates. The effect levels out at higher rates, and, with other factors such as recovery pulse rate tending to limit shoveling rates, values of 18 to 21 scoops/min are quite reasonable. This result can be explained primarily by the ergonomic principle of utilizing frequent and short work–rest cycles to gain maximum benefit from exponential recovery curves.

9.6.1.2 Shovel Load

The consensus on shovel load is not as clear as for shoveling rate. The range for an optimum load is 5 to 11 kg, depending on the decision criterion, the shoveling rate, and the weight of the shovel used (which was not always specified). Thus, based on shoveling performance, Taylor (1913) recommended a 9.7 kg load. Wenzig (1928, 1932), using efficiency as the criterion,

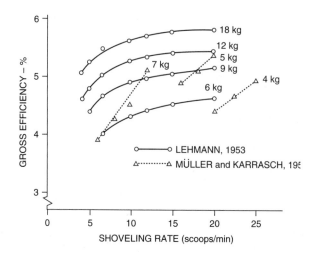

FIGURE 9.13

Efficiency of shoveling as a function of shoveling rate and load. (From Freivalds, A., 1986. *Ergonomics,* 29:3–18. With permission.)

indicated 7 to 8 kg to be optimum for a rate of 8 scoops/min. Kommerell (1929) indicated 11 kg for low rates of 5 to 8 scoops/min. Spitzer (1950) and Dressel et al. (1954) recommended 8 kg for faster rates of 15 to 20 scoops/ min. Müller and Karrasch (1956) indicated 5 kg, based on a heart rate recovery. For constrained mining conditions, Wyndham et al. (1969) specified 6.8 kg at 5 to 6 scoops/min. Adjusted data from the two most complete studies (Lehmann, 1953; Müller and Karrasch, 1956) are also plotted in Figure 9.13. The results are quite different. Lehmann's data indicate increasing efficiency with increasing loads. However, the concomitant increased static load gives rise to increased circulatory stress in the form of increased heart rate. Thus, Müller and Karrasch (1956) used recovery pulse rate as a second criterion. Maximizing efficiency given constrained recovery pulse rates yielded optimum loads between 5 and 7 kg. Thus, for high rates of shoveling (18 to 20 scoops/min), the lower end of the load range (5 to 7 kg) may be more appropriate (which follows the principles of reducing static loading on the circulatory system) while for lower rates (6 to 8 scoops/min), the higher end of the load range (8 kg) may be acceptable (which follows the principles of increasing efficiency with larger loads).

9.6.1.3 Throw Height

Two conflicting decision criteria are found in the literature. Increasing the throw height, especially above 1 m, increased the efficiency of the shoveling task (Wenzig, 1928, 1932; Spitzer, 1950), as shown in Figure 9.14. However, it also increased total energy expenditure rate ($\dot{E}$). Thus, if reasonably possible considering task constraints, the throw height should be reduced, e.g., a reduction in height from 2 to 0.5 m reduced $\dot{E}$ by 50% (Spitzer, 1950). On

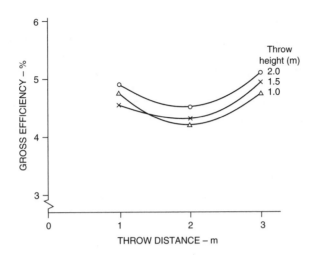

FIGURE 9.14
Efficiency of shoveling as a function of throw height and throw distance. (From Freivalds, A., 1986. *Ergonomics*, 29:3–18. With permission.)

the other hand, as the shoveling performance was reasonably constant to a height of 1.3 m (Stevenson and Brown, 1923), an acceptable throw height may be as high as 1 to 1.3 m.

9.6.1.4   Throw Distance

The same conflicting criteria that apply to throw height also apply to throw distance. Wenzig (1928, 1932) and Spitzer (1950) found minimum efficiency at a distance of 2 m with steadily increasing efficiencies thereafter, as shown in Figure 9.14. Again, however, energy expenditure increased correspondingly. Stevenson and Brown (1923) observed uniform shoveling performance up to a distance of 1.22 m. As these lower distances have a lower $\dot{E}$ and a greater efficiency than at 2 m (due to the incomplete utilization of necessary body movements), then throw distances of up to 1.2 m may be optimum.

9.6.1.5   Posture

Constraining the posture used in shoveling (typically by decreasing the height of the workspace, as in a low-seam mine) increases the energy expended as well as decreases the efficiency of the task. Thus, lowering the working height from 1.2 to 1.0 m increased $\dot{E}$ by 10% (Kommerell, 1929); lowering the height from 1.83 to 0.71 m reduced efficiency by 35% (Wyndham et al., 1969); and reducing the working height from erect to 60% of erect height increased $\dot{E}$ by 13% (Morrissey et al., 1983). The kneeling posture typically requires 6.5% less energy for the same task as a standing posture (Morrissey et al., 1983). A lying posture typically requires 1 kcal/min less than a standing posture (Humphreys et al., 1962).

9.6.1.6 Technique

The technique used in shoveling can also change the amount of energy expended. Thus, Wenzig (1932) recommended standing in front of the destination but facing away and shoveling over the shoulder, rather than standing and shoveling sideways, as the former was 18% more efficient. Dressel et al. (1954) found that scraping the material along the bottom of the pile to fill the shovel is 15% more efficient than digging directly into the pile.

9.6.1.7 Lift Angle

Lift angle was examined by Freivalds (1986b) using an experimental shovel with an adjustable lift of 16° intervals. The energy cost of shoveling sand at a constant rate of 18 scoops/min normalized to the amount of sand shoveled indicated a significantly lower normalized energy cost for lift angles of 16° and 32° as opposed to 0° and 48°. Predicted low back compressive forces were significantly lower at 48° than at the other angles. This suggested that to reduce low back stresses one should use the steepest lift angle. Unfortunately, such a steep angle caused much of the scooped material to slide out during the shoveling motion, resulting in less productive work. Thus a lift angle of 32° appeared to be the best compromise, which corresponded closely to the 37° angle found on most typical shovels.

9.6.1.8 Length of Handle

Wenzig (1932) observed the 0.64 m shovel to be slightly more efficient than a longer or shorter shovel. Kommerell (1929) found a 0.66-m shovel to be 10% more efficient than a 0.9-m shovel, which was very reasonable in his constrained (1.0 and 1.2 m heights) working environment. Lehmann (1953) agreed that short handles were more efficient in constrained environments but felt that there were insufficient data to justify a recommendation for unconstrained environments. Freivalds (1986b) found a significant improvement in efficiency for long-handled as compared to short-handled shovels in an unconstrained environment. Thus, the deciding criterion for shovel length is the amount of headroom and posture used.

9.6.1.9 Handle Material

Traditionally, tool handles have been manufactured from wood, a surprisingly good material in that it is relatively light and resistant to transfer of heat, electricity, and even vibration. However, recently, probably due to the cost of shaping the wood into the appropriate size and shape, there has been a trend to manufacture the handles from other materials such as metal or fiberglass. Metal is a very poor material in that it is heavy and transmits heat, electricity, and vibrations. On the other hand, fiberglass does not seem to have such limitations. Chang et al. (1999) examined shoveling performance, grip force, forearm flexor and biceps brachii EMG, and Borg ratings of perceived exertion for three types of gardening tools, shovel, rake, and hoe, with three different handles, wood, solid fiberglass, and hollow fiberglass. The most effective measure for shovels was shoveling efficiency, i.e., sand shoveled per minute divided by the increase in heart rate per minute. The hollow fiberglass handle was 12% more efficient than either the wood or solid fiberglass handle, probably due to the decreased load handled, as discussed in the next section. Subjective ratings were also significantly lower for the hollow handle, part of which may have also been attributed to the ribbed texture, which provided the subjects with a better tactile feel.

9.6.1.10 Shovel Weight

Kirsch (1939) found that lighter shovels were 20% more efficient than heavier shovels. Müller and Karrasch (1956) recommended a shovel weight of 1.5 to 1.8 kg based on an incomplete study in which shovel weight was dependent on shovel load. Freivalds (1986b) found that subjects gave higher preference ratings to lighter shovels, although there were other shovel parameters that could not be controlled and could have influenced their ratings. Obviously, reducing shovel weight should greatly increase shoveling efficiency, especially if one considers the unproductive weight to be one third to one half of the total shovel load (e.g., Morrissey et al., 1983, used a 4-kg shovel with loads less than 8 kg).

9.6.1.11 Blade Size, Shape, and Thickness

Kirsch (1939) and Lehmann (1953) both agreed that blade size should depend on the density of the material being shoveled: the less dense the material, the larger the blade size. The optimum shape of the blade also depends on the material being shoveled (Kirsch, 1939): for coarse-grained materials (e.g., rock, coal, ore), a square point and flat blade with raised edges and for fine-grained materials (e.g., sand, soil), a round point and curved blade with slightly raised edges. In terms of penetrating the material being shoveled, the coarser and grainier the material being shoveled, the more energy will be expended. Thus, Dressel et al. (1954) observed that shoveling coarse gravel required 37% more energy than sand. Blade thickness (in the range 0.5 to 1.0 mm) was found to be unimportant as long as the blade was properly sharpened (Vennewald, 1939).

Note that there should be a trade-off between blade size and shovel load handled (plus the weight of the shovel itself). For small blades, a relatively small load is handled with comparatively greater energy expenditure for moving the trunk and the shovel itself. For large blades and large loads, excessively high energy expenditures will lead to quick fatigue, for which the individual may compensate by using less than full scoops. This trade-off was examined by Freivalds and Kim (1990) while shoveling sand with various sized blades and shovel weights. The dependent variable, energy expenditure, was normalized to the individual's body weight and load shoveled (including

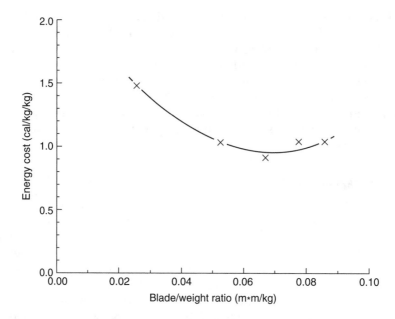

FIGURE 9.15
Energy cost as a function of blade-size/shove-weight ratio. (From Freivalds, A. and Kim, Y.J.,
1990. *Applied Ergonomics*, 21:39–42. With permission.)

shovel weight). The blade size and shovel weight characteristics were combined into one independent variable, the ratio of blade size to shovel weight.
The resulting quadratic functional relationship (shown in Figure 9.15)
yielded a minimum energy cost at a blade/weight ratio of 0.0676 m²/kg,
which for an average-weight subject (77 kg) resulted in an energy expenditure of 5.16 kcal/min, just below the acceptable 8-h energy expenditure rate
of 5.2 kcal/h as recommended by Lehmann (1953). For larger blade sizes
and theoretically larger loads and higher energy expenditures, the subjects
compensated by taking less than full loads. More details on other shovel
parameters may be found in Freivalds (1986a,b).

9.6.2   Axes and Hammers

9.6.2.1   Length and Striking Efficiency

Axes and hammers are striking tools designed to transmit a force to an object
by direct contact and thereby change its shape or drive it forward. The tool's
efficiency in doing this may be defined as the ratio of the energy utilized in
striking to the energy available in the stroke. Using geometric methods,
Drillis et al. (1963) showed that the tool's efficiency could be further defined
by

$$\eta = 1 - \frac{S^2}{\rho_1^2} \qquad (9.17)$$

where η = efficiency; S = distance from the mass center to the line of action (OB in Figure 9.3); and ρ_1 = radius of gyration with respect to the center of action. For the efficiency to be 100%, the center of mass should coincide with the line of action, which is impossible with a shafted tool. In the hand axe of Stone Age humans, the total energy of the stroke movement was converted into useful energy giving maximum efficiency, although the force was fairly weak. The opposite extreme is a uniform rod held at one end, which has an efficiency of only 25% but provides quite a bit more relative force.

Two comparable formulae for tool efficiency were developed by Gorjatschkin (1924, cited in Drillis et al., 1963). The first related tool efficiency to the ratio of S to the tool length, L:

$$\eta = 1 - 1.5\frac{S}{L} \tag{9.18}$$

Again, this indicates that the efficiency increases as the ratio of S to L increases. Physically this is achieved by placing the mass center as close as possible to the center of action, i.e., increasing the mass of the tool head relative to the handle. A second way of expressing the above observation is to relate the mass of the handle to the total mass:

$$\eta = 1 - 0.75\frac{m_1}{m_1 + m_2} \tag{9.19}$$

where m_1 = mass of handle and m_2 = mass of tool head. Drillis et al. (1963) indicated that efficiencies for typical striking tools ranged from 0.8 to 0.95 for axes, from 0.7 to 0.9 for hammers, from 0.55 to 0.85 for scutches, and from 0.3 to 0.65 for hoes.

Regarding impacting tools such as hammers, the efficiency of impact and recoil is very important. When two bodies collide, the ratio between their relative velocity after impact to that before impact is defined as the coefficient of restitution. This can be used to derive the energy of recoil and eventually the efficiency of impact (Drillis et al., 1963).

In the case of forging this can be defined as

$$\eta = \frac{1}{1 + m_0/m} \tag{9.20}$$

where m_0 = mass of hammer; and m = mass of other object (e.g., forging and anvil).

The aim is to transform as much of the kinetic energy of the hammer into deforming the object's shape as possible. Thus, the mass of the hammer should be small relative to the mass of the forging and anvil. On the other hand, in driving a nail the intent is to transform the kinetic energy of the hammer into the kinetic energy of the nail. Then the mass of the hammer should be great in relation to the mass of the nail and the efficiency becomes

$$\eta = \frac{1}{1 + m/m_0} \tag{9.21}$$

The overall efficiency of the system including the operator becomes the product of the efficiency of the tool, the efficiency of the stroke movement, the efficiency of impact, and the physiological efficiency of the human operator. This last factor can range from a low of 3 to 4% for relatively static tasks such as shoveling (Freivalds, 1986b) to a high of 25 to 30% for dynamic tasks such as cycling (Lehmann, 1953). Drillis et al. (1963) computed the overall efficiency of hammering a 6-in. (15-cm) nail into a wooden block as 57%, not counting the physiological efficiency. Using an average value of 15% for physiological efficiency, overall system efficiency reduces to 8.6%.

9.6.2.2 Weight and Striking Efficiency

The effect of the weight of the head on swing characteristics dynamics of striking tools, especially axes, was further investigated by Widule et al. (1978) and Corrigan et al. (1981). Using cinematography they analyzed the dropping motion of the subjects using four axes with head weights of 0.85, 1.6, 2.2, and 3.6 kg. Accelerations as well as kinetic energy for various points of interest were calculated frame by frame from the film.

The results supported the hypothesis that an increase in head weight led to an increase in kinetic energy. However, a noticeable drop-off in angular velocity and kinetic energy was found for the heaviest axe. Thus, there appeared to be a limit to the ability of an individual to achieve rotational inertia and adding additional mass may have been counterproductive in terms of physiological energy costs. The authors concluded that the heavy axes (heads ranging from 2.2 kg and above) used to clear the American forests in the late 1800s, although more taxing in terms of energy expenditure, were more efficient in clearing forests. Rapid bursts of energy were used to chop down a tree, and necessary rest periods could be obtained during preparation of the cut, sharpening the axe, and chopping off branches. The authors also concluded that the American axe, distinguished from the European axe by its possession of a poll (a lump of metal at the rear of the head; see Figure 9.16A), was more efficient. The poll counterbalanced the protruding blade and gave the axe better handling characteristics.

Such observations were confirmed by Drillis et al. (1963) based on his survey of 521 axes used in Latvia. Average head weight was found to be 1.4 kg or about 2% of the user's weight. Average handle length was found to be 0.6 m or about 35% of the user's height. He concluded that these values compared very favorably to folk norms. Optimum swing height to achieve maximum kinetic energy for wood splitting was found to be approximately 1.1 m.

Some variations on these optimum values were noted by German work physiologists. In a study of sledgehammers, Meyer (1930) examined hammers ranging in weight from 4.4 to 10.6 kg. He concluded, however, that to obtain a more lively action (i.e., increased acceleration) one should use lighter

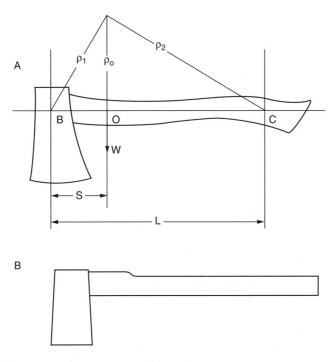

FIGURE 9.16
(A) Determination of striking tool efficiency (American axe); O = mass center, B = center of action, C = center of percussion (ideal point for holding), L = length of the tool, W = weight of the tool. (B) European axe. (From Freivalds, A., 1987. *International Reviews of Ergonomics*, 1:43–75. With permission.)

hammers. Gläser (1933, cited in Lehmann, 1953) investigated axes with head weights under 2 kg for forestry use. He found the opposite and concluded that the "most lively action" was to be achieved using axes weighing 3 to 4 kg. A mitigating factor is that the Germans most likely measured the weight of the whole implement. Subtracting approximately 0.6 to 0.8 kg for the handle yields values more closely in line with the other studies.

9.6.2.3   Other Considerations

Further design principles for striking tools are given by Fraser (1980). The handles should not be cylindrical, but appropriately contoured for a power grip with an enlargement at the end to prevent slippage. Plastic handles are susceptible to fatigue and fracture. Metal handles are only useful if covered with leather or rubber to prevent slippage and reduce shock. Wooden handles, made from ash or hickory, are hard and dense with high shock resistance. The shaft is wedged into the hammerhead with iron wedges to ensure additional security. Handle diameter is in the range of 25 to 40 mm. For more specialized carpentry hammers, handle lengths will be shorter, around 0.3 m (Fraser, 1980).

TABLE 9.4

A Comparison of Sawing Postures and Techniques

	Normalized Cutting Performance (m²/min)	Normalized Energy Expenditure (kcal/min)	Normalized Energy Cost/Output (kcal/m²)
One-handed stooped	100	100	100
Two-handed stooped	130	141	108
Two-handed kneeling	130	120	92

Source: Gläser (1933).

9.6.3   Saws

9.6.3.1   General Considerations

The action of heavy sawing involves a power grip with repetitive flexion and extension at the elbow, while the action of light sawing requires a precision grip with manipulation of the wrist. A large two-man crosscut saw may require use of two hands, one superimposed on the other, although at times one hand can be used. Typical American and European handsaws cut as they are pushed through the wood, while Oriental handsaws cut as they are pulled through the wood (Bleed et al., 1982). For most saws a "pistol grip" is typically used, except for the lightest saws in which a cylindrical screwdriver type handle serves best for a precision grip.

Several studies on sawing have indicated a variety of optimum features. Gläser (1933, cited in Lehmann, 1953) investigated a variety of postures and techniques to be used with two-man crosscut saws in forestry work. Using the one-handed stooped posture as the baseline for relative comparisons, Gläser found the following (Table 9.4). A two-handed action provided more force and better performance, but at a higher energy cost. Most efficient was the kneeling position in which less torso support was needed and less energy was expended. Thus, posture plays an important part in tool usage.

9.6.3.2   Pulling vs. Pushing

The effect of pulling vs. pushing action in sawing, i.e., Oriental vs. American saws, was tested by Bleed et al. (1982). Oxygen consumption was measured while sawing identical beams using the two saws, plus a bow saw that could be either pushed or pulled. Sawing times were not significantly different while oxygen consumption for the Oriental saw was significantly lower than for the American saw (2.59 vs. 3.40 l), and pushing the bow saw was significantly lower than for pulling it (3.28 vs. 4.55 l). The authors indicated that a push stroke is superior to a pull stroke, except that for a Japanese saw a thinner blade and different handle style allowed for more efficient use. However, there is evidence that in a low posture (i.e., 50% of height), an unbraced pull can be stronger than an unbraced push (Ayoub and McDaniel, 1974; Materials Handling Research Unit, 1980), which could also explain the

TABLE 9.5

Characteristics and Performance of Two Hoes Used for Digging Potatoes

Hoe	Angle between Handle and Blade (°)	Weight (kg)	Handle Length (m)	Blade Area (m²)	Performance No. of Potatoes	No. of Strokes	Potatoes/ Stroke
A	72	0.75	1.42	153	179	651	0.275
D	85	1.50	1.28	89	184	1058	0.174

Source: Barnstaet, K. and Kogelschatz, H., 1933. *Landwirtschaftliches Jahrbuch der Schweiz,* 76:861–888. With permission.

Japanese saw's superiority. The differences observed in the bow saw cannot be explained.

9.6.4 Other Agricultural Tools

9.6.4.1 Hoes

Although not really applicable in today's mechanized agriculture, an interesting study with evaluations of a variety of agricultural tools and techniques was performed by Barnstaet and Kogelschatz (1933). Some of the results illustrate general ergonomic concepts that can be applied in modern-day tasks. First, an evaluation of hoes used in digging for potatoes was performed. The characteristics of the two opposite extreme hoes are given in Table 9.5.

Obvious differences in performance can be seen with hoe A 58% more efficient than hoe D in retrieving potatoes and 72% more efficient in hoeing a given area. Decisive factors against hoe D were that the longer blade required greater force and more of a chopping action to penetrate the ground. The shallow blade of hoe A allowed it to be used more in a pulling action.

9.6.4.2 Wheelbarrows

Various techniques have been examined in beet and potato harvesting. Traditional methods use either a stoop posture or crawling on the knees. Barnstaet and Kogelschatz (1933) implemented a cart with wheels to support the torso with a 35% savings in energy expenditure. A similar effect was produced using a stool in potato harvesting. Thus, supporting the torso and eliminating a stooped posture provided large savings in energy expenditure and improved productivity significantly. A third factor of concern not examined in the study is that supporting the upper torso is also likely to alleviate stresses in the low back.

Lehman (1953) also examined the wheelbarrow and found that a typical wheelbarrow was not properly balanced, so either considerable weight was carried by the user or the center of gravity was so high that extra effort was needed to balance the wheelbarrow. Using a proper design and rubber tires a saving of 20% in energy expenditure was obtained, although smoothness of the rolling surface was probably judged to be an even more significant factor, decreasing energy expenditure even more.

For other more obsolete agricultural tools such as the scythe, scutch, flail, etc. please refer to Drillis et al. (1963).

9.7 Industrial Tools

9.7.1 Pliers

Pliers and related tools — wire strippers, pincers, and nippers — are tools with a head in the form of jaws, which can have a variety of configurations, a joint that may be simple or complex, and two handles. Although sometimes the handles are straight, more typically they are curved outward to conform roughly to the position of grasp. The grasp, depending on use, can be of the precision or power type (Fraser, 1980).

In their simple form (Figure 9.10), pliers are a very common tool and, if used casually for short periods of time, will give reasonable performance with little fatigue. However, the relationship of the handles to the head forces the wrist into ulnar deviation (Figure 9.10A), a posture that cannot be held repeatedly or for prolonged periods of time without fatigue or occurrence of tenosynovitis. A further problem is that such a deviation reduces the range of wrist rotation by 50%, thus reducing productivity (Tichauer, 1966). Certain industries, such as the electronics assembly industry, place just such demands on the workers. In the case of pliers a radical ergonomic design has been instituted with remarkable success in reducing medical problems. By bending the handles of the pliers the wrists of the user can be kept straight, reducing stress on the wrist (Figure 9.10B). In the case of two groups of Western Electric Co. trainees, one using conventional straight pliers and the other the redesigned bent pliers during a 12-week training program, there was a sixfold increase in symptoms for the group using the straight pliers as opposed to the group using the bent pliers (Tichauer, 1966, 1976). A similar problem occurred at Eli Lilly and Co. involving diagonal cutting pliers used with considerable wrist extension. After numerous complaints the pliers were redesigned with a similar bend and used successfully (Yoder et al., 1973).

Specifics on modern plier design have been detailed by Lindstrom (1973, cited in Fraser, 1980). Four factors relating to the hand should be considered in the design of pliers: size, strength, endurance, and working position. Lindstrom (1973) recommended a working hand width of 90 mm for men and 80 mm of women and a handle length of 110 mm for men and 100 mm for women. Longer handles would limit the opening of the tool head.

With regard to strength, Lindstrom (1973) cited a maximum grip strength of 588 N for the male dominant hand and 392 N for the female (or approximately

70% of male strength). By age 60 to 65 these values will have been reduced by 30%. For repeated or continuous operations, Lindstrom recommended a working strength of 33 to 50% of the above values. Two-handed operation can increase the force produced by 60 to 70%.

The working posture of the hand is extremely crucial because the finger flexor muscles cross the wrist and are located in the forearm. Thus, when the wrist is flexed, extended, or deviated, the grip force may be reduced by as much as 30%. This phenomenon is another reason to modify the tool to fit the requirements of the user as in the case of the Western Electric pliers.

Lindstrom (1973) also noted that application forces are not always limited by the lack of strength, but also by hand discomfort. For repeated operations by females the pressure should not exceed 100 kPa, and for males the pressure should not exceed 200 kPa with an occasional maximum of 700 kPa. To minimize the applied pressure, it is necessary to enlarge and flatten handles and avoid pressure-producing ridges. Thus, indentation of the handles for the fingers is undesirable. Encasing the basic metal handles in a rubber or plastic sheath provides insulation and improves the tactile feel (Fraser, 1980).

9.7.2 Screwdrivers

The handles of screwdrivers (and similar tools: files, chisels, etc.) can either be used with a precision grip for stabilization or a power grip for torque. The handle must also be capable of being approached equally effectively from all directions. Crucial factors to be considered in screwdriver use are size, shape, and texture of the handle.

Rubarth (1928) examined maximum torque from a power grip on a screwdriver handle. The best shape was cylindrical with a rounded end. Within the range of diameters used, 18 to 40 mm, an increase in diameter allowed for greater force production. Hunt (1934) studied speed of use as a function of handle diameter. The time taken to drive a screw with a 7.6-mm diameter handle was 1.9 s, while with a 16-mm handle it was 3.6 s. Thus, the smaller the diameter, the less the time needed for rotation of the handle. Pheasant and O'Neill (1975) measured torque for various sized cylindrical handles as well as actual screwdriver handles. Again, torque was found to increase with an increase in handle diameter size. Knurled cylinders allow for significantly greater torque production than smooth cylinders. Maximum torque was achieved with knurled cylinders 50 mm in diameter. Actual screwdriver handles compared favorably to knurled cylinder handles. Differences in the precise shape of handles were not significant, as long as the hand did not slip around the handle. Similarly, Habes and Grant (1997a) found increased torque capability and decreased EMG torque ratios (i.e., improved muscle contraction efficiency) with larger diameter handles (3.7 vs. 2.9 cm).

Further studies on the shape of the handle have shown some inconsistencies in results. Fraser (1980) indicated that a tool manufacturer in Germany had introduced a successful version of a screwdriver handle with a triangular cross section. The planes of the sections allowed better use of the fingers in torque application. Magill and Konz (1986) found that a similar screwdriver with three large shallow flutes also produced the largest torque. They confirmed that torque was proportional to grip volume and grip length, and time on task was inversely related to grip volume and length. On the other hand, a new series of ergonomic screwdrivers produced by Ergo in Sweden and marketed by Bahco in the United States use essentially a cylindrical handle with a circular cross section (Bobjer, 1984). Large flutes created pressure concentrations in the palm of the hand and were omitted. To give better frictional characteristics, the handle incorporated 40 axial grooves with cross grooves. A second innovation was that small screwdrivers for precision work were fitted with normal length handles. The lowest part of the handle assisted in finding directions during a precision task. The contradiction in handle shape is not easily explainable and is examined more closely in Section 9.33 on handle shapes.

A final study on screwdrivers and posture (Huston et al., 1984) indicated that greater torque could be produced standing rather than sitting and at the lowest of three body positions: elbow, rather than shoulder or eye height. Similarly, Habes and Grant (1997a) found increased torque capability and decreased EMG torque ratios (i.e., improved muscle contraction efficiency) with a vertical (as opposed to horizontal) orientation of the screwdriver, decreased point-of-operation heights, and decreased reach distances.

9.7.3   Knives

Although a very old tool, the knife has recently reappeared in the literature as a possible cause for the increase in cumulative trauma disorders in the butchering industry. The first study investigated a rash of cumulative trauma disorders in a poultry processing plant (Armstrong et al., 1982). Detailed methods, time and measurement (MTM) analyses, and a frame-by-frame film analysis of the hand motions during cutting were performed. Certain modifications to the currently used boning knife were suggested. A pistol type grip would allow the operator to hold the blade and the forearm horizontal to eliminate ulnar deviation and wrist flexion. A circular or elliptical handle with a larger circumference of 99 mm, as well as a strap, was recommended to allow the hand to relax between exertions without losing grip on the knife. Later research by Habes and Grant (1997b) also confirmed the use of pistol grip knives to promote the use of stab grip as opposed to holding the knife in line with the forearm axis in a slice grip. The stab grip allowed a higher force capability and minimized EMG-to-force ratios in various muscles, indicating more efficient muscle contractions.

The fish canning industry in Sweden has also been plagued by cumulative trauma disorders (Karlqvist, 1984). The common straight knives, which during the cutting action caused large ulnar deviations, were identified as possible causes for the medical incidents. Of the four knives used in different

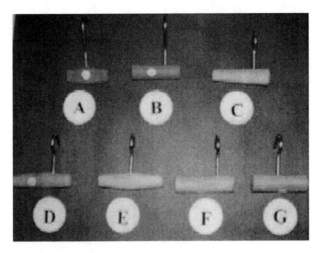

FIGURE 9.17
Different types of meat hooks. Hook A is a traditional design. Hooks B and C have the hook off center. Hooks D and E have a double frustum handle. Hooks F and G have an oval cross section. (From Kong, Y.K. and Freivalds, A., 2003. *International Journal of Industrial Ergonomics,* 32:12–23. With permission.)

operations, one was fitted with a pistol grip similar to Armstrong et al.'s (1982), while the others were fitted with larger diameter handles for better balance and movement.

Knife safety is also of concern during butchering operations. Long hours of static loading on the forearm flexors can result in accelerated fatigue. Because body fluids cause slippery handles, there are frequent instances of the operator's hand, on impact or abrupt stoppage of the knife penetration, sliding down the handle and over the blade, resulting in severe injury. Cochran and Riley (1986a) examined tangs (barriers to the blade projecting perpendicular from the handle) of various heights and found that guard heights of 1.52 cm were optimal for safety with lower heights inadequate.

9.7.4 Meat Hooks

Meat hooks are used to control the accessibility of meat during meat processing operations, typically placed in the nondominant hand (the dominant hand holds a knife or other cutting tool) and are suspected to cause many incidences of tenosynovitis in the nondominant hand ring finger. One currently used model is a 5-mm-thick piece of flat polyethylene with a hook inserted in the middle of the piece (Hook A, Figure 9.17). The thin shape leads to high compressive forces while the location of the hook places high forces on the ring finger (which is only the third strongest finger). Another current model uses a polyethylene frustum with the hook inserted off-center at the smaller end (Hook B, Figure 9.17). Potentially better new designs tested include Hook C, with the hook at the larger end of the frustum, Hook D, a double frustum with

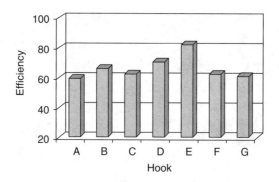

FIGURE 9.18
Efficiency (maximum force per normalized EMG) of meat hooks. (From Kong, Y.K. and Freivalds, A., 2003. *International Journal of Industrial Ergonomics*, 32:12–23. With permission.)

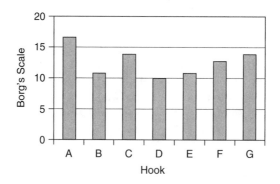

FIGURE 9.19
Borg rating of perceived exertion for meat hooks. (Adapted from Kong and Freivalds, 2003.)

the hook offset (between the two strongest fingers), and Hook E, a double frustum with the hook centered (Kong and Freivalds, 2003).

Force-sensing resistors (FSRs) were used to measure finger forces during simulated meat-pulling tasks. The resulting finger force distributions were compared to the theoretically optimal finger contribution distributions mentioned in Section 9.2.2, with Hook E deviating least from the optimal finger force distribution. Incorporating the empirical FSR forces into the biomechanical hand model (discussed in Section 5.5) produced individual tendon forces, which were normalized per unit external force. This latter measure can be considered as a form of grip efficiency and was best for Hook E (Figure 9.18). The lowest Borg rating of perceived exertion was obtained with Hook D (Figure 9.19). Therefore, a double-frustum-shaped meat hook handle is most efficient for gripping and producing the least amount of tendon forces. The only uncertainty is the placement of the hook.

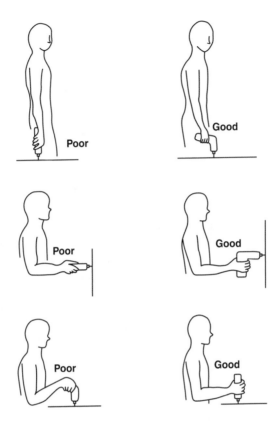

FIGURE 9.20
Proper orientation of power tools in the workplace.

9.7.5 Power Tools

9.7.5.1 *Power Drills*

In a power drill, or other power tools, the major function of the operator is to hold, stabilize, and monitor the tool against a workpiece, while the tools perform the main effort of the job. Although the operator may at times need to shift or orient the tool, the main function for the operator is to effectively grasp and hold the tool. A drill is composed of a head, body, and handle, with all three, ideally, being in line. The line of action is from the line of the extended index finger so that in the ideal drill, the head is off-center with respect to the central axis of the body. Handle configuration is important; the options are pistol grip, in-line, or right angle. As a rule of thumb, in-line and right-angle grips are best for tightening downward on a horizontal surface whereas pistol grips are best for tightening on a vertical surface (Figure 9.20) with the aim of obtaining a standing posture with a straight back, upper arms hanging down, and a straight wrist (Figure 9.8). For the pistol grip, this results in the handle at an angle of approximately 78° with horizontal (Fraser, 1980).

Another important factor is the center of gravity. If it is too far forward in the body of the tool, a turning moment is created, which must be overcome by the muscle of the hand and forearm, creating muscular effort additional to that required for holding, positioning, and pushing the drill into the workpiece. Placing the primary handle directly under the center of gravity, such that the body juts out behind the handle as well as in front, is recommended. For heavy drills, a secondary supportive handle may be needed, either to the side or preferably below the tool, such that the supporting arm can be tucked in against the body rather than abducted (Fraser, 1980).

9.7.5.2 *Nutrunners*

Nutrunners, especially common in the automobile industry, are used to tighten nuts, screws, and other fasteners. They come in a variety of handle configurations (in line, pistol grip, right angle), torque outputs, shut-off mechanisms, speeds, weights, and spindle diameters, and are commercially available from a variety of sources. Torque levels range from 0.1 to 5000 Nm and, for pneumatic tools, are generally lumped into approximately 22 power levels (M1.6 to M45) depending on motor size and gearing required to drive the tool. The torque is transferred from the motor to the spindle through a variety of mechanisms such that the power (often air) can be quickly shut off once the nut or other fastener is tight. The simplest and cheapest mechanism is a direct drive, which is under the operator's control but, because of the long time to release the trigger once the nut is tightened, transfers a very large *reaction torque* to the operator's arm. Mechanical friction clutches will allow the spindle to slip, reducing some of this reaction torque. A better mechanism for reducing the reaction torque is the airflow shut-off, which automatically senses when to cut off the air supply as the nut is tightened. A still faster mechanism is an automatic mechanical clutch shut-off. The most recent mechanisms include the hydraulic pulse system where the rotational energy from the motor is transferred over a pulse unit containing an oil cushion (filtering off the high-frequency pulses as well as noise) and a similar electrical pulse system, both of which, to a large extent, reduce the reaction torque (Freivalds and Eklund, 1993).

Variation of torque delivered to the nut depends on a variety of conditions including properties of the tool, the operator of the tool, properties of the joint, i.e., the combination of the fastener and material being fastened (ranging from soft, with the materials having elastic properties, such as body panels, to hard, when two stiff surfaces, such as pulleys on a crankshaft, are brought together), stability of the air supply, etc. The torque experienced by the user (the reaction torque) depends on the above factors (Figure 9.21) plus the torque shut-off system and is believed to contribute to the development of cumulative trauma disorders. In general, using electrical tools at lower than normal rpm levels or underpowering pneumatic tools resulted in larger reaction torques and more stressful ratings (Figure 9.22). Pulse-type tools produced the lowest reaction torques and were rated as less stressful. It was

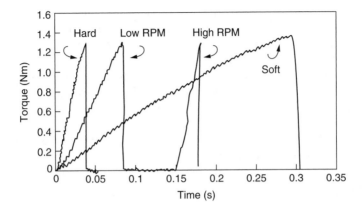

FIGURE 9.21
Nutrunner reaction torques as a function of soft or hard joints and low (100) or high (400) rpm levels. (From Freivalds, A. and Eklund, J., 1993. *Applied Ergonomics*, 24:158–164. With permission.)

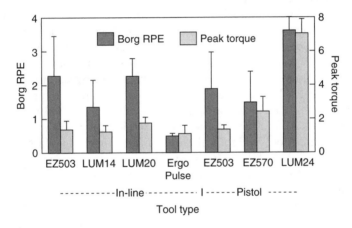

FIGURE 9.22
Comparison of nutrunner torque impulse levels with subjective ratings. (From Freivalds, A. and Eklund, J., 1993. *Applied Ergonomics*, 24:158–164. With permission.)

hypothesized that the short pulses "chop up" or allow the inertia of the tool to resist the reaction torque. Another possibility is to provide reaction torque bars (Freivalds and Eklund, 1993).

9.7.5.3 Handle Sizes

The expectation would be that handle size requirements for power tools should be no different from that of manual tools. Johnson (1988) examined the handle diameter for powered in-line screwdrivers (similar to nutrunners discussed above, except that they tend to have smaller torque levels and are typically either in line or pistol grip) by adding aluminum sleeves to the basic tool. Interestingly larger diameters (5.0 to 6.35 cm) showed decreased EMG levels as compared to smaller diameters (2.86 cm). These numbers would appear to be larger than those recommended for manual circular tool handles (Section 9.3.2). However, there might be a confounding factor in that the additional aluminum sleeve may have absorbed some the vibration or reaction torques discussed above and required less force (i.e., EMG) to grip and control the tool. Oh and Radwin (1993) modified a pistol-grip tool to have an adjustable handle. Larger spans (5 to 6 cm) required the least amount of grip force during the task requirements, which is comparable to the grip span for two-handled tools (Section 9.4.1). Also, as could be expected, extended triggers decreased finger forces and palmar forces during tool operation.

9.7.6   Railroad Tools

Use of large hand tools in the railroad industry has produced many injuries, which are exceeded in number only by injuries from slips, falls, and material injuries. In addition, the injuries are not confined to the hand and wrist, but include a large number (up to 30%) of torso injuries. Striking and leverage tools are possible sources for these problems and thus were examined in a series of studies (Marras, 1986; Marras and Rockwell, 1986; Rockwell and Marras, 1986). The first task involved swinging a 4.5-kg maul about the trunk and hitting a spike (Marras and Rockwell, 1986). This required both strength and skill as the spike surface area was only 3.9 cm^2 and the maul striking surface area was 5.3 cm^2. Six to ten swings were required to drive the spike completely. Three tool weights, three tool striking surface areas, and six spiking methods were utilized in the experimental design. Spiking force was measured by a load cell, and electromyograms of the low back musculature were recorded.

The most obvious results were differences between professional railroad workers and novice subjects. Force levels produced during spiking were greater for professionals and enlarging the striking surface area increased spiking force. The latter effect was due to the worker using a greater ballistic motion because less control was needed to strike the surface. However, too large an area would impede work close to the rails. Thus, the long narrow heads typically used are a compromise. Tool weights in the narrow range selected (3.6 to 5.5 kg) were not significant. The method of tool use significantly affected spiking force for novice subjects but not for professionals, probably because the professionals had already adapted to their preferred techniques. For the novice subjects, methods involving less control, such as back motion alone without hand motion, produced greater ballistic motion and spiking force. The EMG data indicated that using the back alone produced lowest spinal stresses, especially in novice subjects. The overall conclusions were that professionals benefited most from tool changes while novices benefited most from technique changes (Marras and Rockwell, 1986).

In a second experiment, Rockwell and Marras (1986) examined the clawbar used to remove spikes from rails. It is a heavy (12.6 to 13.6 kg) tool leading to injuries when the tool suddenly releases and one operator falls. Two angles of leverage on the claw bar (44° or 66°) and various methods of performing the task were tested. Again, the results indicated significant differences between professionals and novices, with professionals producing 50% greater lifting forces. The best technique involved snapping or jerking the bar downward to create a peak force over a short time. The short impulse was more likely to free a spike and produced less bending in the bar, which could also be a cause of injuries. Tool design in terms of leverage angle was not a significant factor in tool performance. Bar weight and length have some effect, but were not studied (Rockwell and Marras, 1986).

9.7.7 Mining Tools

A significant proportion of underground mining accidents are attributed to the use of hand tools. The worst tools in coal mining in this respect are scaling bars, jacks, pry-bars, hammers, axes, and drills. For metal and non-metal mining the worst tools are jacks, drills, and scaling bars, which account for 85% of the lost days in hand tool accidents (Lavender et al., 1986). In almost all the above cases the injuries either are overexertion injuries to the trunk or result when the tool strikes various body parts. Although the authors did not address specific tools, they suggested that "struck-by" accidents could be reduced by improved lighting, better worksite preparation, and improved training.

9.7.8 Miscellaneous Tools

9.7.8.1 *Soldering Irons*

A variety of other tools have been ergonomically redesigned to fit the human operator. The electronics assembly industry uses many bench-top assemblies that require operators to abduct their arms so that they are nearly horizontal. This is often caused by tools and workspace designs requiring the forearm to angle down into the area of work, such as when soldering wires to terminals on circuit boards lying flat on the workbench. Tichauer (1966) redesigned the soldering iron to include a bend between the tip and the handle, which eliminated the shoulder abduction and lowered the forearm.

9.7.8.2 *Surgical Instruments*

Surgical instruments such as the bayonet forceps have also been examined and redesigned (Miller et al., 1971). The problems with the original forceps included a tendency for it to roll in the fingers while in use, for fatigue to develop in the finger flexor muscles, and for improper passing from nurse to surgeon. Using motion times and EMG recordings of the finger flexors, alternative designs were evaluated until one showed a reduction in grasp times of 25% and in muscle workload of 40%.

9.7.8.3   Dental Instruments

Hoping to improve efficiency in dentistry, dental instruments were evaluated and modified by Evans et al. (1973). Instead of the current dental syringe (providing air, water, and air–water spray with a separate suction device) the authors combined all four into one multifunction instrument. Field tests indicated somewhat improved performance, reducing the number of hand movements required by dental assistants from 64 to 42 and reducing the dentist's cutting time from 91 to 84 s. Energy expenditure, however, did not change. The authors concluded that with more practice time and better control coding, larger improvements would have been obtained.

9.7.8.4   Food Scoops

The design of food scoops was examined by Konz (1975). The traditional food scoop used a thumb-activated clearing mechanism. The control required 17% of mean male thumb strength and could not be shifted to the other hand. Thus, fatigue would be a serious problem and left-handed operators could not use the tool. A second design used a power-grip activator. However, a large force, 10% of male grip strength, was still required. A third alternative design was especially suitable for ice cream, as it eliminated the need for a clearing bar. A liquid center transferred heat from the hand to the scoop melting residual ice cream.

9.7.8.5   Writing Instruments

The ergonomics of writing instruments were examined by Kao (1976, 1977, 1979). Evaluation of writing speed for ballpoint pens, felt-tip pens, fountain pens, and pencils indicated that the ballpoint is best and the fountain pen worst. For least fatiguing writing, i.e., requiring the least pressure, the felt-tip was best and the ballpoint was worst. Considering the trade-offs in speed and fatigue, the felt-tip was judged best overall (Kao, 1979). For any writing instrument, increasing the size of the grip area with a flared design up to a diameter of 13.6 mm should significantly reduce gripping force. This was found to be the case for ballpoint pens as measured by the EMG of the flexor pollicis brevis and pain scores for various hand regions during extended writing (Udo et al., 2000).

9.7.8.6   Scissors

Scissors were evaluated as a means of controlling upper extremity disorders in an automobile upholstery plant (Tannen et al., 1986). Traditional scissors were considered, as well as various blades connected with a C-shaped handle and spring to produce a self-opening scissors. The commercial self-opening blade elicited fewest complaints. However, each instrument had a minority of unsatisfied users. The authors concluded that choice of hand tools appears to be a highly individualized decision, requiring the input of the users.

Scissors used by barbers were redesigned in a study by Bullinger and Solf (1979). Handles were bent 22° with respect to the blades in the plane of the scissors, while the plane of the cutting edges were twisted 30° from the plane of the handles. The redesigned scissors were 50% more efficient than conventional scissors and increased heart rate only 3% as opposed to 21% for the conventional scissors in an experimental shearing task.

9.7.8.7 Toothbrushes

Even the common toothbrush has been redesigned using ergonomic principles (Guilfoyle, 1977). Based on time and motion studies, expert opinions, and survey data, a smaller bristle to concentrate brushing action, an angle handle for easier manipulation, and a contoured thumb area for comfort were incorporated in the new design.

A variety of other interesting tool and handle redesigns are presented in Roubal and Kovar (1962).

Questions

1. Why might there still be need for ergonomic tool design when many of these tools have been in existence for hundreds if not thousands of years?

2. What are some of the basic considerations that all tools need to fulfill?

3. What are the differences between a precision and a power grip? What are the implications for work and resulting injuries?

4. What is a safety margin and what implications does it have for work and resulting injuries?

5. What is a slip reflex and what implications does it have?

6. What may explain the coefficient of friction for skin exceeding the theoretical limit of 1.0?

7. What biomechanical arguments may be used to justify the need to maintain a neutral wrist posture?

8. What biomechanical arguments may be used to justify an "optimum" handle shape?

9. What biomechanical factors are important in designing a two-handled tool such as pliers?

10. Discuss the trade-offs of using gloves with tools.

11. What are some of key factors in designing shovels and a shoveling task for optimum performance?

12. What determines the striking efficiency of a hammer or other striking tool?

13. What factors are important in screwdriver design?

14. What is reaction torque and what power tool and task characteristics will affect it?

Problems

9.1. Plot the relative torque produced as handle diameter increases from practically zero to double the grip span diameter.

9.2. What is the loss in grip strength for an average male using channellock pliers with a grip span of 10 cm held in full ulnar deviation (as would be the case for most work on a horizontal work surface)?

9.3. What is the loss of efficiency for a cheap hammer that is made completely of cast iron as compared to a hammer with a very lightweight handle? (*Hint:* Assume the center of gravity for the first hammer is at the midposition of the handle.)

9.4. Assume that a typical shovel has a blade size of 0.06 m² and weighs 2.2 kg. What effect does doubling the blade size for the same weight have? What effect would reducing the weight of the shovel by 50% have?

References

Aghazadeh, F. and Mital, A., 1987. Injuries due to hand tools, *Applied Ergonomics*, 18:273–278.

Amis, A.A., 1987. Variation of finger forces in maximal isometric grasp tests on a range of cylindrical diameters, *Journal of Biomedical Engineering*, 9:313–320.

An, K.N., Cooney, W.P., Chao, E.Y., and Linscheid, R.L., 1978. Functional strength measurement of normal fingers, *ASME Advances in Bioengineering*, 89–90.

An, K.N., Askew, L.J., and Chao, E.Y., 1986. Biomechanics and functional assessment of upper extremities, in W. Karwowski, Ed., *Trends in Ergonomics/Human Factors III*, Amsterdam: Elsevier, 573–580.

Armstrong, T. J., 1983. *An Ergonomic Guide to Carpal Tunnel Syndrome*, Akron, OH: American Industrial Hygiene Association.

Armstrong, T.J., Foulke, J.A., Joseph, B.S. and Goldstein S.A., 1982. Investigation of cumulative trauma disorders in a poultry processing plant. *American Industrial Hygiene Association Journal*, 43:103–116.

Armstrong, T.J., Radwin, R.C., Hansen, D.J., and Kennedy, K.W., 1986. Repetitive trauma disorders: job evaluation and design. *Human Factors*, 27:325–336.

Athènes, S. and Wing, A., 1989. Knowledge-directed coordination in reaching for objects in the environment, in S.A. Wallace, Ed., *Perspectives on the Coordination in Movement*, Amsterdam: North Holland, 284–301.

Ayoub, M. and LoPresti, P., 1971. The determination of an optimum size cylindrical handle by use of electromyography. *Ergonomics*, 14:509–518.

Ayoub, M.M. and McDaniel, J.W., 1974. Effects of operator stance on pushing and pulling tasks, *American Institute of Industrial Engineers Transactions*, 6:185–195.

Baker, P.T., McKendry, J.M. and Grant, G., 1960. Volumetric requirements for hand tool usage, *Human Factors*, 2:156–162.

Barnstaet, K. and Kogelschatz, H., 1933. Die Untersuchung verschiedener land-wirtschaftlicher Arbeiten mit Hilfe des Respirationsapparatus [Investigation of agricultural work using a respirometer], *Landwirtschaftliches Jahrbuch der Schweiz*, 76:861–888.

Bendz, P., 1974. Systematization of the grip of the hand in relation to finger motor, systems, *Scandinavian Journal of Rehabilitation Medicine*, 6:158–165.

Bennett Ergonomic Labs, 1983. *Why Bennett's Biocurve?* Minneapolis, MN: Bennetts Bend, Inc.

Bleed, A.S., Bleed, P., Cochran, D.J., and Riley, M.W., 1982. A performance comparison of Japanese and American hand saws, *Proceedings of the Human Factors Society*, 26:403–407.

Bobjer, O., 1984. Screwdriver handles design for power and precision, in *Proceedings of the 1984 International Conference on Occupational Ergonomics*, Rexdale; Ontario, Canada: Human Factors Association of Canada, 443–446.

Bobjer, O., Johansson, S.E., and Piguet, S., 1993. Friction between hand and handle. Effects of oil and lard on textured and non-textured surfaces; perception of discomfort, *Applied Ergonomics*, 24:190–202.

Bradley, J.V., 1969a. Effects of gloves on control operation time, *Human Factors*, 11:13–20.

Bradley, J.V., 1969b. Glove characteristics influencing control manipulability, *Human Factors*, 11:21–35.

Brand, P.W., Beach, R.B., and Thompson, D.E., 1981. Relative tension and potential excursion of muscles in the forearm and hand, *Journal of Hand Surgery*, 6:209–218.

Buchholz, B., Frederick, L.J., and Armstrong, T.J., 1988. An investigation of human palmar skin friction and the effects of materials, pinch force and moisture, *Ergonomics*, 31:317–325.

Bullinger, H.J. and Solf, J.J., 1979. *Ergonomische Arbeitsmittelgestaltung II — Handgeführte Werkzeuge — Fallstudien* [Ergonomic improvements to dangerous hand tools], Dortmund: Bundesanstalt für Arbeitsschutz und Unfallforschung.

Bureau of Labor Statistics, 1995. Reports on Survey of Occupational Injuries and Illnesses in 1977–1994, Washington, D.C.: U.S. Department of Labor.

Cannon, L.J., Bernacki, E.J., and Walter, S.D., 1981. Personal and occupational factors associated with carpal tunnel syndrome, *Journal of Occupational Medicine*, 23:255–258.

Chaffin, D. B., Andersson, G., and Martin, B.J., 1999. *Occupational Biomechanics*, 3rd ed., New York: John Wiley & Sons, 355–368.

Chang, S.R., Park, S., and Freivalds, A., 1999. Ergonomic evaluation of the effects of handle types on garden tools, *International Journal of Industrial Ergonomics*, 24:99–105.

Chao, E.Y., Opgrande, J.D., and Axmear, F.E., 1976. Three-dimensional force analysis of finger joints in selected isometric hand functions, *Journal of Biomechanics*, 9:387–396.

Chao, E.Y.S., An, K.N., Cooney, W.P., and Linsheid, R.L., 1989. *Biomechanics of the Hand: A Basic Research Study*, Singapore: World Scientific.

Chen, Y., 1991. An Evaluation of Hand Pressure Distribution for a Power Grasp and Forearm Flexor Muscle Contribution for a Power Grasp on Cylindrical Handles, Ph.D. dissertation, Lincoln: University of Nebraska.

Cochran, D.J. and Riley, M.W., 1982. An evaluation of handle shapes and sizes, *Proceedings of the Human Factors Society*, 26:408–412.

Cochran, D.J. and Riley, M.W., 1983. An examination of the speed of manipulation of various sizes and shapes of handles, *Proceedings of the Human Factors Society*, 27:432–436.

Cochran, D.J. and Riley, M.W., 1986a. An evaluation of knife handle guarding, *Human Factors*, 27:253–265.

Cochran, D.J. and Riley, M.W., 1986b. The effects of handle shape and size on exerted forces, *Human Factors*, 27:295–301.

Cole, K.J., 1991. Grasp force control in older adults, *Journal of Motor Behavior*, 23:251–258.

Cole, K.J. and Abbs, J.H., 1987. Kinematic and electromyographic responses to perturbation of a rapid grasp, *Journal of Neurophysiology*, 57:1498–1510.

Comaish, S. and Bottoms, E., 1971. The skin and friction: deviations from Amonton's laws and the effects of hydration and lubrication, *British Journal of Dermatology*, 84:37–43.

Copley, F.B., 1923. *Frederick W. Taylor*, Vol. II, New York: Harper, 56–67.

Corrigan, D.L., Foley, V. and Widule, C.J., 1981. Axe use efficiency — a work theory explanation of an historical trend, *Ergonomics*, 24:103–109.

Damon, A., Stoudt, H.W., and McFarland, R.A., 1966. *The Human Body in Equipment Design*, Cambridge, MA: Harvard University Press.

Dressel, G., Karrasch, K., and Spitzer, H., 1954. Arbeitsphysiologische Untersuchungen beim Schaufeln, Steinetragen, und Schubkarreschieben [Work physiology studies of shoveling, stone carrying and wheelbarrow pushing], *Zentralblatt für Arbeitswissenschaft und soziale Betriebspraxis*, 3:33–48.

Drillis, R.J., 1963. Folk norms and biomechanics, *Human Factors*, 5:427–441.

Drillis, R., Schneck, D., and Gage, H., 1963. The theory of striking tools, *Human Factors*, 5:467–478.

Drury, C.G., 1980. Handles for manual materials handling, *Applied Ergonomics*, 11:35–42.

Ducharme, R.E., 1975. Problem tools for women, *Industrial Engineering*, September:46–50.

Eastman Kodak Company, 1983. *Ergonomic Design for People at Work*, Belmont, CA: Lifetime Learning Publications, 140–159.

Ejeskar, A. and Örtengren, R., 1981. Isolated finger flexion force — a methodological study, *British Society for Surgery of the Hand*, 13:223–230.

Emanuel, J.T., Mills, S.J., and Bennett, J.F., 1980. In search of a better handle, in *Proceedings of the Symposium of Human Factors and Industrial Design in Consumer Products*, Medford, MA: Tufts University, 34–40.

Evans, T.E., Lucaccini, L.F., Hazell, J.W., and Lucas, R.J., 1973. Evaluation of dental hand instruments, *Human Factors*, 15:401–406.

Fellows, G.L. and Freivalds, A., 1991. Ergonomics evaluation of a foam rubber grip for tool handles, *Applied Ergonomics*, 22:225–230.

Fox, K., 1957. The Effect of Clothing on Certain Measures of Strength of Upper Extremities, Report EP-47, Natick, MA: Environmental Protection Branch, U.S. Army Quartermaster Research and Development Center.

Fraser, T.M., 1980. Ergonomic Principles in the Design of Hand Tools, Occupational Safety and Health Series 44, Geneva: International Labour Office.

Freivalds, A., 1986a. The ergonomics of shovelling and shovel design — a review of the literature, *Ergonomics*, 29:3–18.

Freivalds, A., 1986b. The ergonomics of shovelling and shovel design — an experimental study, *Ergonomics*, 29:19–30.

Freivalds, A., 1987. The ergonomics of tools, *International Reviews of Ergonomics*, 1:43–75.

Freivalds, A., 1999. Ergonomics of hand tools, in Karwowski, W. and Marras, W.S., Eds., *Occupational Ergonomics Handbook*, Boca Raton, FL: CRC Press, 461–478.

Freivalds, A. and Eklund, J., 1993. Reaction torques and operator stress while using powered nutrunners, *Applied Ergonomics*, 24:158–164.

Freivalds, A. and Kim, Y.J., 1990. Blade size and weight effects in shovel design, *Applied Ergonomics*, 21:39–42.

Garrett, J., 1971. The adult human hand: some anthropometric and biomechanical considerations, *Human Factors*, 13:117–131.

Gläser, H., 1933. Beiträge zur Form der Waldsäge und zur Technik des Sägens [Contributions to the design of forestry saws and sawing techniques], dissertation, Eberswalde.

Gorjatschkin, W., 1924. Theory of striking hand tools, *Herald of Metal Industry*, Moscow, No. 4 [in Russian].

Granada, M. and Konz, S., 1981. Evaluation of bent hammer handles, *Proceedings of the Human Factors Society*, 25:322–324.

Grant, K.A., Habes, D.J., and Steward, L.L., 1992. An analysis of handle designs for reducing manual effort: the influence of grip diameter, *International Journal of Industrial Ergonomics*, 10:199–206.

Greenberg, L. and Chaffin, D.B., 1976. *Workers and Their Tools*, Midland, MI: Pendell.

Grieve, D. and Pheasant, S., 1982. Biomechanics, in *The Body at Work*, W.T. Singleton, Ed., Cambridge, UK: Cambridge University Press, 142–150.

Guilfoyle, J., 1977. Look what design has done for the toothbrush, *Industrial Design*, 24:24–38.

Habes, D.J. and Grant, K.A., 1997a. An electromyographic study of maximum torques and upper extremity muscle activity in simulated screw driving tasks, *International Journal of Industrial Ergonomics*, 20:339–346.

Habes, D.J. and Grant, K.A., 1997b. An electromyographic study of strength and upper extremity muscle activity in simulated meat cutting tasks, *Applied Ergonomics*, 28:129–137.

Hall, N.B. and Bernett, E.M., 1956. Empirical assessment of handrail diameters, *Journal of Applied Psychology*, 40:381–382.

Heffernan, C. and Freivalds, A., 2000. Optimum pinch grips in the handling of dies, *Applied Ergonomics*, 31:409–414.

Hertzberg, H., 1973. Engineering anthropometry, in Van Cott, H. and Kincaid, R., Eds., Human Engineering Guide, Washington, D.C.: U.S. Government Printing Office, 467–584.

Humphreys, P.W., Lind, A.R., and Sweetland, J.S., 1962. The energy expenditure of coal miners at work, *British Journal of Industrial Medicine*, 19:264–275.

Hunt, L.I., 1934. A study of screwdrivers for small assembly work, *The Human Factor*, 8:70–73.

Huston, T.R., Sanghavi, N., and Mital, A., 1984. Human torque exertion capabilities on a fastener device with wrenches and screwdrivers, in Mital, A., Ed., *Trends in Ergonomics/Human Factors*, Vol. I, Amsterdam: Elsevier, 51–58.

Hymovich, L. and Lindholm, M., 1966. Hand, wrist and forearm injuries, *Journal of Occupational Medicine*, 8:573–577.

Jackson, D.A. and Clifford, J.C., 1989. Electrodiagnosis of mild carpal tunnel syndrome, *Archives of Physical Medicine Rehabilitation*, 70:199–204.

Johansson, R.S., 1991. How is grasping modified by somatosensory input? in Humphrey, D.R. and Freund, H.J., Eds., *Motor Control: Concepts and Issues*, Chichester, U.K.: John Wiley, 331–355.

Johansson, R.S. and Westling, G., 1984. Roles of glabrous skin receptors and sensorimotor memory in automatic control of precision grip when lifting rougher or more slippery objects, *Experimental Brain Research*, 56:550–564.

Johansson, R.S. and Westling, G., 1987. Signals in tactile afferents from the fingers eliciting adaptive motor responses during precision grip, *Experimental Brain Research*, 66:141–154.

Johansson, R.S., Huger, C., and Bäckström, L., 1992. Somatosensory control of precision grip during unpredictable pulling loads, III. Impairments during digital anesthesia, *Experimental Brain Research*, 89:204–213.

Johnson, S.L., 1988. Evaluation of powered screwdriver design characteristics, *Human Factors*, 30:61–69.

Kao, H., 1976. An analysis of user preference toward handwriting instruments, *Perceptual and Motor Skills*, 43:522.

Kao, H., 1977. Ergonomics in penpoint design, *Acta Psychologia Taiwanica*, 18:49–52.

Kao, H., 1979. Differential effects of writing instruments on handwriting performance, *Acta Psychologia Taiwanica*, 21:9–13.

Karlqvist, L., 1984. Cutting operation at canning bench — a case study of handtool design, in *Proceedings of the 1984 International Conference on Occupational Ergonomics*, Rexdale, Ontario, Canada: Human Factors Association of Canada, 452–456.

Ketchum, I.D., Thompson, D., Pocock, G., and Wallingford, D., 1978. A clinical study of forces generated by the intrinsic muscles of the index finger and the extrinsic flexor and extensor muscles of the hand, *Journal of Hand Surgery*, 3:571–578.

Kirsch, G., 1939. Untersuchungen über die zweckmässigste Gestalt der Schaufelns [Research on an effective shovel shape], dissertation, Berlin-Charlottenberg: Technische Hochschule.

Knowlton, R.G. and Gilbert J.C., 1983. Ulnar deviation and short term strength reductions as affected by a curve handled ripping hammer and a conventional claw hammer, *Ergonomics*, 26:173–179.

Kommerell, G., 1929. Die Schaufelarbeit in gebückter Haltung [Shoveling while in a bent posture], *Arbeitsphysiologie*, 1:278–295.

Kong, Y.K., 2001. Optimum Design of Handle Shape through Biomechanical Modeling of Hand Tendon Forces, Ph.D. dissertation, University Park, PA: Pennsylvania State University.

Kong, Y.K. and Freivalds, A., 2003. Evaluation of meat-hook handle shapes, *International Journal of Industrial Ergonomics*, 32:12–23.

Kong, Y., Freivalds, A., and Kim, S.E., in press. Evaluation of handles in a maximum gripping task, *Ergonomics.*

Konz, S., 1974. Design of handtools, *Proceedings of the Human Factors Society,* 18:292–300.

Konz, S., 1975. Design of food scoops, *Applied Ergonomics,* 6:32.

Konz, S., 1986. Bent hammer handles, *Human Factors,* 27:317–323.

Konz, S. and Johnson, S., 2000. *Work Design,* 5th ed., Scottsdale, AZ: Holcomb Hathaway.

Konz, S. and Streets, B., 1984. Bent hammer handles performance and preference, *Proceedings of the Human Factors Society,* 28:438–440.

Konz, S. and Warraich, M., 1985. Performance differences between the preferred and non-preferred hand when using various tools, in I.D. Brown, R. Goldsmith, K. Coombes, and M.A. Sinclair, Eds., *Ergonomics International 85,* London: Taylor & Francis, 451–453.

Kroemer, K.H.E., 1986. Coupling the hand with the handle: an improved notation of touch grip and grasp, *Human Factors,* 27:337–339.

Kroemer, K.H.E., 1989. Cumulative trauma disorders: their recognition and ergonomics measures to avoid them, *Applied Ergonomics,* 20:274–280.

Kroemer, K.H.E., 1992. Avoiding cumulative trauma disorders in shops and offices, *American Industrial Hygiene Association Journal,* 53:596–604.

Krohn, R. and Konz, S., 1982. Bent hammer handles, *Proceedings of the Human Factors Society,* 26:413–417.

Lavender, S.A., Marras, W.S., Lundquist, R.G., Rockwell, T.H., and Bobick, T.G., 1986. Analysis of hand tool accidents in the underground mining industry, *Proceedings of the Human Factors Society,* 30:1419–1423.

Laveson, J.K. and Meyer, R.P., 1976. Left out "lefties" in design, *Proceedings of the Human Factors Society,* 20:122–125.

Leaky, L.S.B., 1960. Finding the worlds earliest man, *National Geographic,* 118:420–435.

Lee, J.W., and Rim, K., 1990. Maximum finger force prediction using a planar simulation of the middle finger, *Proceedings of the Institute of Mechanical Engineers,* 204:167–178.

Lehmann, G., 1953. *Praktische Arbeitsphysiologie* [Practical Work Physiology], Stuttgart: Thieme, 182–197.

Lindstrom, F.E., 1973. *Modern Pliers,* Enköping, Sweden: Bahco Vertyg.

Lowe, B.D. and Freivalds, A., 1999. Effect of carpal tunnel syndrome on grip force coordination on hand tools, *Ergonomics,* 42:550–554.

Magill, R. and Konz, S., 1986. An evaluation of seven industrial screwdrivers, in W. Karwowski, Ed., *Trends in Ergonomics/Human Factors,* Vol. III, Amsterdam: Elsevier, 597–604.

Marras, W.S., 1986. Measurements of spine loading components during the usage of large hand tools, in W. Karwowski, Ed., *Trends in Ergonomics/Human Factors,* Vol. III, Amsterdam: Elsevier, 693–699.

Marras, W.S. and Rockwell, T.H., 1986. An experimental evaluation of method and tool effects in spike maul use, *Human Factors,* 27:267–281.

Materials Handling Research Unit, 1980. *Force Limits in Manual Work,* Guildford, U.K.: IPC Science and Technology Press.

McCormick, E.J. and Sanders, M.S., 1982. *Human Factors in Engineering Design,* 5th ed., New York: McGraw-Hill, 283–309.

Meagher, S.W., 1986. Hand tools: cumulative trauma disorders caused by improper use of design elements, in W. Karwowski, Ed., *Trends in Ergonomics/Human Factors,* Vol. III, Amsterdam: Elsevier, 581–587.

Meyer, F., 1930. Arbeitsgrösse, Arbeitsaufwand und Arbeitsökonomie beim hantieren schwerer Hammer, *Arbeitsphysiologie*, 3:529.

Miller, G. and Freivalds, A., 1987. Gender and handedness in grip strength, *Proceedings of the Human Factors Society*, 31st Annual Meeting, 906–909.

Miller, M., Ransohoff, J., and Tichauer, E.R., 1971. Ergonomic evaluation of a redesigned surgical instrument, *Applied Ergonomics*, 2:194–197.

Mital, A., 1985. Effects of tool and operator factors on volitional torque exertion capabilities of individuals, in I.D. Brown, R. Goldsmith, K. Coombes, and M.A. Sinclair, Eds., *Ergonomics International 85*, London: Taylor & Francis, 262–264.

Mital, A., 1986. Effect of body posture and common tools on peak torque exertion capabilities, *Applied Ergonomics*, 17:87–96.

Mital, A. and Sanghavi, N., 1986. Comparison of maximum volitional torque exertion capabilities of males and females using common hand tools, *Human Factors*, 27:283–294.

Mital, A., Sanghavi, N., and Huston, T., 1985. A study of factors defining the operator-hand tool system at the work place, *International Journal of Production Research*, 23:297–314.

Monod, H. and Scherrer, J., 1965. The work capacity of a synergic muscular group, *Ergonomics*, 8:329–338.

Morrissey, S., Bethea, N.J., and Ayoub, M.M., 1983. Task demands for shoveling in non-erect postures, *Ergonomics*, 26:297–951.

Müller, E.A. and Karrasch, K., 1956. Die grösste Dauerleistung beim Schaufeln [The longest shoveling work period], *Internationale Zeitschrift für angewandte Physiologie einschliesslich Arbeitsphysiologie*, 16:318–324.

Napier, J., 1956. The prehensile movements of the human hand, *Journal of Bone and Joint Surgery*, 38B:902–913.

Napier, J., 1962. The evolution of the hand, *Scientific American*, 207(12):56–62.

Napier, J., 1963. Early man and his environment, *Discovery*, 24(3):12–18.

Oh, S. and Radwin, R.G., 1993. Pistol grip power tool handle and trigger size effects on grip exertions and operator preference, *Human Factors*, 35:551–569.

Pheasant, S.T. and O'Neill, D., 1975. Performance in gripping and turning — a study in hand/handle effectiveness, *Applied Ergonomics*, 6:205–208.

Pheasant, S.T. and Scriven, J.G., 1983. Sex differences in strength — some implications for the design of handtools, in K. Coombes, Ed., *Proceedings of the Ergonomics Society's Conference 1983*, London: Taylor & Francis, 9–13.

Radhakrishnan, S. and Nagaravindra, M.C., 1993. Analysis of hand forces in health and disease during maximum isometric grasping of cylinders, *Medicine and Biological Engineering and Computing*, 31:372–376.

Replogle, J.O., 1983. Hand torque strength with cylindrical handles, *Proceedings of the Human Factors Society*, 27:412–416.

Rigby, L.V., 1973. Why do people drop things? *Quality Progress*, 6:16–19.

Rockwell, T.H. and Marras, W.S., 1986. An evaluation of tool design and method of use of railroad leverage tools on back stress and tool performance, *Human Factors*, 27:303–315.

Rohmert, W., 1973. Problems in determining rest allowances, *Applied Ergonomics*, 4:91–95.

Rothfleisch, S. and Sherman, D., 1978. Carpal tunnel syndrome: biomechanical aspects of occupational occurrence and implications regarding surgical management, *Orthopaedic Review*, 7:107–109.

Roubal, J. and Kovar, Z., 1962. Tool handles and control levers of machines, *Annals of Occupational Hygiene*, 5:37–40.

Rubarth, B., 1928. Untersuchung zur Festgestaltung von Handheften für Schrauben-zieher und ähnliche Werkzeuge [Research on handles for screwdrivers and similar tools], *Industrielle Psychotechnik*, 5:129–142.

Saran, C., 1973. Biomechanical evaluation of T-handles for a pronation supination task, *Journal of Occupational Medicine*, 15:712–716.

Scheller, W.L., 1983. The effect of handle shape on grip fatigue in manual lifting, *Proceedings of the Human Factors Society*, 27:417–421.

Shock, N., 1962. The physiology of aging, *Scientific American*, 206:100–110.

Silverstein, B.A., Fine, L.J., and Armstrong, T.J., 1987. Occupational factors and carpal tunnel syndrome, *American Journal of Industrial Medicine*, 11:343–358.

Spitzer, H., 1950. Die Rationelle Ausführung der Körperarbeit [Rational organization of physical work], *Stahl und Eisen*, 70:509–515.

Stetson, D.S., Armstrong, T.J., Fine, L.J., Silverstein, B.A., and Tannen, K., 1986. A survey of chronic upper extremity disorders in an automobile upholstery plant, in W. Karwowski, Ed., *Trends in Ergonomics/Human Factors*, Vol. III, Amsterdam: Elsevier, 623–630.

Stevenson, A.G. and Brown, R.L., 1923. An investigation on the motion study of digging and the energy expenditure involved, with the object of increasing efficiency of output and economising energy, *Journal of the Royal Army Medical Corps*, 40:340–349, 423–434; 41:39–45, 99–111.

Swain, A.D., Shelton, G.G., and Rigby, L.V., 1970. Maximum torque for small knobs operated with and without gloves, *Ergonomics*, 13:201–208.

Tannen, K.J., Stetson, D.S., Silverstein, B.A., Fine, L.J., and Armstrong, T.J., 1986. An evaluation of scissors for control of upper extremity disorders in an automobile upholstery plant, in W. Karwowski, Ed., *Trends in Ergonomics/Human Factors*, Vol. III, Amsterdam: Elsevier, 631–639.

Taylor, F.W., 1913. *The Principles of Scientific Management*, New York: Harper & Row.

Terrell, R. and Purswell, J., 1976. The influence of forearm and wrist orientation on static grip strength as a design criterion for hand tools, *Proceedings of the Human Factors Society*, 20:28–32.

Tichauer, E.R., 1966. Some aspects of stress on forearm and hand in industry, *Journal of Occupational Medicine*, 8:63–71.

Tichauer, E.R., 1976. Biomechanics sustains occupational safety and health, *Industrial Engineer*, Feb:46–56.

Tichauer, E.R., 1978. *The Biomechanical Basis of Ergonomics*, New York: Wiley.

Tichauer, E.R. and Gage, H., 1977. Ergonomic principles basic to hand tool design, *Journal of the American Industrial Hygiene Association*, 38:622–634.

Udo, H., Otani, T., Udo, A., and Yoshinaga, F., 2000. A electromyographic study of two different types of ball point pens, *Industrial Health*, 38:47–50.

Vennewald, H., 1939. Über die Zweckmässigkeit der Grabwerkzeugen [On the efficiency of graveyard tools], *Arbeitsphysiologie*, 10:647–667.

Weidman, B., 1970. Effect of Safety Gloves on Simulated Work Tasks, AD 738981, Springfield, VA: National Technical Information Service.

Wenzig, K., 1928. Arbeitsphysiologische Studien VII, Beiträge zur Physiologie des Schaufelns [Contributions to the physiology of shoveling], *Arbeitsphysiologie*, 1:154–186.

Wenzig, K., 1932. Arbeitsphysiologische Studien X, Beiträge zur Physiologie des Schaufelns [Contributions to the physiology of shoveling], *Arbeitsphysiologie*, 5:252–268.

Westling, G. and Johansson, R.S., 1984. Factors influencing the force control during precision grip, *Experimental Brain Research*, 53:277–284.

Westling, G. and Johansson, R.S., 1987. Responses in glabrous skin mechanoreceptors, *Experimental Brain Research*, 66:128–140.

Widule, C. J., Foley, V., and Demo, F., 1978. Dynamics of the axe swing, *Ergonomics*, 21:925–930.

Wyndham, C.H., Morrison, J.F., Williams, C.G., Heyns, R., Margo, E., Brown, A.M., and Astrup, J., 1966. The relationship between energy expenditure and performance index in the task of shovelling sand, *Ergonomics*, 9:371–378.

Wyndham, C.H., Morrison, J.F., Viljoen, J.H., Strydom, N.B., and Heynes, R., 1969. Factors affecting the mechanical efficiency of men shovelling rock in stopes, *Journal of the South African Institute of Mining and Metallurgy*, 70:53–59.

Yoder, T.A., Lucas, R.L., and Botzum, C.D., 1973. The marriage of human factors and safety in industry, *Human Factors*, 15:197–205.

10

The Office Environment

10.1 General Musculoskeletal Problems

Musculoskeletal problems in an office environment have existed as long as writing has been known. The cramping of the writer's hand was a common complaint and became the subject of clinical interest and controversy in England as early as 1855, when it was termed scrivener's palsy or, more typically, *writer's cramp*. With the growth of commerce in the Victorian era, a large number of scriveners were responsible for copying all the contracts by hand using a quill, whose thin shaft had to be gripped firmly. The resulting spasms were first described in detail by Wilks (1878) and later by others (Sheehy and Marsden, 1982) as resulting from the repetitive forceful contractions of the hand with complications induced by co-contractions of the forearm flexors and extensors. This interaction of various aspects of the motor system as well as the sensory system, technically termed, *focal dystonia*, has only recently been counteracted by the use of peripheral sensory stimulation, high-frequency vibrations, and blocking of selected pathways with lidocaine or botulism (Kaji, 2000). In terms of preventing the problem, increasing the size of a ballpoint pen grip area with a flared design to a diameter of 13.6 mm significantly reduced the EMG of the flexor pollicis brevis and pain scores for various hand regions as compared to a common ballpoint pen during extended writing (Udo et al., 2000).

The gradual reduction of writing implements for data entry in favor of faster means by mechanical typewriters, then electronic typewriters, and, eventually, keyboards linked to the personal computer did not eliminate the musculoskeletal problems associated with clerical work. If anything, complaints increased, but for different reasons and in different parts of the body. Whereas overgripping a quill or pen resulted in writer's cramp, the more constrained posture and high force required to operate the keys of mechanical typewriters resulted in tenosynovitis of the fingers (Çakir et al., 1980). Early electronic keyboards were not much better, with a high rate of fatigue and musculoskeletal complaints in Japanese keypunch operators in the 1960s (Komoike and Horiguchi, 1971; Maeda et al., 1982,) leading to neck and upper arm pain, termed the cervicobrachial disorder (Maeda, 1977). Similar problems were later observed in Europe (Çakir et al., 1978; Hünting et al., 1981), in Australia (ACTU-VHTC, 1982; Ferguson, 1984; Hocking, 1987), and in the United States leading to a large NIOSH study of journalists and other office workers (NIOSH, 1981). Many of the early concerns were primarily related to nonbiomechanical outcomes, such as visual fatigue, near sightedness, color vision changes, various occulomotor changes, radiation leakages leading to skin rashes, cataracts, and even miscarriages, resulting primarily from the relatively crude early model visual display terminals (VDTs) with low pixel densities.

Since then, as the electronics of the VDT improved, the emphasis has been primarily on the musculoskeletal disorders (MSDs) related to the constrained postures, physical layout, keyboards designs, etc. Numerous studies have been performed in this area, too many to cite here. However, there are a number of good reviews that summarize these studies and the various occupational factors leading to these MSD of the upper extremities including National Research Council (1984, 2001) and NIOSH (1989, 1995, 1997). Among the most commonly observed biomechanical work-related risk factors are high forces, high repetition, vibration, cold exposure, short cycle times (<10 s), hand tool use, deviated postures, acceleration, and hours of keyboard use. The combination of the two major factors, force and repetition, can increase the risk for injury (odds ratio) up to 30 times greater (Silverstein et al., 1986). There are also numerous psychosocial risk factors than enter into the picture: job satisfaction, work speed, monotony, relations with colleagues and supervisors, work content, and control of work. However, as these are nonbiomechanical, they are not discussed any further here.

10.2 The Seated Workplace

10.2.1 Seated Posture

The most common overall posture found in an office environment is sitting at a computer workstation. That is not to say that there are not some specialized tasks that are performed in a standing posture, such as copying, working with large-sized drawings, using light tables, and handling photographic reproductions, or that some individuals may prefer to work in a standing posture (Thomas Jefferson is the prime historical example; http://standupdesks.com/tj.html) or that standing workstations may be used to increase customer throughput by minimizing the time spent dawdling at library or public computer-laboratory workstations. However, the vast majority of the time will be spent sitting, which causes large alterations to the shape of the spine and increases disc pressure, potentially resulting in increased incidences of low-back pain and injuries in subjects who predominantly work in a sitting posture.

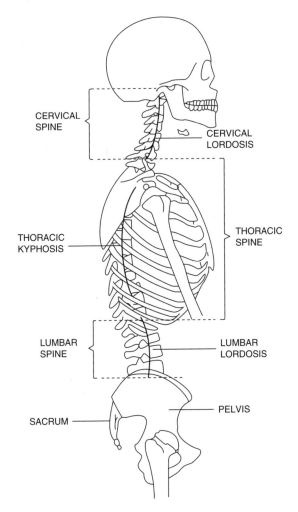

FIGURE 10.1
Anatomy of the human spine. (From Chaffin, D.B. et al., 1999. *Occupational Biomechanics*, 3rd ed., New York: John Wiley & Sons. With permission.)

10.2.1.1   The Spine

The spine or vertebral column is divided into four sections: the *cervical spine* of the neck, the *thoracic spine* of the upper back, the *lumbar spine* of the lower back, and the *sacrum*, primarily fixed within the pelvis. In a standing posture, from the sagittal plane, the spine appears to have an extended-S shape, with several distinctive curves: *lordosis* in the cervical area, *kyphosis* in the thoracic area, and the more critical lumbar lordosis (Figure 10.1). Anatomically, this curve is necessary to maintain the head upright, as the sacrum is tilted considerably down from the horizontal (Chaffin et al., 1999). Functionally, one could argue that such curvature provides dampening of impacts to the brain during locomotion and other physical activity.

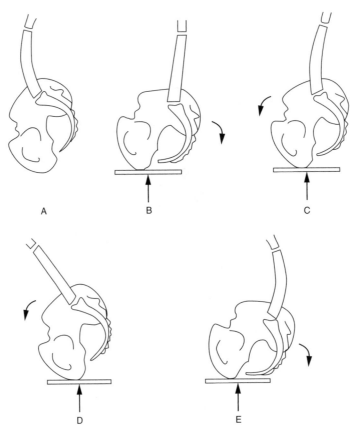

FIGURE 10.2
Posture of the pelvis and the lumbar spine: (A) standing, (B) sitting relaxed, (C) sitting erect, (D) sitting forward, (E) sitting backward. (Note that the head faces left.) (From Andersson, G.B.J. et al., 1974. *Scandinavian Journal of Rehabilitation Medicine*, 6:104–114. With permission.)

More importantly, when one moves from a standing to a seated posture, there is a considerable change to the shape of the spine. Because the lumbar spine is joined to the sacrum, which is practically fixed in the pelvis, a rotational movement of the pelvis also directly affects the shape of the lumbar spine. In the process of sitting down, the pelvis rotates backward, causing the lumbar spine to flatten and lose its lordotic shape (Figure 10.2B,C). Sometimes, as in slouching forward, even a pronounced kyphosis can develop (Figure 10.2D). This lumbar flattening has been verified from radiographic studies and can be prevented by the use of lumbar supports (Andersson et al., 1979) or a more posterior leaning posture (Figure 10.2E; Chaffin et al., 1999).

As described in Section 2.5.4, the spine consists of the bony vertebrae separated by intervertebral discs, each with a gel-filled nucleus pulposus. Such a fluidlike center allows for the insertion of a pressure transducer to directly measure the pressure changes within a disc during various postures

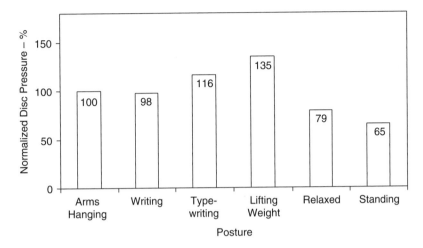

FIGURE 10.3
Mean normalized disc pressures measured in an office chair during simulated work activities (100% = 0.471 MPa or 47.1 N/cm). (Adapted from Andersson and Örtengren, 1974a; Andersson et al., 1974b.)

(Nachemson and Morris, 1964). Later refinements with a strain-gauge transducer needle allowed more detailed experiments on various office and experimental chairs (Andersson et al., 1974a,b; Andersson and Örtengren, 1974a). These results are shown in Figure 10.3, with a resting sitting position with arms handing down normalized to 100% disc pressure. Disc pressures in a standing posture were found to be 35% lower, while, for reference purposes, a supine posture, with minimal effects of gravity on the discs, yielded a pressure of only 10%. When the arms were marginally supported during writing, disc pressures dropped slightly to 98%. When the arms were unsupported, as during typewriting, disc pressure increased to 116%. Holding a 1.2-kg weight with extended arms increased disc pressures to 135%.

10.2.1.2 Disc Compression Forces

In terms of the more commonly used *disc compression forces*, typically calculated from biomechanical modeling (Chaffin et al., 1999), normalized 100% disc pressure corresponds to an absolute pressure of 47.1 N/cm². Given an average lumbar disc area of 17 cm² (Pooni et al., 1986), the disc compression force in a resting sitting posture with arms hanging down is 800 N. The criterion disc compression force used as the basis for the recommended weight limit in the NIOSH lifting equation (Waters et al., 1993) is only four times larger at 3400 N.

Overall, one can conclude that disc pressures increase considerably as the body goes from a standing to a sitting posture and as additional loading is put on the shoulders, i.e., arms not supported. This change in pressure is thought to be due to an increased trunk load moment during the pelvic

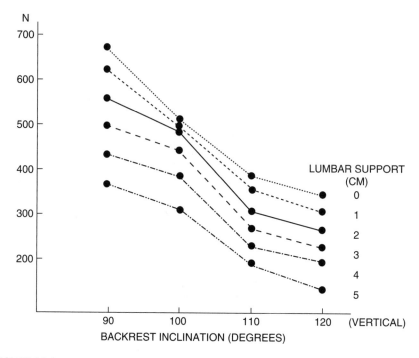

FIGURE 10.4

Disc pressures measured with different backrest inclinations and different size lumbar supports. (From Chaffin, D.B. et al., 1999. *Occupational Biomechanics*, 3rd ed., New York: John Wiley & Sons. With permission.)

rotation and a deformation of the disc itself (Chaffin et al., 1999). On the other hand, adding a lumbar support and inclining the backrest backward decrease disc pressures (Andersson et al., 1974a). This effect is proportional to the thickness of the lumbar support (approximately an 8% decrease for each 1 cm of pad thickness; Figure 10.4) and to the inclination of the backrest (approximately a 1.3% decrease for 1° backward movement). The first serves to maintain lumbar lordosis and transfers some of the load to the support, thus reducing the load on the disc, as was also verified indirectly by the reduction of pressures on the seat pan (Shields and Cook, 1988). The second, similarly, transfers some of the load to the backrest and reduces the load on the discs as measured by spinal shrinkage (Corlett and Eklund, 1984a,b). The use of armrests to reduce the loading on the spine decreases the disc pressures by as much as 16% (Andersson and Örtengren, 1974b).

10.2.1.3   *Electromyography*

Electromyography (EMG) of the back erector spinae muscles has also been used to measure the stresses or loading during a sitting posture. Generally, the EMG levels are low and comparable to a standing posture (Floyd and Silver, 1955; Andersson and Örtengren, 1974a). More forward-leaning postures increase the EMG. However, once forward movement reaches full flexion, i.e., slumping, the EMG levels decrease almost to zero, indicating a relaxation of the erector spinae muscles, with the load supported by ligaments (Floyd and Silver, 1955). EMG levels also decrease when the arms are supported, reducing some of the load on the muscle (Andersson and Örtengren, 1974b). Similar to disc pressure, EMG levels decrease as the angle between the seat pan and backrest is increased and more of the load is supported by the backrest. However, the effect levels off at angles greater than 110° (Andersson et al., 1974b). Coincidentally, at such angles, it would become increasingly difficult to maintain good visibility of the visual task on the working surface.

One consequence of prolonged sitting is the potential for increased risk of low back pain (Magora, 1972; Grieco, 1986), although the results are not conclusive (Svensson and Andersson, 1983). The problem appears to be mainly one of postural rigidity, i.e., of remaining too long in one posture, whether standing or sitting (Grieco, 1986). A large-scale study of 3300 workers by Magora (1972) found that both excessive and minimal time spent in a seated postures are associated with a high frequency of low back pain, while subjects who varied their working postures had negligible frequencies. Unfortunately, with higher use of computer workstations, there is a greater tendency toward postural rigidity as found by Grieco (1986) in the telecommunications industry. Specifically, reorganizing a job to include postural flexibility either through a variety of work activities or the use of chairs that promote movements of the body (Festervoll, 1994) such as a sit-stand chair (discussed in Section 10.2.5) is recommended. For further details and guidelines on sitting postures, please refer to Åkerblom (1948), Grandjean (1969), Zacharkow (1988), and Chaffin et al. (1999).

10.2.2 Seated Posture at a Computer Workstation

In the traditional office workplace of 20 years ago, the wide variety of activities performed by workers precluded any worries about constrained postures. However, with the almost ubiquitous use of personal computers in the office environment, the risk of incurring work-related musculoskeletal disorders (WRMSD) from the static loading of limbs held in constrained postures over long periods of time has increased dramatically. Therefore, the availability of the adjustable computer workstation to fit the anthropometry of differently sized individuals to an optimal is very important. Even more important is that these individuals adjust the furniture to match their needs. However, there remains the question of what is an optimal posture.

10.2.2.1 Standard Posture

A variety of studies were been carried primarily in the laboratory during the early 1980s as computers entered the office environment. These resulted in postures selected by the tested individuals as their preferred postures and are summarized in Table 10.1. Simultaneously, seating design guidelines

TABLE 10.1

Preferred Settings and Design Recommendations for a Computer Workstation (mean values or ranges without wrist support)

Workstation Feature	Brown and Schaum (1980)	Miller and Suther (1983)	Grandjean et al. (1982)	Rubin and Marshall (1982)	Grandjean et al. (1983, 1984)	Weber et al. (1984)	AIHA Guide (Kroemer, 1983)	Human Factors and Ergonomics Society (2002)	Traditional Rule of Thumb
Keyboard height (cm)[a]	74	71	77	71	80	78	47–73	56–72	Elbow rest height
Screen height (cm)	99[b]	93[b]	109[b]	87[2]	103[2]	97[2]	91–130[3]	67–84 est.[3]	Seated eye height[3]
Screen angle (°)[d]	10	3	0	—	5	11	±10[5]	±20°	Small to avoid glare
Screen distance (cm)	59[e]	—	66[e]	—	76[e]	71[f]	—	>40[6]	Resting focus
Seat height (cm)	50	44	47	42	48	47	36–53	38–56 est.	Popliteal height
Type of study	Lab	Lab	Lab	—	Field	Lab	Design Guidelines: 1st per. female to 99th per. male	Design Guidelines: 5th per. female to 95th per. male	Basis for Design Guidelines
No. of subjects	40 females 60 males	15 females 22 males	30 females	—	48 females 20 males	20	—	—	—

[a] Home row from floor.
[b] Center of screen from floor.
[c] Top of screen from floor.
[d] Upward tilted screen relative to vertical.
[e] From center of screen to keyboard edge.
[f] From center of screen to eyes.

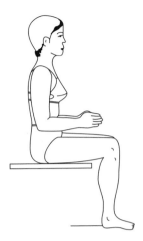

FIGURE 10.5
Standard anthropometric sitting position. (From Webb Associates, 1978.)

were developed independently based on anthropometric measurements taken in a "standard" seating posture, with the trunk vertical and with 90° angles at the elbow, hips, knees, and ankles (Figure 10.5; Diffrient et al., 1974; Branton, 1974; Webb Associates, 1978). These measurements then evolved into various national and international guidelines or standards such as BSR/ HFES 100 (U.S.), BS EN 1135 (U.K.), DIN EN 1135 (Germany), ISO 9241-5 (international), and JIS Z 8513 (Japan). Not unexpectedly, there can be considerable variation in these standards with some of the differences due to ethnic anthropometric differences and others due to trade-offs between interacting parameters assigned different weights. Also, some differences may result from practical considerations, such as the comments of Lueder (1983) that German DIN standards are moving away from excessive workstation adjustability because people tend not to use it. Two of the guidelines for various workstation features are listed in Table 10.1. Specific adjustment ranges for various chair features are given in Figure 10.6 and Table 10.2.

The preferred settings for seat height are quite consistent and fall within the design guidelines of 5th percentile female to 95th percentile male popliteal heights. Keyboard preferences tend to be consistent in the range of 71 to 80 cm above the floor, but tend to be on the high side of the design guidelines based on elbow resting height. Other researches have observed a similar tendency for operators to prefer the home row of the keyboard to be anywhere from 6 to 9 cm above resting elbow height (Grandjean et al., 1983; Life and Pheasant, 1984; Sauter et al., 1991; Liao and Drury, 2000). In such cases, many of the operators actually tended to lean back, acquiring a 104° trunk angle as opposed to the expected 90° vertical trunk position (Grandjean et al., 1983).

10.2.2.2   Screen Height

Preferred screen height also varied considerably and tended to be higher than the recommendation based on the top of the screen being at seated eye

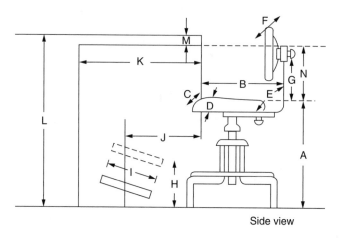

Side view

FIGURE 10.6

Adjustable chair. Specific seat parameter values found in Table 10.2. (From Niebel, B. and Freivalds, A., 2003. *Methods, Standards, and Work Design*, New York: McGraw-Hill. With permission.)

TABLE 10.2

Recommended Seat Adjustment Ranges

Seat Parameter	Design Value (cm)	Comments
A = Seat height	38–56	Too high, compresses thighs; too low, disc pressure increases
B = Seat depth	<43	Too long, cuts popliteal region; use waterfall contour
C = Seat width	>46	Wider seats recommended for overweight individuals
D = Seat pan angle	–3° to +3°	Downward tilting requires more friction in the fabric
E = Seat back to pan angle	90°–120°	<90° leads to fatigue, >120° requires headrest
F = Seat back width	>36	Measured in the lumbar region
G = Lumbar support	15–25	Vertical height from compressed seat pan to center of lumbar support
H = Foot rest height	2.5–23	—
I = Foot rest depth	30.5	—
J = Foot rest distance	42	—
K = Leg clearance	66	—
L = Work surface height	~81	Determined by elbow rest height
M = Work surface thickness	<5	Maximum value
N = Thigh clearance	>20	Minimum value

Sources: A to G from Human Factors and Ergonomics Society (2002); H to M from Eastman Kodak (1983).

height (discounting the Kroemer, 1983, recommendation, which was hard to interpret). In both cases, preferred values obtained after short periods in a laboratory could be vastly different from those that result after many hours of work a day for many months or years.

10.2.2.3 Screen Distance

The preferred screen distance is relatively consistent and corresponds closely to the mean intermediate resting focus of 59 cm found in young adults. This position is hypothesized by Leibowitz and Owens (1975) to provide the least amount of stress for the accommodative system of the eyes and should be the most comfortable reading distance. Preferred screen angles were generally small (i.e., the screen was almost vertical), which is the desired position to reduce reflection from overhead lights and consequent glare.

10.2.2.4 Arm Support

As mentioned previously, if the arms are unsupported, as during typewriting, disc pressure increased to 16% from a normal seated posture with the arms handing comfortably down (Andersson and Örtengren, 1974b). Therefore, the use of a wrist or forearm support during keyboarding would be recommended as long as the support does not impede the activity. Later studies specifically examining keyboards and supports found that the use of a wrist support decreased trapezius EMG activity by 25% and was preferred by two thirds of the subjects (Weber et al., 1984), especially by those with existing shoulder pains and elbows bent at 105° (Erdelyi et al., 1988). Similarly, trapezius EMG activity remained below 1% MVC for almost 50% of the working time with use of wrist supports while the same could be achieved for only 10% of the time without the use of wrist supports (Aarås et al., 1997). The use of wrist supports also significantly decreased wrist flexion (Gerr et al., 2000) and significantly increased the number of keystrokes entered on the second day after practice (Smith et al., 1998). On the other hand, other studies found no improvements with wrist supports (Fernström et al., 1994) with some subjects even reporting an increase in musculoskeletal discomfort (Parsons, 1991). Potentially, the greatest problem with wrist rests may be with the increase of pressures in the carpal tunnel from 14 mmHg in unsupported wrists to 31 mmHg while using wrist rests (Horie et al., 1993). Prolonged pressures of 30 mmHg have been associated with altered nerve function in animal studies (Hargens et al., 1979; Lundborg et al., 1983; Powell and Myers, 1986), which could be the first step in the sequence of events leading to carpal tunnel syndrome (CTS) (Dahlin et al., 1987).

10.2.2.5 Alternate Posture

A cautionary note should be given regarding the traditional 90° seating posture. This posture is not necessarily the posture chosen by all people

(Barkla, 1964; Mandal, 1981) and as few as 10% of individuals will actually sit with the trunk vertical (Grandjean et al., 1983). Also, this approach is based on a static posture and ignores the fact that sitting should be a dynamic activity, which should be further encouraged through job design or the use of sit-stand stools. Similarly, although physical workstation dimensions are important determinants of operator posture, the correlations between specific workstation and anthropometric dimensions are not always very high. For example, Gerr et al. (2000) found highest correlations of $r = 0.7$ for line of sight and monitor height and $r = 0.6$ between keyboard height and elbow resting height. However, monitor height and seated eye height showed only a correlation of $r = 0.18$. Overall, the most critical feature is adjustability of the workstation and its furniture, especially seat height, keyboard height, work surface and thus monitor height, and wrist/forearm support.

10.2.3   Determination of Seated Comfort

Seated comfort is obviously a very subjective issue, very much dependent on each individual preferences as well as the task being performed. Thus, there is no one easy approach to determining a unique value for comfort. Shackel et al. (1969), Branton (1969), Drury and Coury (1982), Lueder, (1983), Zacharkow (1988), and Zhang et al. (1996) have suggested a variety of approaches, including (1) comparison with anthropometric data and guidelines, (2) fitting trials, (3) observation of postural changes, (4) observation of task performance, (5) subjective assessment techniques, and (6) physical measures of comfort.

10.2.3.1   Fitting Trials

In fitting trials, the subjects are allowed to adjust the dimensions of the chair or workplace until subjective comfort is attained (Jones, 1969; Drury and Coury, 1982). These then can be used as a reference point about which the dimensions are varied to establish a tolerable range (LeCarpentier, 1969). The method is reasonably accurate and repeatable in that the selected values compared favorably to anthropometric guidelines (Jones, 1969) and day-to-day variations in mean comfort positions were relatively small, varying only by a few degrees or centimeters (LeCarpentier, 1969).

10.2.3.2   Postural Changes

A variety of body movements occur while sitting, ranging from small involuntary motor responses such as respiration and heart beat to large intentional movements required for the task. Among these are also restless postural changes attempting to compensate for uncomfortable seating conditions. Grandjean et al. (1960) found good correlation between the number of body movements and subjective ratings of seat discomfort. Branton and Grayson (1967) were able to identify differences in train seat designs based on both long-term filming of subjects and short-term observations with a larger sample. Cantoni et al. (1984) found a significant decrease in postural changes, ranging from 44 to 71%, at ergonomically designed chairs and VDT workstations as compared to the traditional switchboard workstation that was replaced for telephone operators. Fenety et al. (2000) found good reliability in using a pressure mat to track a subject's center of pressure as a means of evaluating sitting discomfort. Unfortunately, postural changes are not solely due to uncomfortable chairs. Heat, humidity, general work stress, as well as individual variability and circadian rhythms, can also affect restlessness (Jürgens, 1980). The furniture itself may constrain movements and, thus, further limit the usefulness of postural measures as tool for evaluating seating comfort (Karvonen et al., 1962).

10.2.3.3   Task Performance

Intuitively, there should be a relationship between comfort and task performance. Various office surveys (cited in Lueder, 1983) have found that the majority of office workers felt that increased comfort would enhance their productivity. Operationally, in an office setting, this may be more difficult to prove. Although many studies (Smith et al., 1981; Springer, 1982; Ong, 1984) have shown improved task performance at an ergonomically redesigned VDT workstation, the improvements were probably not solely due to a more comfortable chair, but most likely included all the other improvements: the reduced glare, the copy holders, the arm rests, etc.

10.2.3.4   Subjective Assessment

Subjective assessment of seat comfort is probably the most common evaluation technique due to ease of use and apparent face validity. Typically, overall comfort is elicited through a relatively simple unstructured scale, perhaps with two points (e.g., comfortable/uncomfortable; cited in Drury and Coury, 1982) or three points (uncomfortable, medium, comfortable; Grandjean et al., 1973). More levels — 7 (Shvartz et al., 1980), 11 (Shackel et al., 1969) — or even the use of a continuous visual analogue scale (Drury and Coury, 1982), in principle, may provide greater precision. Five to seven is the optimum number of categories for general psychometric testing (Guilford, 1954). Similarly, a five category scale, but further partitioned into ten scale points, was found to be the most reliable and valid scale for rating seating pressure discomfort (Shen and Parsons, 1997).

Because ratings of overall comfort may be influenced by specific factors of the chair design or even factors beyond the chair itself, it may be useful to focus the ratings on selected features of the chair as well as various regions of the body. In the first case, a chair features checklist (Figure 10.7) was developed by Shackel et al. (1969) and used later by Drury and Coury (1982) to recommend specific design changes in a prototype chair. In the second case, a body discomfort chart, similar to Figure 8.6, has been used to rate

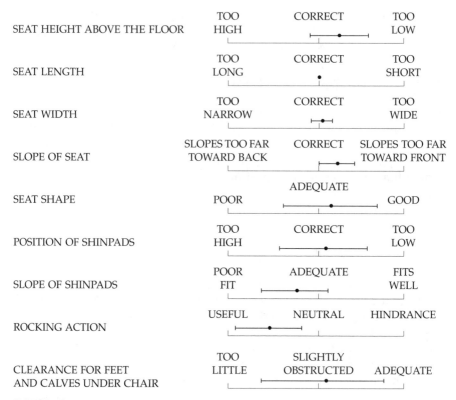

FIGURE 10.7
Chair features checklist. (From Drury, C.G. and Francher, M., 1985. *Applied Ergonomics*, 16:41–47.
With permission.)

specific areas of the body separately using one of the above rating scales
(Drury and Coury, 1982). Later, factor analysis was used successfully on an
expanded list of comfort/discomfort descriptors in quantifying the multidi-
mensional complexity of seating (Zhang et al., 1996; Helander and Zhang,
1997). The combination of all of the above approaches may give the best
overall assessment for a particular chair and especially for the evaluation of
a group of chairs.

In terms of the actual assessment, a smaller number of pretrained testers
may be preferable to a larger sample of untrained subjects, because the
former will be more sensitive to lower levels of discomfort (Jones, 1969).
Subjects having back pain are particularly sensitive discriminators of seating
comfort (Hall, 1972). However, then the ratings might be particularly
weighted by back and buttock comfort as found even in normal subjects
(Wachsler and Lerner, 1960). The duration of assessment has not been specifically established. Although Waschsler and Learner (1960) found no differences in rank ordering at 5 min with ranking at 4 h, most others (Barkla,
1964; Shackel et al., 1969; Drury and Coury, 1982) have advocated and used
longer periods with regular, periodic evaluations.

10.2.3.5   *Physical Measures*

The physical measures discussed in Section 10.2.1 can also be used to assess the comfort of a particular chair. They are especially desirable because of the objective and quantitative nature of the measurements. Although, the correlation between physiological parameters and the overall state of comfort or discomfort is not well understood, first signs of discomfort, imperceptible to the subject, appear in EMG of the back muscles. Once the discomfort becomes perceptible, arousal increases with concurrent signs in heart rate and EMG in other muscles not directly related to sitting (Lueder, 1983). Also the pressure on the buttocks is a common reason for feeling discomfort (Slechta et al., 1959; Wotzka et al., 1969), discussed in greater detail in Section 10.2.4.

There are also disadvantages to physical measures. The measurements can be equipment intensive, costly, time-consuming, and intrusive to the subject, perhaps even changing the person's responses. A low level of EMG activity in one muscle group may not imply comfort, but may show compensation for an increased level in another group, requiring the measurement of a large number of muscle groups, which further increases the cost and complexity of experimentation. Therefore, no one technique yields a good measure of sitting comfort, and, consequently, a variety or combination of approaches may need to be used.

10.2.4   Seat Pressure

During sitting, most of the body weight (65%) is transferred to the seat pan. Some of the weight is also transferred to the floor through the feet (18%), the backrest (4 to 5% at 15° posterior inclination), and the armrests (12%) (Swearingen et al., 1962). The weight transfer to the backrest would be even greater if the backrest included a lumbar support (Diebschlag and Müller-Limmroth, 1980). In an anterior-leaning posture or with forward-sloping seat pans, up to 38% of the weight can be transferred through the feet (Jürgens, 1969).

10.2.4.1   *Seat Pressure Distribution*

Because most of the weight, however, is transferred through the buttocks, it is very important to provide proper seat contour, padding, and shape to achieve an optimum pressure distribution. Within the buttocks and the undersides of the thighs, the major weight-bearing areas are the *ischial tuberosities* or sit bones, which can with stand a pressure of 9 kPa (90 g/cm²) for short periods of time (Rebiffé, 1969). The pressure then decreases as one progresses from these bones to the periphery of the buttocks or thighs, where the values decrease to below 1 kPa (Figure 10.8). Even given such a small area, each ischial tuberosity supports up to 18% of the body weight, while each thigh, with a much larger area, supports up to 21% of the body weight. The sacral area supports roughly 5% of the weight (Drummond et al., 1982).

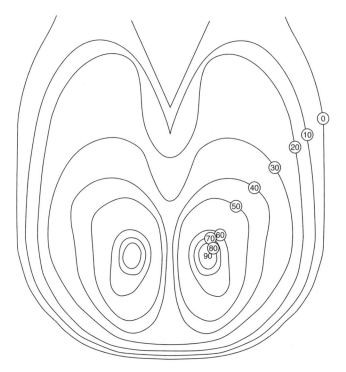

FIGURE 10.8
Seated pressure distribution (g/cm²). (From Rebiffé, R., 1969. *Ergonomics*, 12:246–261. With permission.)

Maintaining such a skewed weight distribution can be aided by the use of slightly contoured seats. On the other hand, overly contoured seats may increase pressure on the softer tissues of the undersides of the thighs, restrict movement, and restrict postural flexibility. Therefore, there must be a compromise design between the different constraints. Similarly, the density and thickness of the seat-pan cushioning will affect the pressure distribution, with most guidelines limiting the thickness to 4 cm, with an outer covering that breathes. Similarly, individuals with their own internal padding in the form of thick gluteal musculature develop discomfort and pain later than individuals with thin gluteal musculature (Hertzberg, 1972). Further details on instrumentation for measuring seat pressure distributions can be found in Section 7.3.

10.2.4.2   Sores and Ulcers

Excessive localized pressure has been linked to pressure sores and *ischemic ulcers*, which are a major problem in long-term health care (Kosiak, 1959). Pressures above 4.7 kPa (35 mmHg) for extended time periods are undesirable because they exceed capillary blood pressure (30 to 35 mmHg), causing ischemia and putting tissues at risk. However, sitting on unpadded flat wooden chairs yields a mean pressure of 43 kPA, exceeding by a magnitude

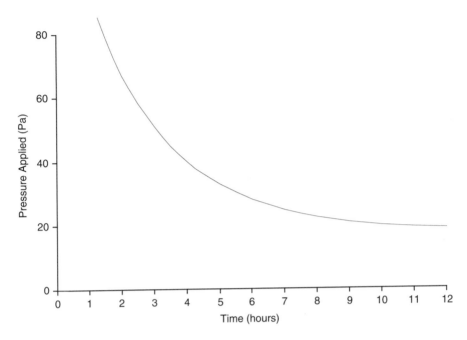

FIGURE 10.9
Pressure–time relationship for the formation of ischemic ulcers. (Adapted from Kosiak, 1959.)

of ten the pressures causing ischemia (Kosiak et al., 1958). Perhaps the continuous variations in pressure patterns observed during restless sitting allow blood to return to the areas that were temporarily ischemic. Such postural flexibility can be purposefully encouraged through task design similar to the approach used in preventing pressure sores for mobility-impaired workers (Swarts et al., 1988). Houle (1969) even suggested using an automatic device to artificially shift pressure concentrations from one area to another. Kosiak (1959) also found a clear inverse relationship between pressure required to start forming ischemic ulcers and time (Figure 10.9). Assuming a reduction in pressures to more tolerable levels, this could serve as the basis for sitting-time guidelines.

10.2.4.3 *Adaptive Seats*

The ultimate approach may be the "intelligent seat system" as prototyped by Ng et al. (1995). Because the buttocks have non-uniform pressure support capability and the material properties of most surfaces have relatively uniform hardness (a hard surface would be very uniform, a softer cushion would be less uniform), it would make logical sense to provide an interactive seat that automatically adjusts itself to the individual's pressure distribution by making pressure-sensitive adjustments. In their design, air-filled bladders embedded in the seat were automatically inflated or deflated to optimize seating comfort based on previously collected data on subjective evaluations and pressure distributions. As the seated subject changed posture or position the system would readjust itself accordingly.

10.2.4.4   Cushioning

Overly contoured and cushioned seats or fluid- or gel-filled seats will tend to distribute pressures uniformly across the seat pan and buttocks. Although advocated by some (Sprigle et al., 1990), this approach allows the prominent areas to sink into the support surface, increases pressures on surrounding softer tissues (Lindan et al., 1965), and impedes transport within tissues (Krouskop et al., 1985). Furthermore, regardless of which type of cushioning material is used, including specialized resin-filled foam cushions designed to reduce ulcerations in wheelchair-bound patients, the pressures on the ischial tuberosities always exceeded capillary blood pressures (Mooney et al., 1971).

10.2.4.5   Two-Stage Seats

Given these potential problems with a uniform pressure distribution, Goonetilleke (1998) presents a contrarian view of purposefully promoting localized force concentrations, even beyond those areas that can withstand them (such as the ischial tuberosities) and cites the popular use of beaded seat covers, massage rollers, and knobby health sandals as examples of this approach. Of course, too high pressure concentrations over extended periods of time will lead to localized ischemia, sores, and ulcerations (Kosiak, 1959). Ultimately, the ideal pressure profile for seats may be a two-stage strategy, with an initial distributed-force comfort, followed by a concentrated-force discomfort that encourages postural flexibility. Undoubtedly, seating comfort also depends very much on individual preferences and further research in the area is needed.

10.2.4.6   Foot Pressure

As mentioned previously, the transfer of up to 25% of the body weight to the feet favors the buttocks, but at the cost of the feet. Over the course of a workday, the legs increase in volume by almost 5% and lead to discomfort in the feet, especially in late afternoon (Winkel, 1981; Winkel and Jørgensen, 1986). A higher seat height with a forward-sloping seat pan increased foot swelling as compared to a lower seat with a slightly upward-sloping seat pan (Bendix et al., 1985). However, modest leg movements every 10 to 15 min, can reduce the swelling by as much as 50% (Winkel and Jørgensen, 1986).

10.2.5   Sit-Stand, Forward-Sloping, and Saddle Chairs

10.2.5.1   Sit-Stand Chairs

The idea of *sit-stand chairs* or stools (no backrest) has been around for some time, first suggested by Staffel (1884) for maintaining lumbar lordosis and

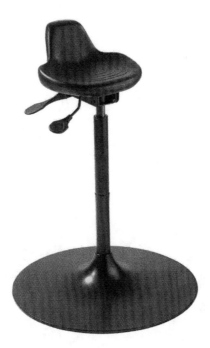

FIGURE 10.10
Industrial sit/stand stool. (Courtesy of Biofit, Waterville, OH.)

then appearing in the design of school furniture as a chair that could be adjusted for supported standing, sitting, and plain standing (Burgerstein, 1915). Later it was promoted for situations when extreme mobility and reach are required (Laurig, 1969), for assembly work on large vertical frames, high workplaces, areas with inadequate leg room, or certain surgical procedures (Bendix et al., 1985). Obviously, the change between sitting and standing postures is quick and simple, and the larger angle between the trunk and thighs preserves lumbar lordosis, even without the use of a backrest (Bendix and Biering-Sørensen, 1983). Similarly, spinal loading as measured by spinal compression was found to be lower than with ordinary office chairs (Eklund and Corlett, 1987; Michel and Helander, 1994). Two necessary features for a sit-stand chair or stool are height adjustability and a large base of support, so that the stool does not tip over when leaning back and sitting down. If the base is large enough, the feet can even rest on and assist in counterbalancing the backward tipping (Figure 10.10). The major disadvantage of sit-stand chairs is the decreased use of the backrest and increased pressure on the feet to avoid sliding out of the seat.

10.2.5.2 *Trunk–Thigh Angle*

The biomechanical advantages of an increased angle between trunk and thigh was first detailed by Keegan (1953) who took radiographs of individuals lying on their sides (Figure 10.11) and concluded that a posture of about

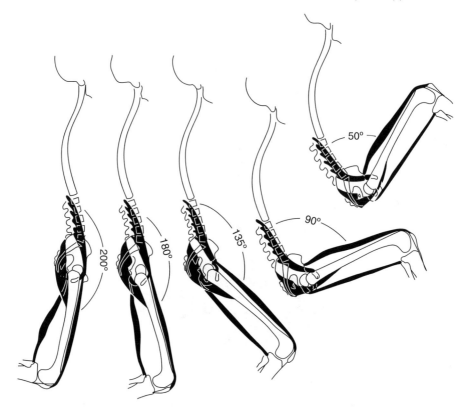

FIGURE 10.11
X-ray drawings on the spine in various postures. Normal lying position of balanced muscle relaxation is with a 135° trunk–thigh angle. (From Keegan, J.J., 1953. *Journal of Bone and Joint Surgery,* 35A:58603. With permission.)

45° hip flexion or 135° trunk–thigh angle to be normal, because that was the posture most typically assumed by individuals when lying relaxed on their side. This is also the posture assumed by individuals under weightless conditions (Figure 10.12). Similarly, Schoberth (1962) analyzed the sacral base angle with respect to horizontal, which for lordosis of a standing posture is typically around 40°. Upon sitting and the loss of lordosis, the sacral angle was almost parallel with the seat. However, when the seat pan was tilted forward 20°, the base angle increased to 20°, with a noticeable lordosis. Similar results from x-ray studies (Burandt, 1969) led to further recommendations of using forward-sloping seats in office chairs (Burandt and Grandjean, 1969). The forward-tilting chair concept was further promoted by Mandal (1976, 1981, 1982) after observing school children tipping their chairs forward and horseback riders exhibiting similar large trunk–thigh angles.

10.2.5.3   *Forward-Sloping Chairs*

Objective comparisons of forward-sloping chairs with more conventional chairs confirmed that kyphosis of the lumbar spine tended to decrease with

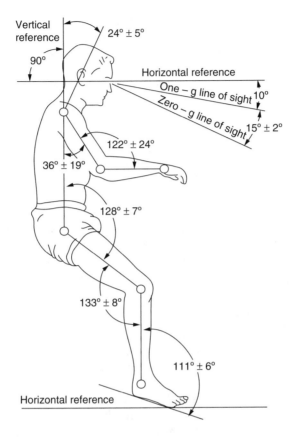

FIGURE 10.12
Typical relaxed posture assumed by individuals in weightless conditions. (From Thornton, 1978.)

increasing forward-sloping seat pans (Bendix, 1984; Bridger, 1988; Bridger et al., 1989). However, as much as two thirds of the body's adaptation to the forward-sloping seat may have occurred in the hip joints, with only one third occurring in the lumbar spine (Bendix and Biering-Sørensen, 1983). Still, increasing seat height, along with the forward-sloping seat, tended to increase lordosis, Coincidentally, subjects preferred freely tiltable rather than fixed forward-sloping seats (Bendix, 1984). In either case, seat heights need to be raised approximately 3 to 5 cm above popliteal height, with a concurrent rise in table heights of 4 to 6 cm above elbow height (Bendix and Bloch, 1986). Note that the same effect can be obtained by using a pelvic support pad, with angles in the range of 4 to 10°, on a conventional chair (Wu et al., 1998).

One of the disadvantages of forward-sloping chairs is the tendency to slide forward in the seat, placing more weight on the feet and increasing foot swelling (Bendix et al., 1985). To avoid this problem, Mengshœl of Norway introduced the Balans stool with a 15° forward-sloping seat pan and a knee-support pad to prevent sliding off (Vandraas, 1981). Because of the forward thigh inclination, he did not think a backrest was necessary, thus resulting in a stool. Initial subjective evaluations elicited mixed responses, with complaints of knee and shin pains and problems of entry and egress (Drury and Francher, 1985). Later, in more objective evaluations, the Balans stool approximated standing lumbar lordosis significantly better than conventional chairs (Frey and Tecklin, 1986; Link et al., 1990). When compared to a forward-tiltable chair, the Balans stool was again significantly better for lumbar lordosis, but produced no significant difference in spinal shrinkage and heart rate (Bendix et al., 1988). Over extended periods of time, the subjects reported greater fatigue in the Balans stool. Similar results were also reported by Lander et al. (1987) with increased cervical and lumbar EMG readings over time as compared to a conventional chair. Finally, Ericson and Goldie (1989) found significantly greater spinal shrinkage with the Balans stool than with a conventional chair, which they attributed to the lack of a backrest. Thus, the Balans stool may have some benefits for some individuals in some situations, but overall may not be the cure for back pain as claimed by the manufacturers.

10.2.5.4　Saddle Chairs

The main disadvantages of forward-sloping chairs (slipping forward and out in conventional designs) and of the Balans stool (increased pressure on the knees) have been eliminated in an alternative design: the saddle chair. Bendix et al. (1985) first introduced a saddlelike sit-stand chair with the operator straddling the seat and allowing the thighs to slope downward 45° from the conventional horizontal position. This approach was extended by Congleton et al. (1985) by adding a pommel to the forward-sloping seat, forming a more sculpted saddlelike seat (Figure 10.13). Specifically designed as a sit-stand chair for surgeons, who rated it superior over conventional surgical stools, the chair was later commercially modified for the office environment.

10.2.5.5　Compromise Seat Pan

A final and, perhaps, simplest alternative is a compromise design that maintains the area under the ischial tuberosities horizontal and slopes the front part of the seat pan forward. This design, first suggested by Jürgens (1969) and later studied by Ericson and Goldie (1989) and Graf et al. (1993), allows most of the body weight to be supported by the area best suited for that, preventing forward slippage, but still opens the trunk–thigh angle to decrease spinal kyphosis. Spinal shrinkage for this design was intermediate between a conventional chair and a Balans chair (Ericson and Goldie, 1989); erector spinae EMG levels and user discomfort ratings were lower than for a conventional chair (Graf et al., 1993). The only disadvantage of the design appears to be a greater percentage of body weight being placed on the feet with concomitant complaints of leg discomfort.

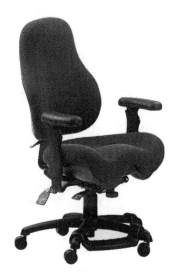

FIGURE 10.13
Saddle chair allowing the operator to straddle the seat. (Courtesy of Neutral Posture, Inc., http://www.igoergo.com/.)

10.2.6 Work Surface and Line of Sight

10.2.6.1 Work Surface Height

The placement of the work surface is critically important in the design of an office environment. If the working height is too high, above the resting elbow height, the shoulders may be elevated with increased activity of the trapezius muscle (Figure 10.14B) or the upper arms may be abducted with increased activity of the deltoid muscle (Figure 10.14C). In either case, eventual fatigue and discomfort to the neck, shoulders, and arms will occur. If the working height is too low, below the resting elbow height, the neck or back will be excessively flexed, resulting in neck and back discomfort. In fact, most of the muscles observed in Figure 10.14B,C are in non-optimum postures and exceed the recommended static muscular loading limit of 5% of maximal voluntary contraction (Jonsson, 1988). At the optimum working height (Figure 10.14A), the home row of the keyboard or the level of the writing surface is set at the resting elbow height. In this posture, muscle activity is at a relative minimum (Hagberg, 1982; cited in Grandjean, 1987) task performance is at a maximum (Ellis, 1951). These studies support the often-cited principle for determining work surface height: upper arms hang down naturally and elbows flexed at 90° so that the forearms are parallel to the ground (Figure 9.8 and Figure 10.14A).

There are modifications to the principle, with the work surface height adjusted to the task being performed (Ayoub, 1973). For difficult-to-see material such as poor-quality typeface or fine assembly, it is advantageous to raise the work surface 10 to 20 cm above elbow height, to bring details closer to

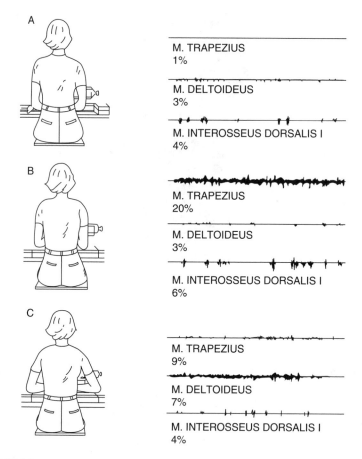

FIGURE 10.14

Electromyographic recordings of shoulder muscle activity: (A) optimal height of home row, (B, C) home row too high, resulting in either elevation of shoulders by trapezius muscle or the abduction of the arms by the deltoid muscle. (From Grandjean, E., 1987. *Ergonomics in Computerized Offices*, London: Taylor & Francis. With permission.)

the normal line of sight (Figure 10.15). Another, perhaps, better alternative is to tilt the work surface approximately 15°. However, rounded parts then have a tendency to roll off the surface. It is also desirable to support the elbow and reduce the previously mentioned static loading. During manual work with heavier parts, the work surface should be lowered up to 10 cm to take advantage of the stronger trunk muscles. However, this distance will be limited by knee height and the thickness of the work surface, and one should consider a standing workplace with the work surface height as much as 40 cm below elbow height. In any case, an easily adjustable work surface to accommodate different sized individuals and various tasks should be the norm. Also, the bottom height of the work surface should allow sufficient leg room for the worker.

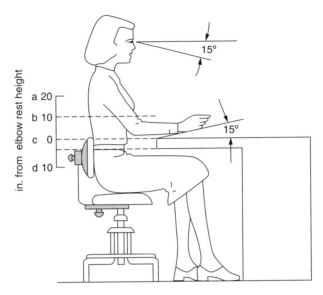

FIGURE 10.15
Tilting of work surface to bring details closer to line of sight.

10.2.6.2 Line of Sight

The *normal line of sight* for seated workers has often been quoted at approximately 15° (±15°) below horizontal (McCormick, 1970; VanCott and Kinkade, 1972; Eastman Kodak, 1983; Grandjean, 1988), but with little definitive research to substantiate these recommendations and without a clear definition of horizontal. Early researchers (Table 10.3) simply related the viewing angle to an undefined "horizontal," whereas later researchers used either the *Frankfurt plane* (FP), the *eye–ear line* (EEL), or *Reid's base line* (RBL) as a reference line (Figure 10.16). The FP is delineated by a line (in the sagittal plane) passing through the *tragion* (notch above the piece cartilage that is just anterior to the auditory passage) and the lower ridge of the eye socket and roughly corresponds to horizontal when the head is held erect (Hill and Kroemer, 1986). The EEL passes through the outer corner of the eyelid and the center of the auditory canal. The two differ by roughly by 13°, 11° as reported by Menozzi et al. (1994), or 15° as reported by Jampel and Shi (1992).

RBL is delineated by a line passing through the center of the auditory canal and the lower ridge of the eye socket, and roughly corresponds to the line created by the FP in the sagittal plane. Unfortunately, in many cases it has been confused with the EEL. There also appears to a difference in the values for normal line of sight obtained from field studies as opposed to laboratory studies. Whereas the latter probably measure the preferred line sight implicitly or explicitly (Heuer et al., 1991) based on resting vergence and resting accommodation, field studies are based on longer time periods and probably take into account musculoskeletal strain due to neck flexion. The true normal

TABLE 10.3

Normal Line of Sight for a 0.5-m Reading Distance

| Ref. | Type of Study | Preferred Line of Sight (°) | | |
		Original	Ref.	Converted to FP
Lehmann and Stier (1961)	Lab	−38	Unknown	—
Grandjean et al. (1983)	Field — VDT	−9	Unknown	—
Kroemer and Hill (1986)	Lab — Landolt rings	−33	FP	−33
Heuer et al. (1991)	Lab — non VDT	−11.3	~10° from FP	−21.3
	Lab — vergence	−13.5		−23.5
Menozzi et al. (1994)	Lab — LEDs	−12.3	FP	−12.3
Villanueva et al. (1996)	Lab — VDT (force positions)	−27.9 to −43.2	EEL	−14.9 to −30.2
Jaschinski et al. (1998)	Field — VDT	−8.6	Unknown	—
Burgess-Limerick et al. (1998)	Lab — VDT	−22 to −27	EEL	−9 to −14
Mon-Williams et al. (1999)	Lab — VDT	−26.8 to −33	EEL	−13.8 to −20
Sommerich et al. (2001)	Lab — VDT	−36.5 (of 3 choices)	EEL	−23.5
Psihogios et al. (2001)	Field — VDT	−24.3	EEL	−11.3

Note: See Figure 10.17; FP = Frankfurt plane, EEL = Eye–ear line, est = estimated.

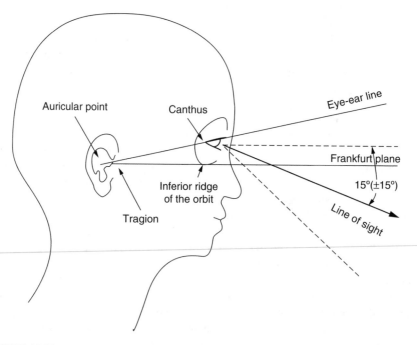

FIGURE 10.16
Normal line of sight with reference to the FP and EEL.

line of sight may depend on the task or workplace situation due to the trade-off of various factors including muscular and visual strain.

Most of the reported values for normal line of vision (Table 10.3) range between –9° and –23.5° (with respect to FP), with a mean of the self-selected positions of approximately –16°. Larger angles of up to –33° were found by Kroemer and Hill (1986) and Villanueva et al. (1996) and may aid vision by improving eye moisture. Sotoyama et al. (1996) reported that larger downward gaze angles decrease the ocular surface area exposed to the atmosphere, potentially reducing the dry-eye problems and the reduced blink rate that arise during VDT use (Yaginuma et al., 1990). However, excessively low screen positions of –40° (defined by center of screen) significantly increased muscle activity in six of ten neck, shoulder, and back muscles studied (Turville et al., 1998) and cannot be recommended for extended periods of time. Thus, overall, the original recommendation of 15° below horizontal is still quite reasonable. Also, given that neck flexion of up to 15° produced no subjective discomfort or EMG changes over a 6-h time period (Chaffin, 1973) and line-of-sight standard deviations having a range of ±13° (Hill and Kroemer, 1986), the recommended range of ±15° is also quite reasonable. In practical terms, this means that the center of the screen should be positioned 15° below horizontal, with the top of the screen roughly at horizontal eye-level (OSHA, 1991).

10.2.6.3   Tilted Work Surface

Tilting the work surface to reduce neck flexion and tension in the neck muscles was recommended as early as the 19th century, especially for school furniture (Staffel, 1984). This practice seems to have decreased over the years, both in the classroom and architectural design studios, but more recent epidemiological (Ferguson, 1976) and biomechanical (Less and Eichelberg, 1976) data have revived interest in tilted work surfaces. A sitting horizontal work surface places strain on the cervical spine due to increased torque from the forward inclination of the head (Less and Eichelberg, 1976), increased kyphosis of the lumbar spine, and lack of elbow support (Andersson et al., 1974a). A 15° sloping tabletop was found to decrease neck flexion angles by approximately 6° (Bridger, 1988) while a 45° sloping desk decreased neck angles by 14° and decreased trapezius activity (Bendix and Hagberg, 1984). This latter steep slope was found to be very acceptable for reading but quite unacceptable for writing, with pencils and paper tending to slide down. Therefore, a compromise design of 10° inclination has been recommended (de Wall et al., 1991; Freudenthal et al., 1991). This resulted in a mean reduction in neck angle of 9°, a mean reduction in trunk angle of 8°, and a decrease in back torque of 29%. A slightly larger desk inclination of 15° (along with a forward-sloping chair) was tested in a primary school setting with very favorable ratings as well as a decrease in neck flexion (4°), an increase in hip angle (12°), and a decrease in muscle activity (Marschall et al., 1995). Whether the ratings were due solely to the inclined desk surface or the combination with the sloping chair was difficult to determine. Coincidentally, university students also preferred a slope of 10 to 15° for a lecture hall desk (Hira, 1980). In any case, the traditional sloping desk may be returning to favor in the classroom.

10.2.6.4   *Working Area*

The work surface should be large enough accommodate the items used for the task, but critical or more frequently used items should be placed within the *normal working area* as defined by the area circumscribed by the forearm when it is moved in an arc pivoted at a fixed elbow (Maynard, 1934). This area represents the most convenient zone within which motions may be made by that hand with minimum muscle action and expenditure of effort. The maximum working area is defined the area circumscribed by the extended arm. This area defined by a pivoting elbow was defined quantitatively by Farley (1955) for an average male and female while Squires (1956) further modified this area into a "windshield wiper" pattern, by allowing the elbow to move along the arc *CD*, with the outer edge limited by 25° lateral shoulder rotation. Because the elbow was allowed to move, the normal working area was increased substantially. Konz and Goel (1969) used Squires (1956) concept to mathematically generate more detailed normal working areas, which, however, did not conform well with the shape of Squires (1956) curve. Therefore, Das and Grady (1983) examined these differences in greater detail, eventually modifying Squires (1956) approach to define coverage on both sides of the body median for 5th, 50th, and 95th percentile males and females (Figure 10.17; Das and Behara, 1995).

10.2.6.5   *Workspace Envelope*

The working area concept can be expanded into a *workspace envelope*, or the three-dimensional space within which an individual can work. This is typically determined for a seated person via functional arm reach, which, as can be expected, will depend on the type of task performed as well as the type of grip or function performed. A fingertip action (e.g., activating a pushbutton) will be roughly 5 cm longer than a thumb tip action (e.g., turning a knob), while a full grip action will be roughly 5 cm shorter than a thumb tip action (Bullock, 1974). In a classic study, Dempster (1955) determined workspace envelopes for different hand actions in various postures (supine, prone, inverted, five angles) for 22 "median and muscular" males. The heavy line is the enveloping outline of many photographic traces of contours of hand movements while the shaded areas depict the region common to all hand motions and postures and, thus, perhaps the optimum region (Figure 10.18). More detailed data on U.S. Air Force personnel were collected by Kennedy (1964).

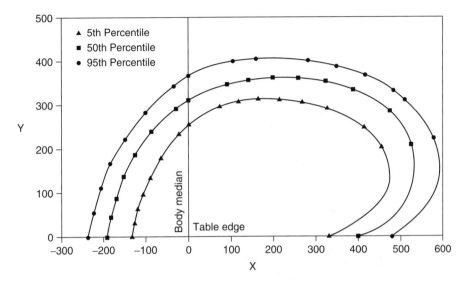

FIGURE 10.17
Normal working area for males. (From Das, B. and Behara, D.N., 1995. *Ergonomics*, 38:734–748. With permission.)

10.3 The Keyboard

10.3.1 Standard Keyboard Features

10.3.1.1 *Keyboard Slope*

The standard computer keyboard evolved, more or less, from the manual typewriter. Characteristics that carried over include the shape, slope, and profile of the keyboard, as well as the size and shapes of the individual keys. The standard keyboard slope of 30° for manual typewriters as reported by Moneta (1960, cited in Alden et al., 1972) appeared to be based on convention rather any data, as Scales and Chapanis (1954) found most individuals preferred slopes in the range of 15° to 25° and Dreyfuss (1959) in his anthropometric tables indicated an optimum slope of 11° and a maximum slope of 20°. Later research on computer keyboards found preferred slopes of 21° (Galitz, 1965, cited in Alden et al., 1972), 18° with higher rates of keystrokes (Emmons and Hirsch, 1982), 10° to 15° (Suther and McTyre, 1982), 18° (Miller and Suther, 1983), and 14.4° to 16.1° (Abernethy, 1984). These results have led to the recommendation of a keyboard slope between 0° and 15°, with an upper maximum at 25° (Human Factors and Ergonomics Society, 2002).

Interestingly, few of the studies show any significant effect of keyboard slope on typing performance. However, preferred keyboard slope was found to correlate inversely and significantly with seat height ($r = -0.71$) with

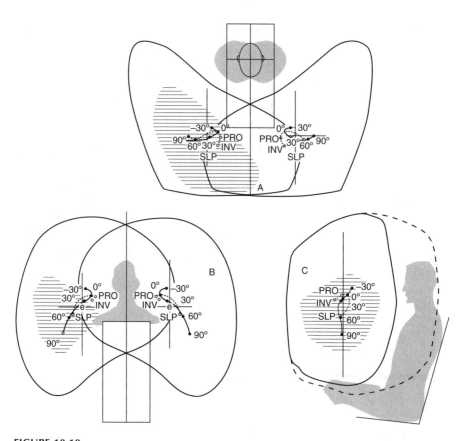

FIGURE 10.18
Optimum (shaded) and maximum (dark lines) workspace envelopes for males in three planes.
(From Kennedy, 1964.)

shorter individuals preferring steeper slopes. Miller and Suther (1983) reasoned that because stature correlates with hand length, a steeper slope makes it easier for shorter individuals to reach all keys. On the other hand, flatter keyboards more easily satisfy work surface height requirements and work better in adjustable keyboard trays. As such, low profile keyboards, defined as having less than 3 cm height at the home row and slope less than 15°, became the standard in Europe and eventually, a *de facto* standard in the United States. Note that for standing workstations, flat and –15° slope keyboards performed significantly better than +15° slope keyboards (Najjar et al., 1988; cited in Lewis et al., 1997).

10.3.1.2   Keyboard Profile

The profile of the keyboard can be stepped, sloped, or dished (Figure 10.19). Although no data were presented, the dished profile was reported to

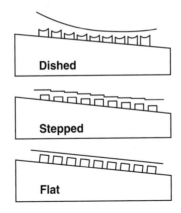

FIGURE 10.19
Keyboard profiles. (From Lewis, J.R. et al., 1997. In Helander, M. et al., Eds., *Handbook of Human–Computer Interaction*, 2nd ed., Amsterdam: Elsevier Science, 1285–1315. With permission.)

improve keying speed for skilled operators (Çakir et al., 1980). Similarly, Paci and Gabbrielli (1984) claimed that performance was better for the dished profile as compared to a stepped profile. However, no data were presented and the two profiles were confounded with different keyboard slopes. Only Magyar (1985; cited in Lewis et al., 1997) indicated statistically significant lower performance on a sloped keyboard as compared to a stepped or a dished profile. However, these results were not sufficient to clearly identify one profile as superior to another. It is, perhaps, more important that the key itself be indented to provide an accurate location of the user's finger, minimize reflections (45% or less), provide a surface for the labels, and prevent accumulation of dirt and dust, either on the key or falling between keys into the mechanism (Çakir et al., 1980). A matte surface will reduce reflections, but an excessively rough surface will tend to accumulate dirt.

10.3.1.3   Key Size, Displacement, and Resistance

In terms of key design characteristics, it appears that as computer input devices came into being during the late 1950s and 1960s, a wide variety of key configurations existed. Key resistances ranged from 0.6 to 2.3 N, key displacements ranged from 0.71 to 1.59 cm, and key sizes were generally around 1.27 cm in width and separated 1.81 cm from center to center, similar to those found on typewriters (Pollock and Gildner, 1963, cited in Alden et al., 1972; Harkins, 1965). Biomechanical and anthropometrical considerations first appeared with the Dreyfuss (1959) recommendations of key resistances in the range of 1.15 to 3.06 N, a 0.47 cm displacement, and key sizes of 1.27 cm in width by 1.11 cm in length. The first reliable experimental data came from the Deininger (1960a,b) study on ten-button key sets for pushbutton telephones. Overall, there were rather small differences in operator responses, but smaller key resistances (around 1 N) were preferable to larger resistances (around 4 N) and intermediate displacements (0.3 cm) were preferable to very small (0.1 cm) or very large (0.5 cm) displacements. Keying times decreased 8% and keying errors decreased from 7.1 to 1.3% as the key size was increased from a 1-cm square to a 1.27-cm square.

Kinkead and Gonzalez (1969, cited in Lewis et al., 1997) found optimum keying performance at low levels of resistance (0.25 to 1.5 N) and travel (0.13 to 0.64 cm). These results were further confirmed by Clare (1976) who recommended 1.27-cm square keys with a 1.9-cm separation distance, by Loricchio and Lewis (1991) who found that keying rates increased 8.8% ($p < 0.05$) in going from 1-cm to 1.4-cm keys, and by Loricchio (1992) who found an 8.2% increase in keying rate in going from a 0.75 N to a 0.5 N ($p = 0.08$) key resistance. However, going to even lower key resistances may be counterproductive in that Akagi (1992) found more errors for 0.35 N resistance than for 0.7 N resistance. Furthermore, 0.5 N seems to be the lower limit for preventing accidental key activation (Rose, 1991). Thus, the 0.5 N value might be optimal and, as such, have led to recommendations of key resistances between 0.5 and 0.6 N with a maximum range of 0.25 to 1.5 N. Key width should be a minimum of 1.2 cm with a horizontal separation of 1.8 to 1.9 cm and a vertical separation of 1.8 to 2.1 cm. Key displacement should be in the range of 0.15 to 0.6 cm but with a preferred range of 0.2 to 0.4 cm (Human Factors and Ergonomics Society, 2002). Later on, more detailed testing and analysis based on Fitts' (1954) law confirmed the 1.9-cm spacing as optimum but found that a smaller key size of 0.8 cm may be more appropriate based on the size of the average finger pad (Drury and Hoffman, 1992).

10.3.1.4 Key Feedback

It would be expected from basic human factors principles that feedback would be necessary for optimum keying performance. However, Deininger's (1960a,b) classic study on pushbutton telephones did not indicate a need for auditory feedback. He reasoned that the force–displacement characteristics of the keys provided sufficient feedback for efficient operator performance. Diehl and Seibel (1962) also found no differences in typing performance under four feedback conditions (none, auditory, visual, and both auditory and visual) and Deininger's (1960a,b) conclusions were supported. On the other hand, Monty and Snyder (1983) found a small but significant improvement with a keyboard having an audible click.

Kinkead and Gonzalez (1969, cited in cited in Lewis et al., 1997) found that keys with a snap-action response caused significantly more errors than without, while Brunner and Richardson (1984) found the linear-spring response to be least preferred and to entail the largest number of errors, followed by the snap-action response. The fewest errors and up to a 6%

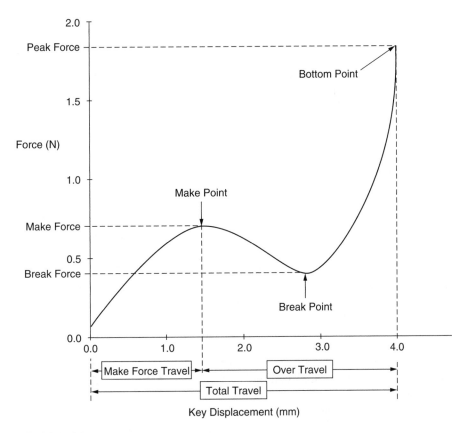

FIGURE 10.20
Optimum force–displacement characteristic in key switches.

faster typing speed was obtained with an elastomer type of response; Figure 10.20). In this type of response there are two force or resistance peaks; the first is the the *make point*, which activates the key switch. The second occurs after a reduction in resistance, the *break point*, which breaks the circuit and deactivates the switch and signals the user that the keystroke has been completed. Because of the inertia of the hand, the key continues to depress until it bottoms out at the *bottom point*. As a consequence, BSR/HFES 100 recommends, at the minimum, tactile feedback with the elastomer type of response (Human Factors and Ergonomics Society, 2002). If possible, auditory feedback should also be provided. Later research showed the even the type of elastomer response can have an effect on performance. Rempel et al. (1999) found that longer times to reach the make point decreased hand pain over 12 weeks of use. The authors hypothesized that this longer lag created a feeling of looseness, less tension, and less fear of accidental activation of the keys in the operators as compared to a short make force travel distance.

10.3.1.5   Keying Forces

Clare (1976) recommended that the force-displacement characteristics for keys should vary depending on finger distance from the base row. However, actual keying forces were not measured until Rempel et al. (1994) instrumented a keyboard with piezoelectric load cells. They identified three distinct phases and forces exerted by the finger in a keystroke corresponding roughly to the pattern of key resistance shown in Figure 10.20: (1) key switch compression to reach *make force,* which preceded the break point in an elastomer key; (2) finger impact on bottoming out, typically registering the peak force; and (3) finger pulp compression as the key is released. Mean keying forces ranged from 1.4 to 2.2 N, or anywhere from 2.5 to 3.9 times greater than the make force or key resistance (Armstrong et al., 1994). Although keying forces were greater for higher key resistances, individuals typed much harder than necessary, with 4.1 to 7.0 times more force than needed, on lower-resistance (0.28 N) keyboards as compared to higher-resistance (0.83 N) keyboards, in which case they exerted 2.2 to 3.5 times more force (Gerard et al., 1996). This effect could either result from a hypothesized motor program of a sequence of fast ballistic movements (Martin et al., 1996) or simply from the inertial properties of the hand (Gerard et al., 1999). In the first case, the authors reasoned that if the two factors, force and speed, could be programmed separately, then, through appropriate training, typing stress levels could be reduced.

In terms of muscle exertion measured by EMG, typists exerted anywhere from 6 to 20% of maximum voluntary contraction (MVC), which is fairly high for a very repetitive task (Martin et al., 1996). Given that Byström and Fransson-Hall (1994) found that fatigue in intermittent hand grip tasks appeared at EMG levels as low 17% MVC, there is the possibility of muscular fatigue arising from keyboarding, especially if key forces are high or the operators overexert. Interestingly, Sommerich et al. (1996) found a significant positive correlation between forced typing speed and keying forces, implying that the problem of muscular fatigue is exacerbated in situations where operators may be attempting to meet deadlines. Preferred typing speed, in less stressful conditions, did not correlate, across subjects, with keying force. Another possible approach to decreasing keying forces is to increase overtravel, which would allow for more time for the finger to decelerate, decreasing the resulting forces. Radwin and Jeng (1997) found a 24% decrease ($p < 0.01$) in peak force as overtravel was increased from 0 to 3 mm. Interestingly, there was a corresponding, although much smaller (2%), but still significant ($p < 0.01$) increase in keying rates. Reducing make force also reduced peak forces, but is limited to the threshold value of 0.5 N in preventing accidental key activation (Rose, 1991).

10.3.2   Split and Sloped Keyboards

10.3.2.1   Standard Keyboard Problems

The standard keyboard creates several biomechanical problems for the operator. First, the hands tend to be ulnarly deviated up to 40° (mean values of

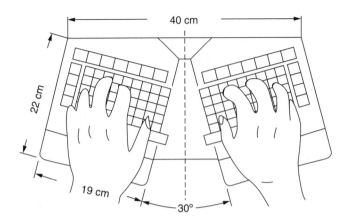

FIGURE 10.21
Split keyboard with improved hand/wrist postures.

25°; Smutz et al., 1994) placing additional loading on the carpal tunnel and increasing the pressure within the tunnel as much as 13% (Werner et al., 1997). Second, to obtain a flat palm, the forearm tends to be pronated close to the anatomical limit (mean values of 76°), which requires the activation of the forearm muscles (mainly pronator teres and pronator quadratus). Such tension over extended time periods can also lead to muscular fatigue. Third, to compensate for this tension, there is a tendency for operators to lift the upper arms laterally and forward, which requires the activation of the shoulder muscles (primarily the deltoid and teres minor). Again, static tension may lead to fatigue. Fourth, depending on the height and slope of the keyboard, there is a tendency for the wrists to be extended up to 50° (mean values of 23°; Serina et al., 1999). Of all the possible wrist deviations, this wrist extension may be the most critical with carpal tunnel pressures increasing to 63 mmHg (for fingertip forces of 6 N), considerably above 30 mmHg, the threshold level for potential injury (Rempel et al., 1997).

Such problems at a typewriter keyboard were noticed as early as 1926 by Klockenberg, who proposed that the keyboard be split into two halves, each angled 15° from the center line (Figure 10.21, included angle is 30°), as well as tilted laterally down (sometimes termed *tented*). Furthermore, Klockenberg (1926) suggested an arching of the key rows for each half of the keyboard to better configure with the natural layout of the fingers. The lateral tilting was more specifically examined by Creamer and Trumbo (1960) with a mechanical typewriter cut into two halves and tilted at five different angles. Keying at the middle position of 44° was 5% significantly faster than at the extremes of 0° (flat) or 88° (nearly vertical). Kroemer (1964, 1965, 1972) performed a more detailed analysis by varying also the upper arm position and found that the subjects preferred a similar hand orientation of 40° for the upper arms hanging down naturally. Although the subjects preferred typing on a split and tilted keyboard over a standard keyboard, typing speed did not show any differences. Error rates, however, decreased by 39%.

10.3.2.2   Optimum Split Angles

Further experimentation by Zipp et al. (1981, 1983) using EMG measurements of the shoulder, arm, and hand muscle indicated optimal ranges of 0 to 60° for pronation and 0 to 15° for ulnar deviation, with the standard position for keyboards of 90° pronation and 20 to 25° ulnar deviation clearly beyond the optimal range. A 13° angulation from the centerline (26° included angle) showed lower EMG than a 26° angulation. In addition, preferred lateral tilt angles of 10 to 20° were smaller than the 44° found by Kroemer (1964, 1965, 1972). Because only three subjects had been utilized in the above experiments, Nakaseko et al. (1985) performed further testing on 20 experienced typists and found similar results with subjective preferences, which led to the first commercial split model standardized at a 25° split (internal angle), a 10° lateral tilt, and a 10° horizontal tilt (far edge higher) (Buesen, 1984). Since then, several other split or tilted models have been introduced and evaluated scientifically to provide better hand and wrist postures (Gerard et al., 1994; Tittiranonda et al., 1999; Zecevic et al., 2000).

10.3.2.3   Performance Effects

Although most research studies confirmed decreased muscular tension with split keyboards, no one examined performance effects until Price and Dowell (1997) found 9.2% slower typing speeds with split keyboards as compared to standard keyboards and Swanson et al. (1997) found a 5.5% decrease in performance with no improvement in discomfort ratings after 2 days exposure. Similar performance decrements were found, 4% by Smith et al. (1998) and 6% by Marklin et al. (1999). The performance decrement in novice users (new to split keyboards) may be due to poor visual feedback from the lateral tilt and in skilled typists, even after prolonged familiarization (7 or more hours), may be due to a difficulty in changing motor patterns (Çakir, 1995). In that case, an adjustable split angle may be preferable to a fixed split angle to allow the user to become accustomed to gradual changes over time (Marklin et al., 1999).

Most of the above studies exposed their subjects, typically healthy typists, to the split keyboards for several hours or, at most, several days. Therefore, although the preferences tended toward the split keyboards, there is the possibility that subjects responded to the novelty effect of the keyboards. Similarly, although postures approached more neutral positions, full adaptation to the new configuration with corresponding changes in motor patterns may not have fully occurred either, as exhibited by the above-mentioned performance decrements. Only Tittiranonda et al. (1999) specifically examined computer users with MSD in a 6-month prospective, observer-blinded, epidemiological study with three different split keyboards and a standard keyboard as a control. At the end of the study, the group with the keyboard with a 24° split angle, 10° lateral inclination, and –2° downward tilt exhibited a significant decrease in pain severity and hand function, but not clinical signs. Satisfaction with keyboards correlated directly with improvement in pain severity. Interestingly, there was a placebo effect for the first week, in which all keyboards, even the standard, but cosmetically altered one, were rated better than a standard keyboard. This further indicates that earlier studies may have been influenced by a placebo effect.

10.3.2.4 Negative-Slope Keyboards

While the split angle and vertical tilt had substantial effects on decreasing ulnar deviation and pronation, respectively, these are not the most critical factors in decreasing carpal tunnel pressures (Rempel et al., 1997). Wrist extension, which increased carpal tunnel pressures more dramatically, was not changed by the split or tilted keyboard designs (Marklin et al., 1999). On the other hand, if an individual's WRMSD has progressed to the point that any postural improvements provide relief of pain and muscle tension, then a 5 to 6% loss in productivity may not be of concern.

Wrist extension has been reduced by the use of negative-slope (i.e., tilted forward) keyboards (Hedge and Powers, 1995). Whereas users on a standard keyboard exhibited 13° of wrist extension, those on a 12° negative-slope keyboard (self-selected by the users) showed a slight 1° wrist flexion. A later field study of 38 typists confirmed decreased wrist extension with increased satisfaction of the negative-slope keyboard as compared to a standard flat keyboard (Hedge et al., 1999).

10.3.3 Layout of Keys

10.3.3.1 Standard QWERTY Layout

The standard layout of keys, termed *QWERTY* because of the sequence of the first six left-most keys in the third row, was patented by C. L. Sholes in 1878 as the eighth of a series of patents on typing machines (Figure 10.22). Although no specific technical claims were made regarding the layout of the keys, it can be hypothesized that Sholes, a printer by trade, used an arrangement similar to that in the printer's type case. Another possible explanation is that the most commonly used keys (or letters) are separated from each other such that they would not jam upon rapid sequential activation (Kroemer and Kroemer, 2001), although a statistical analysis of close typebars (keys typed in succession or less than four intervening keystrokes) shows that the QWERTY keyboard has more close typebars (26%) than a random keyboard (22%) (Noyes, 1998). Also there are some alphabetic patterns found on QWERTY keyboard. In following years, many other variations of and potential improvements to the layout of the keys were patented, including one by F. Heidner in 1915 that included a split and tiltable keyboard.

10.3.3.2 Dvorak Layout

The most notable and scientifically based alternative layout was patented by A. Dvorak in 1936 (Figure 10.22). He allocated the most commonly used keys to the strongest (middle) fingers, more work to the right hand, and the

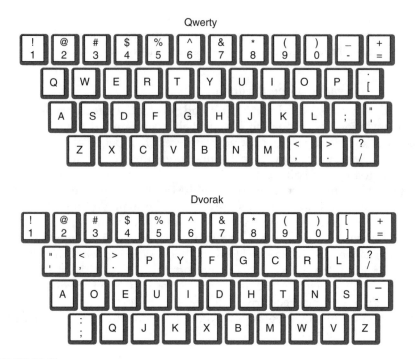

FIGURE 10.22
Standard QWERTY and alternative Dvorak keyboards.

most frequently used letters to the home row such that movement from row to row was minimized (Dvorak, 1943). Extensive investigations into the *Dvorak* layout were carried out by the U.S. Navy in 1944, the Australian Post Office in 1953, and the U.S. National Bureau of Standards (cited in Noyes, 1983a). Unfortunately, although all claimed the superiority of the Dvorak arrangement, especially in the speed of training new typists, none of these studies provided much experimental evidence. The only controlled study, by Strong (1956), found no performance difference on a 1-min typing test and superiority of the QWERTY arrangement both in speed and accuracy on a 5-min test. However, only experienced QWERTY typists were used, who were then retrained on the Dvorak arrangement, which gave them an unfair bias against Dvorak. Also, interestingly, Fox and Stansfield (1964) found that fastest digram keying times occur when successive taps are done with alternate hands, which is precisely what the QWERTY keyboard does.

10.3.3.3   Other Layouts

There have been a variety of other post-Dvorak layouts, either balanced (Griffith, 1949; Maxwell, 1953) or alphabetical (Michaels, 1971) in layout, none of which has received the notoriety of the Dvorak layout; they have failed to show improved performance (Hirsch, 1970) and have suffered the same fate as the Dvorak layout (Noyes, 1983a). Perhaps the best conclusions are given by Norman and Fisher (1982). Performance of alphabetical keyboards is quite slow, at best reaching within 2% of the QWERTY keyboard, because of additional mental processing and visual search requirements. Performance on the Dvorak keyboard shows at best a 5% improvement over the QWERTY keyboard, which is, probably, not great enough to justify switching and retraining millions of people.

10.3.4 Chord Keyboards

Data entry on a typical keyboard is in a sequential manner; i.e., individual characters are keyed in a specific sequence. On the other hand, in a *chord* keyboard entering one character requires the simultaneous activation of two or more keys. The basic trade-off is that with such activation, fewer keys are required and considerably more information can be entered. Research on chord keyboards was conducted primarily in the 1960s for use in post office mail sorting. Using 46 postal employees unskilled in using either a standard typewriter or a chord keyboard and randomly assigned to two groups, Conrad and Longman (1965) found that functional proficiency was achieved roughly 2 weeks more quickly on the chord keyboard. However, the performance in keystrokes per minute was lower because of the shorter practice time. When each group was allowed to continue the keyboarding task for a total of 33 days of effective practice, the chord keyboard group had caught up and surpassed the standard typewriter group by approximately 10 strokes/min (approximately 10% better). However, the learning curve had not yet leveled off and so peak performance had not yet been achieved. The overall error rate, however, for the chord keyboard was double the standard keyboard. Similarly, Bowen and Guinness (1965) found that when memory encoding was required (i.e., specific patterns of keys had to be remembered), subjects could encode up to 55 items/min on the chord keyboards vs. 40 items/min on the standard keyboard. Seibel (1964), based on his previous research of response times for all possible finger pattern (chord) combinations and comparisons of stenotypists (using chord keyboards but confounded in that a shorthand technique is also used) vs. regular typists, estimated that chord keyboards allowed anywhere from 50 to 100% greater data input per time. Perhaps Noyes (1983b) provides the best conclusion regarding chord keyboards. They have distinct advantages of small size and portability and one-handed operation (for a small set of keys), allowing the other hand to perform other tasks. For special tasks, such as stenotyping or mail sorting, where special patterns are remembered, they are especially useful. However, for general usage sequential keyboards fulfill the majority of everyday requirements without the need for additional specialized training.

10.3.5 Numeric Keypads

Of the wide variety of digit arrangements possible on a ten-key numeric keypad, the general characteristic preferred by users is that numerals

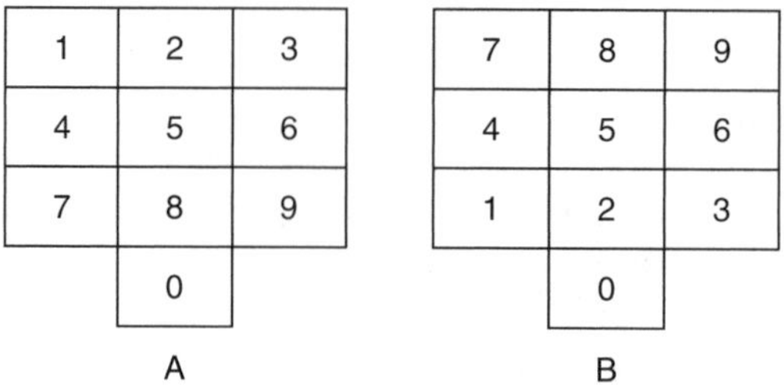

1	2	3
4	5	6
7	8	9
	0	

A

7	8	9
4	5	6
1	2	3
	0	

B

FIGURE 10.23
Numeric keypad arrangements: (A) telephone, (B) calculator.

increase from left to right and then from top to bottom, as shown in Figure 10.23A (Lutz and Chapanis, 1955). In selecting an appropriate arrangement for pushbutton telephones, Deininger (1960a,b) found an average keying time of 4.92 s for the above arrangement as opposed to a slightly longer time of 5.08 s for an alternative arrangement used on calculators in which the numbers increased from the bottom to the top (Figure 10.23B). Interestingly, the pushbuttons arranged in a pattern identical to a rotary dial yielded even faster times. However, because of "engineering advantages" the first layout was selected for pushbutton telephones. In a direct comparison of the two layouts using postal office clerks Conrad (1967, cited in Seibel, 1972) found faster keying rates (0.67 vs. 0.73 s/stroke) and fewer errors (0.55 vs. 1.16%) for the telephone arrangement. Similar advantages for the telephone arrangement were found by Paul et al. (1965, cited in Seibel, 1972) for air traffic controllers.

A study by Conrad and Hull (1968) divided 90 inexperienced "house-wives" into three groups, one to each of the two layouts and a third that alternated layouts while 8-digit codes into the keypads. Not surprisingly, the alternating group had lowest performance at 6.77 codes/min, whereas the telephone layout was best at 7.75 codes/min as compared to 7.41 codes/min for the calculator layout. However, this latter difference was not statistically significant, although the difference between telephone and alternating layouts was significant. More importantly, on all measures of accuracy (% wrong codes, % wrong digits, % codes and digits uncorrected), the telephone layout was significantly better than the calculator layout, contrary to what would have been expected from a speed–accuracy trade-off. A survey of 100 college students in a variety of simulated scenarios found preferences for the telephone layout ranging from 50 to 82% (Straub and Granaas, 1993). A further study of layouts with respect to type of task performed found no significant differences between the two layouts, other than the zero digit should be placed at the bottom of the keypad (Marteniuk et al., 1997). Probably because of the relatively small advantage of the telephone layout, BSR/HFES 100 (Human Factors and Ergonomics Society, 2002) has not come out in favor of either layout, but recommends the use of both. This, however, would produce the worst situation in terms of performance, especially if an office environment included both layouts as could typically be expected, e.g., a telephone next to a PC keyboard having a numeric keypad.

10.4   The Mouse and Other Cursor-Positioning Devices

10.4.1   Cursor Positioning

The primary data entry device for the computer has been the keyboard. However, with the growing ubiquity of graphical user interfaces and depending on the task performed, the operator may actually spend less than half the time using the keyboard. Especially for Windows- and menu-based systems, some type of cursor-positioning device, better than the cursor keys on a keyboard, was needed. For this, a wide variety of devices have been developed and tested. The *touch screen* uses either a touch-sensitive overlay on the screen or senses the interruption of an infrared beam across the screen as the finger approaches the screen. This approach is quite natural, with the user simply touching the target directly on the screen. However, the finger can obscure the target and, in spite of the fairly large targets required, accuracy can be poor (Beringer and Petersen, 1985). The *light pen* is a special stylus linked to the computer by an electrical cable that senses the electron-scanning beam at the particular location on the screen. The user has a similar natural pointing response as with a touch screen, but usually with more accuracy.

A *digitizing tablet* is a flat pad placed on the desktop, again linked to the computer. Movement of a stylus is sensed at the appropriate position on the tablet, which can either be absolute (i.e., the tablet is a representation of the screen) or relative (i.e., only direct movement across the tablet is shown). This then enters tablet size vs. accuracy trade-offs and optimum control-response ratios (Arnaut and Greenstein, 1986). Also, the user needs to look back at the screen to receive feedback. Both displacement and force *joysticks* (currently termed *track sticks* or *track points*) can be used to control the cursor and have a considerable background of research on types of control systems, types of displays, control-response ratios, and tracking performance (Poulton, 1974). The keyboard cursor (arrow) keys can also be utilized, but are slow and poor for drawing. The *mouse* is a handheld device with a roller ball in the base to control position and one or more buttons for other inputs. It is a relative positioning device and requires a clear space next to the keyboard for operation. The *trackball*, an upside-down mouse without the mouse pad, is a good alternative for work surfaces with limited space. For a more detailed review of cursor-positioning devices, refer to Greenstein and Arnaut (1988) or Sanders and McCormick (1993).

When computers first became popular, several studies examined the above-mentioned cursor-positioning devices for performance, typically speed or time to complete various tasks, accuracy, and user preferences. Typically, a limited number of inexperienced subjects were tested. Although, the lack of experience would allow for an unbiased evaluation of the device, learning effects were confounded with performance, and, in one case, perhaps due to inexperience, a subject had to be discarded due to very poor performance (Card et al., 1978). In addition, the small number of subjects would limit generalizability. The results of four such studies are summarized in Table 10.4. A final recommendation for the optimum device is difficult to make because different studies examined different devices and direct comparisons cannot be made. However, overall, there are clear speed–accuracy trade-offs, with the fastest devices (touch screens and light pens) being quite inaccurate. Therefore, consideration may need to be given to the type of task being performed. Keyboard cursor keys were slow and probably are not acceptable. Touch pads were a bit faster than joysticks, but were less preferred by users. The mouse tended to rank high in all studies, both in speed and accuracy, which, probably, indicates why it is so ubiquitous.

10.4.2   The Mouse

Along with the increased use of the mouse, there has been an increase in WRMSDs associated with the mouse. Fogleman and Brogmus (1995) reviewed workers' compensation claims, showing that, although a very small percentage of all claims (0.04%) are related to the mouse, a larger portion of WRMSDs (1%) and computer-related claims (6.1%) are related to the mouse. Furthermore, the problem grew rapidly from 1990 to 1993 and needed further attention.

There are several problems associated with mouse usage. Depending on the placement of the mouse, there are large ulnar deviations (up to 60°) and large lateral shoulder rotations (up to 45°) (Karlqvist et al., 1994) with consequential increased activity in the mouse-side shoulder muscles, primarily the trapezius and the deltoid (Jensen et al., 1998). Depending on the task, pinch and fingertip pressure forces can be quite high. The two main mouse tasks are pointing, i.e., moving and positioning the mouse, sometimes termed *point and click*, and dragging, i.e., manipulating the icons or windows with mouse, sometimes termed *drag and drop*. The mouse has been specifically instrumented with strain gauges to measure the forces during these tasks (Johnson et al., 1997). Mean pinching forces ranged from 0.55 to 1.40 N during pointing tasks and two to three times greater for dragging tasks. The fingertip forces during button operation did not differ significantly (1.51 to 1.99 N) between the tasks (Johnson et al., 1994). Similar fingertip forces were found by Kotani and Horii (2001) in a more complex Fitts' law mouse targeting task, with lowest forces for the highest index of difficulty. However, the forces were up to twice as large as the minimum force necessary to activate the control. Park (1999) also found fingertip forces to exceed the minimum by 2.3 to 2.8 times, which again confirms that individuals tend to

TABLE 10.4

Comparison of Cursor-Positioning Devices

Device	Card et al. (1978)		Albert (1982)			Epps (1987)		MacKenzie et al. (1991)		Average Ranking (two or more entries)		
	Sp	Acc	Sp	Acc	Pref	Sp	Pref	Sp	Acc	Sp	Acc	Pref
Touch screen			1	6.5	2					2	2	
Light pen			2	6.5	2							
Digitizing tablet			3	2	2			1	2			
Joystick, force	2	3	5	3	6.5	6	4			4.3	3	5.3
Joystick, displacement			6	4	6.5	5	3			5.5		4.8
Cursor keys, step	4	4	7	5	5					4.5	4.5	
Cursor keys, text	3	2										
Track ball			4	1	4	2	1	3	3	3	2	2.5
Mouse	1	1				1	2	2	1	1.3	1	
Touch pad, linear gain						3	6					
Touch pad, increasing gain						4	5					
No. of subjects	4		8			6		—		—		

Abbreviations: Sp = speed, Acc = accuracy, Pref = preference; rankings, 1 = fastest, most accurate, or most preferred.

overgrip objects or tools by as much as to five times the minimum necessary force (Lowe and Freivalds, 1999).

One suggestion to reduce at least the pinch forces in the dragging task is for computer manufacturers to include a drag-lock on the mouse similar to that found on trackballs (Johnson et al., 1994). Another approach may be to redesign the mouse with an upright handle gripped with a power grip to provide a more neutral forearm posture and decreased EMG levels in hand, forearm, and shoulder muscles (Aarås and Ro, 1997). An added feature of this particular mouse design (although not specifically discussed by the authors) is that the control button is activated by the thumb, which is 23% stronger than the index finger (Hertzberg, 1973). Furthermore, the button could just as well be placed on the side of the handle, allowing it to be activated directly from the power grip. Later field testing over a 6-month period found a significant reduction in pain intensity and frequency for the wrist/hand, forearm, shoulder, and neck (Aarås et al., 1999).

Keir et al. (1998) measured carpal tunnel pressure during mouse usage and found mean pressures of 33.1 mmHg during dragging and 28.0 mmHg during pointing as compared to 5.3 mmHg during a neutral resting state. The higher pressures during dragging were attributed to the button being depressed for a greater percentage of time and greater pinch forces. Also, mouse usage, in general, promoted wrist extension and forearm rotation, both of which also increased carpal tunnel pressure (Werner et al., 1997; Rempel et al., 1998). Prolonged pressures of 30 mmHg have been associated with altered nerve function in animal studies (Hargens et al., 1979; Lundborg et al., 1983; Powell and Myers, 1986), which could the first step in the sequence of events leading to CTS (Dahlin et al., 1987). Interestingly, Keir et al. (1999) also tested three different mouse designs, each of which promoted slightly different radioulnar deviations. However, there were no significant differences in the carpal tunnel pressures, attributed to the relatively small changes in angle.

Researchers have examined various workstation parameters to reduce the stress of using the mouse. Using forearm supports significantly decreased trapezius muscle activity (Aarås et al., 1997). Considering that the mouse is typically placed to the right of the numeric keypad, the large lateral shoulder rotations and ulnar deviations (Karlqvist et al., 1994) are not unexpected. Removing the numeric keypad and moving the mouse closer to the body median significantly decreased deltoid muscle activity and improved RULA scores (Cook and Kothiyal, 1998). Alternatively, they suggested using the mouse with left hand. Unfortunately, this results in a 30% slower response times for right-handed individuals (Hoffman et al., 1997). Left-handed individuals showed no such decrement, presumably because of previous experiences using the nondominant hand.

Karlqvist et al. (1998) examined several alternative mouse positions, found similar results to Cook and Kothiyal (1998), and recommended an optimum position of a neutral shoulder rotation with a relaxed and supported arm. Park (1999) measured fingertip forces, wrist angles, shoulder abduction angles, and deltoid EMG for a total of 18 different mouse positions, three lateral positions, three heights, and two posterior/anterior positions. The optimum position based on lowest stress for most variables was the lowest height, 90% of the subject's elbow resting height, the most posterior position, at the edge of the keyboard, and the most medial position, 31.5 cm from the body median, centered with the GH keys on the keyboard. Not surprisingly, only wrist extension showed an opposite trend with the highest level yielding the smallest extension angle. Ultimately, as in most ergonomic designs, there will need to be trade-offs, as all variables cannot be optimized.

10.4.3   Mouse Alternatives

The trackball as a similar but alternative devices for the mouse has been reexamined. Harvey and Peper (1997) found lower trapezius and deltoid EMGs with a centrally located trackball, below the center of the keyboard, as compared to a mouse positioned to the right of the keyboard. However, the type of input device was confounded with placement. For the same operating position, to the right of the numeric keypad, Burgess-Limerick et al. (1999) found that a trackball decreased ulnar deviation but increased wrist extension. Given the trade-offs and the large individual variations, they suggested that the use of trackball for interventions be linked to follow-up evaluations of postures. Also there may be concern, not yet examined, with the large amounts of thumb motion.

An early precursor to the *touch pad*, in the form of tiltable pushbutton, was first compared to the mouse and cursor keys by Loricchio (1992). Experienced mouse users did significantly better with the mouse, while non-experienced users had mixed results. However, both experienced and non-experienced mouse users found the pushbutton difficult to use. Çakir et al. (1995) found an improved version of the touch pad to yield performance levels comparable to a mouse within 5 h of usage. Wrist deviations with the touch pad were less than for the mouse with implications (although not tested) of decreased long-term postural discomfort. Latest research by Akamatsu and MacKenzie (2002) indicates that applied forces with a touch pad are significantly lower than for a mouse (1.24 vs. 1.6 N). Interestingly, the applied forces on a touch pad decrease as the operator approaches the target, while the forces on a mouse increase. The authors attributed this effect as a compensatory effect to increase friction with the mouse and consequently improve the precision of the movement. Because the hand and forearm movements used for controlling the mouse are less precise than finger movements used with a touch pad (Langolf et al., 1976), one would suspect that the touch pad should yield more precise movements than a mouse. However, the exact opposite was found. In addition, the touch pad yielded 19% significantly slower movements and 16% lower throughput. The authors alluded to the increased jitter with increased forces in the touch pad, suggesting that the dynamics of the touch pad be altered to be comparable to a mouse for increased precision.

Batra et al. (1998) compared the touch pad to a trackball and a *track point*, an isometric joystick in middle of laptop keyboards. The touch pad and trackball had similar performance on various pointing, box-sizing, and text selection tasks. However, the track point performed consistently worse and was judged not well suited as an input device. Fernström and Ericson (1997) also examined the track point as an alternative to the mouse, but in terms of muscular loading. Shoulder loading decreased significantly, but at the expense of added forearm loading because the forearm was not supported. Subjects were free to use an armrest but only one did so. This again indicates the need for proper training in the adjustment of computer workstation furniture. Also, subjects preferred to use the track point so as to keep their hands on the keyboard; i.e., they resisted the postural variation in reaching for the mouse. Interestingly, highest muscle loading was found for manual handwriting. Thus, overall, the touch pad may prove to be a practical alternative to the mouse, especially for use on notebook PCs.

10.5   Notebooks and Handheld PCs

Portable PCs, or laptop, or notebook computers (earlier distinction based on size, but which is continually changing), are becoming very popular, accounting for 34% of the U.S. PC market in 2000 (Sommerich, 2000). Their main advantage over a desktop PC is reduced size (and weight) and portability. However, with the smaller size, there are distinct disadvantages; smaller keys and keyboard, keyboard attached to screen, and the lack of a peripheral cursor-positioning device. Yoshitake (1995) found that touch typists with wide fingers performed worse on small keyboards (16.7 mm width vs. 19 to 21 mm on standard keyboards) than typists with narrow fingers. Similar results had been found previously (Loricchio and Lewis, 1991) on numeric keypads with narrower interkey spacing and narrow keys. The lack of adjustability in placing the screen has been found to give rise to excessive neck flexion (44° to 50°, beyond the recommended 15°), increased shoulder flexion (22° to 34°, rather than arms hanging naturally), and elbow angles greater than 90° (101 to 110°) (Harbison and Forrester, 1995). Straker et al. (1997) found similar neck flexions (mean of 57°) with greater discomfort after 20 min of work as compared to a desktop PC. This discomfort is most likely due to the increased neck extensor muscle activity as observed by Villanueva et al. (1998) for four different types of notebook computers. Price and Dowell (1998) found that raising the notebook to a higher surface to reduce neck flexion only worsened shoulder flexion. Adding an external keyboard and raising the notebook computer or adding an external monitor improved the body angles comparable to a desktop PC. The problem of an integrated cursor-positioning device was examined by Kelaher et al. (2001) using a Fitts' tapping task with five different locations of a touch pad, top/bottom in combination with center/right side and one attached to the middle of the right side. The top and bottom locations exhibited a trade-off between wrist extension and ulnar deviation. The bottom positions were better than top for elbow and shoulder angles as well as discomfort ratings and performance. However, the right side location proved best, although not significantly, and would require some sort of clip attachment provided by the manufacturer.

Even smaller handheld computers, termed *personal digital assistants* (PDAs), have been developed but are too new to have had detailed scientific evaluations performed. As they are pocket size, they offer much greater portability and flexibility, but at an even greater disadvantage for data entry. Wright et al. (2000) found significant decrements in speed and accuracy when entering text via the touch screen. Most subjects preferred using an external but small keyboard. Older individuals were significantly slower compared to younger individuals, but similar in error rates. The authors recommended alternative input methods such as handwriting or voice input to remedy such an unacceptable form of data entry.

10.6 Control Measures

10.6.1 Rest Pauses

The general principle for the allocation of rest in heavy work, derived from the intermittent work studies of Karrasch and Müller (1951) and Åstrand et al. (1960a,b), is frequent, short rest pauses, as opposed to less frequent but longer pauses. This principle was extended to office work by Çakir et al. (1980) based on cognitive demands and data from Graf (1960; cited in Çakir et al.,1980). Graf found that providing rest pauses of 2, 4, and 6 min after 45, 90, and 125 min in a 3-h task involving arithmetic calculations increased productivity 5.6% over nonstop work, even though the rest pauses decreased working time by 6.7%. Providing the same amount of rest but in shorter, more frequent pauses of 0.5, 1, and 2 min every 15 min increased productivity even more, 9.8% over baseline conditions. Graf's data showing that increasing the length of a rest pause beyond 5 min produced marginal benefits led Grandjean (1987) to generalize the principle for office work as 3- to 5-min rest every hour.

Cognitive work is not the sole factor leading to fatigue in office work. Several studies found degradations in color adaptation and accommodation occurring with prolonged viewing of computer screens, then termed visual display terminals (VDTs), in the ever-increasing computerization of office work (Çakir et al., 1980; Haider et al., 1980; Krueger, 1980). Such degradations were found to be reversed with 15-min breaks (Haider et al., 1980), leading NIOSH (1981) to recommend a 15-min break every 2 h of continuous but moderate VDT work or a 15-min break every hour for very high visual VDT demands or workload. However, these recommendations were made with few detailed studies to support them.

Later research supported the hourly recommendation, with Floru et al. (1985) and Gao et al. (1990) finding that performance on VDT tasks steadily decreased over a 45- to 60-min period, which was then followed by a rebound in performance. This was attributed by Bills (1931) to *blocks* or cycling patterns in mental arousal and, along with associated changes in electroencephalograms and heart rate, indicated a natural point at which a rest pause should be provided. There is some data indicating that these rest pauses should be active (walking or stretching) rather than passive. Sundelin and Hagberg (1989) found that subjects preferred such pauses and experienced less perceived discomfort, although not a statistically significant level. NIOSH researchers (Galinsky et al., 2000) further confirmed the need for breaks every hour, finding significant decreases in perceived discomfort in various body parts in those workers receiving pauses every hour as compared to those receiving pauses every 2 h. Interestingly, although the productivity rate increased slightly, total productivity did not increase, because of the time lost due to the added pauses.

In addition to regular pauses, *micropauses* at irregular, spontaneous intervals may also provide benefit in relieving discomfort and, perhaps, some increase in productivity (Henning et al., 1997; McLean et al., 2001). Previously, Henning et al. (1989) found that self-selected micropauses of 27 s did not completely reduce the steady decline in performance over 40-min work periods and recommended that slightly longer pauses were needed. Also, Henning et al. (1994) found that spontaneous pauses provided just as much benefit as regimented pauses and had the added advantage of eliminating unnecessary task interruptions. Although no specific recommendations for the length of micropauses were ever fully determined, the need for such pauses was supported.

The original recommendation of 15-min rest for every hour for computer data-entry work does not correspond well with the principle of frequent, short pauses and may not be sufficient, based on empirical data. A more flexible schedule of 5- to 15-min rest for every hour, 5 min for good working conditions, 15 min for very poor conditions, with frequent spontaneous micropauses (at least every 10 min) may be a better recommendation (Pheasant, 1991).

10.6.2 Exercises

Although the primary emphasis for control measures has been on proper workstation design, Winkel (1987) and Sundelin and Hagberg (1989) have recommended dynamic rest pauses to relieve the stresses of sedentary work. Although more than 14 exercise programs, specifically designed for VDT users, have been cited in the literature (summarized in Lee et al., 1992), few have been tested for effectiveness in well-controlled laboratory experiments or even well-designed field studies.

Muscle groups that typically fatigue during extended periods at a computer workstation include the shoulder elevators (levator scapulae, trapezius, latissimus dorsi, rhomboid), back muscles (erector spinae), chest muscles (pectoralis, infraspinatus, serratus), and forearm flexors (flexor carpi, flexor digitorum). As a consequence a majority of the exercises (54%) are designated for the shoulders and upper limbs. However, exercises are also suggested for the neck, trunk, back, and legs. At the least the exercises should be (1) practical, i.e., requiring minimum time, causing minimal disruption of work activities and embarrassment to the operator, and corresponding to the ability and motivation levels of the operators, and (2) safe, i.e., should be based on accepted biomechanical and physiotherapy principles and should not pose added risks to the operator. However, some of the exercises were found to require excessive amounts of time and, with considerable flexing, rotation, and extension of joints, may pose risks for those individuals with preexisting WRMSDs of the upper limbs (Lee et al., 1992).

More recent research shows some positive effect from exercises. Although not tested statistically, Sucher (1994) found some improvement in the range of motion for the wrist and an increase in nerve conduction velocities of symptomatic patients. This was attributed to exercises specifically stretching the carpal ligament, which opened the carpal canal. Rozmanryn et al. (1998) divided 197 patients symptomatic with CTS into two groups. Both were treated conservatively, but one group also performed nerve and tendon gliding exercises. Of the control patients, 71% still underwent surgery, while only 43% of the exercising patients underwent surgery, of which 70% remained relatively symptomatic 2 years later. This was a significant ($p < 0.001$) difference, which the authors attributed to the exercise. However, the Seradge et al. (2002) study found that exercise programs work best for mild to moderate cases, with all severe cases still requiring surgery.

Whereas the above studies examined specific exercises as a means of reducing the symptoms for those individuals already diagnosed with CTS, a more critical question is whether exercise programs can prevent or reduce the development of CTS in typical workers subject to occupational stressors. Seradge et al. (2000) introduced an exercise program in a meat-packing plant with 286 production workers. Because no other ergonomic controls were implemented and because the CTS incidence rate decreasing by 45% in 1 year, one could consider the exercise program a success. However, with no control group, the results could also be due to an overall heightened ergonomics awareness or some other extraneous or confounded factor not directly measured.

Disregarding the direct effectiveness of these programs on the individual, there is also the major problem of overall effectiveness. Most such worksite programs attract only a small proportion of a company's workforce (unless they are made mandatory), exhibit high drop-out rates (Song et al., 1982), and provide smaller benefits than predicted from a controlled laboratory setting (Blair et al., 1986). There are many theories of psychosocial factors that either motivate a person or cause perceived barriers to exercise (Godin and Gionet, 1991). However, these factors are no different in the workplace than in a personal setting. Therefore, the same principles that foster exercise in the general population should also guide the promotion of exercise in the workplace (Godin and Gionet, 1991).

Note that, although not specifically tested as an intervention, increased general aerobic exercise and its resultant decrease in percent body fat and increase in peak aerobic capacity have been found to correlate significantly with decreased median nerve sensory latency (Nathan et al., 2001). Consequently, the authors recommended aerobic exercise programs as a means of reducing hand CTS symptoms. Also, one should not excessively overdo strengthening exercise programs, lest the exercise become equivalent to the stressful work of high forces and excessive joint deviations ergonomists are attempting to redesign. Mauer et al. (1991) found that the same CTS symptoms appeared in a group of 30 bodybuilders, especially for those training more than 6 years.

Questions

1. What are some of the factors that may cause musculoskeletal problems in an office environment?
2. How does the spine change in going from a standing to a seated posture?
3. What factors may help reduce the increased disc pressure found in a seated posture?
4. Why may the standard seated posture with 90° angles not be the best posture?
5. How is optimum chair height determined?
6. What are important chair parameters that need to be adjusted for optimum comfort?
7. How can seating comfort be measured? Compare and contrast the approaches.
8. What is the theory behind seat pressure distribution and seat design?
9. What are the advantages of sit-stand chairs?
10. How is work surface height determined and how does it relate to chair height?
11. What is the normal line of sight and how is it determined?
12. How is normal working area determined?

13. What are the trade-offs with a tilted work surface?

14. What are important characteristics of key design for keyboards?

15. Why is feedback important in keystroking? How is it best incorporated?

16. What biomechanical advantages do split and adjustable keyboards provide?

17. What are the trade-offs of a Dvorak layout as compared to the standard QWERTY layout? That is, why have they not become popular in spite of the scientific design?

18. What is a chord keyboard?

19. Compare and contrast different approaches to cursor positioning. Which seems to have the most optimum characteristics?

20. Why are wrist rests not especially recommended in reducing arm fatigue?

21. What are some the problems encountered with laptop or notebook computers?

References

Aarås, A. and Ro, O., 1997. Workload when using a mouse as an input device, *International Journal of Human–Computer Interaction*, 9:105–116.

Aarås, A., Fostervold, K.I., Ro, O., Thoresen, M., and Larsen, S., 1997. Postural load during VDU work: a comparison between various work postures, *Ergonomics*, 40:1255–1268.

Aarås, A., Ro, O., and Thoresen, M., 1999. Can a more neutral position of the forearm when operating a computer mouse reduce the pain level for a visual display unit operators? A prospective epidemiological intervention study, *International Journal of Human–Computer Interaction*, 11:79–94.

Abernethy, C.N., 1984. Behavioural data in the design of ergonomic computer terminals and workstations — a case study, *Behavioural and Information Technology*, 3:399–403.

ACTU-VTHC, 1982. *Guidelines for the Prevention of Repetition Strain Injury (RSI)*, Australian Council of Trades Unions and Victorian Trades Hall Council Health and Safety Bulletin 18, Melbourne, Victoria.

Akagi, K., 1992. A computer keyboard key feel study in performance and preference, *Proceedings of the Human Factors Society*, 36:523–527.

Akamatsu, M. and MacKenzie, I.S., 2002. Changes in applied force to a touchpad during pointing tasks, *International Journal of Industrial Ergonomics*, 29:171–182.

Åkerblom, B., 1948. *Standing and Sitting Posture*, Stockholm: A.B. Nordiska Bokhandeln.

Albert, A.E., 1982. The effect of graphic input devices on performance in a cursor positioning task, *Proceedings of the Human Factors Society*, 26:54–58.

Alden, D.G., Daniels, R.W., and Kanarick, A.F., 1972. Keyboard design and operation: A review of the major issues, *Human Factors*, 14:275–293.

Andersson, G.B.J. and Örtengren, R., 1974a. Lumbar disc pressure and myoelectric back muscle activity during sitting: II. Studies on an office chair, *Scandinavian Journal of Rehabilitation Medicine*, 6:115–121.

Andersson, G.B.J. and Örtengren, R., 1974b. Lumbar disc pressure and myoelectric back muscle activity during sitting: III. Studies on a wheel chair, *Scandinavian Journal of Rehabilitation Medicine*, 6:122–127.

Andersson, G.B.J., Örtengren, R., Nachemson, A., and Elfström, G., 1974a. Lumbar disc pressure and myoelectric back muscle activity during sitting: I. Studies on an experimental chair, *Scandinavian Journal of Rehabilitation Medicine*, 6:104–114.

Andersson, G.B.J., Örtengren, R., Nachemson, A., and Elfström, G., 1974b. Lumbar disc pressure and myoelectric back muscle activity during sitting: IV. Studies on a car drivers seat, *Scandinavian Journal of Rehabilitation Medicine*, 6:128–133.

Andersson, G.B.J., Murphy, R.W., Örtengren, R., and Nachemson, A.L., 1979. The influence of backrest inclination and lumbar support on the lumbar lordosis in sitting, *Spine*, 4:52–58.

Armstrong, T.J., Foulke, J.A., Martin, B.J., Gerson, J., and Rempel, D.M., 1994. Investigation of applied forces in alphanumeric keyboard work, *American Industrial Hygiene Association Journal*, 55:30–35.

Arnaut, L.Y. and Greenstein, J., 1986. Minimizing the touch table: the effects of control-display gain and method of cursor control, *Human Factors*, 28:717–726.

Åstrand, I., Åstrand, P.O., Christensen, E.H., and Hedman, R., 1960a. Intermittent muscular work, *Acta Physiologica Scandinavica*, 48:443–453.

Åstrand, I., Åstrand, P.O., Christensen, E.H., and Hedman, R., 1960b. Myohemoglobin as an oxygen-store in man, *Acta Physiologica Scandinavica*, 48:454–460.

Ayoub, M.M., 1973. Work place design and posture, *Human Factors*, 15:265–268.

Barkla, D.M., 1964. Chair angles, duration of sitting, and comfort ratings, *Ergonomics*, 7:297–304.

Batra, S., Dykstra, D., Hus, P., Raddle, K.A., and Wiedenbeck, S., 1998. Pointing device performance for laptop computers, *Proceedings of the Human Factors and Ergonomics Society*, 42:536–540.

Bendix, A., Jensen, C.V., and Bendix, T., 1988. Posture, acceptability and energy consumption on a tiltable and a knee–supported chair, *Clinical Biomechanics*, 3:66–73.

Bendix, T., 1984. Seated trunk posture at various seat inclinations, seat heights, and table heights, *Human Factors*, 26:695–703.

Bendix, T. and Biering-Sørenson, F., 1983. Posture of trunk when sitting on forward inclining seats, *Scandinavian Journal of Rehabilitation Medicine*, 15:197–203.

Bendix, T. and Bloch, I., 1986. How should a seated workplace with a tiltable chair be adjusted? *Applied Ergonomics*, 17:127–135.

Bendix, T. and Hagberg, M., 1984. Trunk posture and load on the trapezius muscle whilst sitting at sloping desks, *Ergonomics*, 27:873–882.

Bendix, T., Krohn, L., Jessen, F., and Aarås, A., 1985a. Trunk posture and trapezius muscle load whilst work in standing, supported standing, and sitting postures, *Spine*, 54:378–385.

Bendix, T., Winkel, J., and Jessen, F., 1985b. Comparison of office chairs with fixed forwards or backwards inclining, or tiltable seats, *European Journal of Applied Physiology*, 54:378–385.

Beringer, D. and Petersen, J., 1985. Underlying behavioral parameters of the operation of touch–input devices: biases, models, and feedback, *Human Factors*, 27:445–458.

Bills, A.G., 1931. Blocking: a new principle in mental fatigue, *American Journal of Psychology*, 42:230–245.

Blair, S.N., Piserchia, P.V., Wilbur, C.S., and Crowder, J.H., 1986. A public health intervention model for work-site health promotion, *Journal of the American Medical Association*, 255:921–926.

Bowen, H.M. and Guinness, G.V., 1965. Preliminary experiments on keyboard design for semiautomatic mail sorting, *Journal of Applied Psychology*, 49:194–198.

Branton, P., 1969. Behaviour, body mechanics and discomfort, *Ergonomics*, 12:316–327.

Branton, P., 1974. Seating in industry, *Applied Ergonomics*, 1:159–165.

Branton, P. and Grayson, G., 1967. An evaluation of train seats by observation of sitting behaviour, *Ergonomics*, 10:35–51.

Bridger, R.S., 1988. Postural adaptations to a sloping chair and work surface, *Human Factors*, 30:237–247.

Bridger, R.S., von Eisenhart-Rothe, C., and Henneberg, M., 1989. Effects of seat slope and hip flexion on spinal angles in sitting, *Human Factors*, 31:679–688.

Brown, C.R. and Schaum, D.L., 1980. User-adjusted VDU parameters, in Grandjean, E. and Vigliani, E., Eds., *Ergonomic Aspects of Visual Display Terminals*, London: Taylor & Francis, 195–200.

Brunner, H. and Richardson, R.M., 1984. Effects of keyboard design and typing skill on user keyboard preferences and throughput performance, *Proceedings of the Human Factors Society*, 28:267–271.

BS EN 1135, 2000. *Office Furniture, Office Work Chair, Dimensions, Determination of Dimensions*, London: British Standards Institution, available at http://www.bsi–global.com/index.html.

Buesen, J., 1984. Product development of an ergonomic keyboard, *Behaviour and Information Technology*, 3:387–390.

Bullock, M.I., 1974. The determination of functional arm reach boundaries for operation of manual controls, *Ergonomics*, 17:375–388.

Burandt, U., 1969. Röntgenuntersuchung über die Stellung von Becken und Wirbelsäule beim Sitzen auf vorgeneigten Flächen [X–ray study of the position of the pelvis and spin while sitting in forward-sloping surfaces], *Ergonomics*, 12:356–364.

Burandt, U. and Grandjean, E., 1969. Untersuchungen über das Sitzverhalten von Büroangestellten und über die Auswirkungen verschiedenartiger Sitzprofile [Research on seated office workers and on the consequences of various postures], *Ergonomics*, 12:338–347.

Burgerstein, L., 1915. *School Hygiene*, New York: Stokes.

Burgess–Limerick, R., Plooy, A., and Ankrum, D.R., 1998. The effect of imposed and self-selected computer monitor height on posture and gaze angle, *Clinical Biomechanics*, 13:584–592.

Burgess–Limerick, R., Shemmell, J., Scadden, R., and Plooy, A., 1999. Wrist posture during computer pointing device use, *Clinical Biomechanics*, 14:280–286.

Byström, S., and Fransson–Hall, C., 1994. Acceptability of intermittent handgrip contractions based on physiological response, *Human Factors*, 36:158–171.

Çakir, A., 1995. Acceptance of the adjustable keyboard, *Ergonomics*, 38:1728–1744.

Çakir, A. Reuter, H.J., Schmude, L., and Armbruster, A., 1978. *Untersuchungen zur Anpassung von Bildschirmarbeitsplatzen an die physische und psychische Funktionsweise des Menschen* [Research on the adjustment of VDT workplaces and the physical and psychological functioning of workers], Bonn, Germany: Bündesminister für Arbeit und Sozialsordnung.

Çakir, A., Hart, D.J., and Stewart, T.F.M., 1980. *Visual Display Terminals*, New York: John Wiley & Sons.

Çakir, A.E., Çakir, G., Müller, T., and Unema, P., 1995. The Trackpad™ — a study on user comfort and performance, *CHI 95 Conference on Human Factors in Computing Systems*, 2:97–98.

Cantoni, S., Colombini, D., Occhipinti, E., Grieco, A., Frigo, C., and Pedotti, A., 1984. Posture analysis and evaluation at the old and new work place of a telephone company, in Grandjean, E., Ed., *Ergonomics and Health in Modern Offices*, London: Taylor & Francis, 456–464.

Card, S.K., English, W.K., and Burr, B.J., 1978. Evaluation of mouse, rate-controlled isometric joystick, step keys and text keys for text selection on a CRT, *Ergonomics*, 21:601–613.

Chaffin, D.B., 1973. Localized muscle fatigue — definition and measurement, *Journal of Occupational Medicine*, 15:346–354.

Chaffin, D.B., Andersson, G.B.J., and Martin, B.J., 1999. *Occupational Biomechanics*, 3rd ed., New York: John Wiley & Sons.

Clare, R.C., 1976. Human factors: a most important ingredient in keyboard designs, *Electronic Design News*, 21(April):99–102.

Congleton, J.J., Ayoub, M.M., and Smith, J.L., 1985. The design and evaluation of the neutral posture chair for surgeons, *Human Factors*, 27:589–600.

Conrad, R., 1967. Performance with different push–button arrangements, *Hett PTT Bendriff*, 15:110–113.

Conrad, R. and Hull, A.J., 1968. The preferred layout for numeral data-entry keysets, *Ergonomics*, 11:165–173.

Conrad, R. and Longman, D.J.A., 1965. Standard typewriter versus chord keyboard — an experimental comparison, *Ergonomics*, 8:77–92.

Cook, C.J. and Kothiyal, K., 1998. Influence of mouse position on muscular activity in the neck, shoulder and arm in computer users, *Applied Ergonomics*, 29:439–443.

Corlett, E.N. and Bishop, R.P., 1976. A technique for assessing postural discomfort, *Ergonomics*, 19:175–182.

Corlett, E.N. and Eklund, J.A.E., 1984a. How does a backrest work? *Applied Ergonomics*, 15:111–114.

Corlett, E.N. and Eklund, J.A.E., 1984b. Shrinkage as a measure of the effect of load on the spine, *Spine*, 9:189–194.

Creamer, L.R. and Trumbo, D.A., 1960. Multifinger tapping performance as a function of the direction of tapping movements, *Journal of Applied Psychology*, 44:376–380.

Dahlin, L.B., Nordborg, C., and Lundborg, G., 1987. Morphologic changes in nerve cell bodies induced by experimental graded compression, *Experimental Neurology*, 95:611–621.

Das, B. and Behara, D.N., 1995. Determination of the normal horizontal working area: a new model and method, *Ergonomics*, 38:734–748.

Das, B. and Grady, R.M., 1983. The normal working area in the horizontal plane — a comparative analysis between Farleys and Squires concepts, *Ergonomics*, 26:449–459.

de Wall, M., van Riel, M.P.J.M., and Snijders, C.J., 1991. The effect of sitting posture of a desk with a 10° inclination for reading and writing, *Ergonomics*, 34:575–584.

Deininger, R.L., 1960a. Human factors engineering studies of the design and use of pushbutton telephone sets, *Bell System Technical Journal*, 39:995–1012.

Deininger, R.L., 1960b. Desirable push–button characteristics, *IRE Transactions on Human Factors in Electronics*, 1:24–30.

Dempster, W.T., 1955. Space Requirements of the Seated Operator, WADC TR 55-159, Dayton, OH: Wright-Patterson Air Force Base.

Diebschlag, W. and Müller–Limmroth, W., 1980. Physiological requirements on car seats: some results of experimental studies, in Oborne, D.J. and Levis, J.A., Eds., *Human Factors in Transport Research*, Vol. 2., London: Academic Press, 223–230.

Diehl, M.J. and Seibel, R., 1962. The relative importance of visual and auditory feedback in speed of typewriting, *Journal of Applied Psychology*, 46:365–369.

Diffrient, N., Tilley, A.R., and Bardagjy, J.C., 1974. *Humanscale 1/2/3*, Cambridge, MA: MIT Press.

DIN, 1996. DIN EN 1135 Office Furniture — Office Work Chair, Berlin D-10772: Deutsches Institut für Normung, available at http://www.din.de/or http://www2.beuth.de/.

Dreyfuss, H., 1959. *Anthropometric Data*, New York: Whitney Publications.

Drummond, D.S., Narechania, R.G., Rosenthal, A.N., Breed, A.L., Lange, T.A., and Drummond, D.K., 1982. A study of pressure distributions measured during balanced and unbalanced sitting, *Journal of Bone and Joint Surgery*, 64A:1034–1039.

Drury, C.G. and Coury, B.G., 1982. A methodology for chair evaluation, *Applied Ergonomics*, 13:195–202.

Drury, C.G. and Francher, M., 1985. Evaluation of a forward-sloping chair, *Applied Ergonomics*, 16:41–47.

Drury, C. and Hoffman, E., 1992. A model for movement time on data-entry keyboards, *Ergonomics*, 35:129–147.

Dvorak, A., 1943. There is a better typewriter keyboard, *National Business Education Quarterly*, 12:51–58.

Eastman Kodak, 1983. *Ergonomics Design for People at Work*, Vol. 1, Belmont, CA: Lifetime Learning Publications.

Eklund, J.A.E. and Corlett, E.N., 1987. Evaluation of spinal loads and chair design in seated work tasks, *Clinical Biomechanics*, 2:27–33.

Ellis, D.S., 1951. Speed of manipulative performance as a function of work surface height, *Journal of Applied Psychology*, 35:289–296.

Emmons, W.H. and Hirsch, R.S., 1982. Thirty millimeter keyboards: how good are they? *Proceedings of the Human Factors Society*, 26:425–429.

Epps, B.W., 1987. A comparison of cursor control devices on a graphics editing task, *Proceedings of the Human Factors Society*, 31:442–446.

Erdelyi, A., Sihvonen, T., Helin, P., and Hänninen, O., 1988. Shoulder strain in keyboard workers and its alleviation by arm supports, *International Archives for Occupational and Environmental Health*, 60:119–124.

Ericson, M.O. and Goldie, I., 1989. Spinal shrinkage with three different types of chair whilst performing video display unit work, *International Journal of Industrial Ergonomics*, 3:177–183.

Farley, R.R., 1955. Some principles of methods and motion study as used in development work, *General Motors Engineering Journal*, 2:20–25.

Fenety, P.A., Putnam, C., and Walker, J.M., 2000. In-chair movement: validity, reliability and implications for measuring sitting discomfort, *Applied Ergonomics*, 31:383–393.

Ferguson, D., 1976. Posture aching and body build in telephonists, *Journal of Human Ergology*, 5:183–186.

Ferguson, D., 1984. The new industrial epidemic, *Medical Journal of Australia*, 140:318–319.

Fernström, E. and Ericson, M.O., 1997. Computer mouse or trackpoint — effects on muscular load and operator experience, *Applied Ergonomics*, 28:347–354.

Fernström, E., Ericson, M.O., and Malker, H., 1994. Electromyographic activity during typewriter and keyboard use, *Ergonomics*, 37:477–484.

Festervoll, I., 1994. Office seating and movement, in Lueder, R. and Noro, K., Eds., *Hard Facts about Soft Machines: The Ergonomics of Seating*, London: Taylor & Francis, 413–421.

Fitts, P., 1954. The information capacity of the human motor system in controlling the amplitude of movement, *Journal of Experimental Psychology*, 47:381–391.

Floyd, W.F. and Silver, P.H.S., 1955. The function of the erectores spinae muscles in certain movements and postures in man, *Journal of Physiology*, 129:184–203.

Floru, R., Cail, F., and Elias, R., 1985. Psychophysiological changes during a VDU repetitive task, *Ergonomics*, 28:1455–1468.

Fogleman, M. and Brogmus, G., 1995. Computer mouse use and cumulative trauma disorders of the upper extremities, *Ergonomics*, 38:2465–2475.

Fox, J.G. and Stansfield, R.G., 1964. Digram keying times for typists, *Ergonomics*, 7:317–320.

Freudenthal, A., van Riel, M.P.J.M., Molenbroek, J.F.M., and Snijders, C.J., 1991. The effect on sitting posture of a desk with a ten-degree inclination using an adjustable chair and table, *Applied Ergonomics*, 22:329–336.

Frey, J.K. and Tecklin, J.S., 1986. Comparison of lumbar curves when sitting on the Westnofa Balans multi-chair, sitting on a conventional chair, and standing, *Physical Therapy*, 66:1365–1369.

Galinsky, T.L., Swanson, N.G., Sauter, S.L., Hurrell, J.J., and Schleifer, L.M., 2000. A field study of supplementary rest breaks for data-entry operators, *Ergonomics*, 43:622–638.

Galitz, W.O., 1965. *CRT Keyboard Human Factors Evaluation*, Rosemont, IL: UNIVAC.

Gao, C., Lu, D., She, Q., Cai, R., Yang, L., and Zhang, G., 1990. The effects of VDT data entry work on operators, *Ergonomics*, 33:917–924.

Gerard, M.H., Armstrong, T.J., Foulke, J.A., and Martin, B.J., 1996. Effects of key stiffness on force and the development of fatigue while typing, *American Industrial Hygiene Association Journal*, 57:849–854.

Gerard, M.J., Jones, S.K., Smith, L.A., Thomas, R.E., and Wang, T., 1994. An ergonomic evaluation of the Kinesis Ergonomic Computer keyboard, *Ergonomics*, 37:1661–1668.

Gerard, M.J., Armstrong, T.J., Franzblau, A., Martin, B.J., and Rempel, D.M., 1999. The effects of keyswitch stiffness on typing force, finger, electromyography, and subjective discomfort, *American Industrial Hygiene Association Journal*, 60:762–769.

Gerr, F., Marcus, M., Ortiz, D., White, B., Jones, W., Cohen, S., Gentry, E., Edwards, A., and Bauer, E., 2000. Computer users postures and associations with workstation characteristics, *American Industrial Hygiene Association Journal*, 61:223–230.

Godin, G. and Gionet, N.J., 1991. Determinants of an intention to exercise of an electric power commissions employees, *Ergonomics*, 34:1221–1230.

Goonetilleke, R.S., 1998. Designing to minimize comfort, *Ergonomics in Design*, July:12–19.

Graf, M., Guggenbühl, U., and Krueger, H., 1993. Investigations on the effects of seat shape and slope on posture and back muscle activity, *International Journal of Industrial Ergonomics*, 12:91–103.

Graf, O., 1960. *Arbeitsphysiologie*, Wiesbaden.

Grandjean, E., Ed., 1969. *The Sitting Posture*, London: Taylor & Francis.

Grandjean, E., 1987. *Ergonomics in Computerized Offices*, London: Taylor & Francis.

Grandjean, E., 1988. *Fitting the Task to Man*, 4th ed., London: Taylor & Francis.

Grandjean, E., Jenni, M., and Rhiner, A., 1960. Eine indirekte Methode zur Erfassung des Komfortgefühls beim Sitzen [An indirect method for understanding seating comfort], *Internationale Zeitschrift für Angewandte Physiologie einschliesslich Arbeitsphysiologie*, 18:101–106.

Grandjean, E., Hünting, W., Wotzka, G., and Schärer, R., 1973. An ergonomic investigation of multipurpose chairs, *Human Factors*, 15:247–255.

Grandjean, E., Nishiyama, K., Hünting, W., and Pidermann, M., 1982. A laboratory study on preferred and imposed settings of a VDT workstation, *Behaviour and Information Technology*, 1:289–304.

Grandjean, E., Hünting, W., and Pidermann, M., 1983. VDT workstation preferred design: preferred settings and their effects, *Human Factors*, 25:161–175.

Grandjean, E., Hünting, W., and Nishiyama, K., 1984. Preferred VDT workstation settings, body posture and physical impairments, *Applied Ergonomics*, 15:99–104.

Greenstein, J.S. and Arnaut, L.Y., 1988. Input devices, in Helander, M., Ed., *Handbook of Human–Computer Interaction*, Amsterdam: Elsevier/North-Holland, 495–519.

Grieco, A., 1986. Sitting posture: an old problem and a new one, *Ergonomics*, 29:345–362.

Griffith, R.T., 1949. The Minimotion typewriter keyboard, *Journal of the Franklin Institute*, 248:399–436.

Guilford, J.P., 1954. *Psychometric Methods*, New York: McGraw-Hill.

Hagberg, M., 1982. *Arbetsrelaterade Besvär i Halsrygg och Skuldra [Working Report on Neck, Back and Shoulder Disorders]*, Stockholm: Arbetsmiljöinstitutet.

Haider, M., Kundi, M., and Weißenböck, M., 1980. Worker strain related to VDUs with differently coloured characters, in Grandjean, E. and Vigliani, E., Eds., *Ergonomics Aspects of Visual Display Terminals*, London: Taylor & Francis, 53–64.

Hall, M.A.W., 1972. Back pain and car seat comfort, *Applied Ergonomics*, 15:82–91.

Harbison, S. and Forrester, C., 1995. The ergonomics of notebook computers: problems or just progress, *Journal of Occupational Health and Safety, Australia New Zealand*, 11:481–487.

Hargens, A.R., Romine, J.S., Sipe, J.C., Evans, K.L., Mubarak, S.J., and Akeson, W.H., 1979. Peripheral nerve-conduction block by high compartment pressure, *Journal of Bone and Joint Surgery*, 61A:192–200.

Harkins, W.H., 1965. Switch system for consoles, *Industrial Design*, 12(6):39–43.

Harvey, R. and Peper, E., 1997. Surface electromyography and mouse use position, *Ergonomics*, 40:781–789.

Hedge, A. and Powers, J.R., 1995. Wrist postures while keyboarding: effects of a negative slope keyboard system and full motion forearm supports, *Ergonomics*, 38:508–517.

Hedge, A., Morimoto, S., and McCrobie, D., 1999. Effects of keyboard tray geometry on upper body posture and comfort, *Ergonomics*, 42:1333–1349.

Helander, M.G. and Zhang, L., 1997. Field studies of comfort and discomfort in sitting, *Human Factors*, 40:895–915.

Helander, M.G., Billingsley, P.A., and Schurik, J.M., 1984. An evaluation of human factors research on VDTs in the work-place, *Human Factors Review*, 55–129.

Henning, R.A., Sauter, S.L., Salvendy, G., and Krieg, E.F., 1989. Microbreak length, performance, and stress in a data entry task, *Ergonomics*, 32:855–864.

Henning, R.A., Kissel, G.V., and Maynard, D.C., 1994. Compensatory rest breaks for VDT operators, *International Journal of Industrial Ergonomics*, 14:243–249.

Henning, R.A., Jacques, P., Kissel, G.V., Sullivan, A.B., and Alteras-Webb, S.M., 1997. Frequent short rest breaks from computer work: effects on productivity and well-being at two field sites, *Ergonomics*, 40:78–91.

Hertzberg, H.T.E., 1972. The Human Buttocks in Sitting: Pressures, Patterns, and Palliatives, SAE Technical Paper 720005, Warrendale, PA: Society of Automotive Engineers.

Hertzberg, H., 1973. Engineering anthropometry, in VanCott, H. and Kincaid, R., Eds., Human Engineering Guide to Equipment Design, Washington, D.C.: U.S. Government Printing Office, 467–584.

Heuer, H., Brüwer, M., Römer, T., Kröger, H., and Knapp, H., 1991. Preferred vertical gaze direction and observation distance, *Ergonomics*, 34:379–392.

Hill, S.G. and Kroemer, K.H.E., 1986. Preferred declination of the line of sight, *Human Factors*, 28:127–134.

Hira, D.S., 1980. An ergonomic appraisal of educational desks, *Ergonomics*, 23:213–221.

Hirsch, R.S., 1970. Effects of standard versus alphabetical keyboard formats on typing performance, *Journal of Applied Psychology*, 54:484–490.

Hocking, B., 1987. Epidemiology aspects of repetitious strain injury in Telecom Australia, *Medical Journal of Australia*, 147:218–222.

Hoffman, E.R., Chang, W.Y., and Yim, K.Y., 1997. Computer mouse operation: is the left-handed user disadvantaged? *Applied Ergonomics*, 28:245–248.

Horie, S., Hargens, A., and Rempel, D., 1993. Effect of keyboard wrist rest in preventing carpal tunnel syndrome, in *Proceedings of the APHA Annual Meeting*, Washington, D.C.: American Public Health Association, 319.

Houle, R.J., 1969. Evaluation of seat devices designed to prevent ischemic ulcers in paraplegic patients, *Archives of Physical Medicine and Rehabilitation*, 50:587–594.

Human Factors and Ergonomics Society, 2002. *Human Factors Engineering of Computer Workstations*, BSR/HFS 100, Santa Monica, CA: Human Factors and Ergonomics Society.

Hünting, W., Läubli, T., and Grandjean, E., 1981. Postural and visual loads at VDT workplaces, *Ergonomics*, 24:917–944.

ISO 9241–5, 1998. *Ergonomics Requirements for Office Work with Visual Display Terminals, VDTs. — Part 5: Workstation Layout and Postural Requirements*, Geneva, Switzerland: International Organization for Standardization, available at http://www.iso.ch/iso/en/ISOOnline. frontpage.

Jampel, R.S. and Shi, D.X., 1992. The primary position of the eyes, the resetting saccade, and the transverse visual head plane, *Investigative Ophthalmology and Visual Science*, 33:2501–2510.

Jaschinski, W., Heuer, H., and Kylian, H., 1998. Preferred position of visual displays relative to the eyes: a field study of visual strain and individual differences, *Ergonomics*, 41:1034–1049.

Jensen, C., Borg, V., Finsen, L., Hansen, K., Juul-Kristensen, B., and Christensen, H., 1998. Job demands, muscle activity and musculoskeletal symptoms in relation to work with the computer mouse, *Scandinavian Journal of Work and Environmental Health*, 24:418–424.

JIS Z 8513, 1994. *Ergonomics, Office Work with Visual Display Terminals (VDTs)*, Tokyo, Japan: Japanese Industrial Standards Committee, available at http://www.jisc.org/.

Johnson, P.W., Tal, R., Smutz, W.P., and Rempel, D.M., 1994. Fingertip forces measured during computer mouse operation: a comparison of pointing and dragging, *Proceedings of the 12th Triennial Congress of the International Ergonomics Association*, 2:208–210.

Johnson, P., Rempel, D., and Hagberg, M., 1997. Developing and evaluating force sensing mice for use in epidemiological studies, *Proceedings of the 13th Triennial Congress of the International Ergonomics Association*, 5:47–49.

Jones, J.C., 1969. Methods and results of seating research, *Ergonomics*, 12:171–181.

Jonsson, B., 1988. The static load component in muscle work, *European Journal of Applied Physiology*, 57:305–310.

Jürgens, H.W., 1969. Die Verteilung des Körperdrucks auf Sitzfläche und Rückenlehne als Problem der Industrieanthropologie [Distribution of body weight on the seat pan and seat back as an ergonomics problem], *Ergonomics*, 12:198–205.

Jürgens, H.W., 1980. Body movements of the driver in relation to sitting conditions in the car: a methodological study, in Oborne, D.J. and Lewis, J.A., Eds., *Human Factors in Transport Research*, Vol. 2, London: Academic Press, 249–256.

Kaji, R., 2000. Facts and fancies on writer's cramp, *Muscle Nerve*, 23:1313–1315.

Karlqvist, L., Hagberg, M., and Selin, K., 1994. Variation in upper limb posture and movement during word processing with and without mouse use, *Ergonomics*, 37:1261–1267.

Karlqvist, L.K., Bernmark, E., Ekenvall, L., Hagberg, M., Isaksson, A., and Rostö, T., 1998. Computer mouse position as a determinant of posture, muscular load and perceived exertion, *Scandinavian Journal of Work and Environmental Health*, 24:62–73.

Karrasch, K. and Müller, E.A., 1951. Das Verhalten der Pulsfrequenz in der Erholungsperiode nach körperlicher Arbeit [Heart rate recovery during rest after heavy work], *Arbeitsphysiologie*, 14:369–382.

Karvonen, M.J., Koskela, A., and Noro, L., 1962. Preliminary report on the sitting postures of school children, *Ergonomics*, 5:471–477.

Keegan, J.J., 1953. Alteration of the lumbar curve related to posture and seating, *Journal of Bone and Joint Surgery*, 35A:58603.

Keir, P.J., Bach, J.M., and Rempel, D.M., 1998. Fingertip loading and carpal tunnel pressure: differences between a pinching and a pressing task, *Journal of Orthopaedic Research*, 16:112–115.

Kelaher, D., Nay, T., Lawrence, B., Lamar, S., and Sommerich, C.M., 2001. An investigation of the effects of touchpad location within a notebook computer, *Applied Ergonomics*, 32:101–110.

Kennedy, K.W., 1964. Reach Capability of the USAF Population: Phase I. The Outer Boundaries of Grasping-Reach Envelopes for the Shirt-Sleeved, Seated Operator, TDR 64-59, Dayton, OH: U.S. Air Force Aerospace Medical Research Laboratory.

Kinkead, R.D. and Gonzalez, B.K., 1969. *Human Factors Design Recommendations for Touch Operated Keyboards*, Doc. 12091-FR, Minneapolis, MN: Honeywell.

Klockenberg, E.A., 1926. *Rationalisierung der Schreibmaschine und ihrer Bedienung* [Rationalization of typewriters and their operation], Berlin: Springer-Verlag.

Komoike, Y. and Horiguchi, S., 1971. Fatigue assessment on key punch operators, typists and others, *Ergonomics*, 14:101–109.

Konz, S. and Goel, S.C., 1969. The shape of the normal work area in the horizontal plane, *American Institute of Industrial Engineers*, 1:70–74.

Kosiak, M., 1959. Etiology and pathology of ischemic ulcers, *Archives of Physical Medicine and Rehabilitation*, 40:62–69.

Kosiak, M. Kubicek, W.G., Olsen, M., Danz, J.N., and Kottke, F.J., 1958. Evaluation of pressure as a factor in the production of ischial ulcers, *Archives of Physical Medicine and Rehabilitation*, 39:623–629.

Kotani, K. and Horii, K., 2001. A fundamental study on pointing force applied to the mouse in relation to approaching angles and the index of difficulty, *International Journal of Industrial Ergonomics*, 28:189–195.

Krebs, M., Krouskoup, T.A., and Williams, R., 1984. Pressure and relief characteristics of 2 air-flotation beds, *Archives of Physical Medicine and Rehabilitation*, 65:651–661.

Kroemer, K.H.E., 1964. Über den Einfluss der räumlichen Lage von Tastenfeldern auf die Leistung an Schreibmaschinen [Influence of keyboard spatial positioning on the efficiency of typewriters], *Internationale Zeitschrift für Angewandte Physiologie einschliesslich Arbeitsphysiologie*, 20:240–251.

Kroemer, K.H.E., 1965. Vergleich einer normalen Schreibmaschinen-Tastatur mit einer K-Tastatur [Comparison of a standard typewriter keyboard with a K-keyboard], *Internationale Zeitschrift für Angewandte Physiologie einschliesslich Arbeitsphysiologie*, 20:453–464.

Kroemer, K.H.E., 1972. Human engineering the keyboard, *Human Factors*, 14:51–63.

Kroemer, K.H.E., 1983. *Ergonomics Guides, Ergonomics of VDT Workplaces*, Fairfax, VA: American Industrial Hygiene Association.

Kroemer, K.H.E. and Hill, S.G., 1986. Preferred line of sight angle, *Ergonomics*, 29:1129–1134.

Kroemer, K.H.E. and Kroemer, A.D., 2001. *Office Ergonomics*, London: Taylor & Francis.

Krouskop, T.A., Williams, R., Krebs, M., Herszkowicz, I., and Garber, S., 1985. Effectiveness of mattress overlay in reducing interface pressures during recumbency, *Journal of Rehabilitation Research and Development*, 22:7–10.

Krueger, H., 1980. Ophthalmological aspects of work with display workstations, in Grandjean, E. and Vigliani, E., Eds., *Ergonomics Aspects of Visual Display Terminals*, London: Taylor & Francis, 31–40.

Lander, C., Korbon, G.A., DeGood, D.E., and Rowlingson, J.C., 1987. The Balans chair and its semi-kneeling position: an ergonomic comparison with the conventional sitting position, *Spine*, 12:269–272.

Langolf, G.D., Chaffin, D.B., and Foulke, J.A., 1976. An investigation of Fitts' law using a wide range of movement amplitudes, *Journal of Motor Behavior*, 8:113–128.

Laurig, W., 1969. Der Stehsitz als physiologisch günstige Alternative zum Reine Steharbeitsplatz [Sit-standing as a physiologically favorable alternative for a tidy standing workstation], *Arbeitsmedizin, Sozialmedizin, und Arbeitshygiene*, 4:219.

LeCarpentier, E.F., 1969. Easy chair dimensions for comfort — a subjective approach, *Ergonomics*, 12:328–337.

Lee, K., Swanson, N., Sauter, S., Wickstrom, R., Waikar, A., and Mangums, M., 1992. A review of physical exercises recommended for VDT operators, *Applied Ergonomics*, 23:387–408.

Lehmann, G. and Stier, F., 1961. Mensch und Gerät, in *Handbuch der gesamten Arbeitsmedizin*, Vol. 1, Berlin: Urban und Schwarzenberg, 718–788.

Leibowitz, H.W. and Owens, D.A., 1975. Anomalous myopias and the intermediate dark focus of accommodation, *Science*, 189:646–648.

Less, M. and Eichelberg, W., 1976. Force changes in neck vertebrae and muscles, in Komi, P., Ed., *Biomechanics*, Vol. V-A, Baltimore, MD: University Park Press, 530–536.

Lewis, J.R., Potosnak, K.M., and Magyar, R.L., 1997. Keys and keyboards, in Helander, M., Landauer, T.K., and Prabhu, P., Eds., *Handbook of Human–Computer Interaction*, 2nd ed., North Holland/Elsevier, 1285–1315.

Liao, M.H. and Drury, C.G., 2000. Posture, discomfort and performance in a VDT task, *Ergonomics*, 43:345–359.

Life, M.A. and Pheasant, S.T., 1984. An integrated approach to the study of posture in keyboard operation, *Applied Ergonomics*, 15:83–90.

Lindan, O., Greenway, R.M., and Piazza, J.M., 1965. Pressure distribution on the surface of the human body: I. Evaluation in lying and sitting positions using a bed of springs and nails, *Archives of Physical Medicine*, 46:378–385.

Link, C.S., Nicholson, G.G., Shaddeau, S.A., Birch, R., and Gossman, M.R., 1990. Lumbar curvature in standing and sitting in two types of chairs: relationship of hamstring and hip flexor muscle length, *Physical Therapy*, 70:611–618.

Loricchio, D.F., 1992. A comparison of three pointing devices: mouse, cursor keys, and a key-board integration pushbutton, *Proceedings of the Human Factors Society*, 36:303–305.

Loricchio, D.F. and Lewis, J.R., 1991. User assessment of standard and reduced-size numeric keypads, *Proceedings of the Human Factors Society*, 35:251–252.

Lowe, B.D. and Freivalds, A., 1999. Effect of carpal tunnel syndrome on grip force coordination on hand tools, *Ergonomics*, 42:550–564.

Lueder, R.K., 1983. Seat comfort: a review of the construct in the office environment, *Human Factors*, 25:701–711.

Lundborg, G., Myers, R., and Powell, H., 1983. Nerve compression injury and increased endoneurial fluid pressure: a miniature compartment syndrome, *Journal of Neurology, Neurosurgery, and Psychiatry*, 46:1119–1124.

Lutz, M.C. and Chapanis, A., 1955. Expected locations of digits and letters on ten-button keysets, *Journal of Applied Psychology*, 39:314–317.

MacKenzie, I.S., Sellen, A., and Buxton, W., 1991. A comparison of input devices in elemental pointing and dragging tasks, *Proceedings of the CHI 91 Conference on Human Factors in Computing Systems*, New York: ACM, 161–166.

Maeda, K., 1977. Occupational cervicobrachial disorder and its causative factors, *Journal of Human Ergology*, 6:193–202.

Maeda, K., Horiguchi, S., and Hosokawa, M., 1982. History of the studies on occupational cervicobrachial disorder in Japan and remaining problems, *Journal of Human Ergology*, 11:17–29.

Magora, A., 1972. Investigation of the relation between low back pain and occupation, 3. Physical requirements: sitting standing and weight lifting, *Industrial Medicine and Surgery*, 41:5–9.

Magyar, R.L., 1985. *Effects of Curved, Flat, and Stepped Keybutton Configurations of Keyboard Preference and Throughput Performance*, Boca Raton, FL: International Business Machine Corp.

Mandal, Å.C., 1976. Work-chair with tilting seat, *Ergonomics*, 19:157–164.

Mandal, Å.C., 1981. The seated man, *Homo sedens*, *Applied Ergonomics*, 12:19–26.

Mandal, Å.C., 1982. The correct height of school furniture, *Human Factors*, 24:257–269.

Marklin, R.W., Simoneau, G.G., and Monroe, J.F., 1999. Wrist and forearm posture from typing of split and vertically inclined computer keyboards, *Human Factors,* 41:559–569.

Marschall, M., Harrington, A.C., and Steele, J.R., 1995. Effect of work station design on sitting posture in young children, *Ergonomics,* 38:1932–1940.

Marteniuk, R.G., Ivens, C.J., and Brown, B.E., 1997. Are there task specific performance effects for differently configured numeric keypads? *Applied Ergonomics,* 27:321–325.

Martin, B.J., Armstrong, T.J., Foulke, J.A., Natarajan, S., Klinenberg, E., Serina, E., and Rempel, D., 1996. Keyboard reaction force and finger flexor electromyograms during computer keyboard work, *Human Factors,* 38:654–664.

Mauer, U.M., Lotspeich, E., Klein, H.J., and Rath, S.A., 1991. Body building effect on neural conduction velocity of the median nerve in the carpal tunnel [in German], *Zeitschrift für Orthopaedie und ihre Grenzgebiete,* 129:319–321.

Maxwell, W.C., 1953. The rhythmic keyboard, *Journal of Business Education,* 27:327–330.

Maynard, H.B., 1934. Workplace layouts that save, time effort, and money, *Iron Age,* 134(Dec. 6):28–30, 92.

McCormick, E.J., 1970. *Human Factors Engineering,* 3rd ed., New York: McGraw-Hill, 427.

McLean, L., Tingley, M., Scott, R.N., and Rickards, J., 2001. Computer terminal work and the benefit of microbreaks, *Applied Ergonomics,* 32:225–237.

Menozzi, M., von Buol, A., Krueger, H., and Miège, Ch., 1994. Direction of gaze and comfort: discovering the relation for the ergonomic optimization of visual tasks, *Ophthalmology and Physiological Optics,* 14:393–399.

Michaels, S.E., 1971. QWERTY versus alphabetic keyboards as a function of typing skill, *Human Factors,* 13:419–426.

Michel, D.P. and Helander, M.G., 1994. Effects of two types of chairs on stature change and comfort for individuals with healthy and herniated discs, *Ergonomics,* 37:1231–1244.

Miller, I. and Suther, T.W., 1983. Display station anthropometrics: preferred height and angle settings of CRT and keyboard, *Human Factors,* 25:401–408.

Mon-Williams, M., Burgess-Limerick, R., Plooy, A., and Wann, J., 1999. Vertical gaze direction and postural adjustment: an extension of the Heuer model, *Journal of Experimental Psychology, Applied,* 5:35–53.

Moneta, K.B., 1960. Optimum physical design of an alphabetical keyboard, Post Office Research Report 20412.

Monty, R.W. and Snyder, H.L., 1983. Keyboard design: an investigation of user preference and performance, *Proceedings of the Human Factors Society,* 27:201–105.

Mooney, V., Einbund, M.J., Rogers, J.E., and Stauffer, E.S., 1971. Comparison of pressure distribution qualities in seat cushions, *Bulletin of Prosthetic Research,* 10–15:129–143.

Nachemson, A. and Morris, J.M., 1964. *In vivo* measurements of intradiscal pressure, *Journal of Bone and Joint Surgery,* 46A:1077–1092.

Najjar, L.J., Stanton, B.C., and Bowen, C.D., 1988. Keyboard heights and slopes for standing typists, Technical Report 85-0081, Rockville, MD: International Business Machine Corp.

Nakaseko, M., Grandjean, E., Hünting, W., and Gierer, R., 1985. Studies on ergonomically designed alphanumeric keyboards, *Human Factors,* 27:175–187.

Nathan, P.A., Wilcox, A., Emerick, P.S., Meadows, K.D., and McCormack, A.L., 2001. Effects of an aerobic exercise program on median nerve conduction and symptoms associated with carpal tunnel syndrome, *Journal of Occupational and Environmental Medicine*, 43:840–843.

National Research Council, 1984. Video Displays, Work and Vision, Washington, D.C.: National Academy of Press.

National Research Council, 2001. Musculoskeletal Disorders and the Workplace, Washington, D.C.: National Academy of Press.

Ng, D., Cassar, T., and Gross, C.M., 1995. Evaluation of an intelligent seat system, *Applied Ergonomics*, 26:109–116.

Niebel, B. and Freivalds, A., 2003. *Methods, Standards & Work Design*, 11th ed., New York: McGraw-Hill, 189.

NIOSH, 1981. Potential Health Hazards of Video Display Terminals. Report 81-129, Cincinnati, OH: National Institute for Occupational Safety and Health.

NIOSH, 1989. Carpal Tunnel Syndrome: Selected References, Cincinnati, OH: National Institute for Occupational Safety and Health.

NIOSH, 1995. Cumulative Trauma Disorders in the Workplace: Bibliography. Report 95-119, Cincinnati, OH: National Institute for Occupational Safety and Health.

NIOSH, 1997. Musculoskeletal Disorders and Workplace Factors. Report 97-141, Cincinnati, OH: National Institute for Occupational Safety and Health.

Norman, D. and Fisher, D., 1982. Why alphabetic keyboards are not easy to use: keyboard layout doesn't much matter, *Human Factors*, 24:509–519.

Noyes, J., 1983a. The QWERTY keyboard: a review, *International Journal of Man–Machine Studies*, 18:265–281.

Noyes, J., 1983b. Chord keyboards, *Applied Ergonomics*, 14:55–59.

Noyes, J., 1998. QWERTY — the immortal keyboard, *Control & Computing Engineering Journal*, 9(3):117–122.

Ong, C.N., 1984. VDT work place design and physical fatigue: a case study in Singapore, in Grandjean, E., Ed., *Ergonomics and Health in Modern Offices*, London: Taylor & Francis, 484–494.

OSHA, 1991. Working Safely with Video Display Terminals, Washington, D.C.: U.S. Department of Labor, Occupational Safety and Health Administration.

Paci, A.M. and Gabbrielli, L., 1984. Some experiences in the field of design of VDU work stations, in Grandjean, E., Ed., *Ergonomics and Health in Modern Offices*, London: Taylor & Francis, 391–399.

Park, S.K., 1999. The Development of an Exposure Measurement System for Assessing Risk of Work-Related Musculoskeletal Disorders, (WMSDs), Ph.D. thesis, University Park, PA: Pennsylvania State University.

Parsons, C.A., 1991. Use of wrist rest by data input VDU operators, in Lovesey, E.J., Ed., *Contemporary Ergonomics 1991: Proceedings of the Ergonomics Society's Annual Conference*, London: Taylor & Francis, 319–321.

Paul, L.E., Sarlanis, K., and Buckley, E.P., 1965. A human factors comparison of two data entry keyboards, presented at the Sixth Annual Symposium of the Professional Group on Human Factors in Electronics, IEEE.

Pheasant, S., 1991. *Ergonomics, Work and Health*, London: Macmillan.

Pollock, W.T. and Gildner, G.G., 1963. Study of Computer Manual Input Devices, ESD-TDR-63-545, Bedford, MA: U.S. Air Force, Hanscom Field.

Pooni, J.S., Hukins, D.W.L., Harris, P.F., Hilton, R.C., and Davies, K.E., 1986. Comparison of the structure of human intervertebral discs in the cervical, thoracic, and lumbar regions of the spine, *Surgical and Radiologic Anatomy*, 8:175–182.

Poulton, E.C., 1974. *Tracking Skill and Manual Control*, New York: Academic Press.

Powell, H.C. and Myers, R.R., 1986. Pathology of experimental nerve compression, *Laboratory Investigation*, 55:91–100.

Price, J.M. and Dowell, W.R., 1997. A field evaluation of two split keyboards, *Proceedings of the Human Factors and Ergonomics Society*, 41:410–414.

Psihogios, J.P., Sommerich, C.M., Mirka, G.A., and Moon, S.D., 2001. A field evaluation of monitor placement effects in VDT users, *Applied Ergonomics*, 32:313–325.

Radwin, R.G. and Jeng, O.J., 1997. Activation force and travel effects on overexertion in repetitive key tapping, *Human Factors*, 39:130–140.

Rebiffé, R., 1969. Le siège to conducteur: son adaptation aux exigences fonctionelles et anthropometriques [Driver seating: derived from functional and anthropometric requirements], *Ergonomics*, 12:246–261.

Rempel, D., Dennerlein, J., Mote, C.D., and Armstrong, T., 1994. A method of measuring fingertip loading during keyboard use, *Journal of Biomechanics*, 27:1101–1104.

Rempel, D., Keir, P.J., Smutz, W.P., and Hargens, A., 1997. Effects of static fingertip loading on carpal tunnel pressure, *Journal of Orthopaedic Research*, 15:422–426.

Rempel, D., Bach, J.M., Gordon, L., and Tal, R., 1998. Effects of forearm pronation/supination and metacarpophalangeal flexion on carpal tunnel pressure, *Journal of Hand Surgery*, 23A:38–42.

Rempel, D., Tittiranonda, P., Burastero, S., Hudes, M., and So, Y., 1999. Effect of keyboard keyswitch design on hand pain, *Journal of Occupational and Environmental Medicine*, 41:111–119.

Rose, M.J., 1991. Keyboard operating posture and actuation force: implications for muscle over-use, *Applied Ergonomics*, 22:198–203.

Rozmanryn, L.M., Dovelle, S., Rothman, E.R., Gorman, K., Olvey, K.M., and Bartko, J.J., 1998. Nerve and tendon gliding exercises and the conservative management of carpal tunnel syndrome, *Journal of Hand Therapy*, 11:171–179.

Rubin, T. and Marshall, C.J., 1982. Adjustable VDT workstations: can naive users achieve a human factors solution? *International Conference on Man–Machine Systems*, Conference Publication 121, Manchester, U.K.: Institution of Electrical Engineers.

Sanders, M.S. and McCormick, E.J., 1993. *Human Factors in Engineering and Design*, 7th ed., New York: McGraw-Hill, 361.

Sauter, S.L., Schleifer, L.M., and Knutson, S.J., 1991. Work posture, workstation design, and musculoskeletal discomfort in a VDT data entry task, *Human Factors*, 33:151–167.

Scales, E.M. and Chapanis, A., 1954. The effect of performance of tilting the toll-operators keyset, *Journal of Applied Psychology*, 38:452–456.

Schoberth, H., 1962. *Sitzhalten, Sitzschaden, Sitzmöbel* [Sitting Postures, Sitting Disorders, Chairs], Berlin: Springer-Verlag.

Seibel, R., 1964. Data entry through chord, parallel entry devices, *Human Factors*, 6:189–192.

Seibel, R., 1972. Data entry devices and procedures, in H.P. VanCott and R.G. Kinkade, Eds., *Human Engineering Guide to Equipment Design*, Washington, D.C.: American Institutes for Research, 311–344.

Seradge, H., Bear, C., and Bithell, D., 2000. Preventing carpal tunnel syndrome and cumulative trauma disorder: effect of carpal tunnel decompression exercises: an Oklahoma experience, *Journal of the Oklahoma State Medical Association*, 93:150–153.

Seradge, H., Parker, W., Baer, C., Mayfield, K., and Schall, L., 2002. Conservative treatment of carpal tunnel syndrome: an outcome study of adjunct exercises, *Journal of the Oklahoma State Medical Association*, 95:7–14.

Serina, E.R., Tal, R., and Rempel, D., 1999. Wrist and forearm postures and motions during typing, *Ergonomics*, 42:938–951.

Shackel, B., Chidsey, K.D., and Shipley, P., 1969. The assessment of chair comfort, *Ergonomics*, 12:269–306.

Sheehy, M.P. and Marsden, C.D., 1982. Writer's cramp — a focal dystonia, *Brain*, 105:461–480.

Shen, W. and Parsons, K.C., 1997. Validity and reliability of rating scales for seated pressure discomfort, *International Journal of Industrial Ergonomics*, 20:441–461.

Shields, R.K. and Cook, T.M., 1988. Effect of seat angle and lumbar support on seat buttock pressure, *Physical Therapy*, 68:1682–1686.

Shvartz, E., Guame, J.G., White, R.T., Riebold, R.C., and Glassford, E.J., 1980. Effect of the circutone seat on hemodynamic, subjective and thermal responses during prolonged sitting, *Proceedings of the Human Factors Society*, 24:639–642.

Silverstein, B.A., Fine, L.J., and Armstrong, T.J., 1986. Hand wrist cumulative trauma disorders in industry, *British Journal of Industrial Medicine*, 43:779–784.

Slechta, R.F., Forrest, J., Carter, W.K., and Forrest, J., 1959. *Comfort Evaluation of the C-124 Crew Seat (Weber)*, WADC Technical Report 58-136, Dayton, OH: Wright Air Development Center, Wright-Patterson Air Force Base.

Smith, M.J., Cohen, B.G.F., and Stammerjohn, L.W., 1981. An investigation of health complaints and job stress in video display operations, *Human Factors*, 23:387–400.

Smith, M.J., Karsh, B.T., Conway, F.T., Cohen, W.J., James, C.A., Morgan, J.J., Sanders, K., and Zehel, D.J., 1998. Effects of a split keyboard design and wrist rest on performance, posture, and comfort, *Human Factors*, 40:324–336.

Smutz, P., Serina, E., and Rempel, D., 1994. A system for evaluating the effect of keyboard design on force, posture, comfort, and productivity, *Ergonomics*, 37:1649–1660.

Sommerich, C.M., 2000. Inputting to a notebook computer, *Proceedings of the IEA/HFES 2000 Congress*, 671–674.

Sommerich, C.M., Marras, W.S., and Parnianpour, M., 1996. Observations on the relationship between key strike force and typing speed, *American Industrial Hygiene Association Journal*, 57:1109–1114.

Sommerich, C.M., Joines, S.M.B., and Psihogios, J.P., 2001. Effects of computer monitor viewing angle and related factors on strain, performance, and preference outcomes, *Human Factors*, 43:39–55.

Song, T.K., Shepard, R.J., and Cox, M.H., 1982. Absenteeism, employee turnover, and sustained exercise participation, *Journal of Sports Medicine and Physical Fitness*, 22:392–399.

Sotoyama, M., Jonai, H., Saito, S., and Villanueva, M.B.G., 1996. Analysis of ocular surface area for comfortable VDT workstation layout, *Ergonomics*, 39:877–884.

Sprigle, S., Chung, K.C., and Brubacker, C.E., 1990. Reduction of sitting pressures with custom contoured cushions, *Journal of Rehabilitation Research and Development*, 27:135–140.

Springer, T.J., 1982. VDT workstations: a comparative evaluation of alternatives, *Applied Ergonomics*, 13:211–212.

Squires, P.C., 1956. The Shape of the Normal Working Area, Report 275, New London, CT: U.S. Navy Department, Bureau of Medicine and Surgery.

Staffel, F., 1884. Zur Hygiene des Sitzens [Seating health], *Zentralblatt für allgemeine Gesundheitspflege*, 3:404–421.

Straker, L., Jones, K.J., and Miller, J., 1997. A comparison of the postures assumed when using laptop computers and desktop computers, *Applied Ergonomics*, 28:263–268.

Straub, H.R. and Granaas, M.M., 1993. Task-specific preference for numeric keypads, *Applied Ergonomics*, 24:289–290.

Strong, E.P., 1956. A Comparative Experiment in Simplified Keyboard Re–training and Standard Keyboard Supplementary Training, Washington, D.C.: General Services Administration.

Sucher, B.M., 1994. Palpatory diagnosis and manipulative management of carpal tunnel syndrome, *Journal of the American Osteopathic Association*, 94:647–663.

Sundelin, G. and Hagberg, M., 1989. The effects of different pause types on neck and shoulder EMG activity during VDU work, *Ergonomics*, 32:527–537.

Suther, T.W. and McTyre, J.H., 1982. Effect on operator performance at thin profile keyboard slopes of 5°, 10°, 15°, and 25°, *Proceedings of the Human Factors Society*, 26:430–434.

Svensson, H.O. and Andersson, G.B.J., 1983. Low back pain in 40–47 year old men: work history and work environment factors, *Spine*, 8:272–276.

Swanson, N.G., Galinsky, T.L., Cole, L.L., Pan, C.S., and Sauter, S.L., 1997. The impact of keyboard design on comfort and productivity in a text-entry task, *Applied Ergonomics*, 28:9–16.

Swarts, A.E., Krouskop, T.A., and Smith, D.R., 1988. Tissue pressure management in the vocational setting, *Archives of Physical Medicine and Rehabilitation*, 69:97–100.

Swearingen, J.J., Wheelwright, C.D., and Garner, J.D., 1962. An Analysis of Sitting Areas and Pressures of Man, Report 62-1, Oklahoma City, OK: U.S. Civil Aero-Medical Research Institute.

Thornton, W., 1978. Anthropometric changes in weightlessness, in Webb Associates, Eds., Anthropometric Source Book, Vol. 1, NASA RP1024, Houston: National Aeronautics and Space Administration.

Tittiranonda, P., Rempel, D., Armstrong, T., and Burastero, S., 1999. Effect of four computer keyboards in computer users with upper extremity musculoskeletal disorders, *American Journal of Industrial Medicine*, 35:647–661.

Turville, K.L., Psihogios, J.P., Ulmer, T.R., and Mirka, G.A., 1998. The effects of video display terminal height on the operator: a comparison of the 15° and 40° recommendations, *Applied Ergonomics*, 29:239–246.

Udo, H., Otani, T., Udo, A., and Yoshinaga, F., 2000. An electromyographic study of two different types of ball point pens, *Industrial Health*, 38:47–50.

VanCott, H.P. and Kinkade, R.G., 1972. Human Engineering Guide to Equipment Design, Washington, D.C.: U.S. Government Printing Office, 400.

Vandraas, K., 1981. Necessary for some, unusable for others, an alternative for many, *Fysioterapueuten*, 48:546–550 [in Norwegian].

Villanueva, M.B.G., Sotoyama, M., Jonai, H., Takeuchi, Y., and Saito, S., 1996. Adjustments of posture and viewing parameters of the eye to changes in the screen height of the visual display terminal, *Ergonomics*, 39:933–945.

Villanueva, M.B.G., Jonai, H., and Saito, S., 1998. Ergonomics aspects of portable personal computers with flat panel displays: evaluation of posture, muscle activities, discomfort and performance, *Industrial Health*, 36:282–289.

Wachsler, R.A. and Lerner, D.B., 1960. An analysis of some factors influencing seat comfort, *Ergonomics*, 3:315–320.

Waters, T.R., Putz-Anderson, V., Garg, A., and Fine, L.J., 1993. Revised NIOSH equation for the design an evaluation of manual lifting tasks, *Ergonomics*, 36:749–776.

Webb Associates, 1978. Anthropometric Source Book, Vol. I. Anthropometry for Designers, NASA Ref. Pub. 1024, Washington, D.C.: National Aeronautics and Space Administration.

Weber, A., Sancin, E., and Grandjean, E., 1984. The effects of various keyboard heights on EMG and physical discomfort, in Grandjean, E., Ed., *Ergonomics and Health in Modern Offices*, London: Taylor & Francis, 477–483.

Werner, R., Armstrong, T.J., Bir, C., and Aylard, M.K., 1997. Intracarpal canal pressures: the role of the finger, hand wrist and forearm position, *Clinical Biomechanics*, 12:44–51.

Wilks, S., 1878. *Lectures on Diseases of the Nervous System*, London: Churchill, 452–460.

Winkel, J., 1981. Swelling of lower leg in sedentary work — a pilot study, *Journal of Human Ergology*, 10:139–149.

Winkel, J., 1987. On the significance of physical activity in sedentary work, in Knave, G. and Wideback, P.G., Eds., *Work with Display Units 86*, Amsterdam: Elsevier Science, 229–236.

Winkel, J. and Jørgensen, K., 1986. Evaluation of foot swelling and lower-limb temperatures in relation to leg activity during long-term seated office work, *Ergonomics*, 29:313–328.

Wotzka, G., Grandjean, E., Burandt, U., Kretzschmar, H., and Leonhard, T., 1969. Investigation for the development of an auditorium seat, *Ergonomics*, 12:182–197.

Wright, P., Bartram, C., Rogers, N., Emslie, H., Evans, J., Wilson, B., and Belt, S., 2000. Text entry on handheld computers by older users, *Ergonomics*, 43:703–716.

Wu, C.S., Miyamoto, H., and Noro, H., 1998. Research on pelvic angle variation when using a pelvic support, *Ergonomics*, 41:317–327.

Yaginuma, Y., Yamada, H., and Nagai, H., 1990. Study of the relationship between lacrimation and blink in VDT work, *Ergonomics*, 33:799–809.

Yoshitake, R., 1995. Relationship between key space and user performance on reduced keyboards, *Journal of Physiological Anthropology and Applied Human Science*, 14:287–292.

Zacharkow, D., 1988. *Posture: Sitting, Standing, Chair Design and Exercise*, Springfield, IL: Charles C Thomas.

Zecevic, A., Miller, D.I., and Harburn, K., 2000. An evaluation of the ergonomics of three computer keyboards, *Ergonomics*, 43:55–72.

Zhang, L., Helander, M.G., and Drury, C.G., 1996. Identifying factors of comfort and discomfort in sitting, *Human Factors*, 38:377–389.

Zipp, P., Haider, E., Halpern, N., Mainzer, J., and Rohmert, W., 1981. Untersuchung zur ergonomischen Gestaltung von Tastaturen [Research on the ergonomic shape of keyboards], *Zentralblatt für Arbeitsmedizin*, 31:326–330.

Zipp, P., Haider, E., Halpern, N., and Rohmert, W., 1983. Keyboard design through physiological strain measurements, *Applied Ergonomics*, 14:117–122.

Glossary

A

abduction: Raising the arm or thigh away from the body, in the coronal plane; *opp.* adduction.

abscissa: The vertical axis of a coordinate system, also termed the *y*-axis.

accommodation: Adjustment in sensory threshold to a constant-level stimuli, resulting in a decreased rate of firing in the accompanying neuron.

accuracy: The extent to which a measurement is close to the "true value" or has small deviations from the value being assessed.

actin: The globular proteins comprising thin filaments within muscle.

action potential: The active disturbance of nerve and muscle membrane potentials, which creates the means for transmission of information.

activation heat: Heat in muscle tissue coinciding with the active state.

active state: Condition in which there are still some calcium ions left in the myofibrils after a previous muscle contraction, causing a potentiating effect for the following contraction.

adduction: Lowering the arm or bringing the thigh closer to the midline of the body, in the coronal plane; *opp.* abduction.

adenosine triphosphate: The most basic energy molecule in the body, with energy being stored and released with the forming and breaking of its phosphate bonds.

Adson's test: Test for thoracic outlet syndrome in which the patient is seated with the head extended and turned to the affected side; a positive sign is the weakening of the pulse at the wrist while raising the affected arm and taking a deep breath.

aerobic: Requiring oxygen, typically referring to metabolism; *opp.* anaerobic.

afferent: Direction of information flow, typically sensory, from the periphery to the central nervous system; *opp.* efferent.

agonists: Muscles that act as the prime activators of motion; *opp.* antagonists.

algebraic approach: Method for finding the inverse Laplace transform by algebraically manipulating the fractional form of a transfer function.

all-or-nothing response: Once an initial depolarization reaches the threshold level, the production of an action potential cannot be stopped. Also, refers to the fact that once a motor neuron is stimulated all its collaterals will transmit the same action potential to the associated muscle fibers.

anaerobic: Not needing oxygen, typically referring to metabolism; *opp.* aerobic.

anisotropic: Material whose properties vary depending on the direction of applied forces; *opp.* isotropic.

annulospiral: Type of receptor found in the equatorial region of the muscle, sensitive both to changes in length and velocity; also termed primary ending.

annulus fibrosus: The outer onion-like fiber casings of an intervertebral disc.

anode: The positive pole or terminal to which electrons are attracted or current flows.

antagonists: Muscles that counteract the agonists and oppose the original motion.

antenna effect: Tendency for long leads to pick up stray electromagnetic radiation and create noise on top of the desired signal.

anterior interosseous syndrome: Compression of the anterior interosseous branch of the median nerve by the deep anterior forearm muscles, resulting in motor difficulties producing a thumb-index fingertip pinch.

anthropometers: Specialized calipers for measuring body dimensions.

arthritis: Inflammation or degeneration of joint structures; in the form of *rheumatoid arthritis* or *osteoarthritis*.

antidromic: Nerve conduction along an axon in the direction reverse of normal; *opp.* orthodromic.

Atari thumb: *See* de Quervain's disease.

attributable risk: Estimate of the proportion by which the rate of the disease status among exposed individuals would be reduced if the exposure were eliminated.

axial bones: Bones found in the skull, vertebrae, pelvis, etc.

axial rotation: Rotation of a limb or the trunk along the long axis.

axon: The long part of the neuron, which carries the action potential.

B

bandwidth: The amount of information that can be transferred over a channel, defined by the inverse of the Fitts' law slope; also the range of continuous frequencies that can be processed by a system.

basal ganglia: Part of the brain above the brain stem associated with motor processing.

bicipital tendinitis: Inflammation of the long head of the biceps tendon as it passes over the head of the humerus through the bicipital groove caused by hyperabducting the elbow or forceful contractions of the biceps.

biomechanics: The science that deals with forces and their effects, applied to biological systems.

bipennate muscles: Muscles whose fibers are arranged obliquely on both sides of the long axis, as in a complete bird feather.

bipolar: Type of electromyographical recording in which two active electrodes are placed over different areas of the muscle to obtain a differential reading.

bit: Acronym for binary digit, the amount of information obtained from two equally likely alternatives.

block diagram: System representation using block elements.

blocks: Cycling patterns in mental arousal.

Bode plot: Linearized frequency analysis plots on a log-log scale.

body discomfort map: A type of symptom survey in which the worker marks each body part where pain or discomfort is experienced and then rates the level of pain.

bottom point: Point on keystroke travel at which the key mechanically bottoms out.

bowler's thumb: *See* digital neuritis.

brain stem: Part of brain connecting with the spinal cord, associated with a variety of motor and sensory processing.

break force: The minimum force needed to break the circuit and deactivate a key switch; it also signals the user that the keystroke has been completed.

break frequency: A critical value of frequency at which point the plotted values change suddenly.

break point: Point on keystroke travel at which the circuit is broken and the key switch is deactivated; it also signals the user that the keystroke has been completed.

bursae: Closed sacs filled with synovial fluid to reduce friction and facilitate the motion of tendons and muscles over bony protuberances around joints.

bursitis: Inflammation of bursae.

C

cancellous bone: Spongy and less dense bone material found in the center of bone; also termed spongy bone.

capitate: The central wrist bone in the distal row.

carbohydrate loading: Eating increased amounts of carbohydrates two or three days prior to an intense physical activity.

carpal: Refers to the wrist area, typically the eight carpal bones of the wrist.

carpal tunnel: Area of the wrist formed by the eight carpal bones on the dorsal side and the flexor retinaculum on the palmar side of the wrist.

carpal tunnel syndrome: Entrapment of the median nerve in the carpal tunnel, leading to sensory and motor impairment of the middle three fingers.

carpometacarpal joint: The wrist joint.

Cartesian coordinate system: A two- or three-dimensional coordinate system with perpendicular axes, same as the rectangular coordinate system.

cartilage: Connective tissue covering articular bony surfaces or found in the ear and nose.

case-control study: Type of epidemiological study in which individuals are selected based on the presence (cases) or absence (controls) of a disease; then information is collected about earlier exposure to a risk factor of interest.

cases: Individuals having the disease or disorder of interest.

category ratio scale: A scale with verbal anchors for rating muscular exertion, pain, or discomfort.

cathode: The negative pole or terminal from which electrons or current flows.

causality: The extent to which the occurrence of risk factors is responsible for the subsequent occurrence of the disease.

cell membrane: The outer edge of a cell that acts as a selective barrier for the passage of nutrients, wastes, and hormones.

center of gravity: The exact center of an object's mass or equilibrium point of that object, also termed center of mass.

center of mass: *See* center of gravity.

central nervous system: The portion of the nervous system that includes the brain and the spinal cord; *opp.* peripheral nervous system.

centrifugal force: Force acting on the body acting along the radius of the rotation.

cerebellum: Posterior part of the brain that processes feedback control for muscles.

cerebral cortex: Part of the brain that receives sensory information from the neuromusculature and that controls muscle action; also termed sensorimotor cortex.

cervical radiculopathy: Compression of the spinal nerve roots that form the brachial plexus (C5, C6, C7, C8) between the intervertebral openings.

cervical spine: The portion of the spinal column consisting of the seven vertebrae in the neck.

characteristic function: The denominator of a transfer function, the roots of which characterize the system response.

cherry pitter's thumb: *See* digital neuritis.

choice-reaction time: Average time interval for an operator to respond to one or more stimuli with one or more appropriate responses.

chondrocytes: Cartilage cells arranged in a layered zone.

chord: Type of keyboard in which entering one character requires the simultaneous activation of two or more keys.

clasp knife reflex: A reflex involving Golgi tendon organs, in which the limbs collapse due to an overload of force.

clinical trials: Formal intervention study in which individuals are randomly assigned to one of two study groups, an intervention group and a control group, typically to study the effectiveness of a new drug or treatment.

closed-loop system: Type of system in which there is some form of comparison between the system output and the command input, also feedback system; *opp.* open-loop system.

closed-loop transfer function: Complete transfer function representation of a system.

coefficient of friction: A characteristic of the interaction of the material properties of two surfaces, such as the roughness for a grip, the ratio of peak shear force as a function of the normal (perpendicular to shear) gripping force.

coefficient of variability: Simple measure of reliability expressed as the standard deviation of a series of repeat measurements divided by the mean.

cohort study: A type of epidemiological study in which subjects are selected based on the presence or absence of a risk factor; they are then followed over time for the development of the disease of interest.

collagen: Type of fiber providing strength and stiffness to soft connective tissue.

common-mode signal-to-noise rejection ratio: The ability of a device to reject a signal that is common to or applied to both input terminals (typically undesired noise), expressed as the ratio of the differential signal gain to the common-mode signal gain.

compact bone: Denser bone material with higher mineral content, found in the outer edge of the diaphysis; also known as cortical bone.

compression: Loading mode in which the load is applied axially toward the surface, compressing the material.

concentric: A dynamic muscle contraction in which the muscle is shortening; *opp.* eccentric.

congruity: The state of agreement between exposure and disease status.

construct validity: Type of validity that refers to the physiological or psychological construct or characteristic being measured by the test.

content validity: *See* face validity.

contralateral: *See* crossed.

control: Individual without the disease or disorder of interest.

correlation coefficient: A formal calculation of the agreement between two or more sets of measurements; typically the Pearson product moment correlation coefficient.

cortical bone: Denser bone material with higher mineral content, found in the outer edge of the diaphysis; also known as compact bone.

creep: *See* strain retardation.

criterion validity: Type of validity that refers to the relationship of scores obtained using the test and the actual cases incurred.

critically damped: System response for a damping ratio of one.

Cronbach's alpha: An estimate of a test's reliability based on a ratio of the variance of item scores and the variance of test scores.

cross product: Manipulation of vectors using the right-hand rule to calculate the moment of the force, resulting in a vector.

cross-sectional study: Type of epidemiological study in which individuals are sampled at a point in time and then subdivided into distributions of exposures and disease status; *syn.* prevalence study.

crossed: Pertaining to the other side of the body.

crosstalk: A measurement problem in which a signal is communicated from one channel to another channel, where it is not desired.

cubital tunnel syndrome: Entrapment of the ulnar nerve at the ulnar groove or cubital tunnel formed by the two heads of the flexor carpi ulnaris near the elbow, often from direct pressure on that area.

cytoplasm: Cell material other than the nucleus, roughly 80% water.

D

damping element: A dashpot-like element in Hill's muscle model representing the viscous nature of the internal water.

damping ratio: A factor defining the reduction of oscillations in a dynamic system.

delta function: *See* unit impulse.

dendrites: The long branches off the cell body that serve to collect nerve impulses from other neurons.

depolarization: A positive change in the membrane potential.

de Quervain's disease: Tendinitis of the abductor pollicis longus and extensor pollicis brevis of the thumb; sometimes termed Atari thumb or Nintendo thumb due to chronic overuse of the thumb with video games.

diaphysis: The tubular shaft of a long bone.

digital neuritis: Numbness due to direct pressure on the digital nerves while grasping tools or other items with sharp edges; depending on the aggravating task, may be termed also as bowler's thumb or cherry pitter's thumb.

digitizing tablet: A flat pad with a stylus, connected to a computer, the movement of which is sensed at the appropriate position on the tablet and produces input to the computer.

digram: Two-letter keying sequence.

direction: The line of action of a force.

disc compression forces: Compressive forces found in the lumbar discs due to external loads.

disc herniation: The bulging of the intervertebral discs or the even more catastrophic extrusion of the nucleus pulposus gel material.

distal: Referring to the portion of the body that is farthest from the central longitudinal axis of the trunk.

distributed model: Type of modeling approach in which all elements are modeled individually; *opp.* lumped model.

dorsiflexion: Movement of the foot or toes upward; *opp.* plantar flexion.

dose–response relationship: The direct association between the intensity and duration of exposure and the risk or degree of disease status.

dot product: Manipulation of vectors in the same direction resulting in a purely scalar value.

double-crush syndrome: Multiple nerve entrapment, which may lead to multiple and/or conflicting symptoms.

drag and drop: A mouse operation in which an icon the screen is moved and positioned in a new location.

Dupuytren's contracture: Formation of nodules in the palmar fascia, an extension of the tendon of the palmaris longus muscle, leading to permanent contracture of the ring and little fingers.

Dvorak: Type of keyboard layout in which the most commonly used keys are assigned to the strongest (middle) fingers; the home row has the sequence AOEIUDHTNS.

dynamics: Biomechanical principles applied to a system of bodies in motion.

E

eccentric: A dynamic muscle contraction in which the muscle is lengthening; *opp.* concentric.

efferent: Direction of information flow, typically motor control, from the central nervous system to the periphery; *opp.* afferent.

efficiency of electrical activity: A type of analysis for the slope of the EMG amplitude–force curve.

elastic cartilage: Type of cartilage found in the ear and epiglottis of the throat.

elastic region: Initial region of a stress–strain curve that is linear and repeatable.

elasticity: A spring-like property of a material, which enables it to recover from a deformation produced by an external force.

elastin: Type of fiber providing elasticity to soft connective tissue.

electrical impedance: Total resistance to electric current flow.

electromyography: The recording and analysis of the electrical activity of muscles.

endomysium: The inner layer of fascia that covers individual muscle fibers.

energy: The capacity of a system to do work.

enthesopathy: Specific form of tendinitis occurring at the tendon–bone interface.

epidemiology: Branch of medicine that studies the distribution and control of epidemic diseases.

epimysium: The outer layer of fascia covering muscle.

epiphysis: The two enlarged rounded ends of a long bone.

etiologic fraction: *See* attributable risk.

etiology: The study of the cause or development of a disease.

eversion: Moving the sole of the foot outwards; *opp.* inversion.

excitatory postsynaptic potentials: Excitatory inputs that depolarize a section of a motoneuron cell body making it easier to create an action potential.

extension: Joint movement such that the included angle between the two limbs increases, for trunk or neck, bending backward; *opp.* flexion.

external force: Forces acting outside the body, e.g., weight held in hand.

exteroreceptors: Receptors on the body surface that respond to an external sensation.

extrafusal: With reference to the outside of the muscle spindle, typically regular muscle fibers; *opp.* intrafusal.

extrapyramidal tract: Indirect motor control pathway from the sensory cortex, passing through the basal ganglia, cerebellum, and brain stem, with slower processing than the pyramidal tract.

extrinsic: Refers to a mechanism that originates outside the structure on which it acts; typically the finger muscles that are located in the forearm; *opp.* intrinsic.

eye–ear line: Imaginary line passing through the outer corner of the eyelid and the center of the auditory canal.

F

face validity: Type of validity that refers to the content or format of a tool or test, which, on its face level, should measure what it is intended to measure.

failure point: Point at which a material loses its structural integrity.

fascia: Soft connective tissue covering organs and muscles.

fasciculi: A bundle of muscle fibers.

feedback system: *See* closed-loop system.

feed-forward system: *See* open-loop system.

Fenn effect: *See* heat of shortening.

fibrocartilage: Type of cartilage found in the intervertebral discs.

fibromyalgia: Chronically painful and spastic muscles, with tingling sensations, may result in nervousness and sleeplessness; also termed fibrositis.

fibrositis: *See* fibromyalgia.

final value theorem: Method for finding the final value of an output response.

Finkelstein's test: Test for de Quervain's disease in which the patient wraps the fingers around the thumb and deviates the wrist in the ulnar direction; pain at the base of the thumb is a positive sign.

first-class lever: The fulcrum is located between the opposing forces, e.g., a playground teeter-totter.

first-order system: System whose transfer function has only one pole.

Fitts' law: Rule describing the movement time as a function of the difficulty of the movement.

flexion: Joint movement such that the included angle between the two limbs decreases, for trunk or neck, bending forward; *opp.* extension.

flexor digitorum profundus: One of the two major finger flexor muscles; the other is the flexor digitorum superficialis.

flexor digitorum superficialis: One of the two major finger flexor muscles; the other is the flexor digitorum profundus.

flexor retinaculum: The ligament that forms one surface of the carpal tunnel and acts to prevent bowstringing of the flexor tendons; also termed transverse carpal ligament.

flower spray: Type of receptor found in the polar regions of the muscle spindle, sensitive only to change in length.

focal dystonia: *See* writer's cramp.

force: An action that cause bodies to be pushed or pulled in different directions.

force ratio: The ratio of grip force to the tool application force.

Frankfurt plane: Imaginary plane delineated by a line (in the sagittal plane) passing through the tragion and the lower ridge of the eye socket; roughly corresponds to horizontal when the head is held erect.

free-body diagram: The isolation of a body or a part of the body such that it is in static equilibrium.

frequency analysis: A type of signal analysis in which the phase relationship and the ratio of magnitudes of the output to the input are plotted against the frequency characteristics of the input signal.

friction: The interaction between two surfaces when coming into contact as one slides over the other.

frontal plane: Reference plane dividing the body into front and back halves, as observed face to face, *ant.* coronal plane.

fulcrum: The pivot point in a lever system.

fusiform: Spindle shaped, tapering at both ends, usually in reference to muscle spindles.

fusiform muscles: Muscles whose fibers lie parallel to the long axis.

G

gain: The ratio of the output signal to the input signal in a system.

ganglionic cysts: Nodules of synovial fluid that form under the skin of the hand as a by-product of tenosynovitis.

glenohumeral joint: Strictly, the shoulder joint, as opposed to the complete shoulder girdle.

gold standard: The best measurement system that is currently available.

Golgi tendon organs: Receptors at the tendon–muscle junction that respond to tension.

gray matter: The central, H-shaped darker region of the spinal cord containing motoneuron cell bodies.

Guyon canal syndrome: Entrapment of the ulnar nerve at Guyon's canal on the medial side of the hand, leading to tingling and numbness of the little and ring fingers.

H

hamate: The hook-shaped wrist bone in the distal row.

hand-arm vibration syndrome: Tingling, numbness, and loss of fine control due to ischemia of the blood supply to nerves and muscles of the hand; from power tool vibrations, cold temperatures, or direct pressure; *syn.* white finger syndrome.

Haversian canal system: Internal structure of bone formation with repeated layers of collagen fibers and hydroxyapatite crystals.

Hawthorne effect: A phenomenon in which employee-perceived interest by the employer may result in increased productivity; however, more generally, it applies to the difficulty in teasing apart confounded variables in an uncontrolled study, as happened in the original study at the Western Electric Hawthorne Works plant.

heat of shortening: Heat in muscle tissue due to the act of shortening as opposed to a simple isometric contraction; also called the Fenn effect.

heavy meromyosin: The head subunit of the myosin molecule that acts as the rotational bridge between the thick and thin filaments.

Hick–Hyman law: Rule that choice–reaction time is linearly related to the amount of information presented.

hyaline cartilage: Type of cartilage covering articular bony surfaces.

hydrodynamic lubrication: Type of joint lubrication in which translational joint motion creates a wedge effect, forcing synovial fluid between the articular surfaces.

hydrolysis: The splitting of a molecule into two with the use of water.

hydrophilic: Water loving, or allowing water molecules to adhere to the surface.

hydrostatic lubrication: Type of joint lubrication in which loading of the joint forces synovial fluid out of the pores of the cartilage, into the space between the articular surfaces.

hydroxyapatite: A crystalline structure of calcium forming the ground substance within bone.

hypothenar: Muscle group located at the base and acting on the little finger.

hypothenar hammer syndrome: Compression of the ulnar artery against the hypothenar eminence during hand hammering.

hysteresis: A measurement error in which the current value depends on both the present condition and the past conditions.

I

iatrogenesis: An argument that some disorders may result from the course of the professional activities of a physician, such as autosuggestion from discussions, examinations, or treatments.

impulse response: The output obtained by using a unit impulse function for the input, useful in characterizing a transfer function.

in vitro: Muscle preparation maintained in a glass container; *opp. in vivo*.

in vivo: Muscle preparation maintained within a living body; *opp. in vitro*.

incidence rate: The degree of new cases of disease with respect to exposure time.

index of difficulty: The amount of information found in a movement, defined as a function of the distance of movement and target size.

information theory: Theory in which the coding and content of messages can be quantified, typically in bits.

inhibitory postsynaptic potentials: Inhibitory inputs that hyperpolarize a section of a motoneuron cell body, making it more difficult to create an action potential.

initial heat: The combined effect of activation heat and heat of shortening.

initial value theorem: Method for finding the initial value of an output response.

innervation ratio: The ratio of muscle fibers to motoneurons, a measure of motor control.

insertion: Muscle attachment to a bone that is farthest from the midline of the trunk.

integrated: An outdated type of EMG processing in which the raw signal is charged through a capacitor; now typically used in reference to a smoothed signal.

internal forces: Forces acting inside the body, e.g., muscular forces.

interphalangeal: Refers to the joints between the phalanges.

intervention studies: Type of epidemiological study in which the factor of interest is directly manipulated.

intraclass correlation: An estimate of a test's reliability for more than two analysts, based on analysis of variance of the analysts' scores.

intrafusal: With reference to the inside of a muscle spindle, typically intrafusal muscle fibers; *opp.* extrafusal.

intrinsic: Refers to a mechanism located in the structure on which it acts; typically the finger muscles that are located in the hand; *opp.* extrinsic.

invasive: Procedure that breaks the skin; for electromyography, using needle electrodes within the muscle.

inversion: Bringing the sole of the foot inwards; *opp.* eversion.

ischemia: Lack of blood flow.

ischemic ulcers: Inflammation and lesions on the surface of the buttocks due to loss of blood flow from direct pressure of seating for extended periods of time; more typically found in patients with limited mobility.

ischial tuberosities: The major weight-bearing areas of the buttocks; *syn.* sit bones.

isoinertial: A dynamic muscle contraction in which the muscle contracts at a constant acceleration.

isokinetic: A dynamic muscle contraction in which the muscle contracts at a constant velocity.

isometric: Type of muscle contraction in which force production is achieved without changes in muscle length; also static contraction.

isometric experiment: Experiment in which a muscle is contracted isometrically, i.e., with both ends rigidly fixed so that it cannot shorten.

isotonic: A dynamic muscle contraction in which the muscle force remains constant.

isotropic: Material whose properties are independent of the direction of applied forces; *opp.* anisotropic.

J

joystick: A lever-type computer input control device with two degrees of freedom, either proportional to displacement or proportional to force.

K

kappa statistic: An estimate of a test's reliability based on the proportion of agreement observed between analysts but corrected for the proportion of agreement expected by chance.

kinematics: Type of dynamics in which only pure motion, displacement, velocities, and acceleration are studied.

kinetic energy: Capacity of a body to do work associated with linear displacement of the body.

kinetics: Type of dynamics in which the forces that produce a motion are studied in addition to the motion itself.

kyphosis: Distinctive posterior convex curvature of the spinal column in thoracic area; *opp.* lordosis.

L

lactic acid: Breakdown product of anaerobic metabolism, typically associated with fatigue.

lamellar bone: Bone layers formed through repeated deposits of collagen fibers and hydroxyapatite crystals.

laptop computers: Small, portable computers that can be operated while placed in the lap.

latency period: Delay in the rise of muscle tension due to conduction delays.

lateral: Reference direction, farther away from the midline of the body; *opp.* medial.

lateral epicondylitis: Inflammation at the tendon insertion on the lateral epicondyle of the humerus, resulting from forceful, twisting motions; also referred to as tennis elbow.

law of acceleration: Newton's second law: the acceleration of a body is proportional to the unbalanced force acting upon it and inversely proportional to the mass of the body.

law of conservation of mechanical energy: Law of physics stating that energy cannot be created or destroyed, but can only be transformed; i.e., the sum of the various forms will always be constant for any condition of the system.

law of inertia: Newton's first law: a body remains at rest or in constant-velocity motion until acted upon by an external unbalanced force.

law of reaction: Newton's third law: for every action there is an equal and opposite reaction.

lever system: A system of opposing forces acting around a pivot point such that they are in static equilibrium.

ligament: Connective tissue attaching bone to bone.

light meromyosin: The tail subunit of the myosin molecule that serves to bind the long molecules together into a tight filament.

light pen: Special stylus linked to the computer that senses the electron scanning beam at a particular location on the screen allowing for direct manipulation of the screen.

logistic function: Function used for fitting dependent variables with binary values; also termed logit function.

logit function: *See* logistic function.

long bones: Bones found in the extremities, i.e., the femur, the humerus, etc.

longitudinal study: *See* prospective study.

lordosis: Distinctive anterior convex curvature of the spinal column in the cervical and lumbar areas; *opp.* kyphosis.

lumbar spine: The portion of the spinal column consisting of the five vertebrae of the lower back, below belt level.

lumped model: Type of modeling approach in which the elements are treated holistically rather than individually; *opp.* distributed model.

lunate: The half-moon-shaped wrist bone in the proximal row.

M

magnitude: A scalar quantity that indicates the size of the push or pull action of a force.

make force: The peak force needed to break the circuit and deactivate a key switch.

make point: Point on keystroke travel at which a key switch is activated.

matching: The selection of controls such that key characteristics are the same as for the exposed group of individuals.

mechanical advantage: The ratio of the opposing forces in a lever system.

medial: Reference direction, closer to the midline of the body; *opp.* lateral.

metacarpal: Refers to the palm area; typically the bones that connect the fingers to the wrist.

metacarpals: The bones forming the palm.

metacarpophalangeal: Refers to the joint between the proximal phalange and the metacarpal bone.

micropauses: Small rest pauses at irregular, spontaneous intervals.

miniature end plate potential: The depolarization occurring at the motor end plate, as an action potential travels from a neuron to the muscle fiber.

minimum yield strength: The relative material strength at the yield point.

mitochondria: Energy production unit in the cell.

modulation index: The percentage of maximum pinch force utilized as the tool application force modulates between minimum and maximum values.

moment: The tendency of a force to cause rotation about a point when the force is at a distance from the point of rotation; same as torque.

moment of inertia: Quantity resisting rotation in a body.

morbidity: The proportion of individuals within a population having some disease.

motoneuron: An efferent neuron, with the cell body in the spinal cord, carrying information toward a muscle fiber; also motor neuron.

motor unit: Functional unit of muscle, defined as one motor neuron and all of the muscle fibers innervated by collaterals of that motor neuron.

mouse: A handheld computer input device with a roller ball in the base to control position and one or more buttons for other inputs.

multipennate muscles: Muscles whose fibers are relatively short and lie in several different oblique directions.

muscle spindles: Modified muscle fiber receptors that respond to changes in muscle length and velocity.

myalgia: Simple muscle soreness or pain.

myelin: Specialized fatty sheath covering an axon, which forces an action potential to jump between gaps in the myelin, resulting in very high nerve conduction speeds.

myofascial pain syndrome: Chronic muscle strain and myalgia.

myofibrils: Subdivision of a muscle fiber that contains the ultimate contractile mechanism.

myofilaments: The thick and thin protein filaments in a myofibril.

myoglobin: Muscle protein that stores oxygen.

myosin: Long protein molecules with heads comprising thick filaments within muscle.

myositis: Inflammation of muscle tissue.

myotendinitis: Inflammation of the muscle–tendon interface.

N

natural frequency: The characteristic frequency at which a system tends to oscillate with minimal external input.

neuromuscular junction: The interconnection between a neuron and muscle cell.

neuron: Nerve cell consisting of cell body and its dendrites, axon, and collaterals.

Nintendo thumb: *See* de Quervain's disease.

noninvasive: Procedures that do not break the skin; for electromyography, using surface electrodes on the surface of the skin over the belly of the muscle.

normal line of sight: Line of sight assumed by a seated individual in a relaxed posture, roughly 15° (±15°) below horizontal.

normal working area: Region of work surface defined by the area circumscribed by the forearm when it is moved in an arc pivoted at a fixed elbow.

notebook computers: Small notebook-sized computers.

nuclear bag: Intrafusal muscle fibers with swollen equatorial regions.

nuclear chain: Intrafusal muscle fibers with no central swelling.

nucleus: Cell unit containing genetic material.

nucleus pulposus: The gel-like center of an intervertebral disc.

O

odds ratio: The ratio of the odds of a particular exposure among with individuals with a specific disease to the corresponding odds of exposure among individuals without the disease of interest.

onset latency: The time between nerve stimulation and the initial response detected at the active recording electrode; measures the fastest fibers.

open-loop system: Type of system in which the command input is independent of the system output; *opp.* closed-loop system.

open-loop transfer function: Simple representation of a system using only the plant, controller, and feedback element.

opposition: Movement of the thumb to counter the other digits, pulpy surface to pulpy surface.

ordinate: The horizontal axis of a coordinate system; also termed the *x* axis.

origin: The point of intersection of the two axes of a coordinate system from which all points are defined; also the muscle attachment to a bone that is nearest the midline of the trunk.

orthodromic: Nerve conduction along an axon in the normal direction; *opp.* antidromic.

ossification: Bone formation through repeated deposits of collagen fibers and hydroxyapatite crystals.

osteoarthritis: Type of arthritis involving a degenerative process of joint cartilage.

osteoblasts: Bone-forming cells.

osteoclasts: Cells within bone that reabsorb bone structure.

osteocytes: Bone cells that have become mineralized.

overdamped: System response in which oscillations will die out quickly with time.

P

Pacinian corpuscles: Pressure sensitive receptors found in loose connective tissues near joints.

parallel elastic element: Springlike element in Hill's muscle model representing the different types of fascia and membranes that are parallel to the muscle fibers.

Pareto analysis: An exploratory tool in which items of interest are identified and measured on a common scale and ordered in ascending order, creating a cumulative probability distribution; typically a minority (about 20%) of ranked items will account for a majority (about 80%) of total activity.

partial fraction expansion: Method for finding the inverse Laplace transform by manipulating the fractional form of a transfer function.

patellar reflex: A typical stretch reflex created by tapping just below the knee of a free-hanging leg, resulting in it jerking up.

peak latency: Time between nerve stimulation and peak response detected at the active recording electrode.

Pearson product moment correlation coefficient: Type of correlation coefficient based on least-square regression between two variables; the resulting correlation coefficient will range from 0 to ±1, with 0 indicating no relationship, a +1 indicating a perfect relationship, and –1 indicating an inverse relationship.

pennate muscles: Muscles whose fibers are arranged obliquely to the long axis, similar to the fibers in a bird's feather; also termed unipennate.

perimysium: The inner layer of fascia that subdivides bundles of muscle fibers into fasciculi.

peritendinitis: Type of tendinitis with inflammation of only the tendon proper.

personal digital assistants: Small, handheld computers, typically operated with a stylus and touch screen.

phalanges: The bones of the fingers.

Phalen's test: Test for carpal tunnel syndrome in which the patient holds the wrist in hyperflexion for 1 min; pain, tingling, or numbness in the hand is a positive sign.

pisiform: The pea-shaped wrist bone in the proximal row.

plant: A simple transfer function or element that exerts control over the input in a system.

plantar flexion: Movement of the foot downward; *opp.* dorsiflexion.

plastic deformation region: Region of a stress–strain curve in which the material will not return to its original shape when unloaded.

plausibility: The likelihood that an association between exposure and disease status is compatible with a physiological mechanism.

point and click: A mouse operation in which the cursor is moved to a certain location and a command is executed with the activation of a mouse button.

polar coordinate system: A two-dimensional coordinate system using an angle θ and a distance *r*, defined from the origin, to identify points.

pole-zero diagram: A type of plot showing the poles and zeros of a system.

poles: The roots of the denominator of a transfer function.

posterior interosseous syndrome: Entrapment of the interosseous branch of the radial nerve within the supinator muscles of the forearm, resulting in a weakness in extensor muscles for the wrist and little finger.

posture targeting: Procedure for recording joint angle on a body diagram with target-like concentric circle arrangements.

posturegram: System for evaluating posture by plotting the position and angle of each joint with respect to a reference level and independent of other joint positions.

potential energy: Capacity of a body to do work associated with its position in the gravitational field.

power grip: Type of grip in which partly flexed fingers and the palm, with an opposing thumb, forming a clamp around the object; intended for power rather than control.

power spectrum: A plot of the ratio of the magnitudes of the output to the input signals for a given narrow-frequency band, typically expressed in decibels.

precision: The extent to which a measurement shows a small scatter or variance around the "true value"; *syn.* resolution.

precision grip: Type of grip in which the object is pinched between the flexor aspects of the fingers and the opposing thumb; intended for optimal control rather than power.

predictive validity: *See* criterion validity.

predictive value: The ability of a test to predict future occurrences of the undesired state.

pressure: A force distributed over an area rather than a single point of application.

prevalence: The proportion of individuals in a given population that has the disease of interest.

prevalence study: *See* cross-sectional study.

primary endings: *See* annulospiral.

principle of moments: Mechanics principle, which holds the moments of the components must be equal to the moment of the whole body.

pronation: Rotation of the forearm to the palm-down position; *opp.* supination.

pronator teres syndrome: Entrapment of the median nerve at the elbow due to the pronator teres muscle.

proprioreceptors: Mechanoreceptors in the neuromuscular system needed for motor control, e.g., muscle spindles, Golgi tendon organs, etc.

prospective study: A cohort study in which the status of the disease state is followed after the start of the study; *syn.* longitudinal study.

proteoglycan: A polysaccharide composed of hyaluronic acid, proteins, lipids, and water, forming the ground substance of soft connective tissue.

protraction: Drawing the shoulder forward; *opp.* retraction.

proximal: Referring to the portion of the body that is closest to the central longitudinal axis of the trunk.

pyramidal tract: Direct motor control pathway from the sensory cortex to the spinal cord; *opp.* extrapyramidal tract.

Q

quick release: Type of muscle experiment in which the quick release of a stop mechanism exposes the muscle to a constant load.

QWERTY: The standard keyboard in which the sequence of the first six leftmost keys in the third row up is QWERTY.

R

radial deviation: Movement of the hand closer to radius bone in the forearm (toward the little finger); *opp.* ulnar deviation.

radial tunnel syndrome: Compression of the radial nerve at the lateral epicondyle of the radius, resulting in tingling and numbness in the thumb.

radius: One of the forearm bones; the other is the ulna.

radius of gyration: The effective distance from the axis of rotation for which a point mass yields an equivalent moment of inertia to the complete body segment.

ramp function: A function whose whole value increases linearly with time.

rate coding: Theory for EMG signal increase, attributed the increase in frequency of neuronal firing.

Raynaud's syndrome: Constriction of the blood supply to the hand from cold temperatures.

reaction torque: The torque that is transferred from the action of a power tool to the operator's arm due to the time lag in the operator releasing the trigger or due to the delay in the tool's shutoff mechanism.

receiver operating characteristic: The plot of sensitivity as a function of (1 = specificity), showing the power of test in discriminating cases from controls.

reciprocal inhibition: Reflex in which antagonistic muscles are inhibited while the agonists are contracting.

rectangular coordinate system: A coordinate system with perpendicular axes; same as the Cartesian coordinate system.

refractory period: The period of time during which the cell membrane potential returns to normal steady state and cannot be easily stimulated.

Reid's base line: Imaginary line passing through the center of the auditory canal and the lower ridge of the eye socket, corresponding roughly to the line created by the Frankfurt plane in the sagittal plane.

relative risk: *See* risk ratio.

relaxation heat: Heat in muscle tissue observed after muscle contraction; also termed recovery heat.

reliability: Refers to the consistency or stability of a measure; i.e., multiple measurements are in agreement.

reliability coefficient: *See* correlation coefficient.

residue approach: Method for finding the inverse Laplace by differentiating the fractional form of a transfer function.

resolution: *See* precision.

resting heat: Steady-state heat of muscle tissue due to simply being alive.

resting length: Muscle length in a relaxed state, typically yielding maximum tension when contracted isometrically.

reticulin: Bulk filler in soft connective tissue.

retraction: Drawing the shoulders backward; *opp.* protraction.

retrospective study: A cohort study in which the development of the disease state occurred before the start of the study.

rheumatoid arthritis: Type of arthritis involving a generalized inflammatory process.

right-hand rule: Procedure to identify the direction of a vector cross product, the fingers of the right hand pointing in the direction of the first vector are curled toward the second vector so as to cover the included angle between the two vectors, the extended thumb points in the resultant cross-product vector direction, which is perpendicular to both the original vectors.

risk ratio: The ratio of the risk of a particular disease occurring among exposed individuals divided by the corresponding risk among unexposed individuals; also termed relative risk; *syn.* relative risk.

root locus: Analytical procedure for graphing the poles and zeros of the open-loop transfer function for determining system stability.

root-mean-square (RMS) signal: An effective "average" value of a time-varying signal, calculated as the square root of the average value of the signal squared over one cycle.

roots: Solutions of a polynomial function such that the function equals to zero.

rotational equilibrium: Condition in which the net moments about any point in the body due to the external forces are zero.

rotator cuff tendinitis: Inflammation of tendons of various muscles around the shoulder caused by chronically raised or abducted arms.

RULA (rapid upper limb assessment): A posture targeting procedure yielding a rudimentary musculoskeletal injury risk level.

S

sacrum: The portion of the spinal column consisting of five fused vertebrae primarily within the pelvis.

safety margin: The amount of grip force exceeding the minimum grip force required to avoid the object slipping out of the hand.

sagittal plane: Anatomical reference plane dividing the body into right and left halves, as observed from either side of the body.

sarcomere: Repeating unit within the myofibril, delineated by the Z-discs.

sarcoplasmic reticulum: Series of tubules and sacs surrounding the myofibrils from which calcium ions are released into the filaments.

scaphoid: The boat-shaped wrist bone in the proximal row.

second-class lever: A lever system in which the resistance force is located between the effort force and the fulcrum, resulting in a mechanical advantage greater than one.

second-order system: System whose transfer function has two poles, typically used to represent the mass–spring–dashpot systems.

secondary endings: *See* flower spray.

sensitivity: The probability that an individual who actually has the disease will have a positive test result; or a test's ability to identify injurious jobs.

series elastic element: Springlike element in Hill's muscle model representing the tendon in series with muscle fibers.

shear: Loading mode in which the load is applied perpendicular to the surface.

shunt muscles: Muscle with the origin close to the joint and the insertion point far from the joint, creating a large moment arm and a relative stabilizing effect on the joint; *opp.* spurt muscles.

signal-detection theory: A model for explaining the decision-making process for an individual detecting a signal against background noise based on specific criteria provided; similarly applied to a test in diagnosing a disease.

simple-reaction time: Time interval for an operator to respond to a single predetermined stimuli with a single predetermined response.

sit-stand chairs: A fairly high chair or stool that allows the user to easily switch from a semisitting posture to a standing posture, allowing for postural mobility.

size principle: Specific pattern of motor unit recruitment by the size of the neuron, starting with the smallest slow-twitch units and ending with the largest fast-twitch units.

sliding filament theory: Theory of muscle contraction in which the myofilaments slide over one another.

slip reflex: The reflexive increase in pinch force, which occurs approximately 75 ms after the onset of slip between the fingertips and the object being held.

smoothed-rectified signal: Type of EMG processing in which the raw signal is first rectified to all positive values, and then smoothed with a resistor-capacitor circuit to eliminate large spikes.

Spearman–Brown prophecy formula: Method for computing the reliability coefficient for a full test using the split-half procedure.

specificity: The probability that an individual who does not have the disease will have a negative test result; or a test's ability to correctly identify safe jobs.

spherical coordinate system: A coordinates system using distance *r* and two angles θ and φ to identify points from the origin.

split-half procedure: A procedure for establishing the reliability of a test; two halves of the test are scored separately for each person and a correlation coefficient is calculated for the two sets of scores; the reliability coefficient for the full test is computed using the Spearman–Brown prophecy formula.

spurt muscles: Muscles that originate far from the joint of rotation but insert close to the joint, causing the limb to move very rapidly; *opp.* shunt muscles.

squeeze-film lubrication: Type of joint lubrication in which fluid is squeezed out from the areas of high pressure to areas of lower pressure.

stadiometry: Measurement of spinal shrinkage as an indirect assessment of extended spinal loading.

standard anatomical position: Standard reference position of the upright human body with palms facing forward.

static equilibrium: Result of Newton's first law such that bodies are at rest or in constant-velocity motion.

statics: Biomechanical principles applied to a system of bodies at rest.

stenosing tenosynovitis: Acute form of tenosynovitis with localized swelling, a narrowing of the sheath, and the formation of a nodule on the tendon, causing the tendon to be become temporarily entrapped as it attempts to slide through the sheath.

stenosing tenosynovitis crepitans: Extreme form of tenosynovitis, in which the trapped tendon will crackle or crepitate as it is pulled from the entrapment.

strain: Deformation of a material normalized to its initial length.

strain index: An upper limb musculoskeletal injury risk assessment tool that rates six different occupational factors.

strain retardation: The resulting strain response for a unit step input of stress; also termed creep.

stratified sampling: An approach in which the population is divided into mutually exclusive strata with random sampling performed within each stratum.

stress: Load applied per unit area.

stress relaxation: The resulting stress response for a unit step input of strain.

stress–strain curve: A plot of stress as a function of strain during compressive or tensile loading of a material.

stretch receptors: Collectively the annulospiral and flower spray endings of a muscle spindle.

stretch reflex: The contraction of a muscle following a sudden stretch.

striated muscle: Another term for skeletal muscle because of the striated appearance from the various bands.

supination: Rotation of the forearm to the palm up position; *opp.* pronation.

surveillance: Ongoing observation of a population to detect changes in the occurrence of a disease.

survivor bias: The tendency for workers who are resistant to injury to stay on high-exposure jobs, leading to skewed sampling results.

symptom survey: Questionnaire to assess the extent of medical problems.

synapse: The specific gap between a neuron and muscle cell.

synovia: Membranes lining joints and tendons that secrete the low-friction synovial fluid for lubrication.

T

tangential force: Force acting at the center of mass of the body, perpendicular to the radius of rotation.

tarsal: Referring to the instep of the foot.

temporal contiguity: The timeliness of the precedence of an exposure with respect to the disease.

temporality: The fact that the exposure precedes the disease in time.

tendinitis: Inflammation of the tendon, typically due to chronic overuse.

tendon: Connective tissue attaching muscle to bone.

tennis elbow: *See* lateral epicondylitis.

tenosynovitis: Inflammation of the tendon and its sheath, typically due to chronic overuse.

tension: Loading mode in which the load is applied axially away from the surface, stretching the material.

tension-neck syndrome: A type of myofascial syndrome characterized by pain and tenderness in the shoulder and neck region, characteristic of clerical workers and small-parts assemblers, who have contracted the upper back and neck muscles in hunched-forward postures for better visibility.

tented: Term used for a keyboard split in the middle and laterally tilted down.

test-retest reliability: Measurement of the consistency or agreement of measurements with intervening time intervals.

tetanic frequency: The minimum frequency at which the state of tetanus can be achieved.

tetanus: Series of muscle contractions, in which the summation of individual contractions attains a steady level of force higher than the individual contractions.

thenar: Muscle group located at the base and acting on the thumb.

thermocouple: A very sensitive temperature gauge using two dissimilar metals, which, when connected, create an electrical potential proportional to the surrounding temperature.

thermoelastic heat: Heat gained or lost when a material is forcibly stretched or contracted.

third-class lever: A lever system in which the effort force is located between the fulcrum and the resistance force, resulting in a mechanical advantage less than one.

thoracic outlet syndrome: Entrapment of the brachial plexus in one or more shoulder sites: the scalenus muscles in the neck, between the clavicle and first rib and between the chest wall and the pectoralis minor muscle, resulting in numbness or tingling in the arm and hand.

thoracic spine: The portion of the spinal column consisting of the 12 vertebrae of the upper back.

tide mark: Boundary between calcified cartilage and bone.

time constant: The time required for a function to fall to 36.8% (e^{-1}) of its initial value or rise to 63.2% ($1 - e^{-1}$) of its final value.

Tinel's test: Test for carpal tunnel syndrome in which the median nerve at the wrist is tapped; pain, tingling, or numbness in the hand is a positive sign.

torque: The tendency of a force to cause rotation about a point when the force is at a distance from the point of rotation; same as moment.

touch pad: A computer input device located on keyboard that performs similarly to a digitizing tablet but without the special stylus, i.e., direct touch with a fingertip manipulates the cursor.

touch screen: Type of display using a touch-sensitive overlay for direct manipulation of the screen.

trabeculae: The three-dimensional lattice-like structure of fibers in bone, serves to better distribute stress.

track point: A force joystick.

track stick: A displacement joystick.

trackball: A computer input device similar to an upside-down mouse; the rotary displacement of the ball is converted to cursor position.

tragion: The notch above the piece cartilage that is just anterior to the auditory passage.

transfer function: An operator that acts on an input function and transforms it into an output function.

translational equilibrium: Condition in which the net forces on a body are zero.

transverse carpal ligament: *See* flexor retinaculum.

transverse plane: Anatomical reference plane parallel to the ground, as observed directly above the head.

trapezium: A four-sided wrist bone in the distal row.

trapezoid: A four-sided wrist bone (with two sides parallel) in the distal row.

tremor: Involuntary physiological oscillations of a limb, which are smaller than volitional motions.

trigger finger: Stenosing tenosynovitis of the index finger, typically from repeated, forceful activations of a power tool.

trigger points: Small areas of spastic muscle that are tender to touch.

triquetrum: The triangle-shaped wrist bone in the proximal row.

tropomyosin: Thin filament protein that serves to link globular actin molecules together in a chain.

troponin: Thin filament protein that acts as an inhibitor of cross-bridging.

two-point discrimination test: Test for nerve impairment in which individuals are pricked with either one pin or two pins simultaneously; a positive sign is when they cannot distinguish two pricks separated by at least 5 mm.

U

ulna: One of the forearm bones; the other is the radius.

ulnar deviation: Movement of the hand closer to the ulna in the forearm (toward the thumb); *opp.* radial deviation.

ultimate tensile strength: Material strength at the failure point.

undamped: System response for a damping ratio of zero in which the system will oscillate at steady state.

underdamped: System response in which oscillations will die out with time.

unipennate: *See* pennate.

unipolar: Type of electromyographical recording in which one active electrode is attached over the belly of the muscle to obtain the largest signal possible from the greatest number of motor units.

unit impulse: A function in the form of a pulse whose magnitude approaches infinite height as the width of the pulse approaches zero with an area remaining constant and equal to one.

unit membrane theory: Theory in which the cell membrane is modeled as a protein and phospholipid bilayer structure covered with a mucopolysaccharide surface.

unit step function: A function of value zero for time less than zero and value one for time greater than or equal to zero.

V

validity: The appropriateness, meaningfulness, and usefulness of a tool or survey to measure what it is supposed to measure.

vector: The combination of a magnitude and direction into one quantity.

viscoelastic theory: An approach in which a material and its properties can be modeled using springs and dashpots.

viscosity: A dashpot-like property of a material of a material or fluid that resists the force tending to make it flow.

visual analogue scale: Method for indicating the degree of perceived pain by putting a mark on a line, such that the distance indicated is comparable to the pain experienced.

W

Wald statistic: Ratio of regression coefficient to its standard error, used in evaluating the significance of the coefficient.

white finger syndrome: The blanching of skin due to ischemia of the blood supply from hand-arm vibration syndrome or Raynaud's syndrome.

white matter: The lighter outer region of the spinal cord containing the myelin sheaths and axons of descending neuronal tracts.

Wolff's law: "Form follows function" with reference to the trabeculae structure bone adapting to external stress.

work-space envelope: The three-dimensional space within which an individual can work, typically defined by the spherical surface circumscribed by a function arm reach while pivoting about the shoulder.

woven bone: The first layers of bone formation.

writer's cramp: Excessive and repeated muscle contraction while holding a pen or pencil; also termed focal dystonia.

Y

yield point: Point on a stress–strain curve at which the material leaves the elastic region and enters the plastic deformation region.

Z

Z-discs: Myofilament element holding the thin filaments together.

zero drift: A measurement error in which the baseline tends to shift over time.

zeros: The roots of the numerator of a transfer function.

Name Index

Subject Index